Spontaneous Intracerebral Haematomas

Advances in Diagnosis and Therapy

Edited by
H. W. Pia C. Langmaid J. Zierski

With 292 Figures

Springer-Verlag
Berlin Heidelberg New York 1980

Professor Dr. Dr. h.c. Hans Werner Pia
Direktor der Neurochirurgischen Universitäts-Klinik
Klinikstrasse 29, 6300 Giessen (Germany)

Mr. Charles Langmaid, FRCS
174, Lake Road East, Cardiff, CF2 5NR (England)

Dr. Jan Zierski
Neurochirurgische Universitäts-Klinik
Klinikstrasse 29, 6300 Giessen (Germany)

ISBN-13: 978-3-642-95375-0 e-ISBN-13: 978-3-642-95373-6
DOI: 10.1007/978-3-642-95373-6

Library of Congress Cataloging in Publication Data. Main entry under title: Spontaneous intracerebral haematomas. Bibliography: p. Includes index. 1. Hematoma. 2. Cerebrovascular disease--Complications and sequelae. I. Pia, Hans Werner. II. Langmaid, Charles, 1913--III. Zierski, Jan, 1940 – [DNLM: 1. Cerebral hemorrhage Diagnosis--Congresses. 2. Cerebral hemorrhage--Therapy--Congresses. 3. Hematomo--Diagnosis--Congresses. 4. Hematoma--Therapy--Congresses. WL355 S763 1979] RC 394.H35S66 616.8'1 80-22424

Softcover reprint of the hardcover 1st edition 1980

2127/3140-543210

Preface

Spontaneous intracerebral haemorrhages are the most dangerous complication of cerebral vascular disease. Because of their frequency and the fact that they lead to serious injuries, prolonged disabilities and, often, death, they have acquired an enormous significance, both medically and socially.

Their precise diagnosis, location, wide extent and accompanying manifestations were for a very long time uncertain and, in small and deeply situated haematomas, these factors were impossible to determine. Diagnosis was confirmed by the clinical picture, by angiography and sometimes by ventriculography and included, in the main, both lobar and more extensive haematomas.

The results of operative treatment following the first attempt of H. Cushing in 1903 were poor and remained unsatisfactory in spite of the endeavours of numerous authors (Guillaume et al. 1956; Lazorthes 1956; McKissock et al. 1959; Luessenhop 1967 and many others). Especially for the most frequent and typically hypertensive haematomas in the region of the internal capsule, the opinion was often expressed that operative treatment was useless.

My personal interest (Pia) in this topic dates back to 1953, and in the mid-1960s I was joined by the neurologist F. Erbslöh and the internist H. G. Lasch of the Giessen Medical Faculty. We focussed our attention on acute stroke and started as the so-called Giessen Stroke Fire Brigade, with examination and active treatment of every acute haematoma. It soon became obvious that operative treatment in the acute stage of hypertensive haematomas met with very infrequent success, and our attitude became more and more conservative. In addition, computerized tomography and, to a lesser extent, refined angiographic techniques and developments in haematology have considerably influenced diagnosis, conservative and operative treatment, as well as the indications and contra-indications for surgery. Consequently, a discussion of the present state of our knowledge and the possibilities of treatment emerging from new developments was thought absolutely necessary and requiring the participation of neurologists, neuropathologists, neuroradiologists, general physicians, specialists in rehabilitation and neurosurgeons.

To meet this need, a workshop attended by experts from many parts of the world was held in Giessen/Bad Nauheim from 1 – 3 February 1979. This workshop dealt with spontaneous cerebral haemorrhages, especially hypertensive haemorrhages. Topics related to haemorrhages due to coagulopathies, so-called micro-angiomas and diseases of the venous sinuses were added to the programme, as were traumatic intracerebral haematomas, with particular reference to the complexity of the aetiological and pathogenetic factors which are frequently involved.

The workshop followed the format of three previous ones, also held in Giessen, on cerebrospinal-vascular pathology and cerebral angiomas (1973), spinal angiomas (1975) and cerebral aneurysms (1977). Discussions on haematomas related to these vascular anomalies were held and published in three monographs (1975, 1978, 1979). Dr. K. J. Zülch, one of the outstanding figures in brain research, opened the workshop with a special lecture on "Stroke". Reports and discussions on morphology and aetiology, epidemiology, clinical pathology, and aetiological aspects of location formed the basis of the meeting. CT scan findings were discussed in detail as the decisive method for acute diagnosis and follow-up examinations. Quantitative analysis of CT-findings seems likely to give more detailed information on morbid anatomy.

Both conservative and operative treatments were discussed from different points of view, such as aetiology, site, size and clinical findings, as well as the spontaneous course of intracerebral haematomas. The possibilities presented by modern diagnostic procedures have influenced the timing and grading of the lesions, as well as the type of operation to be performed on the individual patient.

Several contributions on personal experiences have shown the present state of our knowledge. The participants in this workshop agreed to start immediately with a prospective co-operative study and to force the creation of interdisciplinary centres for the study of stroke. Such centres in which the problems of prevention, treatment and rehabilitation of cerebral vascular disturbances are attacked on a multidisciplinary basis should open a new chapter in the fight against one of the most devastating diseases of modern man.

The workshop was made possible by the generosity of industry both abroad and in Germany, especially by the support of Codman and Ethicon, FRG., and also of Ciba-Geigy, Wehr, E. Merck, Darmstadt, and Carl Zeiss, Oberkochen.

This volume contains the lectures and discussions that took place at the workshop. The interest it aroused, as in the case of the above mentioned previous monographs, has led to its rapid publication.

The Editors take great pleasure in expressing their thanks to the contributors for their participation and co-operation and understanding in preparing and publishing these proceedings.

Special thanks are due to my co-workers Drs. E. Grote and A. Laun, and also to Mrs. Knappe, Mrs. Wagner and Mrs. Walter for their help during the workshop and in preparing the manuscript.

A special word of thanks is due to Dr. Lore Pia, whose patient assistance and forbearance has been of such great value to all of us, as in the previous books.

We hope that this volume, like the previous books on cerebral angiomas, spinal angiomas and cerebral aneurysms, may contribute to improved diagnosis and treatment of spontaneous intracerebral haemorrhage.

Giessen, February 1980

Hans Werner Pia
Charles Langmaid
Jan Zierski

Contents

1 **Special Lecture**

Stroke (K. J. Zülch, Cologne) 1

2 **Morphology and Aetiology**

2.1 Pathology and Aetiology of ICH (K. Jellinger, Vienna) 13

2.2 Haemorrhage and Haematoma – Morbid Anatomy (H. Güthert, Erfurt) 30

2.3 Diagnosis and Control of Bleeding Disorders (H. G. Lasch and T. Schöndorf, Giessen) 31

2.4 ICH in Clotting Disorders (E. Grote, Giessen) 35

2.4.1 Discussion: Anticoagulants and ICH (J. Iizuka, Bonn) 40

2.5 Micro-angiomas and ICH (H.-P. Jensen, Kiel) 41

2.5.1 Discussion: Micro-angiomas 47

2.6 ICH in Childhood (V. Calatayud-Maldonado, Zaragoza) 48

2.7 Familial Incidence of ICH (W. Luyendijk and G. Th. A. M. Bots, Leiden) 50

2.8 ICH in Sinus and Cerebral Vein Thrombosis (O. Busse, Giessen)........ 56

2.9 Role of Trauma in ICH 58

2.9.1 ICH After Minor Trauma (R. A. Frowein and E. Hamel, Cologne)...... 58

2.9.2 Trauma in Intracerebral Haematomas (D. Parkinson, E. G. Newry, and J. Taylor, Winnipeg) 71

2.9.3 Relationship Between Head Injuries and Intracerebral Haematoma (C. Arseni and A. Gontea, Bucharest) 76

2.9.4 Delayed Traumatic Apoplexy (R. Vara-Thorbeck, Granada) 77

2.9.4.1 Discussion 81

2.10 Haematomas of Unknown Aetiology (W. Luyendijk, Leiden) 82

2.11 Stroke and ICH in Spontaneously Hypertensive Rats (W. Rascher, R. Dietz, H. Haebara, A. Schömig, D. Ganten, and F. Gross, Heidelberg) ... 86

3 Epidemiology

3.1 Epidemiology of ICH in Europe (R. Lorenz, Giessen) ... 91

3.2 Epidemiology of Hypertensive ICH in Japan (H. Kanaya, Morioka) ... 96

3.3 ICH and their Aetiology in India (R. D. Nagpal, Bombay) ... 100

3.4 WHO Statistics of Mortality in ICH (J. Iizuka, Bonn) ... 103

4 Clinical Pathology

4.1 Cerebral Blood Flow in ICH (Is Outcome Determined by Irreversible Haemodynamic Factors?) (J. Overgaard, Odense) ... 107

4.2 Intracranial Pressure in ICH (J. W. F. Beks, Groningen) ... 116

4.2.1 Discussion ... 119

4.3 Sequential Changes in Tissue Surrounding ICH (J. Suzuki and T. Ebina, Sendai) ... 121

4.3.1 Discussion ... 128

4.4 Brain Abscess Following ICH (O. Busse, Giessen) ... 129

5 Aetiological Aspects of Location

5.1 Pathology and Aetiology of Supratentorial Haemorrhage (K. Jellinger, Vienna) ... 131

5.2 Haematomas in Hemispheric Lobes (J. Zierski, Giessen) ... 135

5.3 Intraventricular Haematoma and Haemorrhage (H. W. Pia, Giessen) ... 140

5.3.1 Discussion (C. Arseni and A. Gontea, Bucharest) ... 144

5.4 Correlation Between Ventricular Haemorrhage and Chronic Cerebral Ischaemia in Adult Moya-Moya (J. Suzuki and N. Kodama, Sendai) ... 145

5.5 Cerebellar Haematomas (S. Kunze and W. Schiefer, Erlangen) ... 152

5.5.1 Discussion (L. Calliauw and I. Dehaene, Bruges) ... 154

5.6 Spontaneous Brain Stem (Pontine) Haematomas (K. Sano and C. Ochiai, Tokyo) ... 156

5.6.1 Primary Brain Stem Haematoma (C. Arseni and A. Gontea, Bucharest) . 160

6 Diagnosis

6.1 Angiography in ICH ... 165

6.1.1 Differential Diagnosis of ICH (R. Lorenz and A. Agnoli, Giessen) ... 165

6.1.2 The Role of Angiography in the Neuroradiological Diagnosis of Intracerebral Haematomas (L. Picard, J. Roland, J. Lepoire, and J. Montaut, Nancy) ... 171

6.1.3 Discussion ... 177

6.2 Computerized Tomography (CT) in ICH ... 178

6.2.1 Diagnosis and Differential Diagnosis of Spontaneous ICH with CT Scan (E. Kazner, Munich, W. Lanksch, Munich, T. Grumme, Berlin, and K. Kretzschmar, Mainz) ... 178

6.2.2 Automatic and Quantitative Diagnosis of ICH by CT (M. Nagai and Y. Ueda, Mibu) ... 190

6.2.3 Intraventricular Haemorrhages in CT Scans (A. Laun, A. L. Agnoli, and L. Cristante, Giessen) ... 195

6.2.4 Brain Stem Haemorrhage (A. Laun and A. L. Agnoli, Giessen) ... 196

6.2.5 CT in Traumatic ICH – Measurement of Absorption Values (A. L. Agnoli and J. Zierski, Giessen) ... 202

6.2.6 Natural History and Follow-Up (T. Grumme, Berlin; K. Kretzschmar, Mainz, and W. Lanksch, Munich) ... 216

7 Conservative Treatment

7.1 The Immediate Care of Stroke (W. Dorndorf, Giessen) ... 223

7.2 Conservative Therapy of Spontaneous ICH (H. Reisner, Vienna) ... 225

7.3 Rehabilitation after Acute ICH (K. A. Jochheim, Cologne) ... 228

7.3.1 Rehabilitation after Spontaneous ICH (O. Leitholf, Gailingen) ... 231

7.3.2 Discussion ... 233

7.4 Initial Clinical Course and Prognostic Factors in ICH (F. Regli and D. Jeanmonod, Lausanne) ... 233

7.5 Late Prognosis (H. Gänshirt and R. Keuler, Heidelberg) ... 240

7.5.1 Discussion (F. Danke, Würzburg) ... 243

8 Operative Treatment

8.1 General Surveys ... 247

8.1.1 Experiences with Operation in 149 Cases of Spontaneous ICH (1966 – 1977) (B. Guidetti and F. Gagliardi, Rome) ... 247

8.1.2 Experiences with the Surgical Treatment of 156 ICH (1955 – 1977) (E. Pásztor, D. Áfra, and É. Orosz, Budapest) ... 251

8.1.3 Experience with the Treatment of 48 Hypertensive ICH (1968 – 1978) (A. Erbengi, K. Benli, V. Bertan, S. Saglam, and O. Gurcay, Ankara) ... 257

8.1.4 Surgery in Spontaneous ICH (H. A. D. Walder, Nijmegen) ... 260

8.1.5 Spontaneous ICH – Prognosis and Discussion (W. Piotrowski, Mannheim) ... 262

8.2 Grading and Timing ... 264

8.2.1 Grading and Timing of Operative Treatment (F. J. Gillingham and K. Satyanarayana, Edinburgh) ... 264

8.2.2 Grading and the Indications for Treatment in ICH of the Basal Ganglia (Cooperative Study in Japan) (H. Kanaya, H. Yukawa, Morioka; Z. Itoh, H. Kutsuzawa, Akita; M. Kagawa, Tokyo; T. Kanno, Toyoake; T. Kuwabara, Yokohama; M. Mizukami, G. Araki, Isezaki; and T. Irino, Osaka) ... 268

8.2.3 Grading and Timing of Operation in Putaminal ICH (J. Suzuki and T. Sato, Sendai) ... 274

8.2.4 Discussion (H. W. Pia, Giessen) ... 279

8.3 Aetiology – Indications and Prognosis ... 281

8.3.1 Hypertensive ICH ... 281

8.3.1.1 Possibilities of Operative Treatment and its Limitations (F. Loew and H. Jaksche, Homburg) ... 281

8.3.1.2 Indications and Contra-Indications (R. Lorenz, Giessen) ... 283

8.3.1.3 Discussion (C. Arseni and A. Gontea, Bucharest) ... 287

8.3.1.4 Prognostic Factors in the First 48 Hours in Spontaneous ICH and Spreading Haemorrhages (B. Pertuiset, A. Yacoubi, J. P. Sichez, and D. Gardeur, Paris) ... 294

8.3.1.5 Haemorrhage and Haematoma (C. Arseni and A. Gontea, Bucharest) ... 301

8.3.2 Clotting Disorders ... 308

8.3.2.1 Indications and Prognosis (E. Grote, Giessen) ... 308

8.3.2.2 Haematomas Due to Anticoagulant Treatment (J. Iizuka, Bonn) ... 309

8.3.3 Traumatic ICH ... 310

8.3.3.1 Comparative Study of the Results in Spontaneous and Traumatic ICH (A. Karimi-Nejad and E. Hamel, Cologne) ... 310

8.3.3.2 Indications and Operative Treatment of Traumatic ICH (D. Parkinson, E. G. Newry, and D. Tubman, Winnipeg) ... 317

8.3.3.3 Prognosis in Traumatic ICH (D. Parkinson, E. G. Newry, and M. West, Winnipeg) ... 319

8.4 Location – Indications and Prognosis ... 322

8.4.1 Haematomas in Hemispheric Lobes (J. Zierski, Giessen) ... 322

8.4.2 Intraventricular ICH ... 326

8.4.2.1 Surgical Treatment (F. Loew and H. Jaksche, Homburg) ... 326

8.4.2.2 Location, Indication and Prognosis (H. W. Pia, Giessen) ... 329

8.4.2.3 CT Scan and Treatment (W. J. Stendel, E. Schneider, and H. Becker, Frankfurt) ... 331

8.4.3 Basal Ganglia and Thalamus ... 334

8.4.3.1 Indication for Operative Treatment of Hypertensive ICH in the Basal Ganglia and Thalamus (K. Kitamura and M. Kagawa, Tokyo) ... 334

8.4.3.2 Putaminal ICH with Regard to its Size in CT Scanning (Y. Matsukado and N. Sakurama, Kumamoto) 341

8.4.3.3 Trans-Sylvian Approach in Putaminal ICH with Mild Symptoms (J. Suzuki and T. Sato, Sendai) 345

8.4.3.4 Discussion (J. W. F. Beks, Groningen) 348

8.4.4 Cerebellar Haematomas 348

8.4.4.1 Indications and Prognosis (K. Sano and S. Yoshida, Tokyo) 348

8.4.4.2 Indications and Contra-Indications for Operation in Primary Haematomas of the Cerebellum and Brain Stem (C. Arseni and A. Gontea, Bucharest). 357

8.4.4.3 Operative Treatment (M. Klinger and S. Kunze, Erlangen) 358

8.4.4.4 Intracerebellar Haematoma (T. Banno, M. Shibuya, M. Oda, and N. Kanie, Yokkaichi) 361

8.4.4.5 Operative Treatment (L. Calliauw and I. Dehaene, Bruges) 365

8.4.5 Brain Stem Haematomas 366

8.4.5.1 Clinical Aspects with Reference to Indications for Treatment (K. Sano and C. Ochiai, Tokyo) 366

8.5 Special Technical Problems 371

8.5.1 General Remarks (F. J. Gillingham and K. Satyanarayana, Edinburgh) .. 371

8.5.2 Craniotomy (R. Lorenz, Giessen) 374

8.5.3 Burr-Hole Evacuation (R. Müke, Hamburg) 379

8.5.3.1 Discussion 382

8.5.4 Operative Technique in Putaminal and Thalamic ICH (K. Kitamura and M. Kagawa, Tokyo) 383

8.5.4.1 Trans-Sylvian Approach to Putaminal Haematomas (J. Suzuki and A. Takaku, Sendai) 384

8.5.5 Continuous Ventricular Drainage (E. Grote, Giessen) 386

8.5.5.1 Technical Note (J. Suzuki and A. Takaku, Sendai) 387

8.5.6 Shunt Operations (J. Zierski, Giessen) 389

9 Conclusions

9.1 Conservative and Surgical Management (F. John Gillingham, Edinburgh) 391

9.2 Prospects. The Editors 392

10 References 397

11 Subject Index 000

List of Senior Authors

Agnoli, A. L., Priv. Doz. Dr.: Abt. f. Neuroradiologie, Zentrum für Neurochirurgie am Klinikum der JLU Giessen, Klinikstr. 29, 6300 Giessen (FRG)

Arseni, C., Prof. Dr.: Clinica de Neurochirurgie, Sos. Berceni 10, Bucarest (Romania)

Banno, T., Dr.: Neurosurg. Dep., Yokkaichi Municipal Hospital, Mie 7 – 78, 510 Yokkaichi (Japan)

Beks, J. W. F., Prof. Dr.: Kliniek voor Neuro-Chirurgie, Academisch Ziekenhuis, Oostersingel 59, Groningen (The Netherlands)

Busse, O., Dr.: Zentrum für Neurologie am Klinikum der JLU Giessen, Am Steg 22, 6300 Giessen (FRG)

Calatayud-Maldonado, V., Prof. Dr.: Dep. of Neurosurgery, Avda. de las Torres, 93, 6° F Zaragoza (Spain)

Calliauw, L., Dr.: St. Janshospitaal, 8300 Brügge (Belgium)

Danke, F., Dr.: Psychiatrische Univ.-Klinik, Füchsleinstr. 15, 8700 Würzburg (FRG)

Dorndorf, W., Prof. Dr.: Zentrum für Neurologie am Klinikum der JLU Giessen, Am Steg 22, 6300 Giessen (FRG)

Driesen, W., Prof. Dr.: Neurochirurgische Abteilung der Univ. Tübingen, Calwer Str. 7, 7400 Tübingen (FRG)

Erbengi, A., Prof. Dr.: Department of Neurosurgery, Hacettepe University, Ankara (Turkey)

Frowein, R. A., Prof. Dr.: Neurochirurgische Univ.-Klinik, Joseph-Stelzmann-Str. 9, 5000 Köln 41 (FRG)

Gänshirt, H., Prof. Dr.: Neurologische Univ.-Klinik, Voss-Str. 2, 6900 Heidelberg 1 (FRG)

Gillingham, F. J., Prof.: Department of Surgical Neurology, The Royal Infirmary, Lauriston Place, Edinburgh, EH3 9YW (UK)

Gontea, A., Dr.: Clinica de Neurochirurgie, Sos. Berceni 10, Bucarest (Romania)

Grote, E., Prof. Dr.: Zentrum für Neurochirurgie am Klinikum der JLU Giessen, Klinikstr. 29, 6300 Giessen (FRG)

Grumme, Th., Prof. Dr.: Neurochir. Klinik der Freien Univ. Berlin, Klinikum Charlottenburg, Spandauer Damm 130, 1000 Berlin 19 (FRG)

Güthert, H., Prof. Dr.: Pathologisches Institut der Medizinischen Akademie, Nordhäuser Str. 74, 50 Erfurt (DDR)

Guidetti, B., Prof. Dr.: Istituto di Neurochirurgia dell' Università di Roma, Viale dell' Università, 30, 00185 Roma (Italy)

Haftek, J., Prof. Dr.: Klinika Neurochirurgii WAM, Zeromskiego 113, 90-549 Lódź (Poland)

Iizuka, J., Priv.-Doz. Dr.: Neurochirurgische Univ.-Klinik, Bonn Venusberg, Annaberger Weg, 5300 Bonn 1 (FRG)

Isamat, F., Dr.: Clinica Sagrada Familia, Neurocirurgia, Torras y Pujalt, 1, Barcelona, 6 (Spain)

Jellinger, K., Prof. Dr.: Ludwig-Boltzmann-Institut für Klinische Neurobiologie, Wolkersbergenstr. 1, 1130 Vienna (Austria)

Jensen, H.-P., Prof. Dr.: Neurochirurgische Univ.-Klinik Kiel, Weimarer Str. 8, 2300 Kiel 1 (FRG)

Jochheim, K.-A., Prof. Dr.: Rehabilitationszentrum der Univ. Köln, Lindenburger Allee 44, 5000 Köln 41 (FRG)

Kanaya, H., Prof. Dr.: Department of Neurosurgery, Iwate Medical University, Morioka, Iwate (Japan)

Karimi-Nejad, A., Prof. Dr.: Neurochirurgische Univ.-Klinik, Joseph-Stelzmann-Str. 9, 5000 Köln 41 (FRG)

Kazner, E., Prof. Dr.: Neurochirurg. Klinik der Freien Univ. Berlin, Klinikum Charlottenburg, Spandauer Damm 130, 1000 Berlin 19 (FRG)

Kitamura, K., Prof. Dr.: Department of Neurosurgery, Neurological Institute, Tokyo Women's Medical College, Kawada-cho, 10, shinjuku-ku, Tokyo (Japan)

Klinger, M., Priv. Doz. Dr.: Neurochirurgische Klinik der Univ. Erlangen-Nürnberg, Schwabachanlage 6, 8520 Erlangen (FRG)

Kunze, St., Prof. Dr.: Neurochirurgische Klinik der Univ. Erlangen-Nürnberg, Schwabachanlage 6, 8520 Erlangen (FRG)

Lasch, H.-G., Prof. Dr. Dr. h.c.: Zentrum für Innere Medizin am Klinikum der JLU Giessen, Klinikstr. 36, 6300 Giessen (FRG)

Laun, A., Dr.: Zentrum für Neurochirurgie am Klinikum der JLU Giessen, Klinikstr. 29, 6300 Giessen (FRG)

Leitholf, O., Dr. †: Neurologische Kliniken Dr. Schmieder, 7704 Gailingen (FRG)

Loew, F., Prof. Dr.: Neurochirurgische Univ.-Klinik, 6650 Homburg/Saar (FRG)

Lorenz, R., Prof. Dr.: Abteilung für Allg. Neurochirurgie am Klinikum der J. W. Goethe-Univ., Schleusenweg 2–16, 6000 Frankfurt a. M. 71 (FRG)

Luyendijk, W., Prof. Dr.: Department of Neurosurgery, Academisch Ziekenhuis-Leiden, Rijnsburgerweg 10, Leiden (The Netherlands)

Matsukado, Y., Prof. Dr.: Kumamoto University, Kumamoto 860 (Japan)

Müke, R., Prof. Dr.: Neurochirurg. Abteilung, Krupp'sche Krankenanstalten, Wittekindstr. 30–86, 4300 Essen (FRG)

Nagai, M., Prof. Dr.: Department of Neurosurgery, Dokkyo University, School of Medicine, Mibu, Tochigi (Japan)

Nagpal, R. D. M.S., M.S.: Department of Neurosurgery, K.E.M. – Hospital, Parel, Bombay – 400012 (India)

Overgaard, J., Dr.: Department of Neurosurgery, Odense University Hospital, 5000 Odense (Denmark)

Parkinson, D. D., Prof. Dr.: Department of Neurosurgery, The University of Manitoba, Faculty of Medicine, 700 William Avenue, Winnipeg, Manitoba R3E OZ3 (Canada)

Pásztor, E., Prof. Dr.: National Institute of Neurosurgery, Amerikai u. 57, 1145 Budapest (Hungary)

Penzholz, H., Prof. Dr.: Neurochirurgische Abteilung des Chirurg. Zentrums der Univ. Heidelberg, Gebäude 110, Im Neuenheimer Feld, 6900 Heidelberg (FRG)

Pertuiset, B., Prof. Dr.: Clinique Neuro-Chirurgicale, Hôpital de la Pitié-Salpétrière, 83, Bd. de l'hôpital, 75013 Paris (France)

Pia, H. W., Prof. Dr. Dr. h.c., Zentrum für Neurochirurgie am Klinikum der JLU Giessen, Klinikstr. 29, 6300 Giessen (FRG)

Picard, L., Prof. Dr.: Service de Neuroradiologie, Hôpital St.-Julien, 1, rue Foller, C.H.U., 54037 Nancy Cedex (France)

Piotrowski, W., Prof. Dr.: Neurochirurgische Klinik, Städt. Krankenanstalten, Postfach 23, 6800 Mannheim 1 (FRG)

Rascher, W., Dr.: Pharmakologisches Institut der Univ. Heidelberg, Im Neuenheimer Feld 366, 6900 Heidelberg (FRG)

Regli, F., Prof. Dr.: Service de Neurologie, Centre Hospitalier, Universitaire Vaudois, 1011 Lausanne (Switzerland)

Reisner, H., Prof. Dr.: Neurologische Klinik der Univ., Allgemeines Krankenhaus der Stadt Wien, Lazarettgasse 14, 1097 Vienna (Austria)

Sano, K., Prof. Dr.: Department of Neurosurgery, University of Tokyo, Hongo, Bunkyo-ku, Tokyo (Japan)

Schürmann, K., Prof. Dr. Dr. h.c.: Neurochirug. Klinik der Joh. Gutenberg-Univ. Mainz, Klinikum, Langenbeckstr. 1, 6500 Mainz (FRG)

Stendel, W.-I., Dr.: Abt. f. Allgem. Neurochirurgie, Zentrum d. Neurologie u. Neurochirurgie d. Klinikums der Goethe-Univ., Schleusenweg 2 – 16, 6000 Frankfurt a.M. 71 (FRG)

Suzuki, J., Prof. Dr.: Division of Neurosurgery, Tohoku University, School of Medicine, Institute of Brain Diseases, 5-13-1, Nagamachi, Sendai 982 (Japan)

Vara-Thorbeck, R., Prof. Dr.: Clinica de Patologia Quirurgica II, Hospital Clinico de "San Ceclio", Granada (Spain)

Walder, H. A. D., Prof. Dr.: Kliniek voor Neurochirurgie, Sint Radboudziekenhuis, Reinier Postlaan 4, Nijmegen (The Netherlands)

Zierski, J., Dr.: Zentrum für Neurochirurgie am Klinikum der JLU Giessen, Klinikstr. 29, 6300 Giessen (FRG)

Zülch, K. J., Prof. Dr.: Abt. f. Allg. Neurologie am Max-Planck-Institut für Hirnforschung u. d. Neurolog. Klinik des Städt. Krankenhauses Köln-Merheim, Ostmerheimer Str. 200, 5000 Köln 91 (Merheim) (FRG) [illegible], Prof. Dr., [illegible] Neurologie, [illegible] 1011 Lausanne (Switzerland)

[illegible], Prof. Dr., [illegible] der [illegible] Wien, [illegible]gasse 14, 1090 Wien (Austria)

[illegible], Prof. Dr., [illegible] Japan)

[illegible]

[illegible]

[illegible]

[illegible]

[illegible]

1 Special Lecture

Man findet so mancherley Meinungen über die Natur und Heilung der Schlagflüsse und Lähmungen, daß es ein wichtiger Gegenstand ist, sich mit der Untersuchung derselben zu beschäftigen.

Carl Christlieb Bethke: Über Schlagflüsse und Lähmungen, Leipzig, 1797

One meets many concepts of the nature and cure of stroke and palsies, therefore it seems important to occupy oneself with their investigation.

Stroke*

K. J. Zülch, Cologne

When discussing our subject we have first to define the term "stroke". Yet, to define it semantically seems to be difficult. In modern terminology "stroke" may be classified as an "abrupt, sudden, or progressive neurological defect syndrome (of consciousness motor, sensory, neuropsychological and/or other systems) on a vascular basis". Apparently this goes further than the semantic content of the term "stroke", which means literally that some individual is struck down to the ground. This is also expressed by "apoplexy" from the Greek *apoplexia* or *apoplettein*, while the German *Schlaganfall* expresses actually the same as stroke. A page of a doctoral thesis from 1840 (Ludovico Josepho Melicher) will show you the many terms for stroke, partly in Latin, partly reproduced in European languages, as for instance in Italian: *percossa, colpo, cocciolra, apoplessia, accidente* (Melicher, p. 1).

How difficult it was for the doctor at that time to differentiate between the various types of apoplexy may be deduced from the following (Table 1). But even today the problem of stroke has not lost any of its importance, as WHO figures on stroke as a cause of death will show us (death rate for 1955, 167.6 per 100000; in 1967, 175.2 per 100000).

Cause and Pathogenesis. The first half of the following discussion will deal with the cause and pathogenesis of stroke. The causes for such an "ictus" or stroke which brings someone down to the ground, are manifold and they are well known to you. It would be too time-consuming to deal with all these forms of stroke. Therefore, I will restrict this part of my discussion to "cerebral haemorrhage by vessel rupture", and I shall treat this from the standpoint of an "acquired disease", thereby omitting the malformative lesions. Because of this restriction I will show only the most common causes of intracranial haemorrhage (Table 2). However, I remind you that for some decades even intracerebral hypertensive striatal haemorrhage was – and still is in some parts of the world – of interest to

Table 1. Types of apoplexy

1) Apoplexiam sanguineo-serosam	4) Apoplexiam seroso-nervosam
2) Apoplexiam sanguineo-nervosam	5) Apoplexiam nervoso-sanguineam
3) Apoplexiam seroso-sanguineam	6) Apoplexiam nervoso-serosam

* Supported by a grant of Frau Andrea Möller, Hamburg

Table 2. Pathogenetic classification of cerebral haemorrhage

1)	Hypertensive cerebral haemorrhage
2)	Rupture of saccular aneurysm
3)	Rupture of angioma
4)	Traumatic haemorrhage
5)	Internal disorders (leukaemia etc.)
6)	Undetermined
7)	Haemorrhage into brain tumour
8)	Haemorrhage into haemorrhagic infarction
9)	Haemorrhage into brain stem in axial shift
10)	Various causes of so-called brain purpura (avitaminoses, toxic, allergic causes, fat embolism, etc.)
11)	Inflammation
12)	Iatrogenic (heparin, acetylsalicylic acid, dicumarol)

neurosurgeons with the aim of emptying the blood clot. When I delivered a special lecture 12 years ago to one of the neurosurgical meetings in Bad Ischl (unpublished), and also in Leipzig (Zülch 1961) on this particular topic, I emphasized that the rationale of such an operation could only be (1) to decrease the increased intracranial volume, (2) thereby avoiding or removing raised intracranial pressure with lateral (hypothalamus!) and axial (caudal brain stem!) shifts, and finally (3) avoiding or decreasing perifocal brain oedema, which increases volume and furthermore destroys the infiltrated brain tissue (oedema necrosis). However, since my task here is to define hypertensive mass haemorrhage, I will start by considering a statement by Luginbühl (1966), an outstanding Swiss veterinary pathologist. He said that "this unique type of haemorrhage is not known to occur in animal species and could not be reproduced experimentally" (see Globus and Epstein 1953). In other words, cerebral haemorrhage (in the hypertensive) is essentially a human phenomenon (see also the contribution of Rascher, Sect. 2.11).

Discussion of the pathogenesis of cerebral haemorrhage goes far back into the nineteenth century. Then the two great pathologists of the first half, namely Cruveilhier and Virchow, already had very sound ideas about most of the types of haemorrhage. Cruveilhier, for instance, stated distinctly that there were two forms, one in which the blood clot was in the middle of the damaged brain tissue, whereas in the other case there had been a diffuse infiltration of blood into the softened brain substance, a lesion which he called "capillary apoplexy" (which corresponds naturally to "haemorrhagic infarction" in our terminology). Virchow gave a similar description and emphasized moreover the importance of vascular disease as a cause of haemorrhage.

When Cruveilhier postulated haemorrhage from a ruptured vessel he only followed the Swiss author Wepfer (1658) to whom we owe an excellent book on stroke, and the famous Morgagni (1769).

Although, as mentioned, pathologists then had a very sound interpretation and classification of the pathogenesis of intracerebral haematomas, the clinicians, on the other hand, followed the wrong path for more than 100 years. They regarded the second mentioned entity, described so well by Cruveilhier (1829) and Virchow (1856), namely pericapillary bleedings (e.g. "haemorrhagic infarction"), and not the rupture of a diseased artery, as the primary cause of the final clot. However, some pertinent illustrations may show you that it is sometimes difficult to distinguish between these two forms.

The first clinicians who postulated a primary softening with pericapillary bleeding from which the haemorrhage later developed, were Rouchoux (1814) and later Durand-Fardel (1854). However, only a little later, one of the highlights of pathogenetic discussion was started by

Charcot and Bouchard (1868); they described "miliary aneurysms" which could be seen on the ruptured vessels by the naked eye when washing out the blood clot in all their 77 observations. We will return later to a discussion of these famous aneurysms (Fig. 1).

I will refrain from historically dividing the investigators of haemorrhage in the nineteenth century into two groups according to the aforementioned two concepts in pathogenesis, but will move on to this century. In 1918, Rosenblath developed the theory of an unknown damaging factor possessing extremely potent chemical properties and which probably stemmed from the kidneys. This, he postulated, would destroy a focus of brain tissue to such an extent that haemorrhages from capillaries and veins resulted; these would then coalesce into real haematomas, the origin of the future massive haemorrhage.

This concept was accepted and enlarged by the internists Westphal and Bär (1926), two prominent members of the von Bergmann school. They assumed angiospastic ischaemia as the cause of the softening, but otherwise followed Rosenblath's ideas. Here, the older members of the audience will recall that von Bergmann and his school expressed the opinion that spasm of the smooth musculature was the starting point of many internal diseases.

The pathogenetic theory endured in this form, both in Germany and France, until the 1950s and even as late as 1952, it formed the basis of the chapter written by the famous French neurologist, Jean Lhermitte (1949). This is particularly surprising, since a basic discussion on pathogenesis had already been started anew 12 years previously by the contributions of Spatz (1939) and Anders and Eicke (1940) at the meeting of the German internists in Wiesbaden in

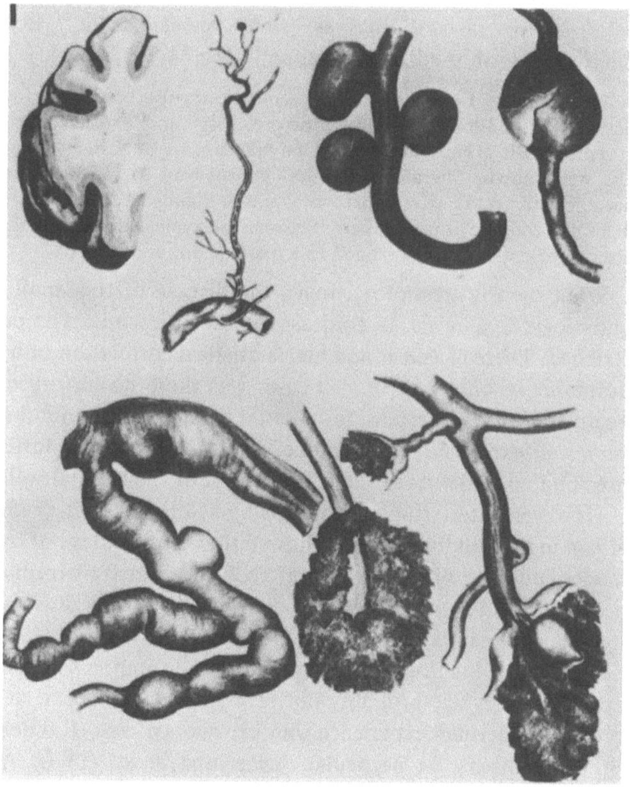

Fig. 1. Reproduction of Charcot-Bouchard's drawing of the "miliary cerebral aneurysms"

1938. Here Spatz successfully launched the concept of a rupture of the basal ganglia arteries. Moreover these authors were right in emphasizing the importance of a hyalinoid change in the small arteries of the basal ganglia. However, Spatz included one surprising statement that the cortical *Kugelblutung* could be considered a model in miniature of mass haemorrhage. Yet, *Kugelblutung* (Hiller 1936) is acutally encountered very rarely in neuropathology. Pabelick (1967) found it twice in our 70 cases. Therefore, it would seem highly risky to base a theory more or less on one very pronounced case which the authors apparently had seen.

Here in Cologne, Volland, who came from the school of Hallervorden and Spatz and was very familiar with the pattern of *Kugelblutung* saw only two cases in his life, although he performed all the autopsies for Professor W. Scheid's stroke cases. I have seen perhaps four to five in more than 1000 vascular cases other than in brains after leukaemia, in which small similar haemorrhages – of any size – are not infrequent.

In all our 70 cases of striatal mass haemorrhages (Pabelick 1967), which are the particular basis of my contribution to pathogenesis, we came to the conclusion that cortical *Kugelblutung* cannot serve as a model for pathogenesis of hypertensive mass haemorrhage.

Summarizing this part, we may state with a high degree of probability that this typical type of hypertensive bleeding stems from the rupture of one of the arteries of the "striatum" (80.5%), the thalamus (3.1%), the dentatum (5.4%) or pons (11%), although the pathogenesis has still to be completed. For this reason I would like to show you our observations in our work with serial sections from many cases and I shall start with the problem of hyalinosis, mentioned by Spatz (1939) and by Anders and Eicke (1940).

Hyalinosis. What then is hyalinosis, a term most frequently met in the German literature and better known in cardiology as "small vessel disease"? Both terms correspond to arteriolosclerosis, a term used by general pathologists.

At this point, I come again into semantic trouble and, therefore, I must first clarify the correlation between arteriolosclerosis and atherosclerosis and arteriosclerosis. In German, arteriosclerosis and atherosclerosis are usually used synonymously. In English-speaking countries the term arteriosclerosis is less well known. Therefore, it seems appropriate to follow the suggestions made by German general pathologists, to use arteriosclerosis as a more comprehensive term for any gross arterial disease, thereby including the two forms, atherosclerosis, the typical disease of the major arteries seen with aging, and arteriolosclerosis, mostly related to hypertension, and directly by name a "small vessel disease".

What then is arteriolosclerosis, the disease of the small vessels, or as it called in cerebral pathology, hyalinosis, in contrast to atherosclerosis. The pathogenesis is here not sufficiently clarified. There is a clear and high statistical correlation of hyalinosis with hypertension of long duration. In only 7 of our 70 cases was there no history of hypertension. Eicke (1952) once postulated that hypertension must be of at least six months duration in man. It has not been very well explained how hyaline, a plasmaprotein is infiltrated by the raised pressure and precipitated underneath the endothelium of the arterial wall.

However, interesting experiments by Muirhead et al. (1951) and Montgomery and Muirhead (1954) in the Goldblatt model showed that after 10 days of hypertension an acute necrosis of the media could be produced and after 20 days, a transformation into hyaline; after 70 days a perfectly genuine hyalinosis of the arterial wall was present. Similarities were also seen in the hypertensive rat experiments of Ooneda et al. (1965), of Yamori et al. (1976) and of Rascher (Sect. 2.11). One thing seems to be clear and important, namely that once hyaline changes are apparent, they are probably *not* reversible. In contrast, atherosclerosis may be reversible, as proved by German experience with prisoners of war (Randerath) and the experimental evidence of many others, in particular Armstrong et al. (1970), Wissler and Vesselinovitch (1975), Wissler (1977) and Betz and Schlote (1979). This reversibility holds at least as regards the calcareous and lipid content.

"Miliary Aneurysms". We must now focus our attention on a second feature of cerebrovascular pathology and ask: What is the nature of the famous Charcot-Bouchard aneurysms and their significance in intracerebral haemorrhages? Aneurysm means to the general pathologist, in its restricted sense, a saccular widening of an artery, but fusiform or ampullary types are also included.

To this end we have to discuss the nature of the structures described by Charcot and Bouchard (1868). I am able to show you the original drawings of these aneurysms thanks to the kindness of Dr. Castaigne of Paris. Charcot and Bouchard (1868) saw these miliary aneurysms with the naked eye in all of his 77 cases.

Rokitanski (1844) had already described similar structures, Kölliker and Hasse (1846) also saw pear-like ectasias and Pestalozzi (1849) called these "dissecting aneurysms". Subsequently, scientists studied these phenomena as described by Charcot and Bouchard (1868) and we find that Zenker (1872) described a size of 0.2 – 1 mm, the same size as seen by Charcot. Nothnagel (1879) described measurements of 2 – 4 mm. In a modern description we find that Cole and Yates (1967) in Manchester – two authors very familiar with the subject – report sizes *below* 250 μm. Their investigation of 53 of 200 brains showed that "... some 15 – 25 aneurysms were found in each brain ..."; "... not one was found on the main striate vessel e.g. Charcot's artery of cerebral haemorrhage ...". (Lancet 1967). Ross Russell (1963) in England found the size to be between 300 and 900 μm. Finally, Matsuoka (1952) examined serial sections from 146 brains and found aneurysms measuring 200 – 700 μm, which is smaller than "miliary", and they were strictly correlated to hypertension. The arteries had a lumen of 70 – 200 μm and there was no correlation to atherosclerosis. Haemorrhages were by no means always a consequence of such aneurysms.

From the very beginning, the concept of these aneurysms being the cause of bleeding has been accepted with great reluctance. Virchow had seen similar structures and called them "ampullary ectasias". He and Robertson (1900), Zenker (1872) and Eppinger (1888) objected to the name of true aneurysms as suggested by Charcot. Rightly, Pestalozzi (1849) and Virchow (1856) called them *aneurysma spuria,* meaning dissecting aneurysms, as did Ellis (1909) and Pick (1910), in Berlin, who described them beautifully. At that time each author had to illustrate them and we find many illustrations in the literature (see Gowers 1892, 1893). We should now define the real nature of aneurysms. Were they, in fact, real aneurysms? Russell (1963) had found them at points of branching where they were often multiple, but such an excellent connaisseur of cerebrovascular problems as Miller Fisher (1971) could not find aneurysms at the site of rupture when making serial sections, and Moossy (1966, 1971) found them also in normotensives.

From the foregoing brief discussion it becomes obvious that findings and interpretations are contradictory from the very beginning. I personally have doubted the "single" nature of the aneurysm-like out-pouchings seen by the naked eye (Zülch 1961, 1966). Therefore, together with Pabelick, we went into a detailed morphological study (1967), but we chose a somewhat different approach. We examined the side contralateral to the bleeding and not the area of the haemorrhage itself, where the tissue was destroyed. We thereby made the premise that the lesions should be equally developed on both sides, since mass bleedings have no side of predilection.

Our observations will now be listed:

1) Hyaline spheres as outpouchings in the arteries of the basal ganglia, corresponding in size to the Charcot aneurysms (Figs. 2a, b, 3a, 4);
2) Local ectatic widenings of the vessels, simulating aneurysms and corresponding to Virchow's ampullary ectasias (Fig. 5b);
3) Local, more "balloon-like", outpouchings of the arteries which one could possibly compare with the true Charcot type (Fig. 5b);

4) Small old and new periarterial haemorrhages which could correspond to the *Kugelblutungen* of Spatz (Figs. 3b, 6);
5) Local arterial necrosis of the hyalinotic arteries, both older – occurring in the area of the most pronounced changes, and fresh – and necrosing the arterial wall considerably, as described by many general and neurological pathologists (Figs. 3b, 6); and
6) Not infrequently, signs of true atherosclerosis in the proximal segment of intracerebral arteries (Fig. 5a).

It will be immediately stated that the atherosclerotic changes occurred predominantly in a deeper basal plane than the hyalinotic alterations, e.g. below a horizontal section through the anterior commissure and, therefore proximally, where the lumen of the artery was wider.

It was mentioned above that atherosclerosis, together with a more frequent hyalinosis (58 of 70 cases), occurred in this catalogue of pathological phenomena in massive haemorrhage. What was its share in the pathogenesis of the bleedings? The following statement is important: Hyalinosis occurred on the contralateral side in the majority of the haemorrhage cases that we have examined in serial sections, but hyalinosis is patchy and sometimes one needs 20–40 serial sections before one encounters it. Intracerebral atherosclerosis occurred in about the same percentage of cases as was seen in the basal arteries, that is, in the circle of Willis. This distribution corresponded to the incidence of atherosclerosis in a normal population of the same older age group. We cannot therefore conclude that atherosclerosis may be neglected in the discussion of the pathogenesis of massive haemorrhage.

From our observations we conclude that structures corresponding to the macroscopical description of Charcot's "aneurysms" do occur. Microscopically, however, according to our own findings and those of other authors, they correspond to processes different from those described above.

Instead of discussing at length our concepts about the origin of hypertensive haemorrhage, the following arguments for our theory regarding arterial rupture will now be presented:

1) The walls of the lenticulostriate and other paramedian arteries are relatively thin as compared with others. Pabelick (1967) has measured the lumen of 500 intracerebral arteries and found a "constitutionally thin wall in these end arteries". They are very frequently tortuous.
2) Massive haemorrhage is closely correlated to hypertension and hyalinosis.
3) Massive bleeding is seldom encountered without hypertensive arterial disease, e.g. hyalinosis, old and fresh periarterial haemorrhage, arterial necrosis etc.
4) In a high percentage of cases terminal massive haemorrhages are correlated clinically with an acute hypertensive crisis.
5) Frequently there are premonitory neurological signs in a milder hypertensive crisis some time before the large bleeding; the older periarterial haemorrhages and the arterial necroses could be correlated pathogenetically with this.
6) Hyalinosis often leads to occlusion of an artery with micro-infarcts in the form of lacunae, as shown by M. C. Fisher (1969). These occlusions must raise the pressure locally in the proximal arteries.
7) It can be shown that the striatal arteries in cadavers of hypertensive patients can only rarely be ruptured (two cases!) even if high pressures (1520 mm Hg) are applied (Lampert and Müller 1926).
8) According to macroscopical observations – as well as in the excellent chapter of Hiller (1936; Fig. 90) – ruptures probably start near the knee of the lenticulostriate arteries. Pabelick (1967) found old small haemorrhages in three cases and nine cases of relatively recent periarterial haematomas.

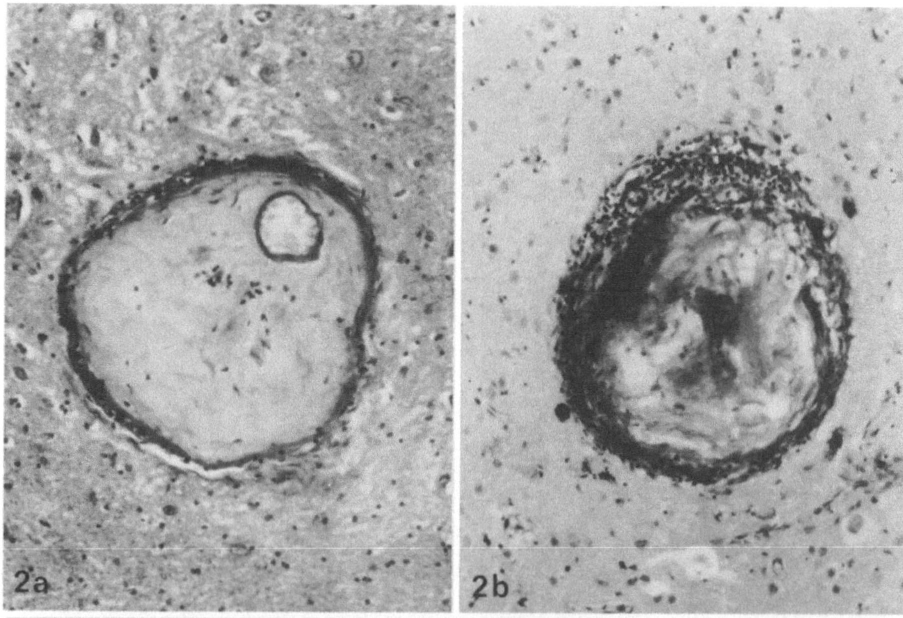

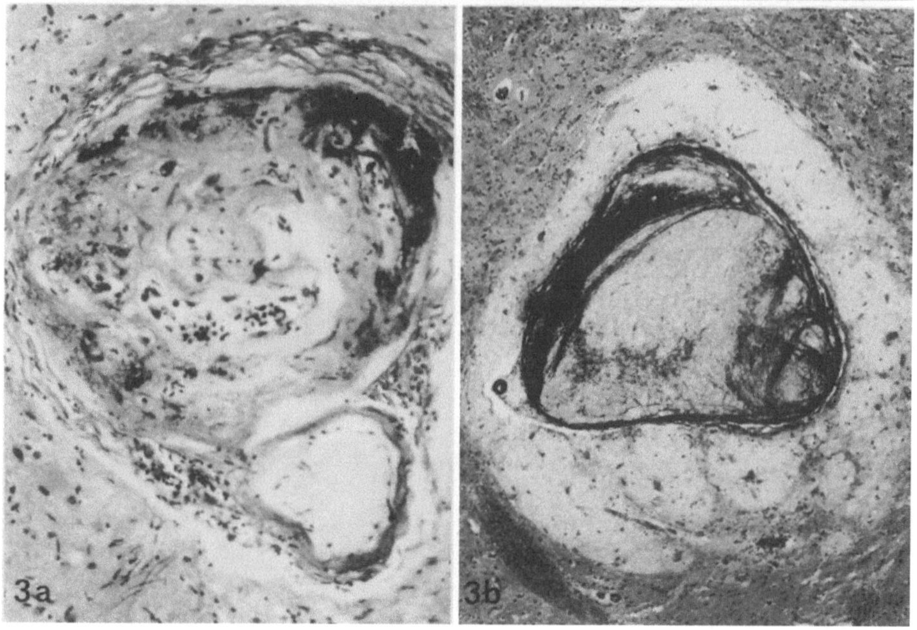

Fig. 2. a Transformation of the entire media into hyaline with thickening and high-grade stenosis of the artery. Masson's trichromic stain × 150. **b** Total change of an artery into a hyaline mass with lymphoid infiltration and macrophages (so-called arterionecrosis). H and E × 125

Fig. 3. a Almost complete occlusion of an artery by hyaline masses, which stain either red (dark) or blue (light) by Masson's stain. × 125. **b** Almost complete digestion of a hyalinized artery by periarterial bleeding. Van Gieson's elastic stain. × 50

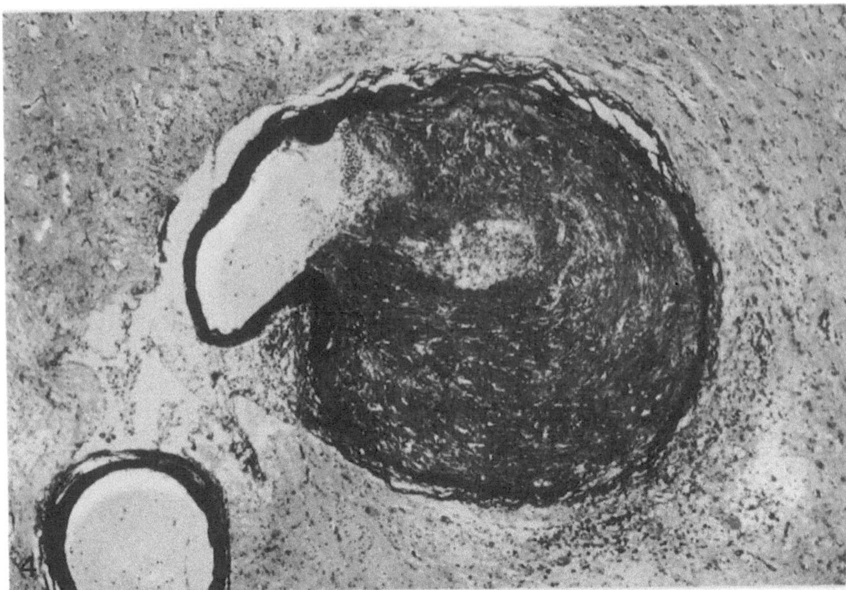

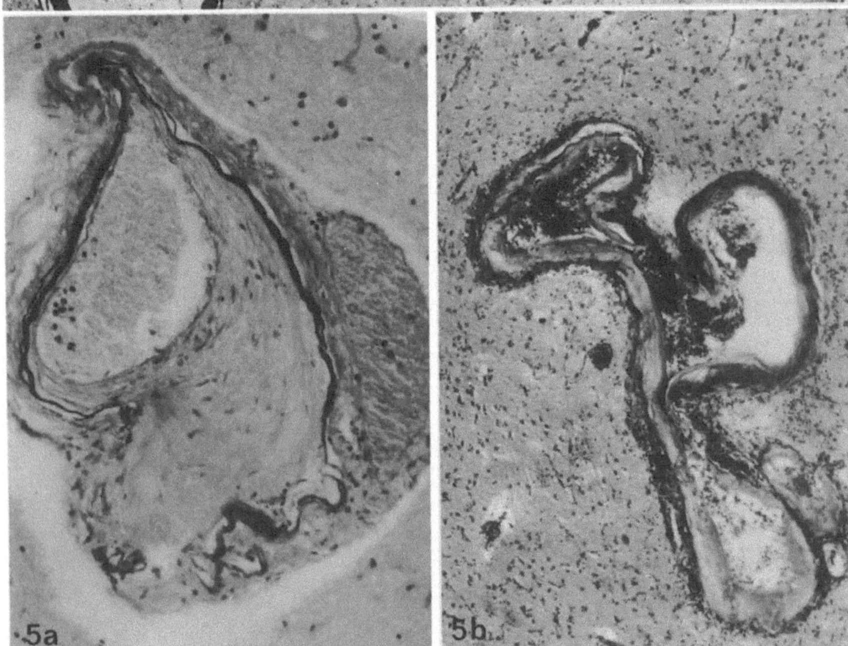

Fig. 4. Tearing of an arterial wall and formation of a small haemorrhage with halfmoon-shaped fibrin mantle. Also, subendothelial bleeding is seen. Van Gieson's elastic stain × 50

Fig. 5. a Transverse section through a lenticulo-striate artery (proximal segment), typical arteriosclerotic changes. × 250. **b** The lenticulostriate artery shows coils and outpouchings. These are partly due to ectasia, partly to hyalinotic changes both Van Gieson's elastic stain × 125

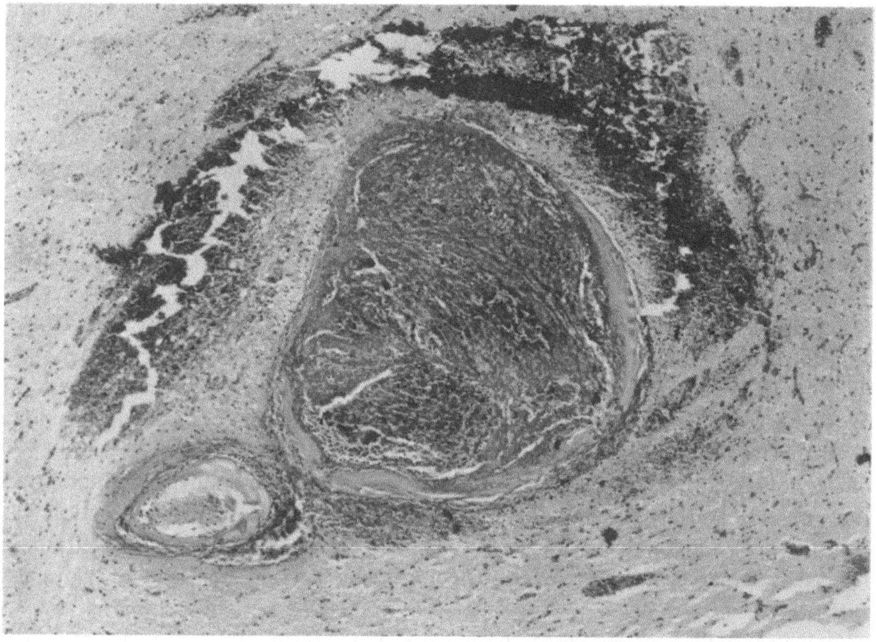

Fig. 6. Splitting of an arterial wall with "digestion" of some of the lamellae within a periarterial bleeding. The innermost lamellae consist of hyaline. H and E × 125

Our deductions are as follows: If the arterial pressure, at some stage of the development of an acute hypertensive crisis, is higher than the necrotic vessel wall, weakened by hyalinosis and arterial necrosis, can withstand, then rupture occurs. Once bleeding commences, other vessels in this zone will be ruptured and "additional bleeders" will be initiated in an avalanche fashion, as C. M. Fisher has formulated. Within a few minutes this may disrupt the inner capsule and surrounding brain tissues.

This interpretation of the facts and observations seems fairly convincing. However, it still seems hard to understand how, from such a small artery or arteries, a fist-sized or larger haematoma can arise in an intracranial cavity which is not elastic, although there are many reserve spaces in the intracranial cavity around and within the aged brain.

Clinically, hypertensive haemorrhage is definitely on the decline because of prevention and better treatment of hypertension. Patients with haemorrhage were received only in the ratio of 1:10 in our intensive care unit (Zülch and Gehlen 1972). This is quite different from the figures given in earlier times (Lyager 1955, 19 haemorrhages, 14 infarctions in 331 cases, 10:7; Zimmerman 1949, in 183 cases, 4:7; Reisner 1954, 11:13; Aring and Merrit 1935, 11.5:13; Fahr 1937, in 800 cases, 11:13; Fisher and Adams 1951, 157 cases, 2:9; and Böhne 1931, 1:9!). According to data I obtained recently, the ratio in Shanghai, China was 1:3.

It is to be hoped that within some decades, hypertensive intracerebral haemorrhage will no longer play a role in the pathogenesis of stroke.

Since the title of this discussion is "stroke", the most common cause of stroke which is cerebral infarction, must be at least briefly discussed although its pathogenesis has been elucidated even less.

In contrast to haemorrhage the pathogenetic discussion on infarction is still lively because of the numerous experimental models (Sundt and Waltz 1971; Symon et al. 1974; Heiss et al. 1976;

Heiss et al. 1977) and investigations particularly on its biochemistry. This was stimulated by the surprising data obtained in our laboratory by K.-A. Hossmann (1977), working on experimental prolonged global ischaemia of the brain.

Serial angiography and rCBF measurements on one side and the biochemical studies about the recirculation and reversibility of nervous tissue ischaemia on the other have stimulated the discussion. Therefore, I shall give here, in a very abbreviated form, some purely personal reflections on a possible concept of cerebral infarction in man.

The following factors seem of importance to me:

1) A well-functioning general circulation, as a *vis a tergo,* expressed by heart action and flow (peripheral resistance blood pressure!);
2) Local obstacles in the vasculature, mainly by atherosclerotic stenoses and/or occlusions;
3) Primary and secondary thromboses and subsequent macro- or micro-thrombo-embolism;
4) An undisturbed microcirculation mainly dependent on the viscosity of the blood; and
5) The possibility of a collateral circulation dependent on pre-existing anastomoses and a sufficient perfusion pressure.

Our conception for most cases of regional cerebrovascular insufficiency and infarction is still that of a disturbance of general circulation by failure of heart action (arrhythmias, insufficiency) and/or decreasing resistance with falling blood pressure predominantly in the hypertensive patients, where local obstacles in the arteries then lead to regional decrease of flow.

Only in a smaller percentage (perhaps 3% – 5%) to the contrary, e.g. a hypertensive crisis can lead to arterial phenomena inducing cerebrovascular insufficiency. This consists of angiospasm (according to the Bayliss principle) and vaso-dilatation associated with a breakthrough of the blood brain barrier.

The simple haemodynamics of the process of cerebral infarction are easily defined, when one knows about the stenoses and occlusion on one side, the possible and actually operating anastomoses on the other and, in addition, the state of the general cardiovascular system. Here the laws of the uneven distribution of the circulating blood in the terminal supply areas, either of one source artery or of two source arteries (last field and watersheds, Zülch 1963, 1977), have made us understand the more complex patterns of cerebrovascular insufficiency or infarction. Sometimes one can predict the likely location in a given case. This notion is based on some work done with Gessaga (Zülch and Gessaga 1972) on the location and predilection of 700 cerebral infarcts.

However, one has to hesitate when calling the haemodynamics "simple". It is well known now that "simple" haemodynamics are only part of the pathogenetic process. Since 1967 we have emphasized a "multiple factor theory" of cerebrovascular insufficiency and have indicated for instance, the results of Swank and Bartsch (1971) who observed aggregation of platelets and erythrocytes after having induced hypotension in the dog. The importance of these disturbances of microcirculation are well known after the research on the action of acetyl-salicylic acid and dipyridamole in preventing thrombosis. Lately the importance of the fibrinolytic enzymes in the process of infarction has been shown by V. Hossmann (1977) in our intensive care unit. Viscosity and even the process of thrombosis seems to depend widely on these systems.

Thrombosis frequently develops on an atherosclerotic plaque; thus, in a final act stenosis progresses into occlusion, after primary sludging. However, thrombosis may often develop in a virgin artery, particularly in young people, as we have noticed several times. Here thrombo-embolism has been observed during an anovulation regime. Another form of thrombo-embolism is considered to be the pathogenetic basis of transient ischaemic attacks (TIAs). In vogue is the concept that on the ulcerated surface of an atherosclerotic plaque at the carotid bifurcation in the neck, for instance, thrombotic material will develop and be thrown into the blood stream as micro-emboli, thus inducing transient disturbances. This concept has followed the undoubted observation of micro-emboli in the retina in cases of amaurosis fugax. In our team we have always been reluctant to accept this as the common basis of TIAs and have collected many arguments, particularly in the light of our experience with hundreds of micro-embolization experiments (Zülch and Tzonos 1965; Zülch et al. 1976; Zülch 1977; Schuier et al. 1978).

One of the basic questions investigated with success in the experiment, although not yet of any assistance clinically, is the problem of reversibility of nervous tissue ischaemia. K.-A. Hossmann's (1977) experience with prolonged (1 h!) global ischaemia showed that the old rule of thumb was basically no longer valid in the experiments, namely that after 6 – 8 min of ischaemia, tissue necrosis would follow.

However, the experience of Opitz and M. Schneider (1950) is still valid in man although the experiments – and up to now only experiments – show that this is not correct for the animal. Nevertheless, in the ward we still have to accept the old statement. Moreover, there is up to now no symptom or test analysing the state of the nervous tissue involved, e.g. whether the ischaemic damage is reversible. Intensive therapy therefore usually has to be prolonged until the outcome shows that the damage is irreversible.

Finally, other clinical problems have to be discussed. The first question which has to be answered is: Where is the stroke patient to be received? We believe that a neurological department needs its own intensive care unit (Zülch 1972). We opened such a unit in Cologne-Merheim at the beginning of 1968 and until 31 July 1978, that is, in a period of 10.5 years, we have treated 2701 patients and gave preliminary reports on the results in 1971 and 1972.

It is our opinion that the neurologist should be trained in intensive care medicine so that he can run the unit with the aid of his anaesthetist and medical colleagues. Patients with stroke comprised 50% of all ICU cases during the first few years, but they have increased over recent years. A final report of the results is in preparation.

The diagnostic steps in the intensive care unit include taking the history of the period before and of the time of stroke; cardiovascular and neurologic examination, in addition to EEG with frequency analysis and computer tomography and/or conventional technetium scan. The latter can be combined with a global flow study by a Lassen-Ingvar (1963) device with 10 – 16 detectors directed in a vertex view. rCBF studies by an intracranial approach are performed in any case if angiography is indicated.

The results of the various methods now allow the condensation into an exact localization of the ischaemic lesion on an artificial grid which can be adapted to a brain chart containing the convolutions and architectonic areas. This seems to be the best possibility of precisely localizing an ischaemic focus (Zülch et al. 1978). A therapeutic programme comprises the following suggestions:

Table 3. General therapeutic programme

Blood volume	Myocardium	Cardiovascular		
Antioedematous treatment			Blood pressure	Electrolytes
Dextrans Sorbitol Frusemide	Glycosides Anti-arrhythmic drugs	Hydergine Dihydroergotamine Theophylline derivatives	Arterenol Nor-Ephedrine – Antihypertensive agents	Substitution

A final question is whether the results of an intensive care unit for stroke merit the tiring, time-consuming and exhausting forms of treatment. This cannot easily be answered. In the beginning with the stroke patients, we had a 50% mortality rate. However, this figure can hardly be compared with data in the literature (S. E. Pitner and C. J. Mance 1973; around 30%!), since it depends on the type of lesion in the patients in the ward. We reported at the Giessen-meeting of the German Society of Neurology in 1973 about particularly satisfying results in single patients.

As an example of this series (Zülch et al. 1973), we mention the instance of a 52-year-old woman who had an occlusion of the middle cerebral artery with aphasia and hemiparasis, but is now living 15 years later without any deficit and is executing tiring social activities.

At the end a statement may be allowed: Around 16% of deaths annually can be attributed to cerebrovascular problems most frequently caused by vascular disease such as atherosclerosis. Of coronary patients, 25% die from the same cause. More than 50% altogether die from the sequelae of atherosclerosis (if we also take into account renal disease and vascular problems of the extremities; see Notabene Medici, 2/1978. Arteriosklerose: Todesursache Nr. 1 in den Industrieländern).

We have a cancer institute in our country, as in many other countries, and support for cancer research is growing. But where are the parallel institutions for atherosclerosis research correlated with the necessary satellite hospitals for cardio- and cerebrovascular and angiological conditions?

I have asked this question for years without provoking any response from the public. However, I am happy to announce that at last Max-Planck-Gesellschaft and the City of Cologne have decided to continue my former department and clinical wards as a unit for cerebrovascular research, supported by a new ward for stroke patients in the Merheim Hospital.

2 Morphology and Aetiology

2.1 Pathology and Aetiology of ICH

K. Jellinger, Vienna

The term spontaneous intracerebral haemorrhage refers to all varieties of bleeding into the cerebral parenchyma in which trauma or other exogenous factors do not play an essential part (D. Russell 1954) although haemorrhages from ruptured aneurysms and arteriovenous malformations have also been excluded by some authors (Johansson and Melin 1960; Walter and Schütte 1965; Vanderark and Kahn 1968; Benes et al. 1972), as have intracerebral haematomas from brain tumours by others (Grote et al. 1970). Although modern CT methods permit accurate identification of small intracerebral bleedings, only significantly large haemorrhages exceeding 2 – 3 cm in diameter in the cerebrum and cerebellum and 1.5 cm in the brains stem which are not due to trauma or neonatal damage will be considered (Russell 1954; Jellinger 1977).

Natural History

The annual mortality rates from cerebral vascular disease (CVD) range from 95 to 300 per 100000, and show great regional and racial differences (Wylie 1972; Sahs 1975; Kurtzke 1976). CVD accounts for about 15% of all deaths, subdivided into 2% – 8% from infarctions and 2% – 9.7% (average, 3% – 4%) from haemorrhage (Table 1). While in clinical statistics the ratio of cerebral infarction to haemorrhage is estimated as 10:1 – 2, bleedings are considered to account for 15% – 30% of all deaths attributed to CVD (Zülch 1971; Wylie 1972). The proportion of cerebral haemorrhages is 10% – 40% in large clinical materials and 37% – 83% in

Table 1. Incidence of spontaneous cerebral haemorrhage in autopsy series

Author, year	Autopsies	Haemorrhages	Infarcts
Michael (1932)	15257	1112 (6.5%)	
Rose (1948)	7057	227 (3.2%)	
Zimmerman (1949)	4240	107 (2.5%)	75 (1.7%)
Courville (1950)	40000	1135 (2.8%)	
Fisher & Adams (1951)	925	28 (3.0%)	72 (7.8%)
Staemmler (1958)	4532	129 (2.8%)	92 (2.0%)
Marks (1960)	adults	3.0%	
Rey & Bellet (1960)	4625	224 (4.9%)	
Dinsdale (1964)	19093	511 (2.7%)	
Brewer et al. (1968)	5187	503 (9.7%)	281 (5.4%)
McCormick & Rosenfeld (brain) (1973)	3372	144 (4.2%)	
Inst. Path. Univ. of Vienna (1969 – 1971)	5553	166 (3.0%)	
Jellinger (neurolog. hospital) (1977a)	1743	87 (4.9%)	149 (8.5%)
Personal series (neuropath. material) (1965 – 78)	8380	430 (5.1%)	570 (6.8%)

autopsy series (Jellinger 1972). The acute mortality from intracerebral haemorrhage ranges from 37% – 75% with a close relationship to the location (Sahs 1975; Hier et al. 1977), while mortality rates after surgical treatment are between 5% and 7% (Luyendijk 1972; Schiefer 1972).

Course and Tissue Reaction

With regard to clinical development cerebral haematomas have been divided into acute, subacute and (sub)chronic forms (Luyendijk 1972). Gross examination of the brain soon after a massive haemorrhage reveals a clot which is soft and like red currant jelly. When the clot is removed, the walls of the cavity are ragged, and small vessels are often found projecting into it. Around the main clot, numerous petechial haemorrhages are visible in the adjacent tissue, which is soft and swollen. A massive haemorrhage has a tendency to track along tissue planes, separating rather than destroying the nervous substance. The haematoma usually results in large intracranial displacements, or ruptures directly into an adjacent ventricle or less often into the subarachnoid space (Figs. 7, 11, 13). Many major haemorrhages produce death before there is much tissue reaction. The early reaction is that of oedema of adjacent tissues and exudation of neutrophils. Later, macrophages undertake the slow process of digestion, and the resultant cavity is encapsulated after a period of some weeks and finally walled off by a scar which usually has a fairly prominent collagenous component in addition to astrocytes. The final result is a large single or multilocular cavity filled with serous fluid, and a brownish capsule (Fig. 5), where haemosiderin-loaded macrophages may persist for many years (Zülch 1968; Ule and Kolkmann 1972; Yates 1976).

Aetiology

There are many causes of intracerebral haemorrhage, the proportion of which varies considerably from series to series. In post-mortem studies, over 50% of all massive haemorrhages are associated with hypertension. Almost 20% are due to ruptured berry aneurysms, while blood dyscrasias and angiomatous malformations rank third in frequency as the cause of spontaneous intracerebral haemorrhage. A lesser number occur in association with cerebral tumours, other vascular diseases and anticoagulation therapy, while in 3% of intracerebral haemorrhage no cause can be demonstrated (Table 2). In clinical records, vascular malformations (aneurysms and angiomas) are almost as frequent causes as hypertension, while in a considerable proportion of cases the aetiology of the bleeding is not clear (Table 3).

Hypertensive Cerebral Haemorrhage

In whites this has a Gaussian age distribution curve with maximum occurrence during the 6th and 7th decades, although 25% – 30% are present under the age of 50, with a much higher frequency in young hypertensives and blacks (Wylie 1972). After the age of 65 there are no significant differences in the incidence of lethal intracerebral haemorrhages (Freytag 1968; Kane and Aronson 1969).

Site. About 80% of hypertensive haemorrhages occur in the cerebral hemispheres, and of these 60% – 80% rupture into a ventricle. Bleeds into the basal ganglia account for 65% of all

Table 2. Causes of spontaneous cerebral haemorrhage in autopsy series

Author Cause	Zimmerman 1949	Russell 1954	Staemmler 1958	Mutlu et al. 1963	Schaafsma 1968	Brewer et al. 1968	Blackwood 1969	McCormick 1973	Personal series	Total	Percent
Hypertension	81	232	119	135	26	503	143	37	160	1436	57.4
Aneurysm	–	96	–	44	1	–	246	20	69	476	19.0
Blood disorders	2	36	5	30	4	23	2	30	34	166	6.6
Angioma	3	21	2	6	–	2	25	15	63	137	5.6
Tumours	5	9	1	2	2	4	14	13	44	94	3.3
Mycotic aneurysm	–	28	–	–	–	–	1	1	3	33	1.4
Arteritis	–	13	–	2	1	–	–	5	4	25	1.0
Anticoag. tr	–	–	–	–	8	–	–	4	10	22	0.9
Phlebo-thrombosis	–	–	–	–	–	–	–	4	8	12	0.5
Infarcts	–	1	–	3	1	–	–	2	5	12	0.5
Eclampsia	–	–	2	3	–	–	–	1	4	10	0.4
Amyloid angiopathy	–	–	–	–	–	–	–	–	10	10	0.4
Unknown, others	–	19	–	–	8	–	18	12	16	73	3.0
Total	91	455	129	225	51	532	449	144	430	2506	100.0

Table 3. Causes of spontaneous cerebral haemorrhage (clinical series)

Authors	Hyper-tension	Aneurysm	Angioma	Tumour	Blood diseases	Antico-agulants	Angiitis, phlebo-thrombosis	Unknown and others	Total
Margolis et al. 1951	55	29	9	–	–	–	–	14	107
Lazorthes et al. 1956	92	78	40	10	–	–	–	134	354
Weber 1963	16	1	2	2	–	–	2	21	44
Krayenbühl et al. 1964	24	64	68	–	–	–	–	–	156
Odom et al. 1966	56	56	17	3	4	–	–	15	151
Luessenhop et al. 1967	64	49	13	2	–	–	–	2	130
Riishede 1967	55	13	5	–	–	–	–	–	73
Paillas 1968	126	–	19	–	–	–	–	24	169
Vanderark-Kahn 1968	22	–	8	–	–	–	–	–	30
Grote et al. 1970	117	40	46	(x)[a]	8	8	3	22	244
Gargand et al. 1971	59	8	5	–	5	–	–	2	79
Pia 1972	63	48	89	28	–	–	–	25	253
Scott 1975	43	5	8	8	1	–	1	14	80
Pers. ser. (biopsies)	8	3	61	12	2	2	5	19	112
Total	800	394	390	65	20	10	11	292	1982
Percent	40.0	19.7	19.5	3.3	1.0	0.5	0.5	14.5	100.0

[a] Not included

hypertensive haemorrhages; of these the majority are located in the putamen, while only about 13% are primarily in the thalamus (Table 4). The cerebral hemispheres and white matter are the sites of haemorrhage in about 16% of the cases, the pons and midbrain in 10% – 12% and the cerebellum in 8% – 9%, while multiple hypertensive bleeds are rare (Table 4).

The classification, extension and aetiology of supratentorial haemorrhages are discussed elsewhere (see Sect. 5.1). Spontaneous cerebellar haematomas, which in 33% – 90% of adults are associated with hypertension, but in younger subjects usually result from small "cryptic" vascular malformations (Meienberg et al. 1972; Hollin et al. 1977; Mauersberger et al. 1977), originate mainly in the deep paradental white matter, presumably from rupture of a branch of the superior cerebellar artery. They may rupture into the subarachnoid space (Fig. 3).

Primary haemorrhages of the brain stem, almost 90% of which occur in hypertensive patients (Silverstein 1972; Collomb et al. 1973), usually originate in the centre of the pons at the junction of the tegmentum and basis where the anterior and posterior pontine vessels converge. They often extend to the mid-brain and only rarely to the medulla (Fig. 1); isolated involvement of the medulla oblongata is extremely rare (Fig. 6).

Pathogenesis. The crucial importance of hypertension in the origin of massive brain haemorrhage is documented by significant correlations between hypertension, cardiomegaly, hypertensive cerebral vascular disease and cerebral haemorrhage (Brewer et al. 1968; Kane and Aronson 1969; Zülch 1971; Wylie 1972; Yates 1976). Long-standing hypertension has been found to be the most important factor for the development of intracerebral arterial degeneration (Fig. 3). It manifests its greatest influence upon the frequency of cerebral haemorrhage in younger age groups.

There are several theories explaining the mechanism of injury that produces intracerebral bleeding (see Zülch 1971; Jellinger 1972; Luyendijk 1972; Yates 1976).

a) The functional hypothesis suggests that a pre-haemorrhagic episode of vasospasm associated with a hypertensive crisis might induce ischaemic necrosis of the vessel wall and/or adjacent brain tissue thus resulting in a sudden extravasation of blood (Rosenblath 1918; Schwartz 1972).

b) The almost inevitable finding of fairly severe atherosclerosis in hypertensive patients has suggested to many that large intracerebral haemorrhage may be no more than an extensive haemorrhagic infarct or at any rate haemorrhage from poorly "supported" arteries transversing ischaemically softened areas (Rouchoux 1842; Globus et al. 1949). The coneept that a pre-existing area of cerebral softening with re-establishment of flow provides a milieu in which both haemorrhagic infarct and haemorrhage may occur has some experimental support (Laurent et al. 1976). In the vasoproliferative stage of mature infarction produced by occlusion of the proximal middle cerebral artery in monkeys, a rapid rise of mean arterial pressure induced by a cerebral vasoconstrictor caused a haemorrhagic infarct, while cerebral vasodilatation caused intracerebral haematomas. Whether or not the hypothetical mechanisms schematically suggested in Table 5 pertain to the natural history of spontaneous cerebral haematomas in man remains debatable.

c) Structural changes of the cerebral vasculature due to hypertension, and rupture of small aneurysmal dilatations of the arteries, first described in 1868 by Charcot and Bouchard, are now the most widely accepted aetiological explanation for the occurrence of hypertensive brain haemorrhage. These vascular lesions, referred to as hypertensive or fibrinoid angiopathy, hyalinosis, lipohyalinosis, fibrinoid or hyaline arterial necrosis or angionecrosis, etc. (Scholz and Nieto 1938; Anders and Eicke 1941; Staemmler 1958; Fisher 1971; Ooneda et al. 1973; Rosenblum 1977), are characterized by marked thickening with deposition of fibrinoid or

Table 4. Location of hypertensive cerebral haemorrhages

Author	Striatum	Basal ganglia	Thalamus	Cerebral hemispheres	Cerebellum	Pons	Multiple	Total
Aring-Merritt (1935)		58		40	2	4	12	116
Russell (1949)		151		21	18	32	4	226
Staemmler (1958)		73		44	6	16		139
Johansson-Melin (1960)		107		36	8	11		162
Mutlu et al. (1963)	83		11	33		8		135
Freytag (1968)	165		60	38	47	63	20	393
Brewer et al. (1968)		333		72	36	62		503
Schaafsma (1968)		21			4	1		26
Wiedersberg (1970)		36		18	6	15		75
Zülch (1971)	102		4	–	7	14		127
Personal material	93		17	15	15	6	4	150
Subtotal		1314 (64.0%)		317 (15.45%)	149 (7.6%)	232 (11.6%)	40 (1.95%)	2052
			Supratentorial		Infratentorial		Others	
Courville (1950)			938		124	73		1135
Adams-Eecken (1953)			131		21	12		164
Blackwood (1959)			26		3	3		32
McKissock et al. (1961)			82		22	19		123
Total			2808 (80%)		319 (9.0%)	339 (9.9%)	40 (1.1%)	3506

Table 5. Schematic representation of hypotheses explaining haemorrhage into mature infarction (modified after Laurent et al. 1976)

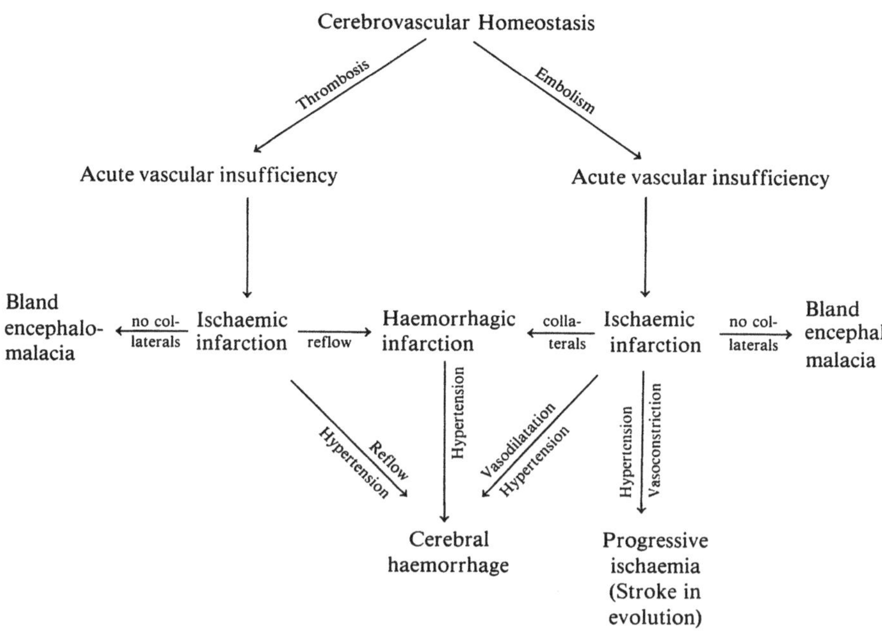

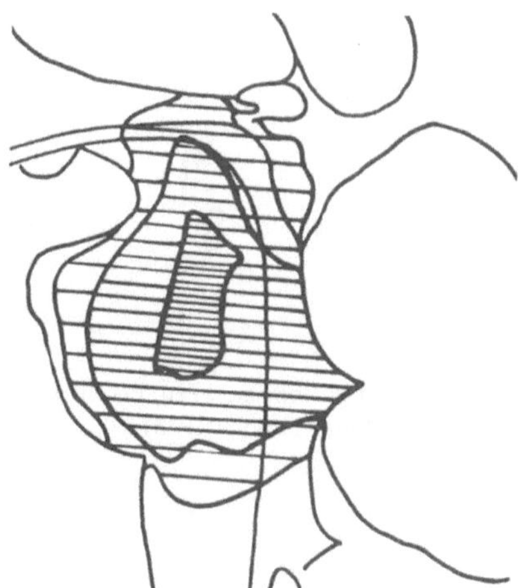

Fig. 1. Centre and extension of spontaneous brain stem haemorrhage

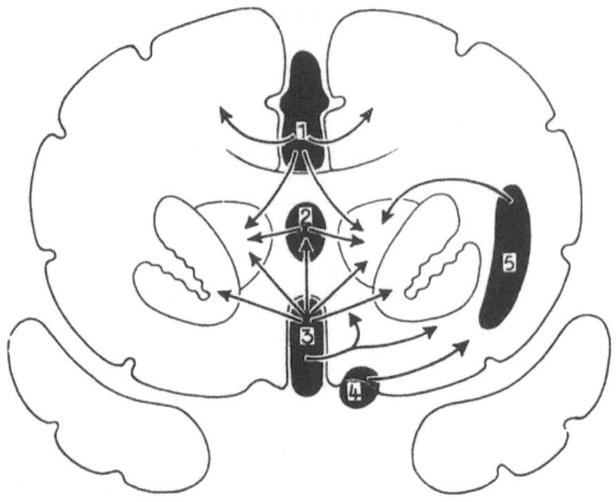

Fig. 2. Extension of haemorrhages arising from ruptured aneurysms

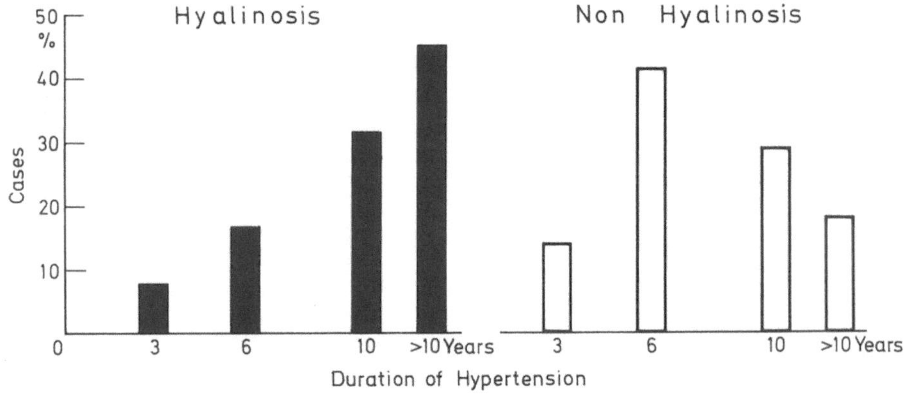

Fig. 3. Correlation between cerebrovascular hyalinosis and duration of hypertension in 170 cases (Rothemund and Frische 1973)

hyalin material and subsequent fibrosis (Fig. 8). They may be associated with local or diffuse aneurysmal dilatation of the vessel wall, although existing fibrinosis may not be a pre-requisite for miliary aneurysm formation (Rosenblum 1977). Experimental and electron microscopic studies indicate a subintimal onset with plasma exudation between the opened endothelial junctions, enlargement of the subendothelial spaces with ensuing atrophy or necrosis of medial smooth muscle cells, and disruption of the internal elastic lamina (Rapoport 1976; Shinkai et al. 1976; Nag et al. 1977). Scanning electron microscopic studies on cerebral vessels in spontaneously hypertensive rats revealed both progressive changes in the endothelial cells, e. g. increased plasmalemmal pits, numerous microvilli and well-developed marginal folds, and regressive changes including balloon-like protrusions and crater-like concavities (Hazama et al. 1978). These regressive changes may contribute to increased permeability of the vessel wall and to platelet adhesion on the injured endothelial surface of arteries (Amano 1977). Recent data suggest that the proliferating factor of platelets may play a role in the cellular hyperplasia of the arterial wall seen in hypertension (Hazama et al. 1978). While hypertrophic hyalinotic vessels show thickened subendothelial space with intercellular deposition of fibrin and collagen fibres, the areas of aneurysmal dilatation reveal thickened basement membranes and media lacking delimitation from the adventitia, with accumulation of collagen, fibroblasts and granular material (Cervos-Navarro and Iglesias Rozas 1976).

The ready demonstration of fibrinoid degeneration or miliary aneurysms in many cases of intracerebral haemorrhage suggests but does not prove that these changes lead to vessel rupture and the haemorrhage itself, although these changes may occur in the absence of any hypertension (Yates 1976; Rosenblum 1977; Fig. 4). The hypothesis that brain haemorrhage was due to rupture of intracerebral arterial micro-aneurysms, put forward by Charcot and Bouchard 1868, discredited by subsequent authors, was confirmed by recent studies in man (Cole and Yates 1967; Fisher 1972; Ooneda et al. 1973; Rosenblum 1977) and hypertensive animals (Santos-Buch et al. 1976; Lee and Berry 1978). Post-mortem X-ray micro-angiography

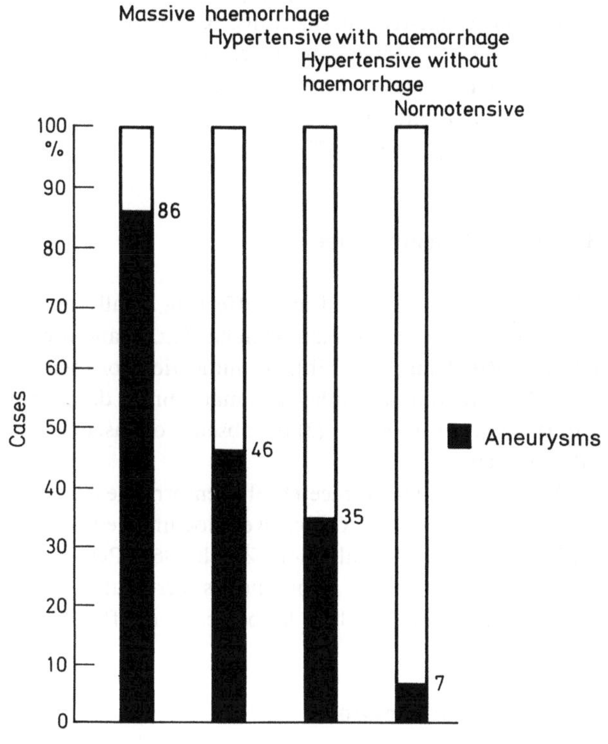

Fig. 4. Percentage of intracerebral micro-aneurysms in 200 normo- and hypertensive cases with and without haemorrhage (Cole and Yates 1967)

in hypertensive individuals revealed, in addition to "pseudo-aneurysms" due to perivascular blood clots, true miliary aneurysms made up of hyaline-fibrinoid material in close apposition to brain haemorrhage. Their presence is clearly related to age (Cole and Yates 1967). They are found most frequently within the basal ganglia on the branches of the striate vessels at points of bifurcation, beneath the cortical grey matter and on leptomeningeal surface vessels, and less frequently in the pons and cerebellum. They involve small arteries and meta-arterioles of 150 – 300 μm in diameter, showing severe hyaline or fibrinoid degenerative changes. Microscopic serial sections indicate that hypertensive haemorrhage results from rupture of such a small damaged artery, and the bleeding secondarily disrupts other adjacent small vessels, giving rise to an expanding bleeding, whereas primary, rupture of several arteries appears less reasonable (Fisher 1971). The predilection for both haemorrhage and hypertensive angiopathy and/or atherosclerosis in the areas of perforating arteries in the lenticular nucleus and pons is likely to be related to vascular morphology and haemodynamic factors:

1) The transitional arteries (meta-arterioles) of the brain have a sparse smooth muscle coat, a poorly defined internal elastic lamina and lack of prominent adventitia.
2) There is a relatively high arterial pressure and transverse tension to the vessel wall existing in the small perforating lenticulostriate (and pontine) branches which originate at a right angle from the main trunks of the middle cerebral (and basilar) artery.
3) The predilection for hypertensive haemorrhage in the basal ganglia was related to their location between the two great arterial circulations, the peripheral (meningeal) and the central (basal) branches of the circle of Willis. Margolis et al. (1968) hypothesized that prolonged vasospasm in the striate arteries, the terminal branches of the central system, leads to fibrinoid arteriopathy with subsequent vascular rupture.
4) Other suggested mechanisms: Capsulolenticular haemorrhages may occur in young hypertensive individuals, in eclampsia or after renal transplantation where the presence of micro-angiomas and hyalinosis are both uncommon; other causes, such as small vascular malformations, acute angionecrosis, oedema or vasospasm are also to be considered (Burger and Vogel 1977).

Traumatic Haemorrhage

This is due to shearing strains affecting small vessels at the time of impact and they not infrequently occur in the basal ganglia (Fig. 5) and other common sites of spontaneous bleeding (Peters 1969; Jellinger 1977b). An indication for their traumatic origin is (1) severe head injury with skull fracture and other traumatic brain damage; (2) manifestation of the haemorrhage shortly after the injury; or (3) the absence of vascular and hypertensive disease or malformation (Peters 1969).

Delayed traumatic intracerebral haemorrhage (early and late forms) developing days or weeks after head injury is a rare, but well documented event, the pathogenesis of which is not clear and deserves critical evaluation (Zülch 1968; Peters 1969; Barathan and Dennyson 1972).

On the other hand, spontaneous cerebral haemorrhage may cause head injury, and distinguishing between these lesions can be difficult, e.g. in forensic cases.

Vascular Malformations

These represent another source of intracerebral bleeding, but the frequency of haematomas caused by ruptured saccular aneurysms and angiomas varies widely from series to series. While in clinical studies, intracerebral haemorrhage is noted in 8% – 15% of ruptured berry aneurysms (Krayenbühl and Yasargil 1972; Luyendijk 1972) and in 40% – 68% of angiomas (Perret and Nishimoto 1966; Pia et al. 1979), its incidence in acute death from ruptured aneurysm is 43% – 79% (Freytag 1968) and was 66% in our autopsy series of 170 cases (Jellinger 1978).

a) Ruptured saccular aneurysm has been found to be the cause in 20% of intracerebral haemorrhages in both clinical and post-mortem series (Tables 2, 3). They most commonly cause death during the 4th and 5th decades, about two-thirds becoming manifest after the age of 40 (Krayenbühl and Yasargil 1972). Our youngest case was a boy, aged 4 years, with tuberous sclerosis, renal cysts and frontal haemorrhage from ruptured congenital aneurysm arising at Heubner's recurrent artery (Jellinger 1977a). About 85% of aneurysms occur on the circle of Willis (Jellinger 1979). Those in the Sylvian and interhemispheric fissures, embedded in the cerebral structures, are favourably located for the production of intracerebral haematomas, the site and extension of which are related to the site of the aneurysm. Haemorrhage arising from aneurysm of the anterior communicating and anterior cerebral arteries ploughs through the frontal lobe to enter the ventricle. Bleeds arising from the carotid bifurcation area and the middle cerebral artery enter the temporal lobe and lentiform nuclei, occasionally mimicking spontaneous capsulolenticular haemorrhage (Fig. 2). Intracerebellar haemorrhage may result from ruptured aneurysm of the posterior inferior cerebellar artery. Intracerebral haemorrhage caused by a ruptured aneurysm without an extension of the bleed into the subarachnoid space is very rare (Housepian et al. 1958), e.g. localized frontal haemorrhage resulting from intracavernous saccular aneurysm of the internal carotid artery (Fig. 9). The prognosis and mortality of ruptured aneurysms mainly depend on the location of the haemorrhage, entering of the ventricles and acute intracranial pressure. Some aneurysms giving rise to fatal intracerebral haemorrhage are not easily detected: A boy, aged 15 years, 5 days after an uncomplicated fall on the occiput, developed acute headache and lapsed into coma. In spite of bilateral craniotomy he died the next day. There was a large haematoma in the frontal lobe and basal ganglia the source of which was a ruptured aneurysm of the anterior cerebral artery. Fibrous organization with haemosiderin and lymphocytic infiltration around the ruptured sac suggested previous leakage as the cause of the initial fall (Fig. 10).

b) Mycotic aneurysms, the development of which is related to septicaemia, were the source of intracranial haemorrhage in 6% of Russell's series, but their incidence has markedly diminished (Molinari et al. 1973). We saw three such instances: a cerebellar bleed after valvulotomy with endocarditis, a ruptured mycotic aneurysm of the vertebral artery due to post-traumatic meningitis; and another one on the middle cerebral artery in coincidental infection caused by Candida albicans after kidney transplantation. Carotico-cavernous sinus aneurysms (fistulas) and dissecting aneurysms are extremely rare sources of intracerebral haemorrhage.

c) Angiomas have been found to be responsible for 1% – 6% of cerebral haematomas found at autopsy (Table 2) and for 10% – 40% (average 20%) of surgically treated intracerebral haemorrhages (Table 3). In our material, 14.6% of haemorrhages found at autopsy, and 55% of those in the neurosurgical specimens, were of angiomatous origin. About three-quarters of haemorrhages occur in younger age groups with a peak in the second and third decades (Krayenbühl and Yasargil 1972; Pia et al. 1979), although in our case series ranging in age from 2 to 72 years, about 15% were over age 60. The relatively high incidence of haemorrhage from angiomas in older age groups may be of importance for differential diagnosis. The angiomas have been classified by size (small "cryptic", medium-sized and large), location, and by morphological appearance, comprising (a) capillary telangiectasis, (b) cavernomas, (c) arteriovenous malformations and (d) venous angiomas (McCormick et al. 1973; Jellinger 1975). All types of vascular anomalies are capable of producing intracerebral haemorrhage, but in the case of telangiectasias and Sturge-Weber's disease this is extremely rare. Very large angiomas show less tendency to rupture than small cryptic vascular malformations (micro-angiomas) up to cherry size, which are undetectable by clinical methods (Pia et al. 1979). The site of the angioma has considerable bearing on the occurrence of bleeding. It is more frequent in centrally located angiomas than in the peripheral ones, although "atypical" hemispheral haematomas may also arise from small superficial pial malformations. Arterio-venous malformations are the most frequent types which are estimated to represent 1% – 4% of all intracranial space-occupying processes (Pia et al. 1979). Haemorrhage arising from large arteriovenous angiomas and cavernomas may be confined to the cerebral hemispheres and basal ganglia or enter the ventricles. Haemorrhages into the brain stem (Fig. 15) and cerebellum with or without ventricular rupture have a much poorer prognosis, e.g. a large cerebellar haemorrhage from a ruptured A-V malformation in a girl aged 13 (Figs. 13, 14). Cryptic malformations or micro-angiomas (Krayenbühl and Siebenmann 1965) are a frequent source of haemorrhages. The disclosure of these small lesions which include all morphologic types, though chiefly A-V malformations, is dependent on careful microscopic examination, although some of them are destroyed by the haemorrhage (Russell 1954). Cryptic malformations have been found in all parts of the CNS (McCormick et al. 1973; Jellinger 1975), but those located in the periventricular areas are of particular interest. Autopsy of a 70-year-old female revealed a small A-V angioma in the thalamus as the cause of apoplexy (Figs. 11, 12). Vascular malformation in the choroid plexus (Fig. 12) reported as the source of intracerebral haemorrhage in both neonates and adults (Butler et al. 1972; Doe et al. 1972); Pia et al. 1979) were seen in 5.2% of our autopsies and in 3.6% of the biopsy cases of cerebral vascular malformations (Jellinger 1975). The age of the patients ranged from 7 weeks to 50 years, most of them presenting with intraventricular haemorrhage. It is suggested that more instances of ventricular angiomas will be found on routine histological examination.

"Atypical" Spontaneous Haemorrhage

This includes a wide variety of disorders including blood dyscrasias, coagulation defects and vascular diseases.

a) Intracerebral bleeds, ranging from multiple microhaemorrhages to large haematomas, are frequent complications or terminal events in leukaemias (about 50%), lymphomas, blood marrow depression and coagulation defects, including polycythaemia, haemophilia, thrombocytopaenia or thrombocytopathies, fibrinolysis, etc. (Jellinger 1971; Luyendijk 1972; McCormick et al. 1973; Seeler et al. 1973). Recent widespread use of anticoagulants has resulted in the fact that a not inconsiderable proportion of neurosurgically treated or fatal intracerebral haematomas result from this treatment (Grote et al. 1970; Sreerama 1973). Intracerebral haemorrhage after cardiac surgery, with intraoperative coagulation and episodes of hypertension is well documented (Nelson et al. 1973; Humphreys 1975).

b) All types of vascular disease must be included as potential causes of cerebral haemorrhage. Polyarteritis nodosa and necrotizing angiitis are rare causes of massive bleeding (Jellinger 1972;

Fig. 5. Traumatic haemorrhage in corpus striatum
Fig. 6. Hypertensive haemorrhage in medulla oblongata
Fig. 7. Hypertensive putaminal haemorrhage
Fig. 8. Fibrinoid (hyalin) degeneration of striatal meta-arterioles in hypertension. H and E × 30
Fig. 9. Frontal and intraventricular haemorrhage due to ruptured intracavernous aneurysm of internal carotid artery without subarachnoid haemorrhage
Fig. 10. Ruptured aneurysm of anterior cerebral artery in boy, aged 15, with fibrinous organization around ruptured sack and recent haemorrhage into cerebral parenchyma

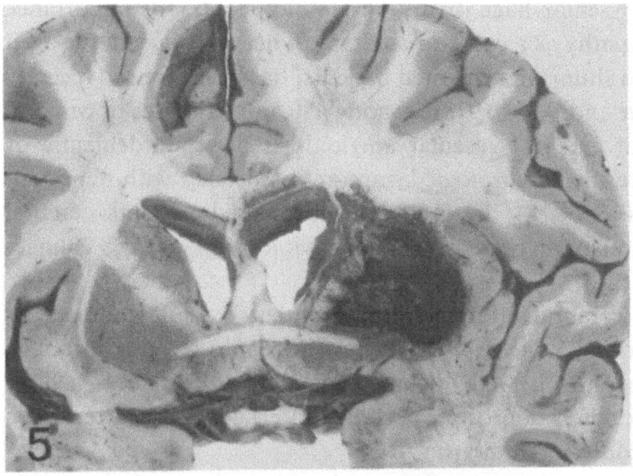
5

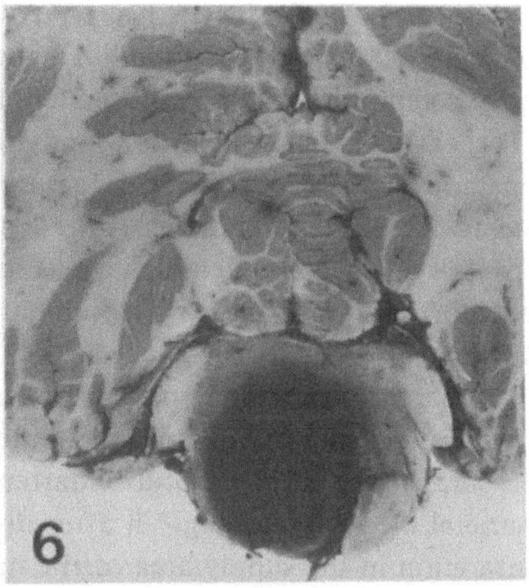
6

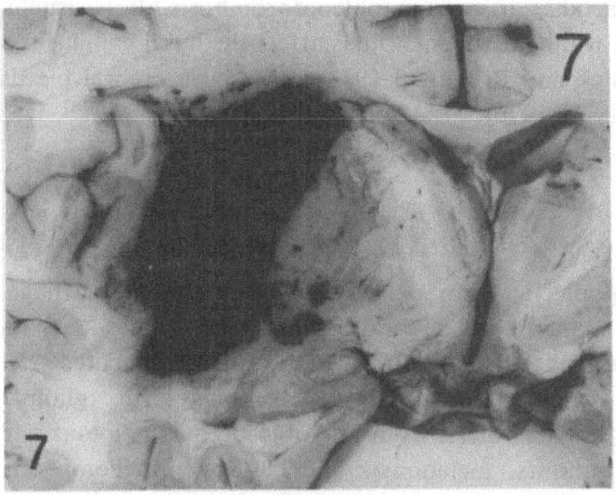
7
7

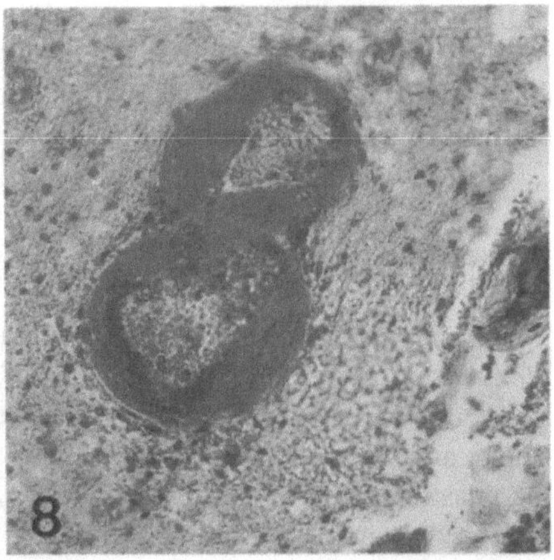
8

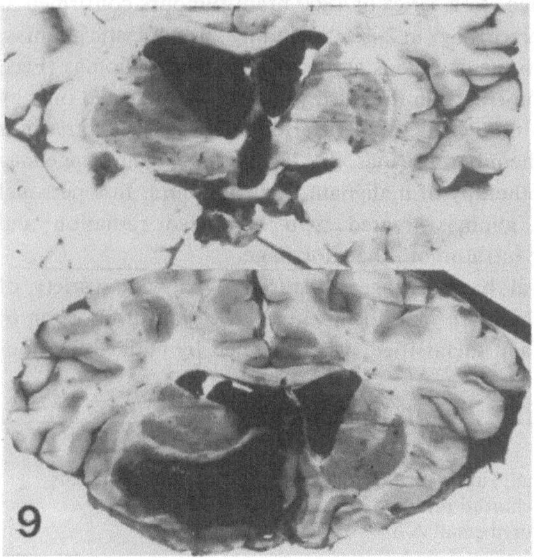
9

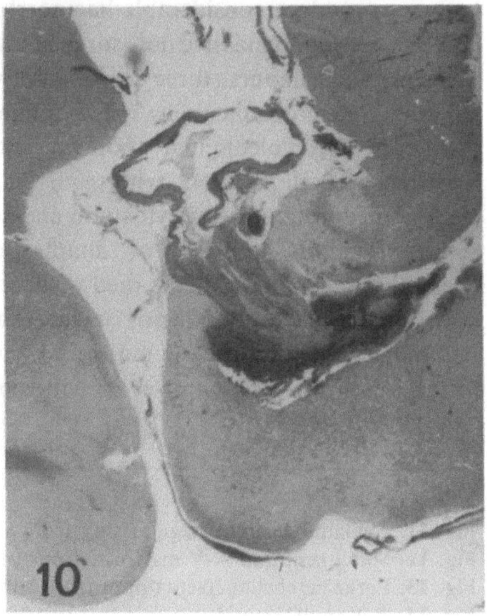
10

Yates 1976). While the cortical type of haemorrhage is very rare in old people, the importance of cerebral amyloid (congophilic) angiopathy as a cause of an atypical haemorrhage in the aged or of cerebral haematoma subsequent to shunts in demented patients, has been stressed recently (Torack 1975; Jellinger 1976; Mandybur and Bates 1978). Among 430 autopsy cases of cerebral haemorrhage we observed ten cases of cerebral vascular amyloidosis in senile dementia or subacute Alzheimer's disease with acute focal neurologic symptoms associated with temporal, frontal or striatal haemorrhage (Figs. 16–18). In other old, demented patients cerebral haemorrhage was due to a combination of hypertensive and amyloid angiopathy (Jellinger 1977c).

c) Large haematomas may arise in cerebral infarcts from secondary vascular damage or rupture, oedema or vasospasm (Burger and Vogel 1977). Haemorrhage into recently infarcted cerebral tissue after carotid endarterectomy is well documented (Wylie 1972), e.g. a large parietal bleed developing 7 h after disobliteration of an occluded internal carotid artery with infarction in the supply area of the middle cerebral artery.

d) Haemorrhage may, however seldom, also arise from phlebothrombosis. It is usually subcortical and can be removed surgically, while rare haematomas affect the basal ganglia and may rupture into the ventricles (McCormick and Rosenfeld 1973). Rare intracerebral bleeds occur in Moya-Moya syndrome (Mauersberger 1976).

Intracranial Tumours

These can manifest themselves in an apoplectic form or may give rise to haemorrhage, representing 2%–10% (average, 3%) of spontaneous cerebral haematomas (Tables 2, 3). In large tumour series, the frequency of haemorrhages is 1.4–7.6% (Padt et al. 1973; Scott 1975). They arise particularly from highly vascularized tumours, i.e. anaplastic gliomas (glioblastomas) and metastases (Fig. 21), but less often from angioblastic meningiomas and pituitary adenomas. Among metastatic tumours, melanomas and chorionepitheliomas are known to produce considerable haemorrhage. In a series of 1800 brain tumours confirmed at autopsy, we found massive non-surgical haemorrhage in 2.4%, including 20 anaplastic gliomas, 17 metastatic tumours, three sarcomas, two meningiomas and two oligodendrogliomas (Figs. 19, 20). A meningioma giving rise to a haemorrhage in the third ventricle was detected only by histology. Capsulolenticular apoplexy was mimicked by diffuse reticulum cell sarcoma in a hypertensive male, aged 45, with recurrent hemiparesis (Figs. 22, 23). Lethal haemorrhage may also occur during or after cytostatic chemotherapy of malignant brain tumours. In a personal series of about 40 cases of anaplastic gliomas treated with combined radiation and chemotherapy, three patients died of acute intratumoral haemorrhage.

In conclusion, spontaneous intracerebral haemorrhage is caused by a wide variety of pathological conditions, the majority of which are well documented. A certain proportion of intracerebral bleedings, however, will remain unclassified, when studied by clinical methods

---

Fig. 11. Thalamic haemorrhage arising from small ruptured A-V malformations of choroid plexus ▶

Fig. 12. Small ruptured A-V malformations of choroid plexus

Fig. 13. Large cerebellar haematoma from ruptured small A-V

Fig. 14. A-V malformation

Fig. 15. A-V malformation with recent lethal haemorrhage in mesencephalic tegmentum

Figs. 16–18. Haemorrhage in senile dementia arising from ball-like haemorrhage around arteriole (*17*) and amyloid angiopathy of cortical vessels (*18*). PAS. × 250

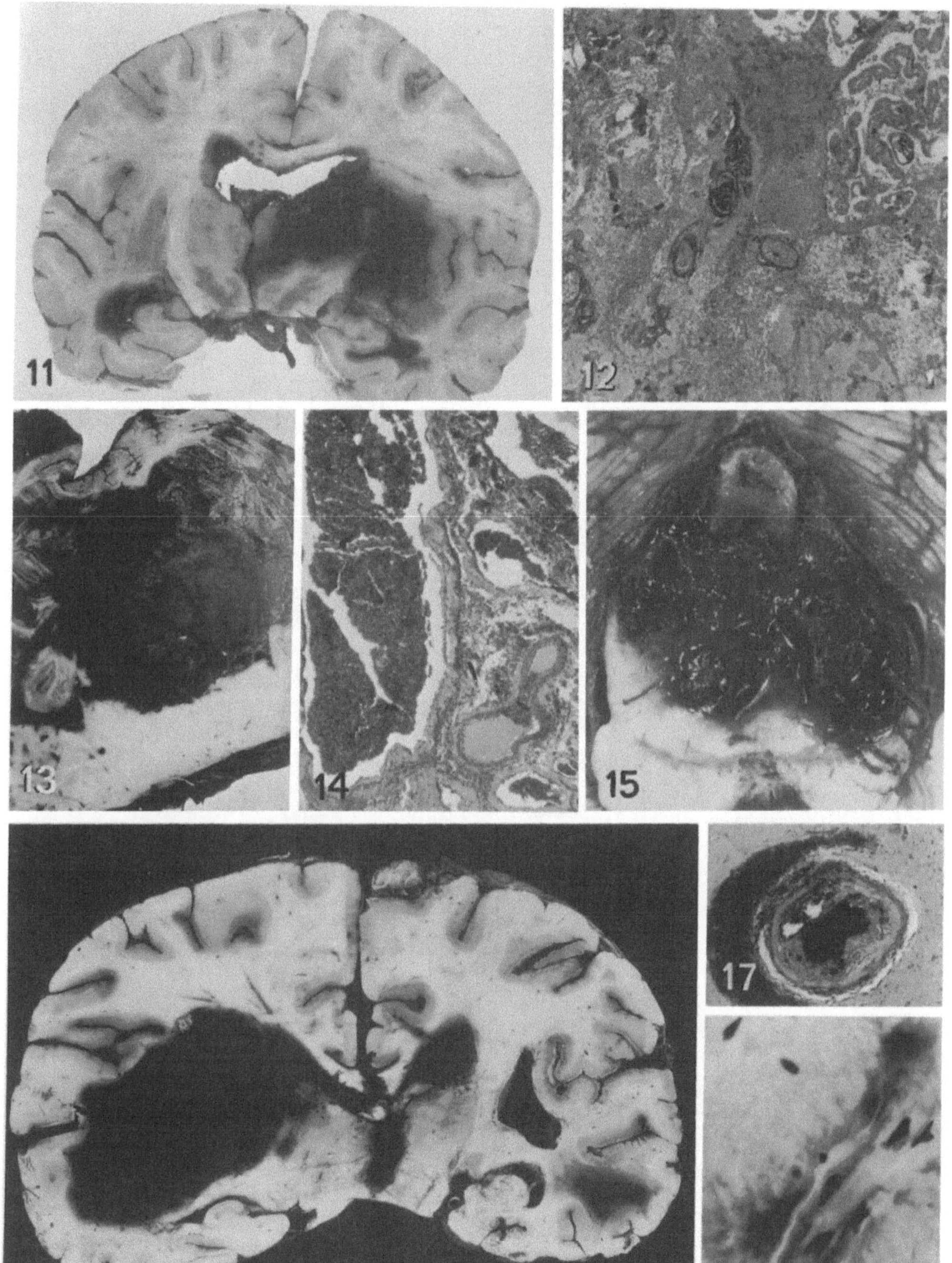
11
12
13
14
15
16
17
18

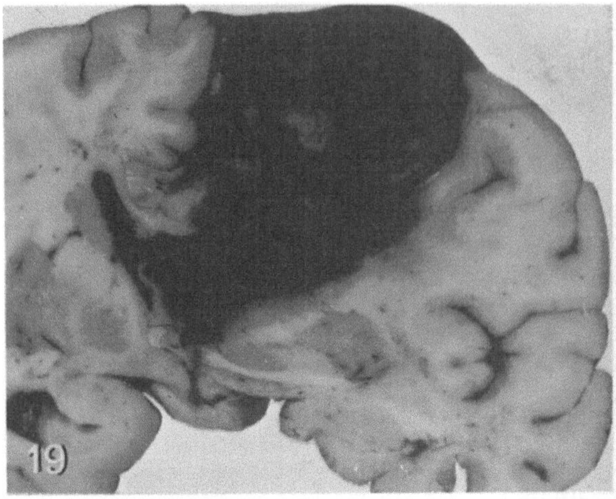
19
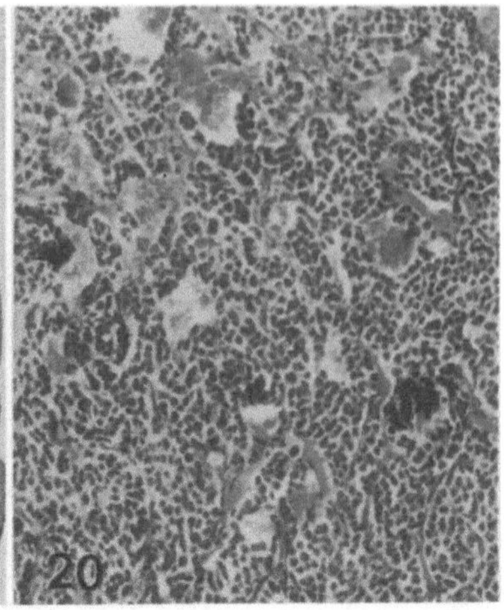
20
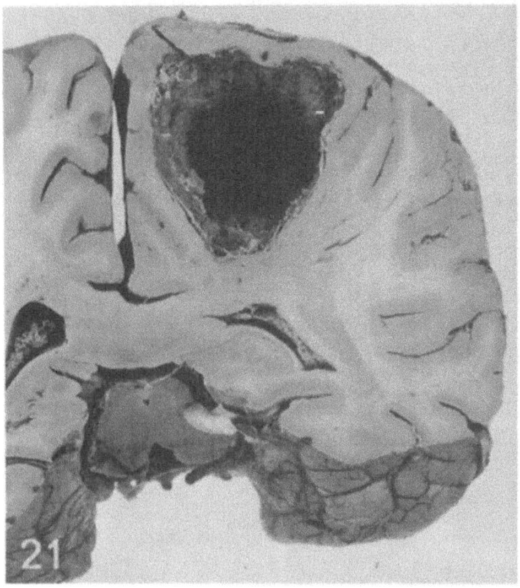
21
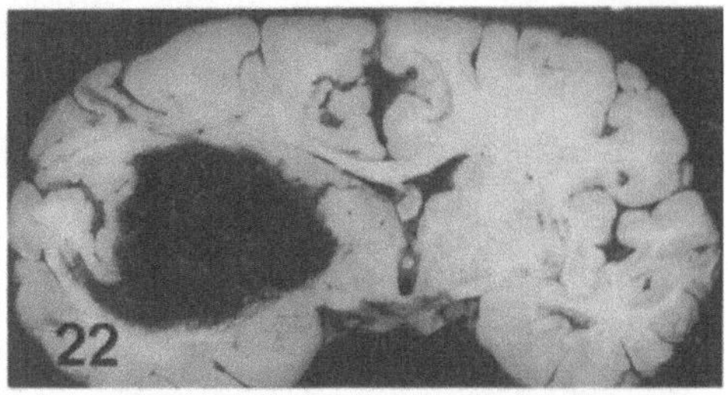
22
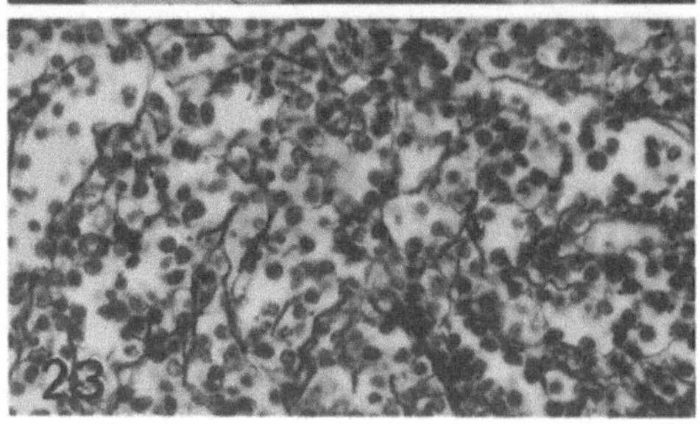
23

alone. The study of the pathology and pathogenesis of intracerebral haemorrhage emphasizes the importance of early diagnosis and may lead to a rational therapy, particularly if it is neurosurgical, as it can show the predilection sites, the source of the bleeding and its secondary complications.

Summary

Spontaneous, non-traumatic intracerebral haemorrhage accounts for 15% – 30% of all deaths attributed to cerebrovascular disease, and to 2.5% – 9.7% (average 4% – 5%) of all autopsies. Aetiologically, in autopsy series, over 50% of all massive haemorrhages are related to hypertension, 20% are due to ruptured aneurysms and about 6% each to blood dyscrasias and A-V malformations, while a lesser number occurs in coagulopathies or other vascular diseases, and 3% remain undetermined. In clinical series, vascular malformation is almost as frequent a cause as hypertension (40% each), while in a considerable proportion of cases (14.5%), the cause remains undetermined. In both autopsy and clinical material, about 3.3% of haemorrhages occur in brain tumours. Of the hypertensive haemorrhages, 80% occur in the cerebral hemispheres, the majority being located in the basal ganglia, with about 16% in the cerebral lobes. Pontine and cerebellar haematomas are each found in 8% – 10%. Among the various pathogenetic theories explaining the origin of hypertensive haemorrhage, hypertensive fibrinoid or hyaline angiopathy with rupture of miliary or micro-aneurysms is the most widely accepted explanation. The basic mechanism of hypertensive angiopathy and the morphological and haemodynamic bases for the predilective location of hypertensive haemorrhages in the putamen and pons are discussed.

Ruptured saccular aneurysms are the cause of 20% of intracerebral haemorrhage in both clinical and post-mortem series, while mycotic aneurysms are rare. Vascular malformations (angiomas) were the source of intracerebral haemorrhages in 14.6% of autopsy cases and in 55% of the surgically treated haematomas. The importance of small ("cryptic") malformations, in particular those in the choroid plexus for the origin of intracerebral and intraventricular haemorrhages is emphasized. Blood dyscrasias and anticoagulation treatment are increasing causes of intracerebral bleeds. Among other vascular diseases giving rise to intracerebral haemorrhages, senile cerebrovascular amyloidosis and phlebothrombosis must be considered. Among 1800 cerebral tumours, massive haemorrhage was found in 2.4%, mainly in anaplastic gliomas and metastases. Lethal haemorrhage may also occur during or after cytostatic treatment of malignant brain tumours.

◀ **Figs. 19, 20.** Large frontal haemorrhage in recurrent oligodendroglioma
Fig. 21. Parietal haemorrhage in metastasis of lung carcinoma
Fig. 22, 23. Recent putaminal bleeding due to malignant lymphoma (reticulum cell sarcoma). Gomori. × 100

2.2 Haemorrhage and Haematoma – Morbid Anatomy

H. Güthert, Erfurt

As far as possible in any discussion between clinicians and neuropathologists, clear definitions and an efficient nomenclature should be ensured at the beginning. This clarification is more necessary in the German language where the possibility of confusion seems to exist.

A "haemorrhage" is an active process in the course of which a haematoma develops. In the brain (and in no other organ) one has tended to call this a "haemorrhage" (in German, *Massenblutung*). This suggests that the terms haemorrhage and haematoma are used synonymously, so that we should possibly be more self critical. However, the term haemorrhage is so firmly established in the German neurological sciences that only with difficulty can the correct term – haematoma – be substituted. A cerebral haemorrhage can develop (as a primary lesion) in the presence of arteriosclerosis as a sequel to a vascular rupture (rhexis) in the course of which a raised blood pressure, through the hyalinosis of the vascular wall, actually prepares or helps not only the arteriosclerosis, but also the vascular rupture. It should be added that severe arteriosclerosis of the basal cerebral vessels and their branches can exist without any vascular rupture and also that the existence of a raised blood pressure is not a regular precursor of a haematoma. On the other hand, such haematomas can develop without any morphological changes being detectable in the vessels by traditional light microscopy. All haematomas that develop without any vascular rupture are the result of diapedesis. This involves an extravasation, first of all of the fluid, and later of the corpuscular elements of the blood, from morphologically intact vessels. The disturbances of permeability responsible for these haemorrhages are "functional", and their extent is related directly to the blood pressure, the speed of circulation and the vessel diameter, as well as depending on a series of complex metabolic disturbances. Disturbances of permeability arise from an oxygen deficiency, which can be direct or indirect.

Haematomas which develop from any of these causes are nowhere so impressive as in the brain. In every other organ there are rigid mesenchymal structures which more or less circumscribe, restrict and mould a haemorrhage; in the brain its extent depends only on the blood pressure and the site of the bleeding (particular sites of predilection are well known). The adjoining white matter is torn through by the bleeding and completely destroyed. In the other parts of the brain, such as the thalamus, pons and medulla, haemorrhages are a sequel to disturbances of permeability arising after the fall of blood pressure. These tend to be multiple and suggest a haemorrhagic infiltration rather than a solitary haematoma. Their shape and extent are dependent on the basic structure of this part of the brain, and they should be clearly distinguished from haemorrhagic infarcts.

If the bleeding is associated with a fall in blood pressure there is limitation of the haematoma, but if not, it may rupture into the adjoining spaces, i.e. the ventricle and occasionally the subarachnoid space.

An infarction of the brain develops usually as a result of gradual arteriosclerotic occlusion of an artery (with or without thrombosis). Although in the past, brain arteries were regarded functionally as end-arteries, it has been known for some considerable time that collaterals do exist in the brain, especially through the meningeal vessels. These come into play particularly when there is a small infarct, and after a complete arterial occlusion they can maintain a reduced supply. As regards the close relationship between the circulation and the metabolism of the brain, there is a range of functional disturbances which behave clinically as an infarct, although they precede its actual development and cannot be confirmed morphologically. Here we can only mention such details as disturbances of respiration, of transport function, nutrition and of the acid-base balance which may well play a prominent part in the genesis of an infarct.

The complex disturbances of the balance of flow back and forth between vessels and tissues, particularly of the concentration of acid ions in the tissues, leads to a vasodilatation. This produces a hyperaemia which can be regarded as superfluous because the nerve cells are already irreversibly damaged. The infarct therefore starts with an initial hyperaemic phase which is followed by the final anaemic phase. Bleeding can occur secondarily into the infarcted area through collaterals. As a result of this, one may see combined white, red and/or mixed infarcts.

Small or larger haemorrhages present in the vicinity of an infarct must be regarded as a disturbance of permeability of the collateral circulation arising as a result of the metabolic disturbances. They are almost always present and, in case of doubt, are a definite diagnostic point of distinction between haemorrhagic infarcts and haematomas, in which such peripheral haemorrhages are absent.

While in theory it would seem conceivable that a haematoma could develop secondarily in an infarct, in practice this is never encountered.

2.3 Diagnosis and Control of Bleeding Disorders

H. G. Lasch and T. Schöndorf, Giessen

Specific plasma proteins – the coagulation factors, a sufficient number of functionally intact platelets and the vascular integrity are the three major components of an equilibrated haemostasis. Under physiological conditions there is a dynamic balance between the three components. A disturbance of haemostasis caused by a procoagulatory stimulation which clinically results in thrombosis or bleeding may develop spontaneously or after trivial traumas when any of the three components required for normal haemostasis is qualitatively abnormal or quantitatively deficient. The haemostatic process is divided into phase 1, the vascular phase with the interaction and exposure of the blood to collagen, vasoconstriction and the release of tissue thromboplastin; phase 2, characterized by platelet aggregation and various platelet release reactions; and phase 3, the coagulation phase, in which a firm impermeable coagulum or clot, the thrombus, is formed to arrest bleeding.

Bleeding disorders can be thus classified according to these three physiological factors: (1) vascular abnormalities; (2) disorders of platelets; and (3) coagulation disorders.

As there is no single laboratory test which can show the exact nature of a disturbance of haemostasis, the diagnosis of bleeding disorders depends on the history of bleeding, the clinical features of the bleeding, including the diagnosis of the underlying disease, and on the results of certain laboratory coagulation tests.

Abnormal haemorrhage may be the result of hereditary or acquired bleeding disorders. Hereditary bleeding disorders are caused by genetically determined abnormalities which either diminish quantitatively the haemostatic component or by a qualitative aberration of the biochemical structure which disturbs the function of normal coagulation. The relative incidence of the forms of inherited coagulation disorders varies greatly, depending on the population studied. The most common inherited bleeding disorders are: (1) classic haemophilia A, a factor VIII deficiency; (2) haemophilia B; both disorders have a sex-linked recessive inheritance;

(3) von Willebrand's disease, which has an autosomal dominant trait; and (4) dysfibrinogenaemia, which results from a defective fibrin molecule causing retarded clot formation.

Thrombasthenia, or Glanzmann's disease, is the most common hereditary platelet disorder and is characterized by diminished clot retraction and deficient platelet aggregation.

Vascular disorders are most often encountered in Osler's disease, telangiectasis, various forms of inborn haemangiomas and vascular purpuras.

Inherited bleeding disorders are clinically characterized by a lifelong history of "spontaneous" bleeding episodes, bruises and increased tendencies to bleed after minor injuries or surgery. The basic therapy when severe bleeding occurs or for the prevention of intraoperative bleeding is an adequate substitution of the deficient coagulation factors (transfusion of antihaemophilic globulin, PPSB preparation, (Cohn-I fraction) or the transfusion of functional normal platelets, if necessary, complement by erythrocyte transfusion.

In acquired bleeding disorders, there is a quantitative reduction of several coagulation factors. Acquired bleeding disorders can be classified as follows:

1) Retarded coagulation due to deficiency of vitamin K-dependent coagulation factors;
2) Disseminated intravascular coagulation or consumption coagulopathy;
3) Acquired inhibitors of coagulation, the circulatory anticoagulants;
4) Platelet disorders, e.g. malfunction of the platelets induced by immune processes or drugs such as acetylsalicylic acid (aspirin); and
5) Hypocoagulation induced by anticoagulants.

Various other diseases such as uraemia, leukaemia or dysproteinaemia are often linked with a bleeding tendency.

The coagulation factors – prothrombin, factor VII, factor IX and factor X, summarized as the prothrombin complex – are synthesized in the liver by a process which requires vitamin K. A deficiency of these vitamin K-dependent coagulation factors occurs in diverse clinical conditions affecting the liver. Damage to the hepatic cells can reduce the synthesis of the factors of the prothrombin complex to various degrees, despite the presence of adequate amounts of vitamin K. In severe liver diseases the synthesis of factor V and fibrinogen, neither vitamin K-dependent, can also be affected. Liver cirrhosis with portal hypertension, pathological proteolysis, blockade of the RES, followed by an accumulation of activated coagulation factors, may lead to intravascular coagulation accompanied by a decrease of platelets. Vitamin K absorbed only in the presence of bile salts is consequently lacking in all forms of bilary tract obstruction. Vitamin K has to be administered to prevent abnormalities of the prothrombin complex during sterilization of the gut by means of a prolonged broad-spectrum antibiotic therapy and should be substituted during long-term infusion therapy.

Indirect anticoagulants, such as the warfarin-like drugs, interfere with the synthesis of normally functioning factors of the prothrombin complex (PIVKA = protein induced vitamin K absence).

Diffuse intravascular coagulation with the consumption of coagulation factors is one of the most serious acquired coagulation disorders. Diffuse intravascular coagulation has to be considered as a syndrome of an underlying disorder and cannot itself be regarded as a disease. Many pathological processes have the capacity to activate the coagulation mechanism to such a degree that the physiological haemostatic balance is overwhelmed.

The main features of disseminated intravascular coagulation are: diverse haemorrhages as a result of a persistent consumption of the plasma coagulation factors and platelets. The bleeding is often accentuated by a secondary fibrinolysis. Thrombin is persistently elaborated within the circulation followed by a severely disturbed microcirculation due to disseminated fibrin deposits. These fibrin deposits can cause hypoxia and profound changes in most organ systems, eventually leading to necrosis. The changes in the coagulation and circulation can not only initiate but also perpetuate all forms of shock.

Acquired inhibitors of coagulation (circulatory anticoagulants) are rare. Specific inhibitors are most commonly directed against factor VIII. Non-specific inhibitors may arise in association with collagen diseases, particularly in systemic lupus erythematosus. Acquired bleeding complications may be also caused by numerous drugs which interfere with platelet function. Acetylsalicylic acid (ASA), dipyridamole and sulphinpyrazone decrease platelet function and inhibit release reactions by interfering with the prostaglandin metabolism. Such medication should be interrupted 3 – 4 days before any operations to avoid any increased bleeding tendency.

Anticoagulants are administered to induce hypocoagulability in the prevention of thrombo-embolic diseases. The coumarin-like drugs, the direct anticoagulants, interfere with the synthesis of the vitamin K-dependent coagulation factors. The hypocoagulatory effect of these drugs does not start until 2 or 3 days after the beginning of the medication. Warfarins are used for long-term anticoagulant prophylaxis after myocardial infarction, arterial emboli and venous thrombo-embolic complications.

Heparin exerts a direct and immediate inhibitory effect on the coagulation of the blood. Low doses of heparin are now widely used as prophylaxis against thrombo-embolism in general surgery and in internal medicine. Because of the possibility of inducing small postoperative haematomas, low doses of heparin are not recommended in brain and spine operations.

Low doses of heparin inhibit the conversion of factor X inactive to factor Y active and, consequently, the generation of greater amounts of thrombin. High concentrations of heparin are required to inactivate already generated thrombin in thrombotic processes.

As no single laboratory test enables one to evaluate the whole haemostatic situation, some basic screening tests (Table 1) have to be performed to distinguish primary coagulation from platelet disorders. The partial thromboplastin time (PTT), the prothrombin time (Quick) and the thrombin time should be performed routinely for the laboratory screening of any plasmal defect (Table 2). The platelet count and bleeding time are the basic methods for determining antihaemostatic defects caused by platelets.

Table 1. Basic laboratory tests

Coagulation system	Platelets
PTT	Platelet count
Prothrombin time (Quick)	Bleeding time (Duke-Ivy)
Thrombin time	Aggregation
a) Determination of single clotting factors b) Fibrinogen-Fibrin conversion	

Table 2. Prolongation of PTT/prothrombin time (Quick)

PTT abnormal Quick normal	Haemophilia A/B, von Willebrand's disease (rare factor XI or XII deficiency)
PTT normal Quick abnormal	deficiency of factor VII (rare)
PTT abnormal Quick abnormal	1) consumption coagulopathy 2) heparin 3) coumarin further laboratory analysis required

The PTT gives information about the pathway of the intrinsic contact activation (Fig. 1). Since this test bypasses the tissue-activated extrinsic pathway, it is unaffected by factor VII. The PTT will be prolonged if the level of any of the required factors is below 20% – 30% of normal, and it thus detects patients with hereditary coagulation disorders, e.g. haemophilia and von Willebrand's disease, or acquired coagulation deficiencies, e.g. disseminated intravascular coagulation. The test is also prolonged by heparin and by acquired circulatory inhibitors of any of the essential factors.

The plasma prothrombin time (Quick) measures the fibrinogen production via the extrinsic pathway (see Fig. 1).

Since the test is more sensitive to factors VII, X and prothrombin than to fibrinogen, it is most widely used to control the vitamin K-dependent factors in liver disease and the hypocoagulatory effect of the warfarin drugs.

The thrombin time is prolonged when the fibrinogen level is low, or when the fibrinogen is functionally defective, but the thrombin time is unaffected by the levels of the other coagulation factors. It is very sensitive to heparin and prolonged by abnormal amounts of other antithrombins.

The reptilase or thrombin coagulation time should also be included in the basic diagnostic programme now that heparin is increasingly in use. The reagents measure the fibrinogen conversion as well as the thrombin time, but they are not influenced by heparin. The thrombin time, the reptilase time and the determination of fibrinogen are usually sufficient for obtaining basic information on the fibrinolytic activity of the plasma and supervising fibrinolytic therapy. Detailed information on hyperfibrinolysis can be obtained by the determination of the fibrinogen-fibrin degradation products. They can be identified by more elaborate methods such as the water-agglutination test and staphylococcus clumping test (TRHI).

In disseminated intravascular coagulation most coagulation factors are diminished in such a way that those with a short half-life decrease first. In addition to the disturbance of the plasmatic coagulation, a fall in the platelet count is of diagnostic importance. Repeated laboratory controls of coagulation are of the utmost importance in disseminated intravascular coagulation.

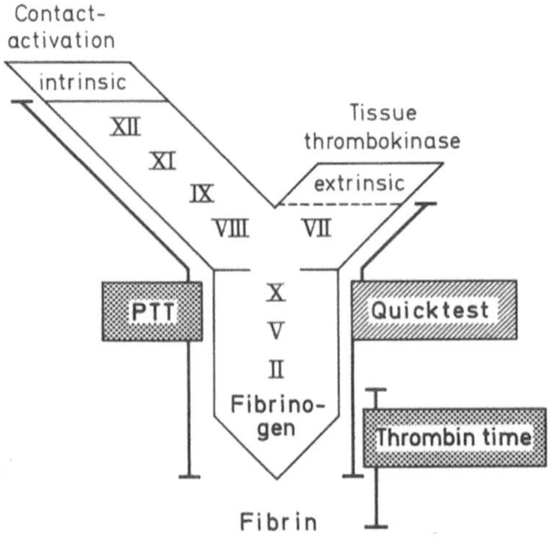

Fig. 1. Diagnosis and supervision of haemostatic disturbances. Schöndorf, T. H. (1978)

Table 3. Control of anticoagulant therapy

Medication	Control methods
Heparin	Thrombin time (TT), PTT
Coumarin	Prothrombin time – Quick (10% – 25%)
	Thrombotest (7% – 12%)
Streptokinase	Fibrinogen, TT, reptilase time
Acetylsalicylic acid (ASA)	Aggregation (collagen-induced)
Substitution therapies	
Haemophilia A/B	PTT (factors VIII/IX)
von Willebrand's disease	PTT (factor VIII)
	Bleeding time

A thrombotic process cannot be shown by laboratory tests. There is often an increase of coagulation factors and/or hypercoagulability can be demonstrated even in the blood system. Hypercoagulability is caused by increased thrombin generation and results in a shortened PTT, an increase of factors VIII and V, of fibrin monomers and a decrease in antithrombin III. Suitable laboratory tests for controlling anticoagulant therapy or a substitution therapy of the most common coagulation defects are shown in Table 3.

Summary

The diagnosis of bleeding disorders is based on adequate information about the family and/or individual history of the patient and on the clinical manifestation of the bleeding, including the diagnosis of underlying diseases, and is supplemented by a basic programme of laboratory tests. According to the results and constellation of the basic laboratory data most hereditary or acquired causes of acute bleeding disorders can be diagnosed so as to initiate the necessary treatment. The basic diagnostic programme can be expanded according to the individual requirements, but highly specialized coagulation analyses are not usually necessary in acute emergencies.

2.4 ICH in Clotting Disorders

E. Grote, Giessen

Some years ago we summarized 244 spontaneous intracerebral haemorrhages from the neurological and neurosurgical University Clinics of Giessen and Göttingen to evaluate the incidence of those due to haemostatic problems (Grote et al. 1969, 1971). Of these, 19 (8%) were shown to belong to this group; 9% were of undefined aetiology; about one half were in hypertensive patients and the rest arose from aneurysms and angiomas.

We will first discuss those patients with a spontaneous or iatrogenic clotting disorder leading secondarily to intracerebral bleeding. The physiology and pathology of clotting and fibrinolysis is summarized in the diagram. Clotting may be initiated both by circulating coagulation factors as well as by enzymatic action from injured tissues (Fig. 1); this is true for fibrinolysis as well (Fig. 2). These two enzymatic cascade systems run parallel and in equilibrium (Fig. 3). This homeostasis may be disturbed by various diseases and by specific and non-specific drugs. A decrease in the coagulation factors and in the number of thrombocytes will lead to impaired coagulation. An increase in fibrinolysis from some other cause will dissolve existing clots. The net result of either process may be intracerebral bleeding.

Extrinsic system	*Intrinsic system*
Tissue thromboplastin	Factor XII
Factor VII	Factor XI
Factor X	Factor VIII
Factor V	Factor X
Ca^{++}	Platelets
	Ca^{++}

Prothrombin activator 1

↓

Prothrombin + Ca^{++} → Thrombin 2

↓

Fibrinogen → Fibrin 3

Fig. 1. Activation of haemostasis

Tissue
(i.e. uterus)

Blood cells
(i.e. granulocytes)

Plasma
Proactivator 1

+ Lysokinase
(i.e. ascites)

or

+ Bacterial kinase
(i.e. streptokinase)

Activator

↓

Plasminogen → Plasmin 2

↓

Fibrin → Fibrin degradation products 3

Fig. 2. Activation of fibrinolysis

In most of our cases, the action of specific drugs inhibiting the production of coagulation factor was responsible for intracranial haematomas. Uncontrolled drug administration and, in many instances, the simultaneous intake of other drugs, affecting the efficacy of dicumarol, were the reasons for lowering the coagulative potential. In all cases the diagnosis was easily made and the coagulative disorder treated before and during operation. Some of the patients had suffered a mild head injury, while others had not. From our cases of haematoma it is not conclusive, whether a head injury is of any importance in the aetiology.

We have observed that many coagulative disorders are complicated by subdural haematomas and, in contrast to the hypertensive lesions, they spare the ventriculostriate area. Apart from this they do not show any particular location or form. However, they often demonstrate a tumour-like course with a history extending over days or weeks.

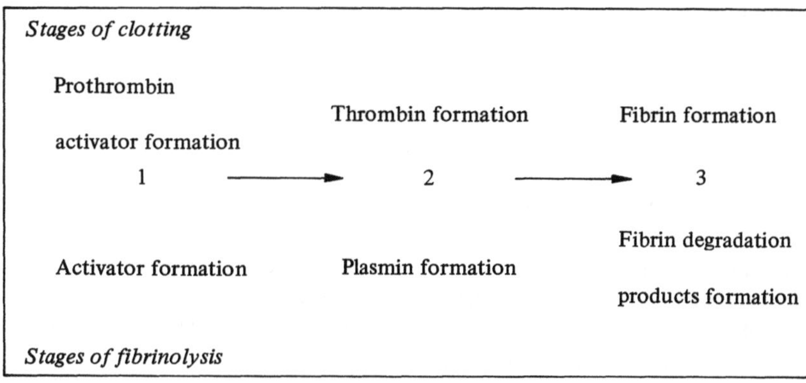

Fig. 3. Action of haemostasis and fibrinolysis

Two patients known to be haemophilic of type A were seen. One was a 9-year-old boy with a clinical course of some days after a minor head injury. At autopsy, however, no single haemorrhage was found, but rather multiple small haematomas indicating that the head injury was not a significant factor. A 36-year-old man who also showed slow progression of symptoms was found to have a huge intracranial haematoma.

Multiple haematomas scattered through the brain were found in two children with thrombocytopenia caused by leukaemic bone marrow infiltration. Another child suffered from multiple haematomas after streptokinase therapy for peripheral thrombosis. In comparison with hypertensive bleedings, the whole group of coagulation disorders is characterized by a peak of incidence in the lower age group (Fig. 4) and by a pattern of development suggestive of a tumour. The diagnosis of a clotting defect was established in every case and adequate therapy started.

However, there are special diagnostic problems in some cases of spontaneous haematoma that show coagulation troubles in peripheral organs as well.

Generalized hyperfibrinolysis of undetermined aetiology is of particular interest. Leukaemia, liver cirrhosis, metastatic disease of prostate, stomach and pancreas, as well as precocious separation of the placenta are known to cause increased fibrinolytic activity. A patient with a

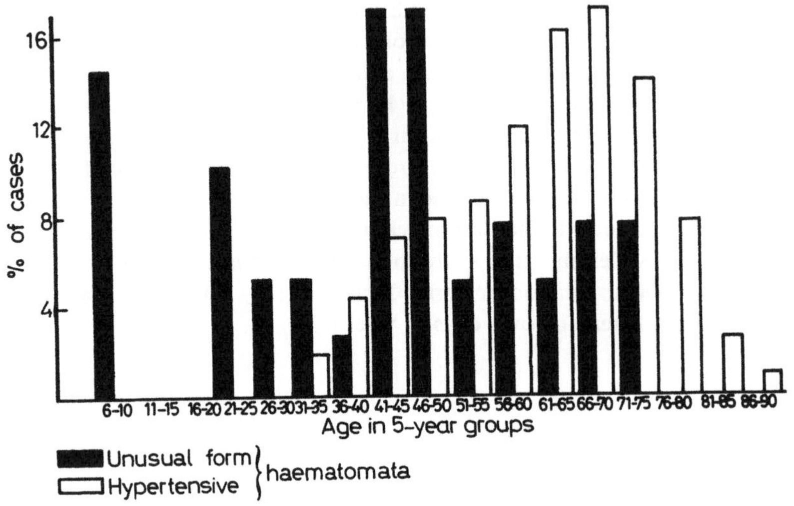

Fig. 4. Age distribution: haematomas of hypertensive origin and in coagulation defects

history of skin effusions and a course suggesting a tumour was found to be suffering from hypofibrinogenaemia caused by hyperfibrinolysis (Fig. 5) (Grote et al. 1970). Large amounts of fresh blood, epsilon-aminocaproic acid and fibrinogen given before, during and after surgery were necessary to ensure haemostasis. Therapy was interrupted after months and, once again, hyperfibrinolysis resulting in decreased levels of fibrinogen occurred. Medical follow-up did not succeed in establishing any cause for this.

Locally increased fibrinolytic activity in brain tissue was suspected many times. Experimentally, both dura and normal brain tissue show high levels of plasminogen activity. This is also true for mesenchymal tumours and medulloblastomas. A 15-year-old boy with chronic, partially calcified subdural effusions (Fig. 6) may be an example of high fibrinolytic activity of dura and brain tissue. After evacuation, resection of dural membranes and bone,

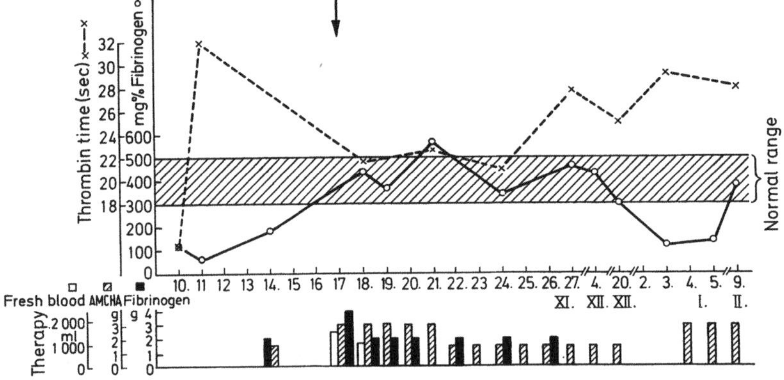

Fig. 5. Hyperfibrinolysis of unknown origin

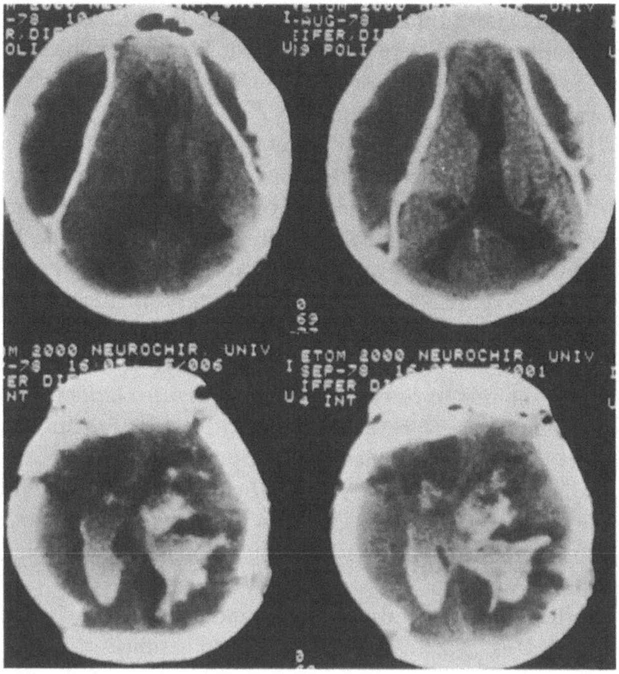

Fig. 6. Partially calcified chronic subdural haematoma

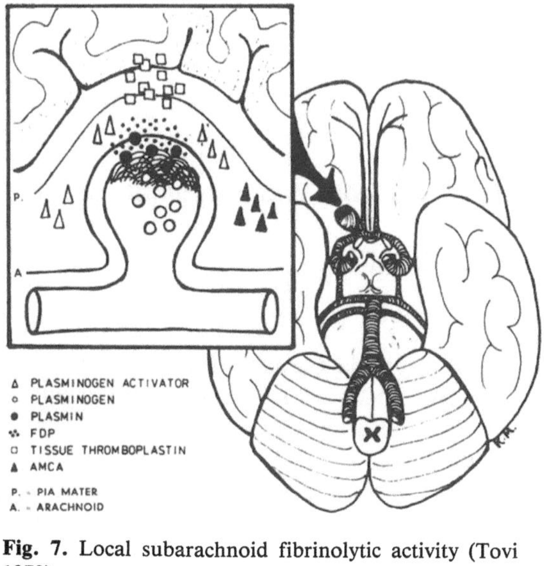

Fig. 7. Local subarachnoid fibrinolytic activity (Tovi 1972)

uncontrollable hyperfibrinolysis resulted in hypofibrinogenaemia. In spite of energetic specific therapy with epsilon-aminocaproic acid, heparin and coagulation factors, fibrinolysis could not be interrupted. Multiple bleedings occurred from the wound, trachea and GI tract, and intraventricular haematomas were detected. At autopsy, bilateral haematomas in the frontal and temporal lobes were demonstrated. We are convinced that large amounts of plasminogen activator from un-resected thickened dural membranes were responsible for uncontrollable hyperfibrinolysis.

This assumption is supported by the experimental investigations of Tovi (1972), who found high spontaneous fibrinolytic activity in the form of plasminogen activator in the choroid plexus, in the meninges and in big arteries. In addition, after experimental intracerebral haematomas, not only local and CSF fibrinolytic activity, but also its activity in the peripheral blood was increased. His concept of an interplay between coagulation and fibrinolytic factors may be exemplified by a case of an aneurysm (Fig. 7). After bleeding, injured brain tissue releases thromboplastin leading to coagulation and clot formation. This is followed by activation of plasminogen from the meninges and blood vessels resulting in fibrinolytic activity. If the dissolution of clot is extensive and occurs before there is tissue repair, bleeding will recur.

In summary, peripheral diseases and external factors, resulting in depletion of coagulation factors and thrombocytes, may cause spontaneous intracerebral haematomas. Further investigations are necessary to confirm the theory that there are primary conditions of the brain, meninges and vessels, besides aneurysms and a.v. angiomas, which might be responsible for intracerebral haematomas without there necessarily being any disorder of haemostasis in the peripheral blood.

Until recently, because of this tumour-like course, many intracerebral haematomas were diagnosed as avascular space-occupying lesions and were operated upon. Now, computer tomography can show in every case the nature of the process before operation. Diagnostic investigation of coagulation and fibrinolysis will clarify the situation in time, before such procedures as transfusion, administration of dextran and anaesthesia have blurred haematological diagnosis.

2.4.1 Discussion: Anticoagulants and ICH

J. Iizuka, Bonn

At the meeting of the German Neurosurgical Society in Giessen in 1969, I reported five cases of so-called iatrogenic ICH in patients on anticoagulants which I had seen in a period of 11 years. I have been keeping my eyes open ever since and now present the results of my observations during the last nine years.

It appears that the incidence is increasing because of the extensive use of phenprocoumon (Marcumar) by general practioners. We have seen a further nine cases. The introduction of adequate checking and follow-up of the entire range of clotting factors by haematologists has contributed towards a significant improvement of conditions in patients after surgical removal of haematomas. This has been seen particularly among those patients suffering from vascular insufficiency when they have been kept on heparin without any risk of recurrence, even in cases where the ICH was removed just a couple of hours prior to the administration of heparin. We are absolutely convinced that a grave risk of cerebral or coronary infarction has been reduced to a minimum by means of anticoagulant therapy during the time of after-care.

From the study of case histories it is obvious that a considerable number of cases developed either among alcoholics or during alcoholic intoxication, and from the aetiological viewpoint I feel that this is more responsible than anticoagulant drugs for the ICH.

The high incidence of haematomas among diabetics may suggest that a vascular factor, like an angiopathy or arteriosclerosis, may well be the most important among the three main factors, i.e. blood clotting, blood pressure and blood vessels.

When one considers that haematogenetic or haemodynamic factors may be easily corrected by attention to the clotting time or the blood pressure, I am afraid that no adequate treatment is available for the malformation or degeneration of the cerebral vessels, and these may cause a cerebral infarction and an intracranial haematoma at the same site and even at the same time. In conclusion I feel that medical treatment in general and anticoagulants in particular should be considered both beneficial and encouraging, and no blame should be placed upon this treatment as long as close control of clotting time is maintained and overdosage is avoided.

2.5 Micro-angiomas and ICH

H.-P. Jensen, Kiel

Micro-angiomas are significant in the aetiology of intracerebral haematomas as first reported by Margolis et al. (1951). But what is the definition of micro-angioma?

Dorothy Russell (1954) introduced the term "cryptic arteriovenous and venous hamartomas" to designate angiomatous malformations that are clinical silent, measure less than 2–3 cm and which may cause intracerebral haemorrhage.

Margolis et al. (1961) have drawn attention to the fact that clear recognition is difficult due to the small size of the malformation and its frequent partial destruction by the haemorrhage. This causes some difficulty in histological examination, but even more in examinations of surgical specimens from the whole haematoma.

With regard to clinical diagnosis, Gerlach and Jensen (1958) reported ten cases of intracerebral haematoma in patients aged 14–39 years (average age, 28), in which "minute" vascular malformations could be detected by careful analysis of the individual vessels on angiography (Fig. 1). In some surgical specimens, histological telangiectasis, extremely small venous, cavernous or arteriovenous malformations were detected that corresponded to the arteriographic findings. Clinically, the malformations were termed "capillary angiomas".

In later analysis (1960) of 21 similar cases, the term "micro-angioma" was selected to avoid encroaching on the morphological classification.

As the lower limit for definition of micro-angioma, we accepted histological identification, while the upper limit was not sharply defined, but included malformations up to the size of several millimetres visible in angiography (Fig. 2). The crucial point, however, was that micro-angiomas only cause clinical symptoms when they lead to haemorrhage and thus to intracerebral haematoma. Therefore, the cryptic hamartomas described by Russell as measuring up to 3 cm could definitely be included in the clinical term micro-angioma (Fig. 3).

The introduction of computer tomography has thrown new light on the diagnosis of intracerebral haematoma. We diagnosed a large number of haematomas (Table 1) which, according to clinical history and findings, size, shape and location, could not be ascribed to any

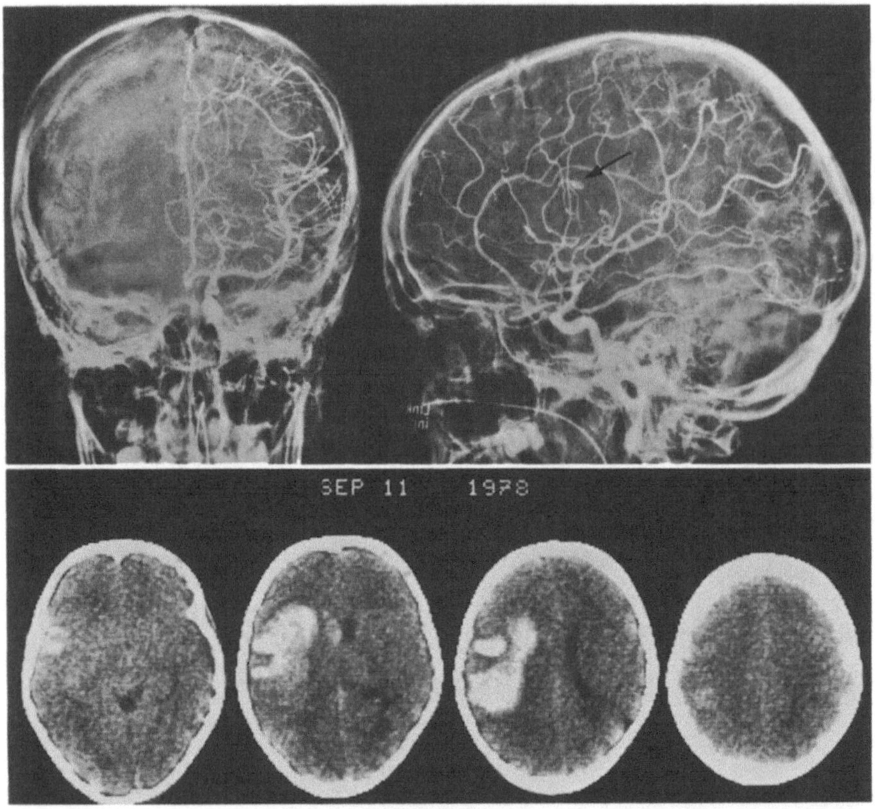

Fig. 1

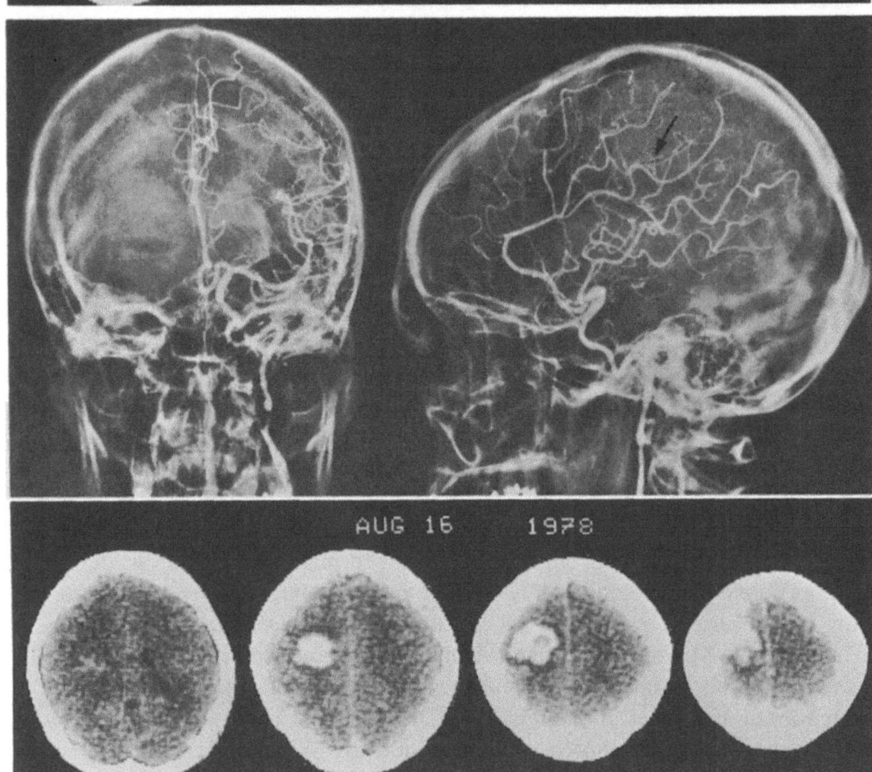

Fig. 2

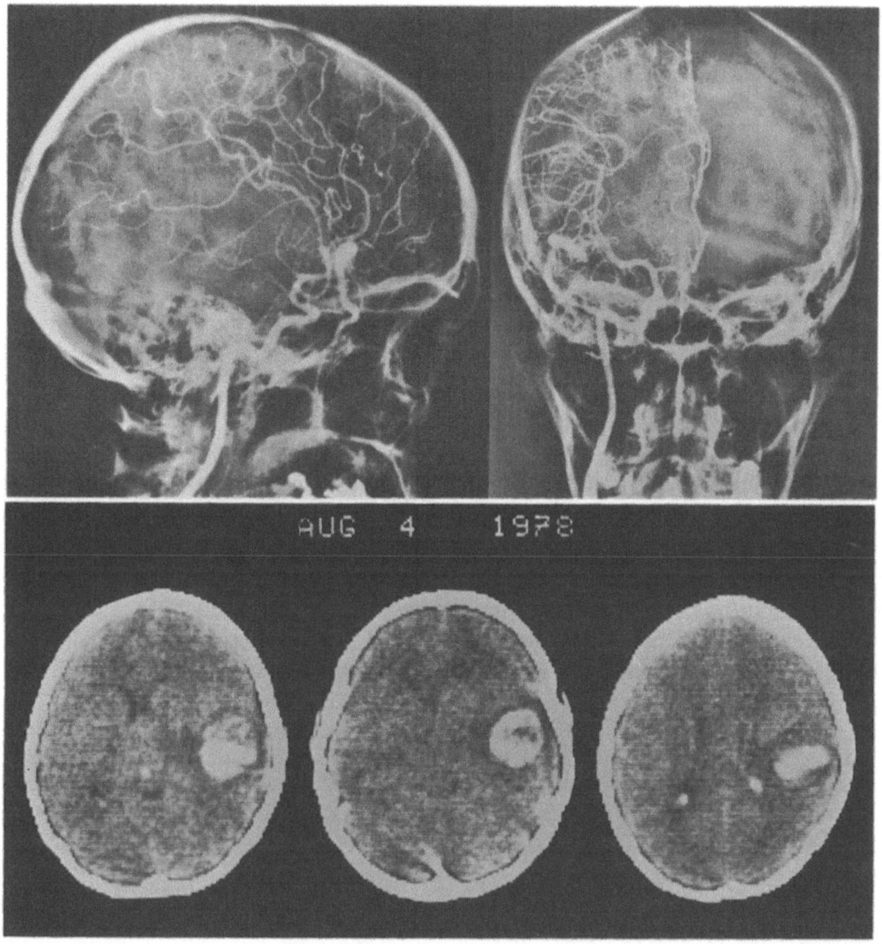

Fig. 3. CT scan of a 45-year-old female. Micro-angioma, 15-mm diameter, in the course of the right middle cerebral artery. Clinically silent prior to sudden onset of headache

well-known pathogenesis. Micro-angioma could be demonstrated arteriographically only in some of these cases (Fig. 4).

Since operation is not indicated in many cases, especially in cases of unfavourable location, we often observe, with continuous CT control, good absorption and simultaneous clinical improvement in these cases (Fig. 5).

The term "spontaneous" haematoma seems to be unsatisfactory, because spontaneous bleeding is simply unlikely in an absolutely healthy vascular system, just as healthy bones do not

◀ **Fig. 1.** CT scan of a 13-year-old male. Micro-angioma in the course of a frontal branch of the left middle cerebral artery. Haematoma in the Sylvian sulcus and the left precentral region. Clinically silent prior to sudden onset of unconsciousness; right hemiparesis and conjugate deviation to left side

Fig. 2. CT scan of a 35-year-old female. Left parietal haematoma. Micro-angioma in the course of the left pericallosal·artery suspected, histologically proved

Table 1. Intracerebral haematomas detected in CT examinations[a]

Cause	Number
Unknown	64
Micro-angioma	8
Marcumar	14
Aneurysm	29
A.-V. angioma	17
Total	132

[a] University Neurosurgery Clinic, Kiel, 1976–1978

break spontaneously. It would undoubtedly be better to refer to such haematomas as of an unknown source, or of a "cryptic origin" or even perhaps as "cryptic malformations".

On the basis of their investigations McCormick et al. (1966) have stated, "No one knows exactly what percentage of cerebral haemorrhages are actually due to 'cryptic' vascular malformation, but we believe that the relationship is significant."

With computer tomography, perhaps the term "cryptic hamartomas" gains still another, completely different meaning. I would like to demonstrate this with two cases.

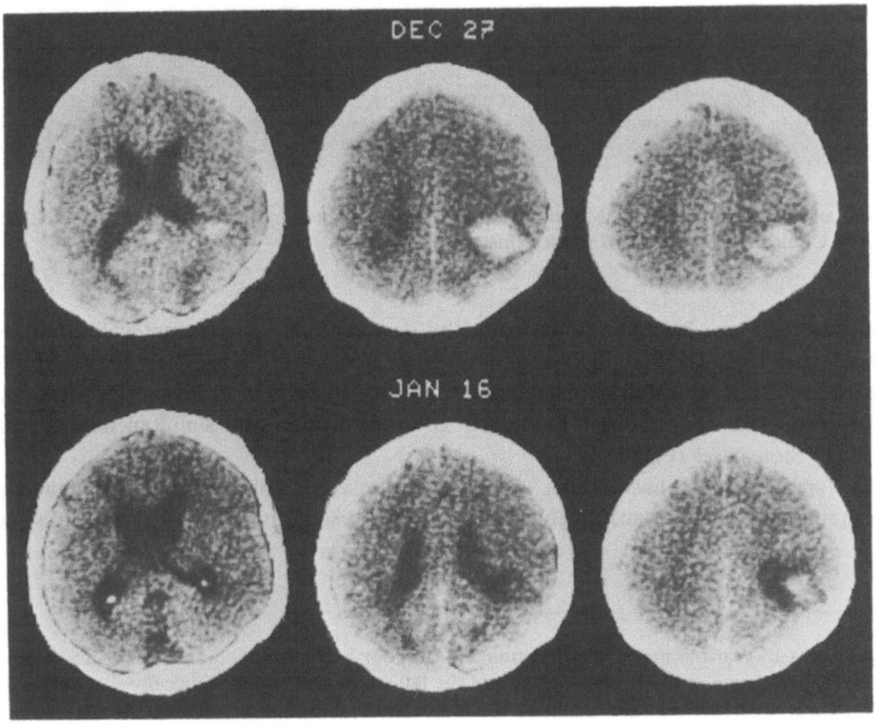

Fig. 4. Intracerebral haematoma of unknown cause. CT controls revealed good absorption

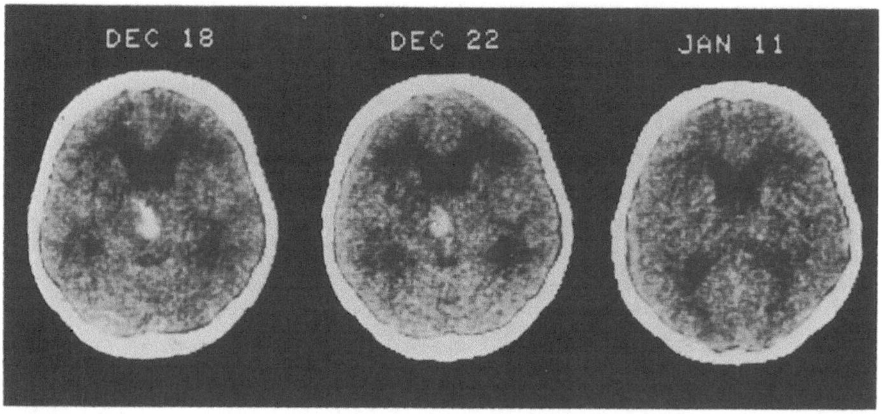

Fig. 5. Good resorption and clinical improvement of a left thalamic haematoma

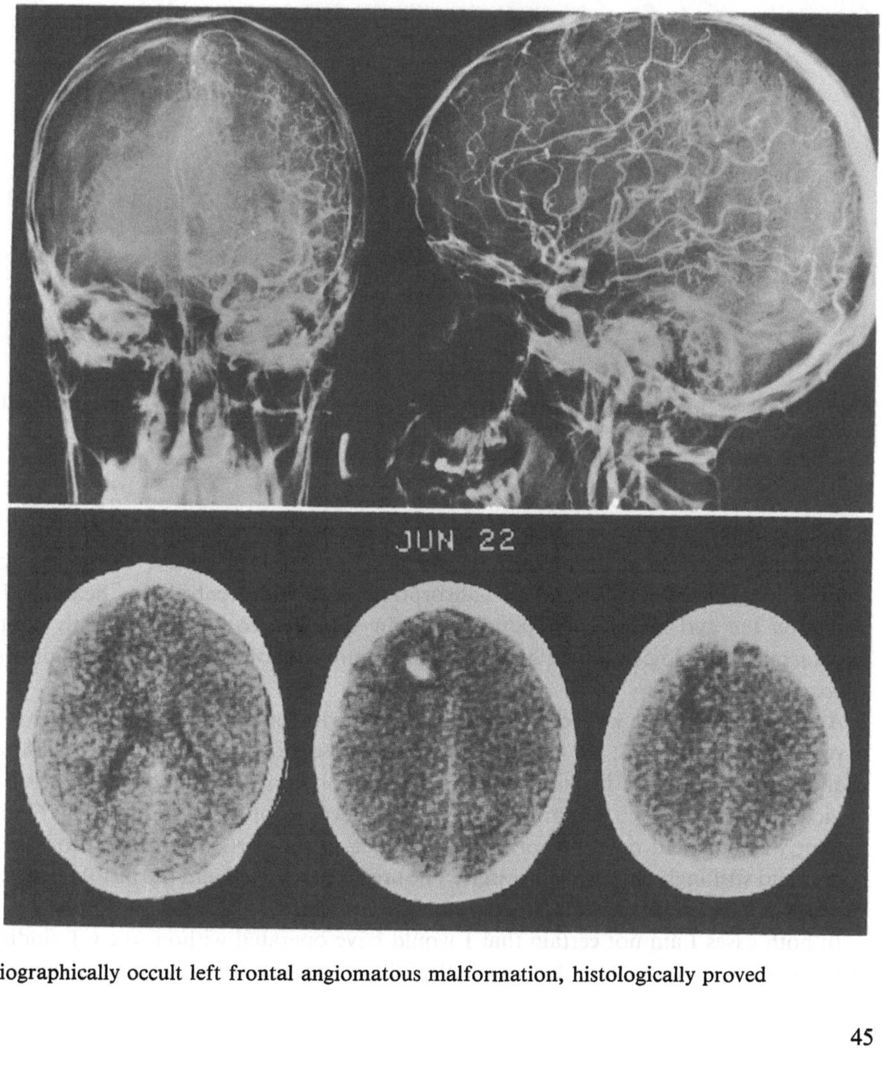

Fig. 6. Angiographically occult left frontal angiomatous malformation, histologically proved

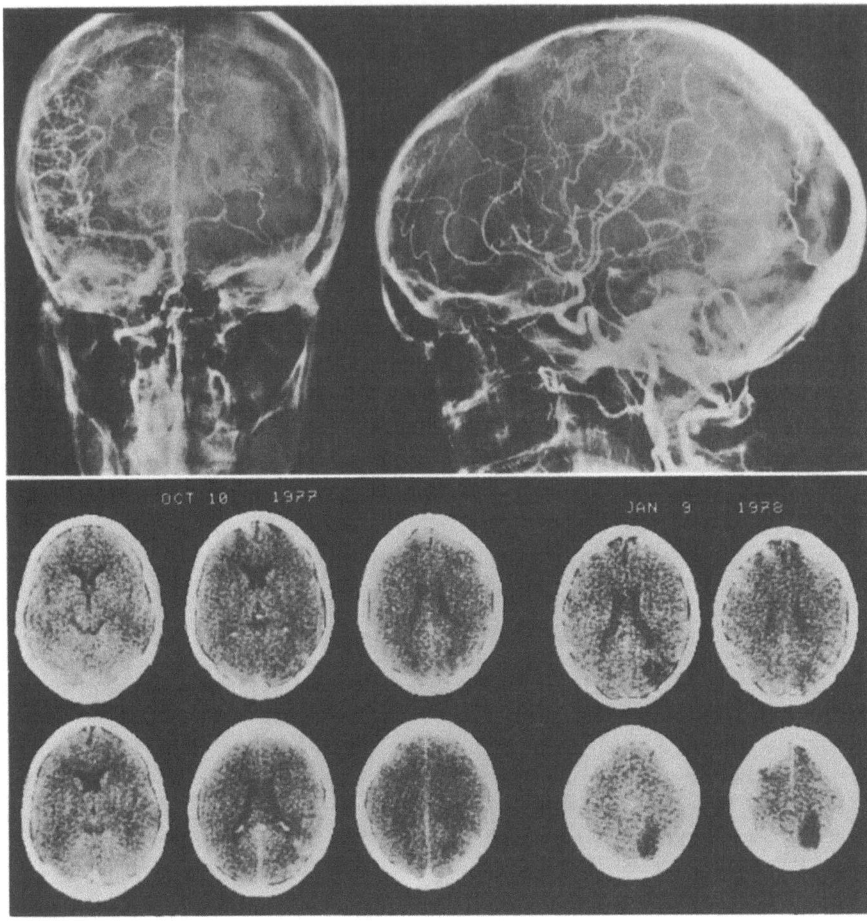

Fig. 7. Increase of a low-absorption area in the right occipital region. Angiographically "cryptic" angiomatous malformation, histologically proved

A 22-year-old male was examined because of occasional focal cerebral seizures. Left carotid angiography revealed a distal shift of the anterior cerebral artery. Computer tomography showed a localized left frontal low-absorption area with central calcification (Fig. 6). At operation the gyri in the corresponding region appeared to be more sharply contoured and hyperaemic. Histological investigations of the removed tissue revealed an angioma *capillare et venosum.*

A 46-year-old female was referred by her psychiatrist for computer tomography for suspected psycho-organic changes. A localized right low-absorption area was found. A visual field examination showed an incomplete left-sided homonymous hemianopia. Right-sided brachial angiography showed no abnormality (Fig. 7). Because of later additional CT findings, the patient was operated on. The corresponding area in the cortex was found to have an altered colour and strikingly thin-walled vessels. The area was resected and the histological examination revealed a haemangioma with lamellar cortical necrosis.

In both cases I am not certain that I would have operated without the CT findings. On the other hand, I am quite sure that my clinical diagnosis would not have been angioma.

In conclusion:

1) Micro-angiomas are small cryptic hamartomas. They are clinically silent as long as they do not cause an intracranial haemorrhage. They are not recognizable by CT scan, but sometimes they may be detected by careful analysis of angiograms.
2) Intracerebral haemorrhages may easily be detected by CT scan. In haematomas of apparently unknown aetiology, a micro-angioma should always be considered, even if angiography fails to prove it.
3) Angiomatous malformations of larger size may be seen in CT examination as an area of altered density. In some cases contrast enhancement may not change their absorption values, and in addition they might not be visible on angiography. A diagnosis of this kind of vascular malformation can only be proved by histological examination.

2.5.1 Discussion: Micro-angiomas

W. Driesen, Tuebingen: The frequent occurrence of small arteriovenous angiomas (so-called micro-angiomas) associated with haematomas may be due to the fact that angiomas tend to enlarge with the passage of time or as the patient grows older. However, many of them remain silent and show no striking symptoms.

We had two patients, in whom abnormal behaviour was the presenting symptom. The angiograms were negative and the CT scan only demonstrated the typical findings of a haematoma 10 days later. Diagnosis was confirmed by the histological examination.

Question:

What is your definition of micro-angioma?

H.-P. Jensen, Kiel: The general pathologist should certainly be able to diagnose and to measure any kind of malformation or tumour in his specimen. He does not need terms like "micro-angioma".

The neurosurgeon deals with patients having "spontaneous" intracerebral haemorrhage. Sometimes he discovers a small "irregularity" on the course of an artery in the angiogram, like a tiny scalloped fleck of contrast material, which he believes might be the cause of the haemorrhage. Sometimes at operation he is able to resect a small suspicious area from the wall of the haematoma, which again might have been the cause of the haemorrhage.

From the onset of symptoms and signs, until the correct histological diagnosis of an angiomatous malformation by the pathologist, the neurosurgeon uses the term "micro-angioma" to describe circumstantially the findings that are suspected as being the likely cause of the haemorrhage.

In the clinical term "micro-angioma", the prefix denoting smallness does not mean a "microscopic" angiomatous malformation or tumour.

B. Pertuiset, Paris: In two cases of so-called micro-angiomas we were surprised to find in the control angiograms quite large angiomas supplied in part by the vertebral arteries. I think that control angiogram of both the vertebral and carotid territories is mandatory.

M. Samii, Hannover: We are not able in every case to make the diagnosis of micro-angioma pre-operatively. Angiomas which are compressed by haematomas are not seen on angiograms. If we wait and there is a reduction of haematoma, a repeat angiography may reveal an angioma. If the malformation can be seen on an angiogram it should not be called "micro-angioma".

K. J. Zülch, Cologne: The majority of atypical haematomas are caused by malformations. For a long time we have very carefully examined the peripheral zone of every atypical haematoma. By atypical I mean haematomas without relation to the arteries of the basal ganglia. We have practically never seen an angioma. On the other hand we have found micro-angiomas just by chance, spontaneous, without bleedings or with microbleedings. These seem to have a predilection for the thalamomesencephalic region.

F. Isamat, Barcelona: If you can see an angioma on angiogram it is not a micro-angioma. However, sometimes it is only with subtraction technique that an angioma can be demonstrated. I do not like the term micro-angioma. The terminology is very confusing.

K. J. Zülch, Cologne: Micro-angioma is a clinical and arteriographic definition. We would probably never speak of micro-angiomas because we would define them morphologically and more precisely as capillary, ectasias, teleangiectasia, cavernoma or arteriovenous types of malformation.

J. Gillingham, Edinburgh: I think there is still some confusion between the clinicians and neuropathologists. Everybody seems to have his own term for micro-angiomas. As has been said, a micro-angioma from the clinical viewpoint cannot be seen in the angiogram, even by using magnification or subtraction. If we removed the haematoma and make a postoperative angiogram showing a very small angioma, this is not a micro-angioma. On the other hand a neuropathologist, after examining the haematoma with material from the peripheral zone, may say there was a vascular abnormality, a teleangiectasia. It is quite possible that depending on the timing of surgery, you can have a peripheral vascularized zone which under the microscope then gives the impression that it is an angioma or teleangiectasia but which, in fact, reflects vascular regeneration in the tissue.

H. Güthert, Erfurt: After discussing the subject with Professors Zülch, Jellinger and Frowein we arrived at the following conclusions. From the pathological point of view it does not matter whether the malformation is small or large. It is therefore up to the clinicians to agree whether they want to speak about micro- or macro-angioma. The demand for the prefix "micro-" comes from the clinical language, because there is an obvious necessity for it. One speaks about microcarcinoma of the duodenum or stomach and, in recent times, about microcarcinoma of the breast. This nomenclature is a response to the necessity of achieving the highest precision in diagnosis and treatment of these lesions.

2.6 ICH in Childhood

V. Calatayud-Maldonado, Zaragoza

The causes of intracerebral haemorrhage in children are quite different from those in adults, as certain factors do not apply to any significant extent; these include vascular hypertension, craniocerebral trauma and disturbances of the clotting mechanism.

Angiomas were the most frequent cause, so that these lesions were not truly spontaneous. Four patients with myeloid leukaemia had massive diffuse haemorrhages which involved not only the white matter, but also the ventricles. One of the tumours, a metastasis from a neuroblastoma presented with a massive haemorrhage into the lateral ventricles, with obstruction of the foramen of Monro. The second case, a pituitary adenoma developed as an apoplexy

Table 1. Intracerebral Haemorrhage in Childhood (1975 – 1978)

Aetiology	
Aneurysms	3
Angiomas	7
Blood disorders	4
Brain tumours	2
	16

with spread of the bleeding into the right frontal lobe. In the cases of leukaemia and the metastatic tumour, the rapid onset did not allow investigation by angiography, and the diagnosis was confirmed at autopsy.

Angiography was done in the remaining cases, but in the absence of a CAT scanner the value of radio-isotope angiography is pointed out. This is a simple, rapid and safe method and allows an investigation not only of the tumour mass, but also of the cerebral circulation. Of the seven angiomas three were shown in the posterior projection and four in the anterior projection. In five cases it showed the typical isotope angiographic appearances of an A-V malformation, and in two cases there were arterial/vascular shifts. One thrombosed angioma and an A-V fistula could not be demonstrated. Only in two cases did the morphological studies show changes related to the malformation; however, in five cases, there was a zone of increased activity corresponding to the presence of the intracerebral haematoma and not related to the vessels.

Two of the three patients with giant aneurysms showed changes in the isotope angiogram. Both cases showed similar findings, viz. an increase in focal perfusion apparent during the arterial phase, combined with reduced perfusion in the hemisphere ("steal"-syndrome on the side of the aneurysm).

Two aneurysms were also identified in the static pictures. Two of the three intracerebral haematomas produced changes in the static pictures, in one of which the haematoma had invaded the ventricles. The four patients with haemorrhages secondary to blood disorders were not investigated by isotopes.

Discussion

In a series of intracerebral haemorrhages, 6.25% occurred in childhood. A comparative study shows that they occur twice as frequently in adults. These are serious lesions, which in most cases show a rapid course which demands early diagnosis and urgent treatment (Pia 1968). Those associated with blood disorders, including leukaemia, had a fatal outcome as pointed out by McCormick and Rosenfield (1973) and Robson and Anderson (1973). There is also a poor outlook in haemorrhages associated with tumours, as in the majority of cases they are associated with malignant primary tumours or a metastasis. This is reflected in the statistics of McCormick and Rosenfield (1973), Goutelle et al. (1969), and Mandybur (1977). The prognosis is more favourable in the cases of angioma and aneurysm, and this depends on the site of the lesion, its extent and progress, whether acute, sub-acute or chronic.

In all these lesions the diagnosis must, of course, be confirmed by angiography. In many cases isotope angiography provides a correct diagnosis and gives indications for operation.

It may also be possible to recognize the nature of the lesion which has caused the bleeding. Aneurysms are better shown in the early pictures because of the progressive drop of the isotope level in the blood. On the other hand, a positive dynamic investigation can appear normal in the sequential study.

In many cases of bilateral carotid aneurysms or giant midline aneuryms, we can only demonstrate a single basal midline lesion. This occurred in one of our cases with unilateral findings, where it was difficult to distinguish between the aneurysm itself and the changes caused by the haematoma which surrounded it.

Isotope angiography is valuable for the information it provides about the effects of an aneurysm on the cerebral circulation in its immediate neighbourhood, as well as the changes in the general circulation, which are caused by the rupture itself (Rockett and Moinnuddin 1976; Stein and Winter 1974).

The serial dynamic cerebral study combined with carotid angiography (Goodman and Hayes 1974) is a suitable procedure for deciding the correct time for surgical intervention. It is also possible to monitor the cerebral circulation post-operatively in surgically treated patients. It is in these cases that the analysis of the activity-time curve over the lesion, before and after operation, has been shown to be of great value (Binet and Lomen 1970).

Landmann and Ross (1979) reviewed 200 cases to determine the accuracy of isotope angiography in the diagnosis of A-V malformations. They made a correct diagnosis in 77% of cases with static pictures and in 92% with dynamic studies, figures comparable to those of Tyson et al. (1979) who achieved 96% correct diagnosis with dynamic studies. In angiomas of smaller size and those which are deeply situated, the lesion is only demonstrated with difficulty, and usually only in those that have caused a haemorrhage.

Summary

1) Intracerebral haemorrhages in childhood are uncommon, and when they occur it can usually be explained by A-V malformations or blood disorders.
2) The apoplectic onset and subsequent course urgently demand an early diagnosis and, if necessary, surgical intervention. However, there is no place for this in the most common lesions – the blood disorders.
3) Even if cerebral arteriography offers the greatest certainty as a diagnostic measure, isotope angiography is also of considerable significance in the diagnosis and management of these lesions. At the same time it allows one to study the main circulation and that in the affected zone without, however, being able to achieve the precise diagnosis of computer tomography.

2.7 Familial Incidence of ICH

W. Luyendijk and G. Th. A. M. Bots, Leiden

Verjaal (1958, 1964), while still working in the Hague, drew our attention to a family from Scheveningen, many members of which died from intracerebral bleeding between the ages of 40 and 50. Wattendorff (personal communication, 1978) collected data on six members of this family, who between 1950 and 1965 suffered from haematomas and haemorrhages occurring between the ages of 43 and 57. The fifth decade was recognized as especially dangerous, and family members who reached the age of 55 knew that they had escaped the familial threat.

Figure 1 shows brain sections revealing a large haematoma in the left frontocentral region of one of these siblings. In the left temporal lobe a cleft is seen, due to a temporal haematoma, as demonstrated by arteriography 2 years earlier.

From our material, examples of familial intracerebral haematomas can be presented as follows:

1) The first case is a rather restricted one and concerns a 14-year-old male who was completely healthy until the beginning of December 1972, when spells of right-sided headache, accompanied by nausea and vomiting, started spontaneously without any causative evidence. Neurological examination revealed slight left-sided clinical signs. Carotid angiography showed a characteristic avascular space-occupying lesion in the right temporal lobe, with no sign of a vascular anomaly, however.

   At operation 3 weeks after the onset of his complaints, an old intracerebral haematoma was removed. Biopsy of the wall of the haematoma showed no pathological abnormalities, except for an enveloping layer of granulation tissue and reactive gliosis.

   The boy recovered completely and was submitted to another angiography, 6 months later, which showed no abnormalities at all.

   The daughter of a brother of the patient's mother was also operated on for an intracerebal haemorrhage. From Noordenbos and Van der Werf we learned that at the age of 15, this girl had suffered from a comparable quasi-spontaneous intracerebral haematoma located in the left frontoparietal region. In this case, as in the previous one, no vascular anomalies or other causes could be established.

   Although the incidence is very low, the two cases are remarkable examples of quasi-spontaneous intracerebral haematoma of unknown aetiology occurring at the ages of 14 and 15 in first cousins.

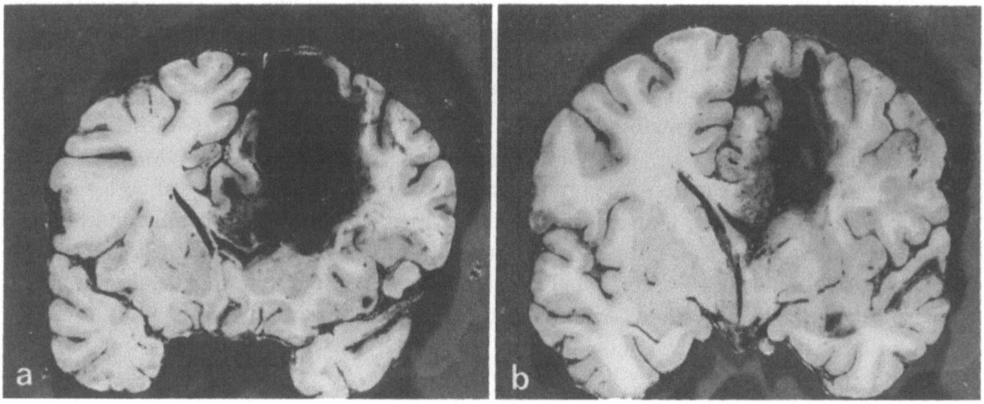

Fig. 1a, b. Brain sections demonstrating a large haematoma in the left frontocentral region. In the left temporal lobe a cleft is seen due to a temporal haematoma established by arteriography 2 years before death

2) The second case concerns an extensive family living in Katwijk, a fishing village on the North Sea near Leiden. This family has lived there for centuries and bears a name which is characteristic of that region. As most of these native families, their offspring and interrelations are quite numerous, offering, on the one hand, attractive circumstances for studying hereditary and familial pathology – and on the other an excess of data. The latter aspect has prevented us from presenting as complete a history as we would have wished. The members of this family are all fully aware of their possible fate in their fifth and sixth decades, as was evident once more in our last case which was operated on 2 weeks ago.
   Figure 2 shows aspects of the pedigree of this family. These parts are undoubtedly interconnected, but so far it has been impossible to complete the full chart with certainty. Anyhow, the diagrams show a remarkably high incidence of verified intracerebral haematomas amounting to a total of 18 cases. This finding is parallel with the available histories which indicate that many other family members died from stroke, mostly in their fifth and sixth decades. None of the surgically treated patients suffered from pre-existing hypertension, as far as was known, and after recovery and discharge from hospital, the blood pressure appeared to be normal.
   As far as can be seen in this survey, the sex ratio shows a female preponderance of 1:2, which is completely different from the next family (family 3).
   Pathological examination has shown a thickening of the arterial vessel walls, especially of the tunica media. In contrast to the next family the pathological process does not seem to have such a systematic localization.
3) The third case also concerns a family from Katwijk for which a pedigree beginning in 1836 has been more or less completed, showing the characteristic features previously mentioned (Fig. 3). Among the 65 siblings, 20 died from intracerebral haemorrhage; the incidence is extremely high in the third generation. The diagnosis could be verified in the majority of the siblings of the third and fourth generation. In this group 17 cases are found, 11 of which appear to be intracerebral haematomas. The lesion occurs mostly during the sixth decade, but the patients may be younger. The youngest one died at the age of 37. The sex ratio shows a male preponderance of 3 to 1, which is different from the family previously described.
   Seven cases were surgically treated in our department. All haematomas manifested themselves quasi-spontaneously. The blood pressure was normal except for one case with a slight hypertension of 170/100. Arteriography revealed no vascular abnormalities. Three patients died as a consequence of their haematomas, and another one died 2 years later because of a recurrence. Neuropathological examination of the wall of the haematoma was performed in all operated cases.
   In addition to our four fatal cases, autopsy has been done in eight other patients who died from an intracerebral haematoma. In all these cases a remarkable arteriolosclerosis was found, which appeared to be strictly localized to the grey matter of the brain. In contrast, the vessels of the white matter, the brain stem, the cerebellum and the spinal cord show no arteriolosclerotic changes. Outside of the brain, vascular pathology was not found in any other organ. Figures 4, 5 and 6 shows these concentrically thickened vessels and clearly illustrate their systemic character. One of the arteriolosclerotic vessels had ruptured and is enveloped by satellite bleeding. Although the same pathological changes may be found in cases of arterial hypertension, only one of our patients had a slightly elevated blood pressure (170/100).

One comparable report has been found in the literature. Gudmundsson et al. (1972) have described a family from Iceland in which a high incidence of cerebral haemorrhages and haematomas exists. According to his study, which includes their histories, 54% of its members have been struck by this lesion at a rather early age. Pathological amyloidosis of the cerebral

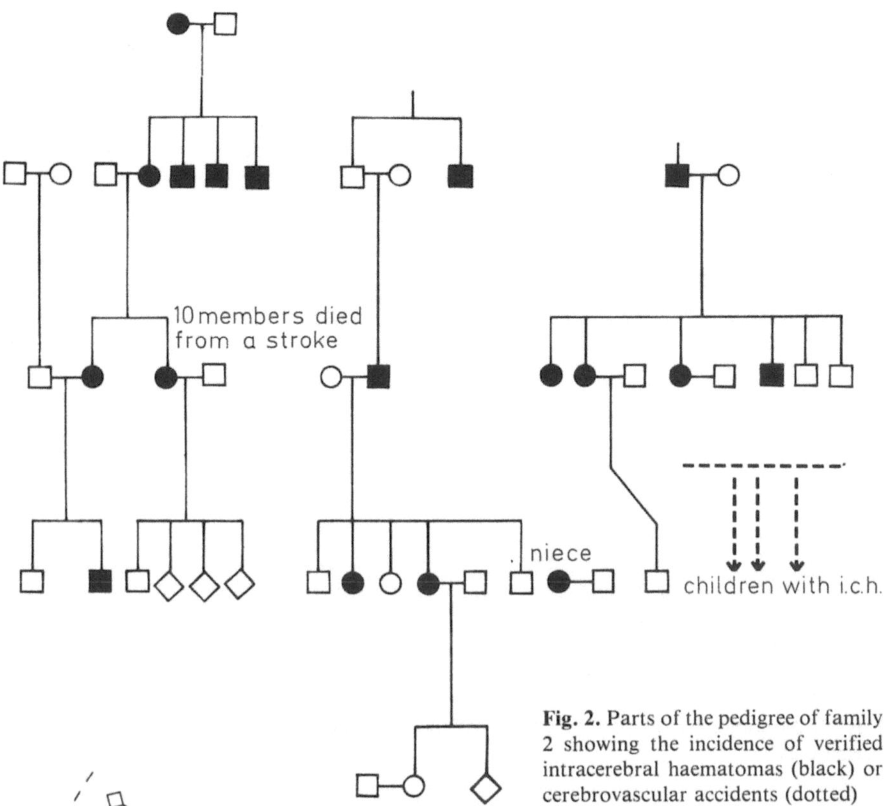

Fig. 2. Parts of the pedigree of family 2 showing the incidence of verified intracerebral haematomas (black) or cerebrovascular accidents (dotted)

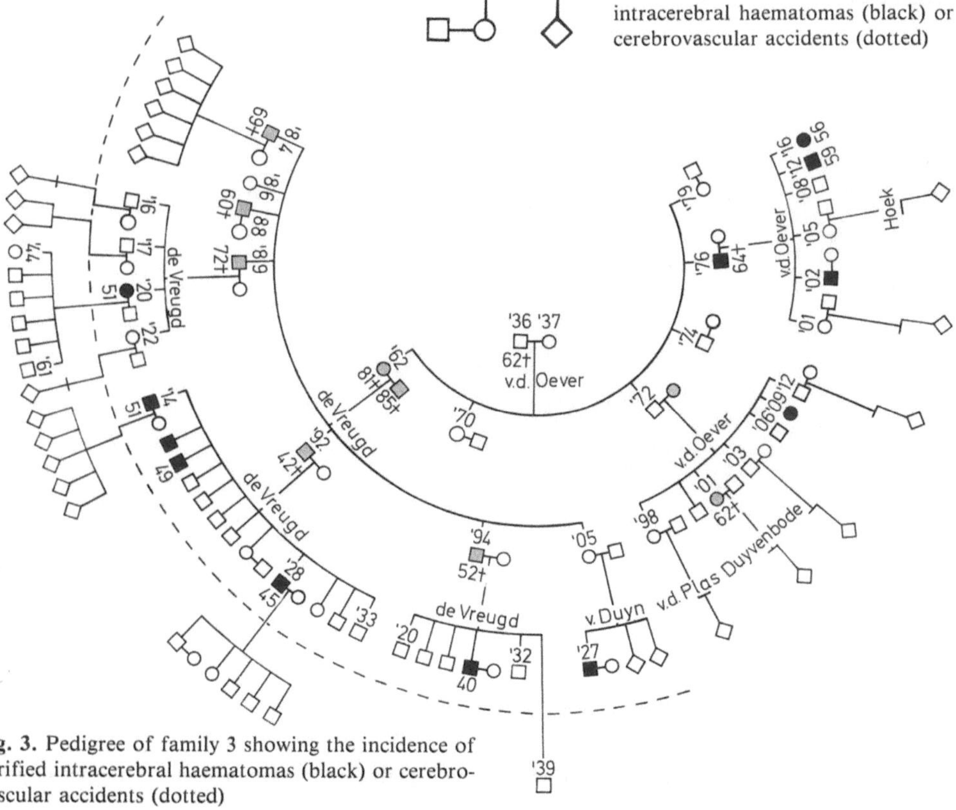

Fig. 3. Pedigree of family 3 showing the incidence of verified intracerebral haematomas (black) or cerebrovascular accidents (dotted)

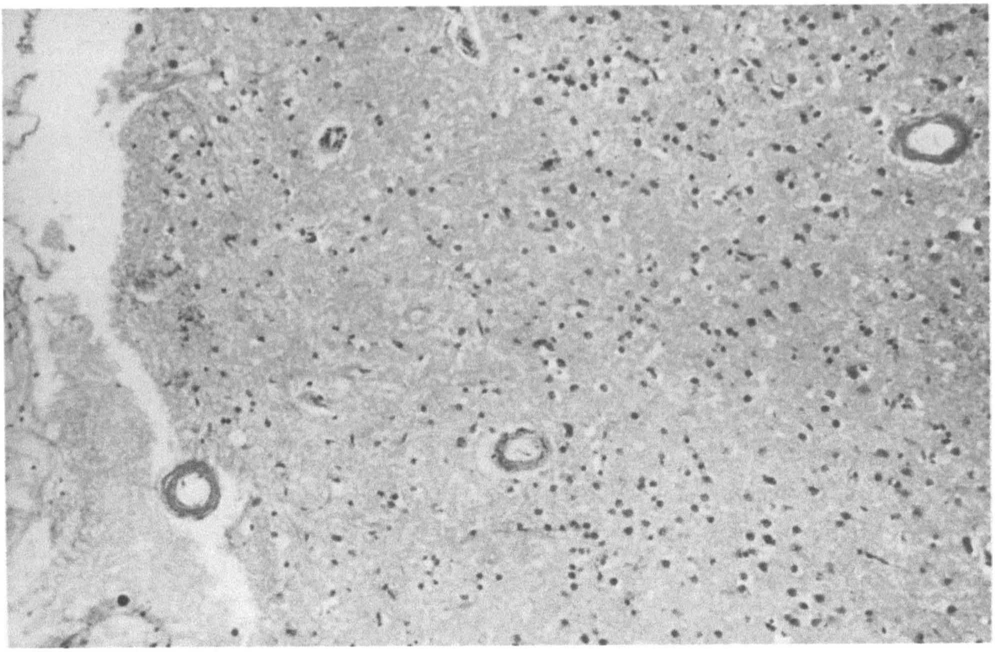

Figs. 4. Arteriolosclerosis of the cortical arteries, with perivascular haemorrhages in the vicinity of a haematoma

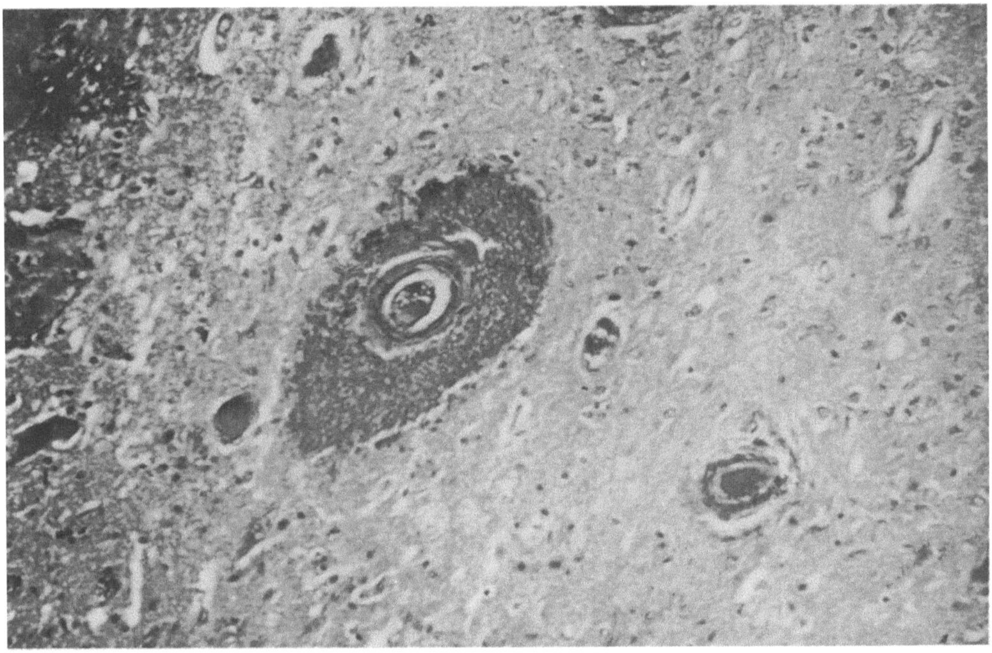

Fig. 5. Arteriolosclerosis of the cortical arteries, with perivascular haemorrhages in the vicinity of a haematoma

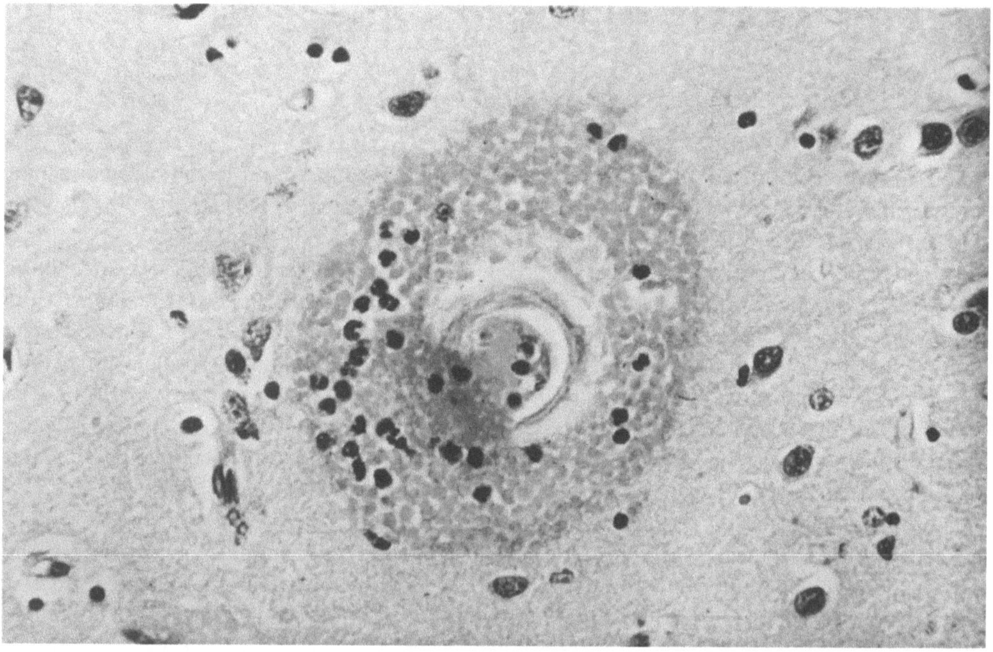

Fig. 6. Arteriolosclerosis of the cortical arteries, with perivascular haemorrhages in the vicinity of a haematoma

arteries appeared to be an associated factor. This seems to be different from the systemic hyalinosis of the arteriolosclerotic vessels in the third family we have described here. No other example of this kind has so far been found in the literature.

However, it appears evident that intracerebral haematomas can show a high incidence in certain families, especially during the fifth and sixth decades, and that systemic arterial pathology may be a causative factor (Luyendijk 1972; Luyendijk and Schoen 1964).

Acknowledgement

The authors are very much indebted to Dr. L. N. Went and Mrs. M. Vegter-van der Vlis (Department of Anthropogenetics) for their kind assistance and provision of family histories.

Addendum

"Recent pathological examinations (Dr. Bots) have clearly revealed that amyloidosis of the tunica media is also present in our cases from Katwijk, as well in those of Dr. Wattendorf concerning the case from Scheveningen.

This finding of a familial occurrence of intracerebral haematomas along the coast of the North Sea and Iceland suggests that they may be considered as group having a genetical factor in common."

2.8 ICH in Sinus and Cerebral Vein Thrombosis

O. Busse, Giessen

Thrombosis of cerebral veins or sinuses is an extremely rare cause of intracerebral haematoma. In autopsy material the incidence of haemorrhages is estimated to be between 2% and 3% (McCormick and Rosenfield 1973; Jellinger 1977).

The disturbances of venous drainage occurring in the case of sinus and large vein thrombosis are, at the beginning, compensated by venous collaterals. The insufficiency of the latter results in oedema and small bleedings by diapedesis, which may finally result in a haemorrhagic infarction of the white and grey matter (Huhn 1965, 1972; Noetzel and Jerusalem 1965). The extent and location of the haemorrhagic infarction are related to the territory of the venous drainage and the adequacy of the venous collateral circulation. Rupture of engorged and distended veins can produce an actual haematoma, which acts as a space-occupying lesion and may rupture into the CSF spaces (Noetzel and Jerusalem 1965; Krücke 1971).

The clinical diagnosis of cerebral vein and sinus thrombosis may be quite difficult owing to lack of clear-cut clinical symptoms and often uncertain angiographic signs. Before the introduction of computerized tomography, intracerebral bleeding complicating venous thrombosis was rarely diagnosed. Small bleedings could not be demonstrated, and large vascular space-occupying lesions were interpreted either as a haematoma of other aetiology or as a tumour, depending on the clinical picture. Demonstration of a cerebral mass in the arterial phase of angiography, combined with a delay in the circulation time caused by oedema, tended to distract attention from the possible venous obstruction.

Case reports

A 32-year-old patient presented with a progressive left-sided hemiparesis, Jacksonian-type fits and clouding of consciousness. Carotid angiography showed a right parieto-occipital mass. The venous phase of the angiogram was normal. Craniotomy was performed and blood clot mixed with necrotic brain tissue was removed. The autopsy showed thrombosis of cortical veins with cortico-subcortical haemorrhagic infarction and haemorrhage not only in the right, but also in the left parietal lobe (Fig. 1). In computerized tomography very small haemorrhages were demonstrated. Multiple uni- or bilateral areas of increased density in computerized tomography have been reported as reflecting small haemorrhagic infarcts (Barnes and Winestock 1977; Buonanno et al. 1978; Kazner et al. 1975; Lavin et al. 1978).

In another patient with clinical and angiographic signs of cerebral vein and sinus thrombosis, computer tomography was performed on the 6th day after the onset of symptoms. The CT scan showed diffuse oedema with areas of increased density corresponding to bilateral parietal and temporal haemorrhages (Fig. 2). After some days the patient died, and at autopsy extensive haemorrhagic infarcts and haematomas were found in the frontoparietal areas on both sides (Fig. 3).

In view of such findings it is obvious that anticoagulation therapy is contra-indicated in such cases. Serial computerized tomography will show the further evolution of such bleedings,

---

Fig. 1. Large haemorrhagic infarction with destruction of white and grey matter in the parietal region. Multiple small haemorrhagic infarcts on the opposite side ▶

Fig. 2. Bilateral small haemorrhages, temporal and parietal, in a patient with sinus and cerebral vein thrombosis

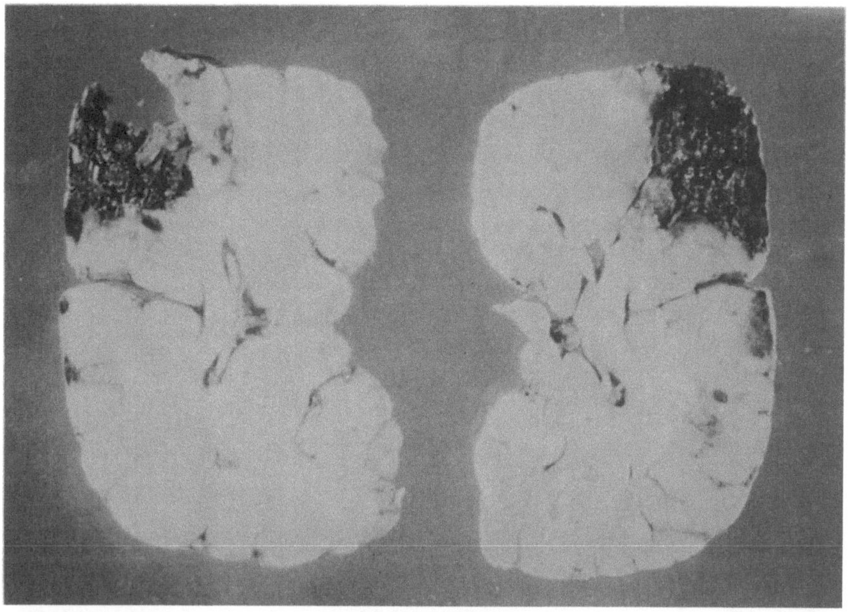

Fig. 1

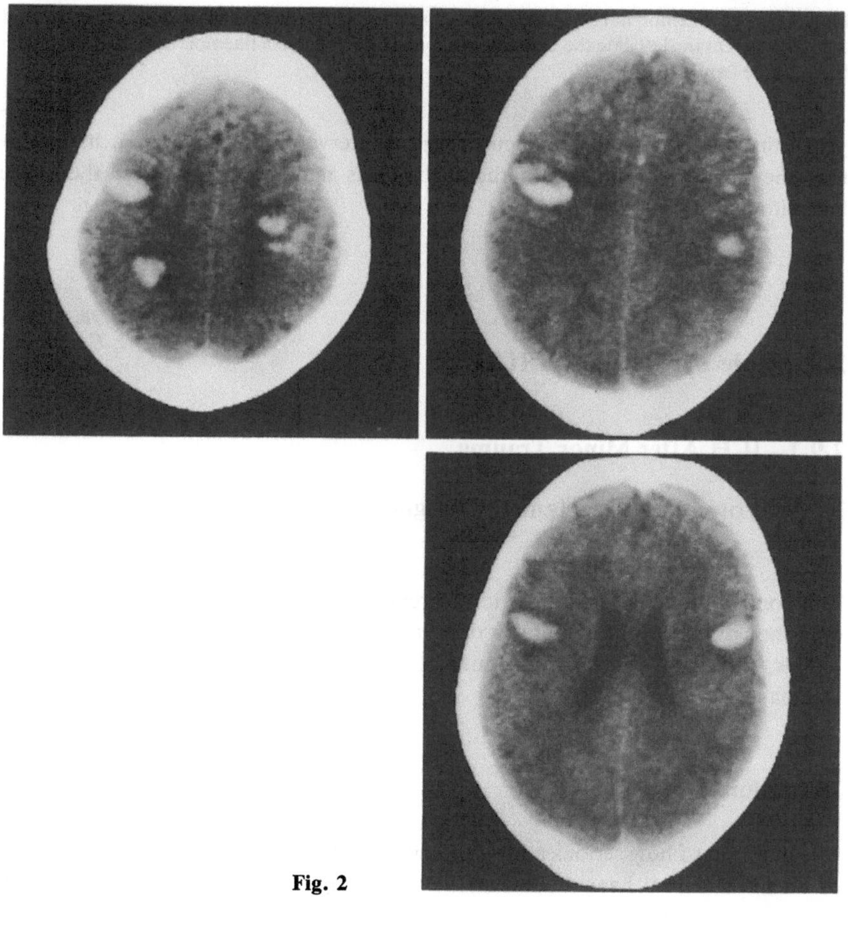

Fig. 2

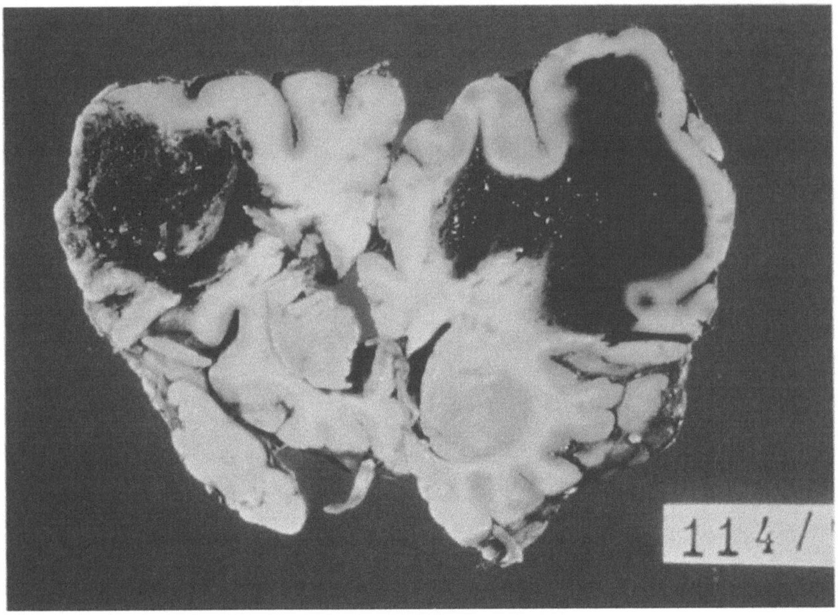

Fig. 3. Large haemorrhages in the frontoparietal white matter in a case of sinus and cerebral vein thrombosis. On the left side the haematoma looks like a massive haemorrhage, because macroscopically no brain tissue can be seen

permitting the best timing for neurosurgical intervention. However, it has to be remembered that the disease continues and the thrombosis may propagate after the evacuation of the haematoma.

2.9 Role of Trauma in ICH

2.9.1 ICH After Minor Trauma

R. A. Frowein and E. Hamel, Cologne

This contribution concerns those intracerebral haematomas in which a head injury plays a role, even though this injury is minor or does not immediately give rise to serious brain disturbances.

This, therefore, will be an account of intracerebral haematoma following minor or trivial trauma.

Definition

The question of how serious a head injury must be for us to be relatively certain that it will lead to an intracerebral haematoma has never, to my knowledge, been investigated. I found no references to this matter in the publications of Gögler (1968). Therefore, I have no choice but to rely on personal clinical experience.

One hundred and forty-nine cases of traumatic intracerebral haematomas treated in our hospital (Hamel and Karimi-Nejad 1978) are entered on this chart according, on the one hand, to the nature of the accident and, on the other, to the syndromes which developed in the course of the day following the accident. No disturbances of consciousness, or clouding of consciousness, or coma stages I – IV, according to the Brussels definition of 1976, were found (Brihaye et al. 1978) (Fig. 1).

We were interested primarily in those cases where no disturbances of consciousness at all or only slight clouding of consciousness occurred.

In our division of different causes of head injury, we tried to differentiate lesser and greater degrees of impact to the head:

1) Brain injury is likely to be minor if a not too heavy object falls on or hits the head, if the head is banged against some solid object, if a person falls but manages to save himself, or if a person is knocked down by someone else.
2) Falls from a ladder or down stairs, falls from a bicycle or falls from a moderate height can result in varying degrees of brain injury, but the driver or the pedestrian in a traffic accident is likely to suffer more serious injuries.

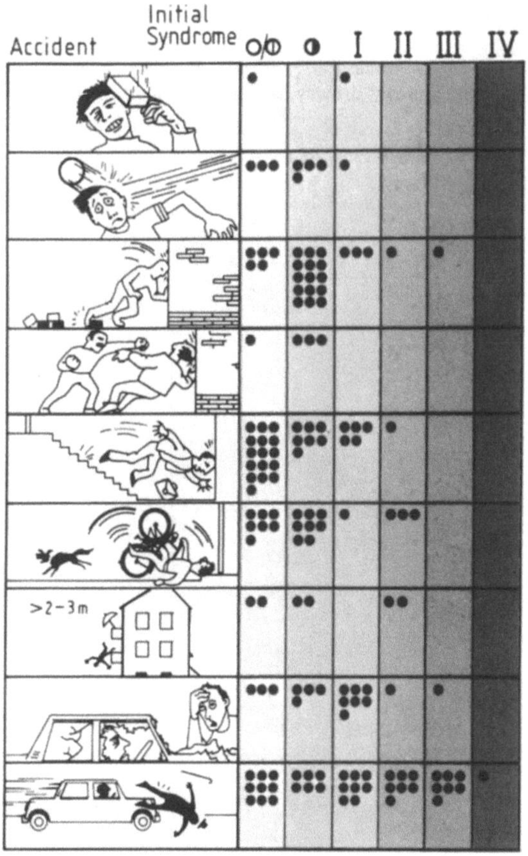

Fig. 1. 149 cases of traumatic intracerebral haematomas after different degrees of impact to the head

Only 27 of the total of 149 cases of traumatic intracerebral haematomas were minor enough for our analysis. These are entered in Table 1. I shall return later to the question of whether the patient's condition resulted only from the trauma or whether his condition was influenced by other factors, such as alcohol or vascular disease.

In addition to the first group of 27 patients, we included in our study a further 15 patients with arterial aneurysms, arteriovenous angiomas and patients under treatment with anticoagulants.

In the past 10 years, 343 cases of arterial aneurysms have been treated in our clinic. Only eight of these cases suffered rupture of the aneurysm followed by intracerebral haematoma after minor trauma, either alone or influenced additionally by alcohol or vascular disease.

Among 176 cases of arteriovenous angiomas there were only four cases of intracerebral bleeding following minor trauma of the skull. Among 25 patients receiving treatment with anticoagulants three intracerebral haematomas were observed.

Case Reports

The following case reports provide examples of these different groups of haematoma after minor trauma:

Minor Trauma Plus Alcohol

A 25-year-old male (5633/56) was involved in a fight in a bar. The following day he complained of a headache and was drowsy, but he was not admitted to hospital until at least 15 days after the trauma. There

Table 1. Distribution of cases according to aetiology

Trauma				
Tr. only	b. 5, s. 14			
Alcohol		6		
Vasc. D.			2	
				27
Aneurysm				
Tr. only	4			
Alcohol		1		
Vasc. D.			3	
				8
Angioma				
Tr. only	4			
Alcohol				
Vasc. D.				
				4
Anticoagul.				
Tr. only				
Alcohol				
Vasc. D.			3	
				3
	27	7	8	42

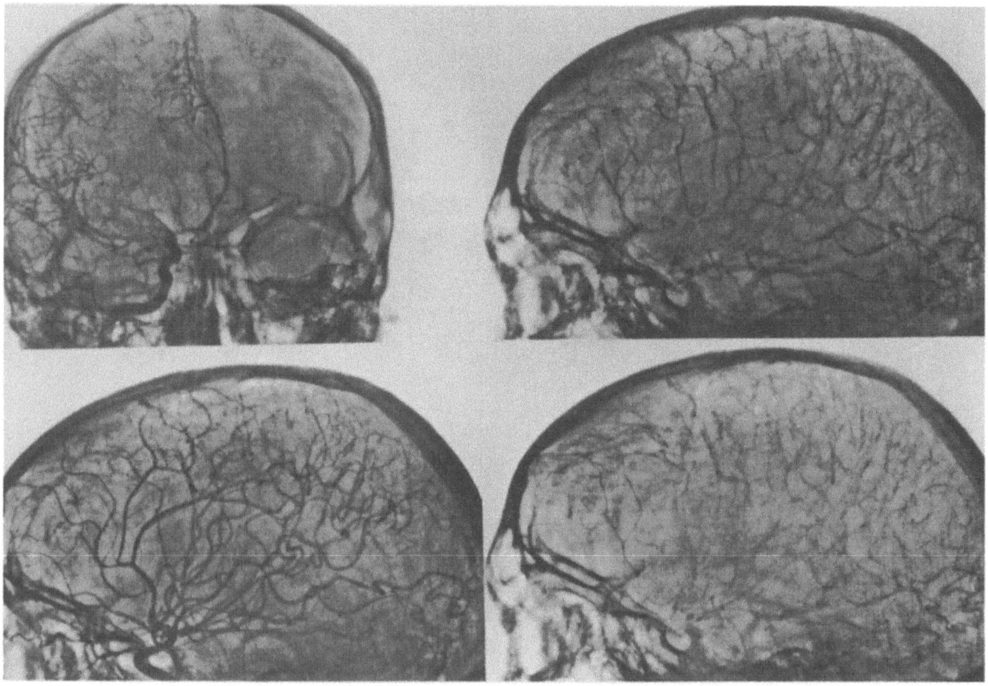

Fig. 2. Right frontal intracerebral haematoma 15 days after a fight (5633/56)

was no external wound or fracture of the skull. The EEG showed a focus in the right frontal region, and angiography (Fig. 2) revealed an avascular space-occupying lesion in the same area. At operation, W. Tönnis evacuated a large intracerebral haematoma. Nevertheless, although the patient regained full consciousness and seemed to be recovering, he was unable to work and died 4 months later.

Minor Trauma and Vascular Disease

A 30-year-old Spanish worker (14529) was hit on the bridge of his nose by a metal spring; 10 days later he suddenly became comatose. Angiography revealed an intracerebral haematoma in the left temporal region (Fig. 3). The haematoma was evacuated through a burr-hole, but the patient died the following day. The autopsy showed a haemorrhagic diathesis.

Aneurysm

A 45-year-old male (171/74) suffered a concussion in a car accident. While the formalities were being attended to after the accident, he developed a right-sided hemiparesis. Angiography (Fig. 4) showed a large aneurysm at the bifurcation of the internal carotid artery. The temporal intracerebral haematoma was evacuated and the aneurysm surrounded with muscle. The patient died in coma.

A 42-year-old male (935/77) was involved in a fight. Afterwards he complained of a persistent headache. Examination 2 weeks later revealed a right frontal intracerebral haematoma, the result of the rupture of an aneurysm of the anterior communicating artery.

In these cases the head injury had only an indirect effect on the aneurysm.

A direct effect might occur on aneurysms of the internal carotid artery at the origin of the posterior communicating artery, if the sac of the aneurysm is in contact with the tentorium,

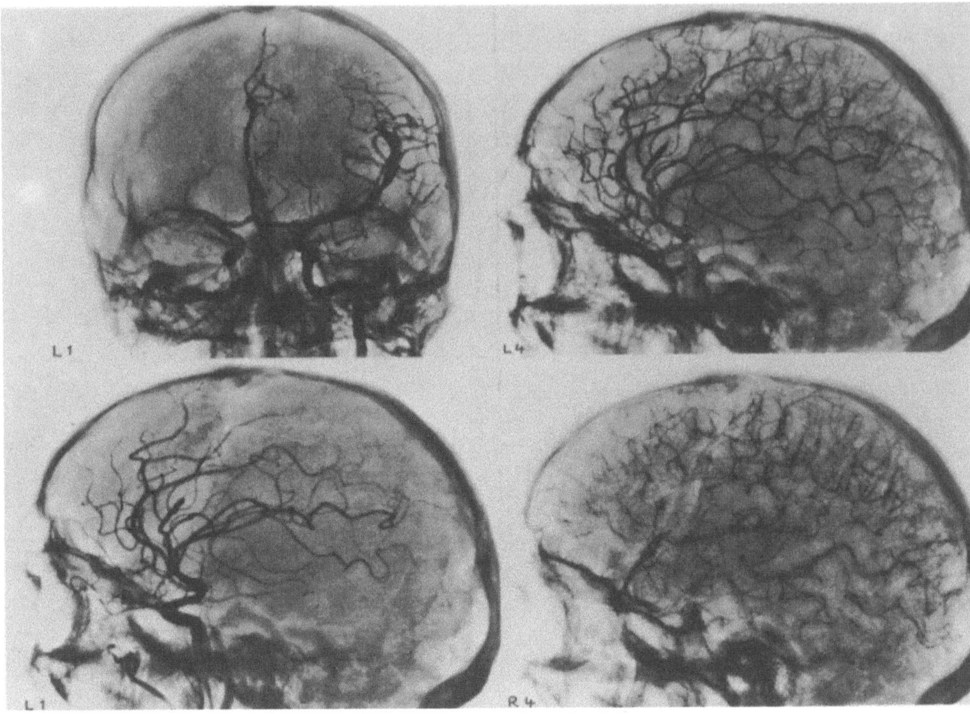

Fig. 3. Left temporal intracerebral haematoma 10 days after a hit on the bridge of the nose (14529)

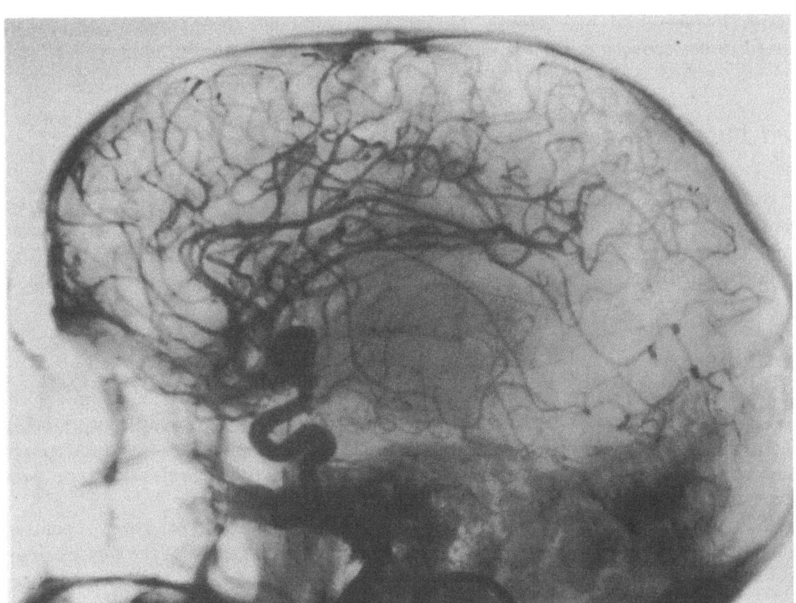

Fig. 4. Temporal intracerebral haematoma with an aneurysm of the bifurcation of the internal carotid artery, 6 h after concussion in a car accident

or in rare cases of aneurysms of the pericallosal artery (Laun 1978). Here are two such cases:

A 55-year-old female (1382/78) was hit on the head by a swing-door. Vomiting was followed the next night by a persistent headache. Nine weeks later she had to enter hospital. CT scan (Fig. 5), angiography and operation showed a giant aneurysm of the pericallosal artery, with a left-sided frontal intracerebral haemorrhage, which was evacuated; the aneurysm was surrounded by muscle. The patient recovered.

The bleeding of such an aneurysm of the pericallosal artery in the case of a 6-year-old boy (270/72) proved fatal. He was struck by a car, was comatose for 4 h and then regained consciousness. Nineteen days later he fell into coma. The circulation time in the angiography was extremely slow (Fig. 6). At operation the sac of the aneurysm was firmly attached to the edge of the falx. Evacuation of the blood did not ameliorate the coma of the child. It is difficult to know whether the sac of the aneurysm was damaged at the time of the head injury and gave rise to a haemorrhage 19 days later, or whether the haemorrhage occurred spontaneously.

Smith and Bardenheier (1968) were able to disclose the development of an aneurysm on the right pericallosal artery within 3 weeks of a closed head injury. Laun (1978), in his review of 70 cases of traumatic aneurysms, also mentioned one case after closed head injury.

Angioma

A 32-year-old male (112/71a) with a right frontotemporal angioma died as a result of an intracerebral haemorrhage following a trivial head injury caused by a football. The operation was performed 5 days after the injury.

Birth Trauma

Too late for inclusion in the statistical tables was the case of a baby with intracerebral haematoma after birth trauma caused by vacuum extraction (Fig. 7).

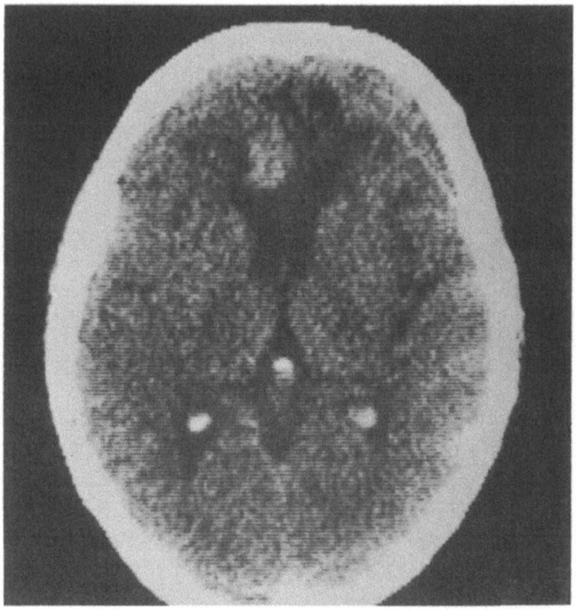

Fig. 5. Left frontal intracerebral haematoma with an aneurysm of the pericallosal artery, 9 weeks after a hit on the head by a swing-door (1382/78)

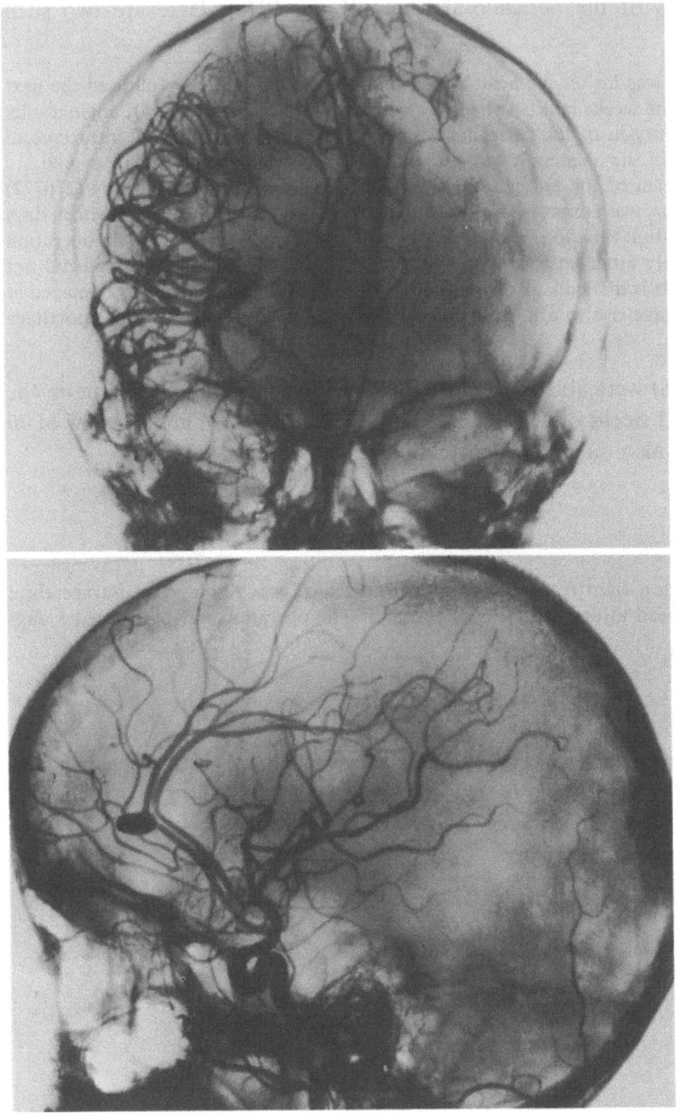

Fig. 6. Intracerebral and subdural haematoma with an aneurysm of the pericallosal artery 19 days after a car accident (270/72)

To summarize: in two-thirds of all the cases in our sample the main cause of intracerebral bleeding was trauma. Bleeding as a result of aneurysm, angioma or anticoagulative treatment occurred in only one-third of our 42 patients (Fig. 8). Alcohol was a factor in 7 of the 42 patients, i.e. one in six, or 17%. Vascular disease played a part in eight cases, that is about 19%.

Age

The age distribution of our patients is worth examining. In Fig. 9, I have made a distinction between particularly minor traumas, which I label trivial trauma, and other minor traumas; the

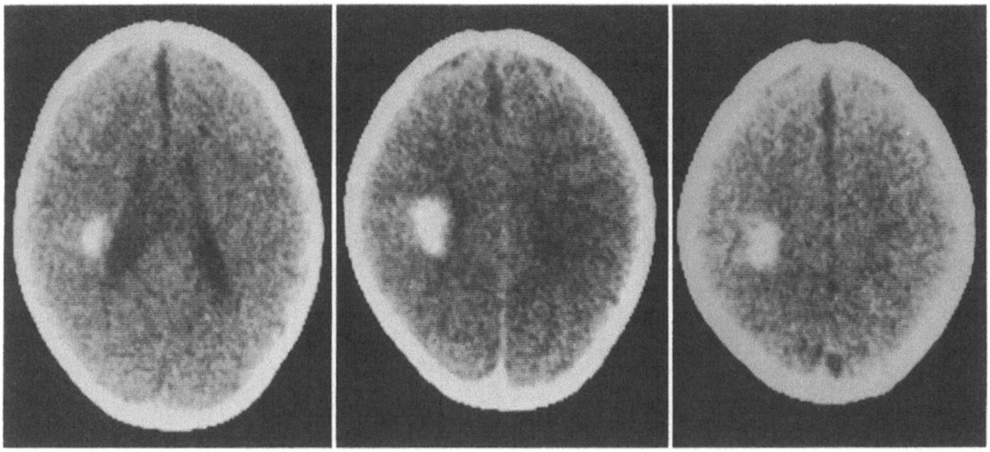

Fig. 7. Left central intracerebral haematoma after birth trauma caused by vacuum extraction (26. 10. 78)

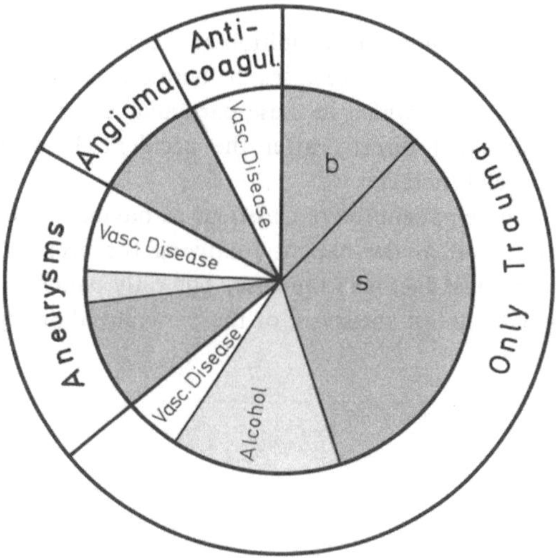

Fig. 8. 42 cases of intracerebral haematoma after minor trauma

trivial injuries are entered on the left of each column, the other minor traumas on the right. The trivial trauma patients were, with one exception, under 45 years of age; ten patients were under 20. The effects of alcohol begin to appear from the age of 20, of vascular disease from the age of 45. In this chart patients who died are indicated by filled-in circles.

The 42 patients on which this analysis is based is so small a number that a statistical evaluation is not possible. One can only point to some of the trends which seem to emerge. For instance, whereas only one-half of the patients under 50 years of age died, two-thirds of those over 50 died.

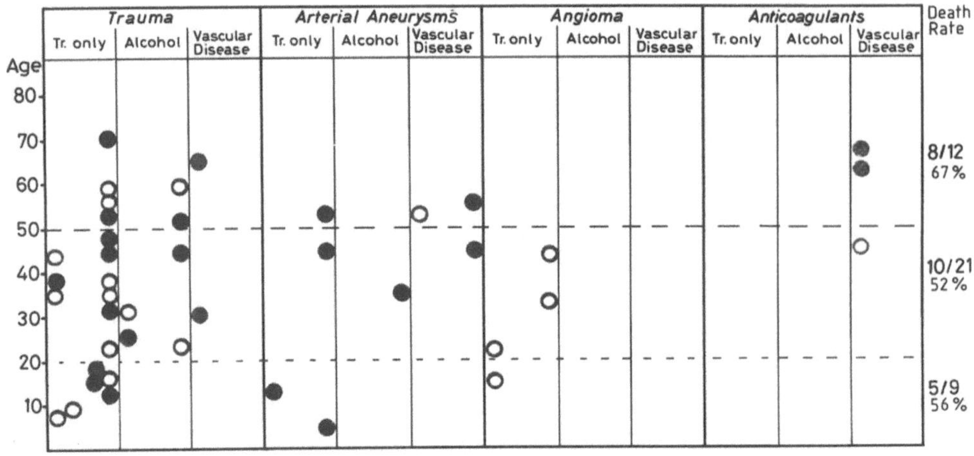

Fig. 9. Age distribution of our patients with intracerebral haematoma after minor trauma

Initial Syndrome

Figure 10 shows the condition of the patients immediately following the accident, insofar as this was known. In three cases the actual cause of the accident was not determined. By definition, the trauma, which in these particular cases led to intracerebral haematoma, seemed to be so minor that directly after the accident 38 of the 42 patients suffered no disturbances of consciousness.

Three patients were classified as having clouding of consciousness, either because the exact condition of the patient following the accident was not known or because alcohol was an additional factor in the case. The only patient who was unconscious at an early stage was the child with an aneurysm of the pericallosal artery. He regained consciousness 4 h later.

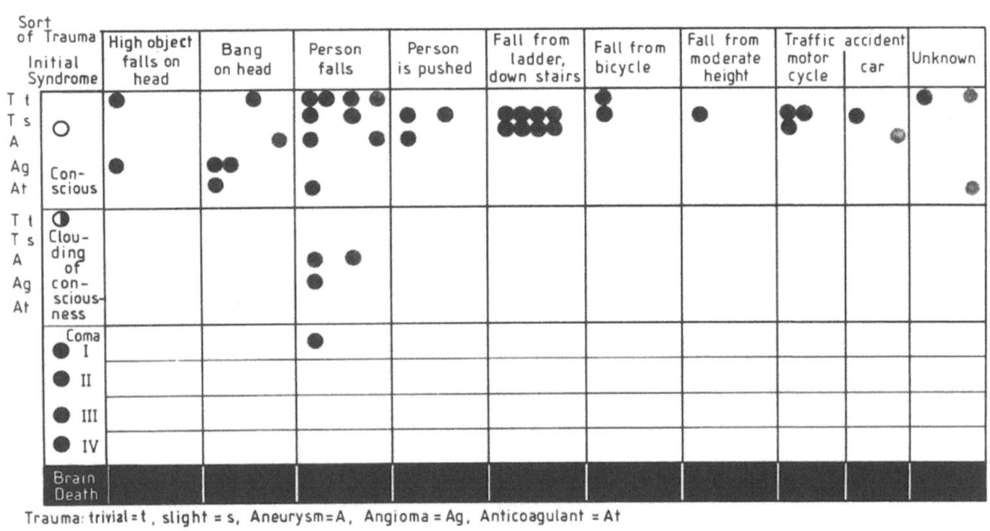

Fig. 10. Initial syndrome in 42 cases of intracerebral haematomas after minor trauma

Latency Between Trauma and Onset of the Haematoma Symptoms

To examine both the connexion between trauma and haematoma and the further development of the condition, we need to analyse the period between the trauma and the actual onset of the symptoms of intracerebral haematoma (Fig. 11).

After a short symptom-free period of 2–24 h, 21 of our 42 patients developed clear symptoms of haematoma. Most of these patients suffered clouding of consciousness. One third of the 21 cases suffered coma, four of them stage I, and relatively few of them stages II, III or IV.

Only two patients retained full consciousness for 2 months and then suffered fits or similar manifestations.

Where the symptoms of haematoma develop in the course of the 1st, 2nd or 3rd day, a relationship between trauma and bleeding is easy to understand (Brown et al. 1978). But an interval of 5 or more days, or 1 or several weeks, or even 1 or more months makes the matter more problematical.

In a few cases, of course, delayed diagnosis was involved. In three other cases, some days, weeks, or months later, bleeding or fits recurred. The extremely long course of all such cases will certainly become rarer with the increased use of computerized tomography, and it will also become easier to arrive at early judgements on such cases.

To summarize, a period of weeks can separate the minor trauma from the development of symptoms of haematoma.

Progress of Patients who Survived

After the haematoma symptoms had been recognized, 38 of the 42 patients were operated on. The progress of the 18 patients who survived is shown in Fig. 12.

Seven of the 18 patients who survived were fully conscious before the operation. The symptoms of the remaining 11 patients became suddenly more acute shortly before the operation, which led to a diagnosis and to the operation itself. Of particular importance in the

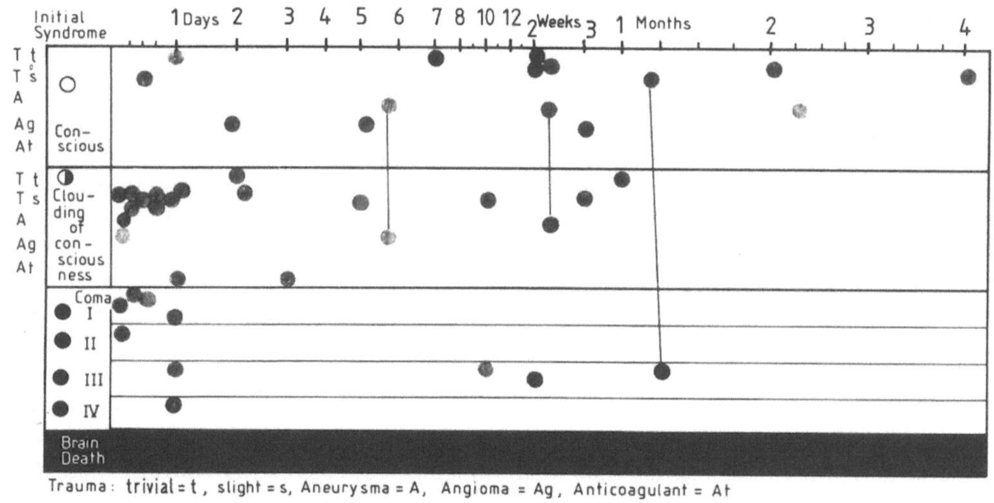

Fig. 11. Latency between trauma and beginning of haematoma symptoms or operation

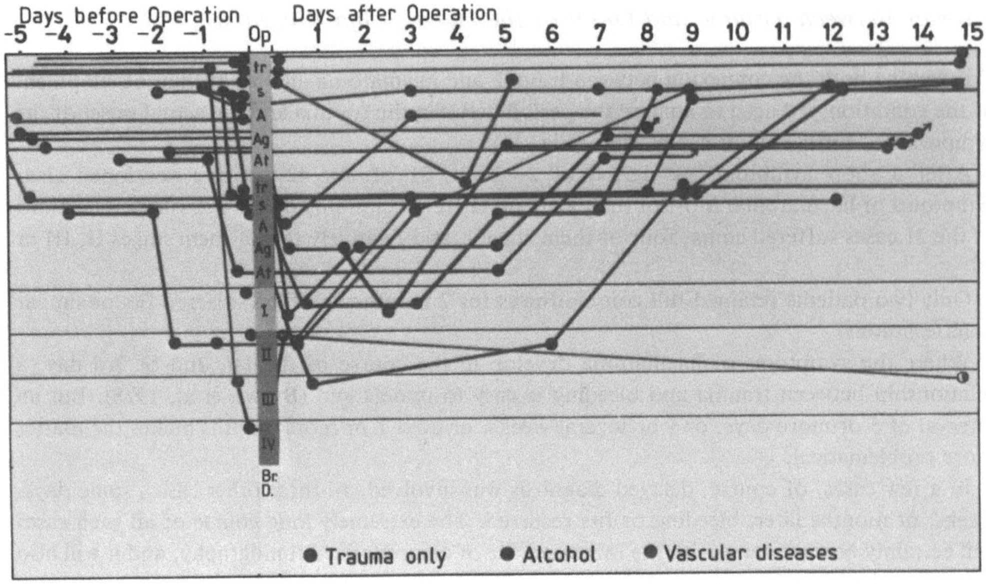

Fig. 12. Syndrome time diagram of intracerebral haematoma after minor trauma; progress of survivors

case of the survivors is that only four cases were in coma pre-operatively, and after the operation this quickly became a clouding of consciousness. After 5 – 7 days clear consciousness had returned. The only exception was a case where bleeding occurred after the operation, necessitating a second operation. This pattern, therefore, conforms to our own previously described experience: The chances of recovery for young people and adults are relatively good if the stage of coma has not lasted more than 5 – 7 days (Frowein et al. 1978).

Fatal Cases

The syndrome/time diagram of the fatal cases shows a different pattern of progress (Fig. 13). Here, too, the symptoms of most of the patients suddenly became much more acute. Half of the patients suffered clouding of consciousness and the other half fell into coma. In spite of surgery, improvement was partial or inadequate. In a few cases an initial improvement was followed by a later relapse. Three patients died much later, that is 3 weeks, 4 months and 5 months, respectively, after the operation.

In one of these cases the cause of death remained unclear. This was the case mentioned earlier of the young man involved in a fight. This case also confirmed our earlier experience that where coma has lasted more than 5 – 7 days, a permanent recovery is unlikely.

This analysis of clinical progress shows that there were 20 patients fully conscious with a pre-operative history of more than 1 day; nine of them remained fully conscious up to the operation and after it, whereas 11 deteriorated before surgery, after which seven, that is one-third of these patients, died. The crucial question is, in what way it might be possible to distinguish those who remain stable and those who will deteriorate. This seems very important in view of some reports in which conservative therapy under CT control is chosen.

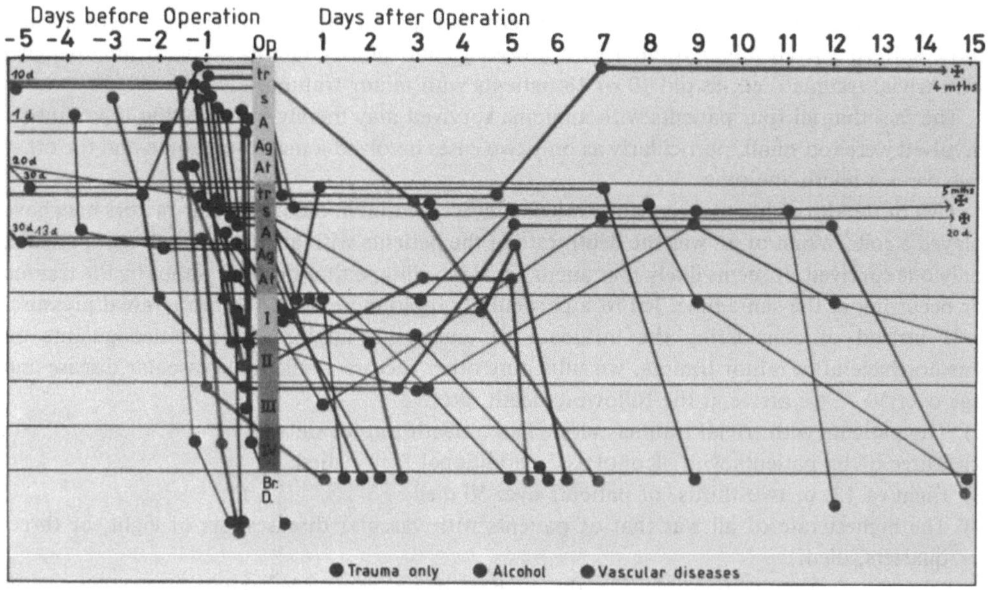

Fig. 13. Syndrome time diagram of intracerebral haematoma after minor trauma; progress of non-survivors

Assessment of Outcome Taking into Consideration Primary and Secondary Aetiological Factors

Finally, I have attempted to analyse how the various causes of bleeding affected the course of these haematomas. Survivors and non-survivors were divided into groups according to whether trauma alone or trauma in conjunction with aneurysm, angioma or anticoagulative treatment was the cause of the bleeding (Fig. 14).

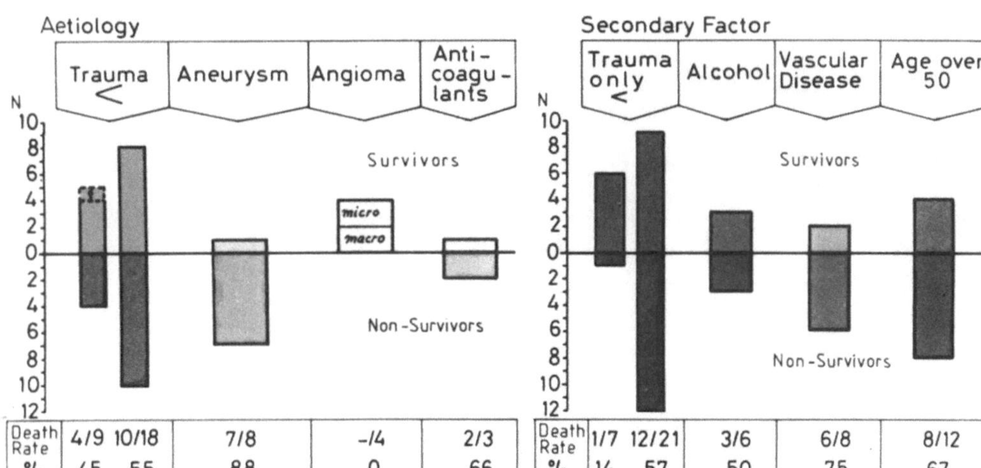

Fig. 14. Outcome in cases of intracerebral haematomas

No great differences in death rate were discernible between patients suffering from trivial and those suffering from minor trauma with no other contributory factors; four of nine patients with trivial trauma died, as did 10 of 18 patients with minor trauma.

The fact that all four patients with angioma survived may merely indicate that the numbers involved were too small, particularly as only two cases involved a macro-angioma and the other two cases a micro-angioma.

Two of the three patients receiving anticoagulative treatment died; vascular factors may have played a role. Worst of all was the death rate of the patients with aneurysms; of eight patients, only one survived. It seems likely that aneurysmal bleeding, either brought about by the trauma or occurring at the same time, led to a particularly rapid increase in the intracranial pressure.

If instead of considering the influence of aneurysm, angioma and anticoagulants on haemorrhage after minor trauma, we substitute other factors – alcohol, vascular disease and age over 50 – we arrive at the following death rates:

1) The patients with trivial traumas alone had a death rate of only 14%.
2) Three of six patients with alcohol as an additional factor died.
3) Eight of 12, or two-thirds, of patients over 50 died.
4) The highest rate of all was that of patients with vascular diseases: six of eight, or three-quarters, died.

Thus the factors responsible for the highest death rates are traumatic bleeding from aneurysms and age over 50, together with vascular disease.

These factors are ones that neither doctor nor patient can influence to any great degree.

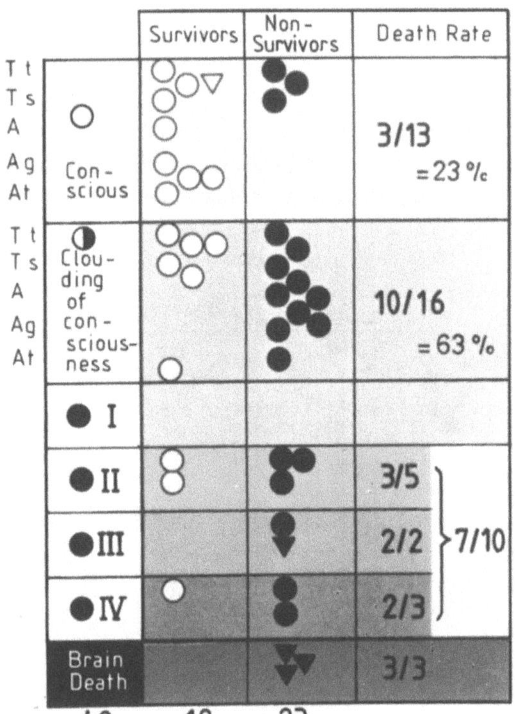

Fig. 15. Outcome in relation to pre-operative syndrome in cases of intracerebral haematoma after minor trauma

Influence of Pre-operative Syndromes

Figure 15 illustrates the varying death rates when pre-operative syndromes are taken into account.

The lowest death rate of 23% was found among patients who were fully conscious before operation. When clouding of consciousness was present before the operation, two-thirds of the patients died.

Only three of the 13 patients who were in coma before the operation survived, and of these one still demonstrated an apallic syndrome 2 weeks after the operation. The death rate in this group was 77%.

It seems possible that timely diagnosis could have prevented deterioration to such a poor pre-operative condition.

2.9.2 Trauma in Intracerebral Haematomas

D. Parkinson, E. G. Newry, and J. Taylor, Winnipeg

Introduction

It is nearly 90 years since the term *Spätapoplexie* was coined to describe the sequence of injury-interval-apoplectic deterioration believed by Bollinger (1891) to result from the delayed or renewed haemorrhage from the originally damaged intracerebral vessels. The few series in the intervening years reporting on this rare condition have done nothing to clarify the two questions raised by Bollinger's concept viz. the role of surgery and the length of the interval beyond which a fresh haemorrhage may no longer be attributed to the original injury. By contrast the nominally similar sequence of injury-interval-deterioration associated with the extracerebral clot and described by the term "lucid interval" has engendered innumerable reports of huge series, leaving no doubt as to either the advisability of operation or the relationship of the injury to the clot. However, even a cursory study of reports of both conditions emphasizes that the clinical courses may mimic each other throughout (Lanerhans 1903; Naffziger and Jones 1928; King and Chambers 1952; Pia 1959, 1968; Bender 1960; Parkinson and Chochinov 1960; Hemmer 1965; Parkinson et al. 1971).

Definitions

The CT scan will pick up intracerebral clots as small as 1 cm in diameter, and we must accept this measure in future reporting. Such small lesions previously would be undetected with the investigations then available and would be diagnosed merely as swollen hemispheres or contused temporal lobes.

Material

There is currently under way a prospective computerized study which is storing, processing and retrieving up to 185 variables for each of the 1100 head injuries admitted annually to our centre. (This study is supported by research grant from the Manitoba Medical Services Foundation, Inc.) A 4-year survey has retrieved 70 intracerebral haematomas which form the material for this report. There are few significant differences in our series from the reported series, where comparison is possible. Browder's (1942) 80 cases were from a 5-year survey with no background figures given. Bender (1960) reported 65 cases over a 10-year period. McLaurin's (1956) 16 cases were retrieved from a 6-year review averaging 300 head injuries per year. Courville's (1940) 36 cases were from 439 fatal head injuries. Galbraith (1976) had 35 cases from a total of 307 intracranial traumatic clots. Jamieson's (1972) 63 operated cases were from 11 000 admissions over an 11-year period. Kozniewska's (1965) averaged 0.5% of the head injuries.

Incidence

The incidence of these lesions must be divided into two categories, i.e. the pre- and post-CT scan eras. The papers published before the CT scan indicate that less than 1% of head injury admissions have intracerebral haematomas, diagnosed only by surgery or autopsy. Since the introduction of the CT scan the incidence in our own series has risen to 1.59% of all head injury admissions. Thus, the incidence will be increasing with the addition of more small and otherwise incidental clots picked up by the increasingly routine use of the scanner (Figs. 1, 2). These cases will reduce the mortality rate overall and also in the non-operative series.

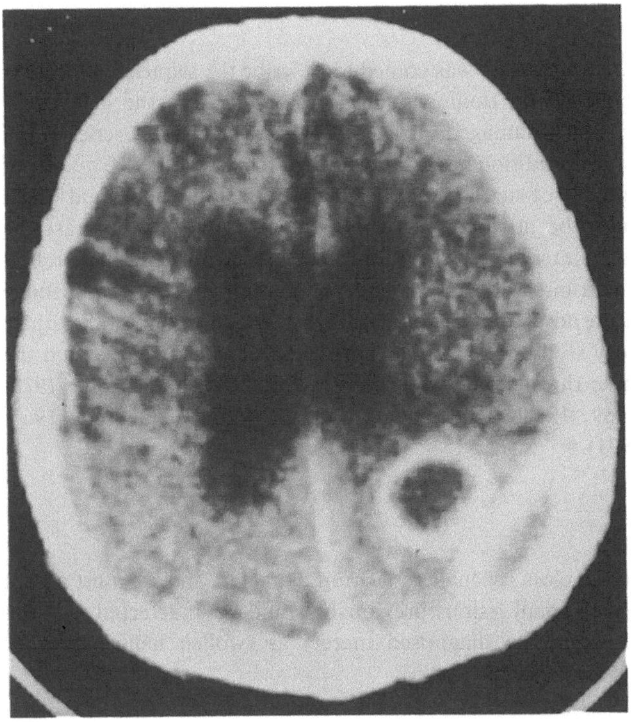

Fig. 1. Enhanced CT scan showing intracerebral haematoma adjacent to a subdural haematoma in the right occipital region of a patient who was entirely asymptomatic

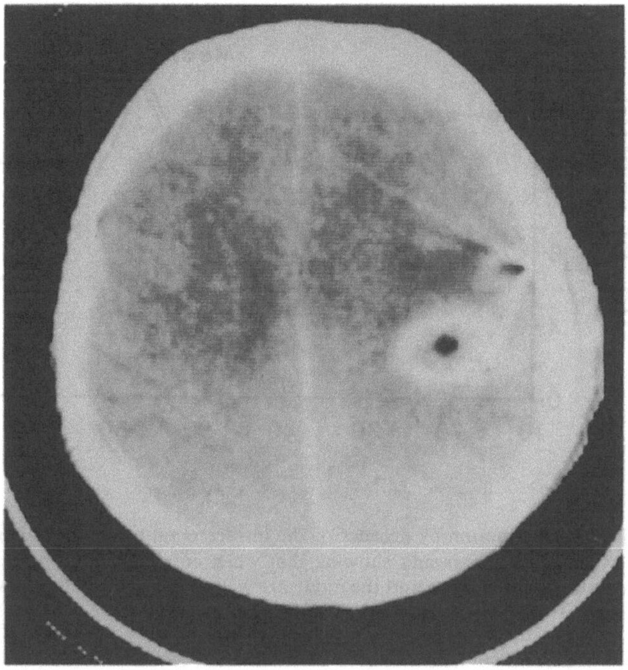

Fig. 2. Enhanced CT scan showing unsuspected intracerebral haematoma with a small amount of air beneath a depressed fracture (Courtesy of Dr. Rankin Hay)

Aetiology

The principal factors involved are the force and direction of the blow, but we are unable to measure these with any accuracy in the human patient with his enormous propensity for a wide variation of mishaps, as well as an equal (understandable) unwillingness to participate in controlled head injury experiments. None of the series emphasizes severe violence as a cause, and our own series would indicate that most occur as a result of a force no greater than that of a fall from standiang height or less. However, force is very difficult to evaluate when a car crash at 50 mph can produce a very mild concussion, while a fall backwards from a sitting position may cause a fatal head injury with multiple cerebral lacerations and haematomas. Age stands out as an important factor. Our range was from 1 to 93 years, with a corrected mean just over 56 years (Fig. 3). Apart from one infant dropped on his head by the babysitter there is a gap in the first decade. The population mean is about 39 years, and the mean of our overall head injury admission series is just over 30 years. McLaurin's average of 50 years is somewhat altered by his high rate in the third decade with motorcycle riders crashing at high speed under the influence of alcohol. Our climate mitigates against a preponderance of motor cycle riders, although there were two in our series. The male-female ratio is 3 to 1, compared with nearly 2 to 1 in the overall head injury series (Table 1). The average male was slightly younger than the average female.

In the overall head injury series motor vehicle accidents account for approximately 33% and assaults for 27%, with alcohol a factor in over 70% of both these groups. The remaining accidents were household and sporting events. About an equal percentage of the intracerebral haematomas subgroup resulted from motor vehicle accidents, but alcohol was a factor in less than a quarter of those accidents. Falls from no higher than a standing height accounted for

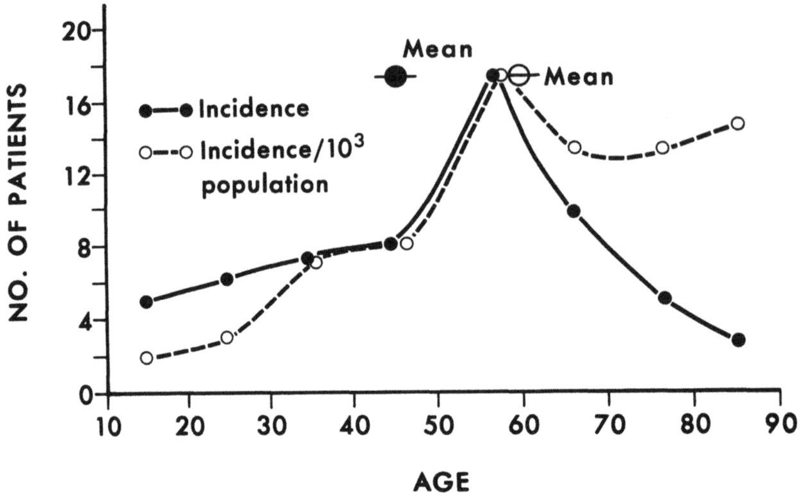

Fig. 3. Distribution by decades of the intracerebral traumatic haematomas, omitting the two extremes of 1 year and 93 years and showing that when corrected for a percentage of the population alive in each decade both the mean and the mode are well to the right of 30 years which is the population mean and the mean of the overall head injury admission group

nearly two-thirds of the intracerebral haematomas subgroup, with alcohol a factor in approximately one-half of those (Tab. 2).

Pre-existing vascular disease does not appear in our series as a demonstrable factor beyond the obvious association of progressive atherosclerosis with age. None of our patients was on anticoagulants or suffering from bleeding diathesis, although these would seem self-evident if present. The use of tobacco becomes suspicious with its known deleterious effect on the blood vessels throughout the body.

The typical case thus seems to emerge as a 56-year-old male falling from no more than a standing height while intoxicated ($p > 0.05$ for these three factors). This could be interpreted to mean that the intoxicated 56-year-old male is susceptible to an intracerebral haematoma from any given head injury or that the 56-year-old intoxicated male is likely to have the type of head injury productive of an intracerebral haematoma. The latter seems more probably.

There have been very few reports that would meet Bollinger's (1891) criteria for *Spätapoplexie* (Langerhans 1903; Bailey 1904; Naffziger and Jones 1928; Jamieson and Yelland 1972). We had only one, a male re-admitted 2 weeks after discharge with a normal interval followed by apoplectic deterioration. Bollinger's (1891) longest interval was 50 days and his shortest, 12. Three of his had fourth ventricle clots and one a paraventricular clot. It is evident that we are dealing with two mechanisms, namely one that immediately produces a haematoma

Table 1. Four-year survey of head injuries admitted to the Health Sciences Centre and the intracerebral haematomas subgroup from the same group

	Number	Mean age	Male: female	Extracerebral haematomas
Head injuries admitted	4400	30–40	2:1	177
Intracerebral haematoas	70	56	3:1	27

Table 2. Comparison of the entire head injury group with the subgroup of intracerebral haematomas

	Motor vehicle accidents	Falls	Assaults	Sports	Other	Use of alcohol [a]
Head injuries admitted	33%	30%	27%	7%	3%	60%
Intracerebral haematomas	34%	60%	5%	–	–	35%

[a] Alcohol was a factor in over 70% of the motor vehicle accidents of the entire head injury group, in less than 25% of the intracerebral subgroup and in nearly 50% of the falls in the intracerebral subgroup ($p > 0.05$)

and another that will produce delayed bleeding (or enlargement of an existing haematoma). The mechanisms cannot be proved for either category but only assumed. Evans's (1946) concept of coalescing petechial haemorrhages does not seem plausible as it assumes minute bleeders with sufficient force to continue and destroy the intervening feltwork of brain structure. An initial shearing force appears as the most likely mechanism destroying cerebral structure while at the same time tearing many minute vessels which are free to bleed into the resulting cavity. If a sufficiently large vessel is torn it probably continues bleeding, with a fatal outcome. The smaller and relatively elastic torn and stretched vessels may cease bleeding from a combination of spasm and thrombosis or equalization of pressure.

The subsequent deterioration may be due to progressive enlargement of the residual, otherwise static, clot as a result of breakdown products and osmotic factors, but we have no proof. Careful follow-up with a CT scan may be informative in this area, noting the mass effect. It must be remembered that clots may become isodense and seemingly disappear for a few days.

Delayed haemorrhage may be the result of original direct damage to the vessel wall with formation of a false aneurysm, a proven circumstance in one of our cases. Cerebral softening with eventual lysis and haemorrhage is put forth as a mechanism, but no one has specifically mentioned damage to the vasa vasorum, a mechanism that results in vessel wall necrosis elsewhere. However, Stebbens (1972) states that the intracerebral vessels have no vasa vasorum until such time as atherosclerotic changes develop. This would be compatible with the mean age of these lesions. Softening of the original occluding thrombus may also account for a recurring haemorrhage. Any of the above mechanisms could account for the appearance of an apoplectic haemorrhage after an interval of 2 – 3 weeks, but if a fresh haemorrhage is demonstrable after this interval, it is increasingly likely that the original accident was a coincidence. Factors that favour trauma are the multiplicity of lesions, the coup-contracoup locations, distance from the basal ganglia and internal capsule, and the absence of any other demonstrable cause. On the other hand, factors favouring spontaneous haemorrhage are proximity to the centrum and, in particular, to the posterior limb of the internal capsule, solitary lesions, pre-existing hypertension or blood dyscrasias and a demonstrable vascular anomaly (Courville and Blomquist 1940; Browder 1942; Pia 1959, 1968; Bender 1960; Benes et al. 1972; Jamieson and Yelland 1972). It should be remembered that trauma may cause an intracerebral vascular anomaly to bleed and, in the very young, this should be strongly suspected (Ameli 1968).

2.9.3 Relationship Between Head Injuries and Intracerebral Haematoma

C. Arseni and A. Gontea, Bucharest

There are four possibilities:

1) The Injury Is Primary and the Haematoma Secondary. The injury produces contusion or laceration of the brain and, subsequently, an intracerebral haematoma. Surgery or necropsy may reveal bruising of the scalp, a fracture of the skull, with or without rupture of the dura, and the pathological finding of contusion or laceration of the brain and an intraparenchymatous haematoma.

2) Primary Haematoma and Secondary Head Injury. A cerebral vascular accident with the patient falling down. The cause of the ictus may be cerebral circulatory insufficiency, arterial hypertension, etc.; following loss of consciousness the patient falls down and hits his head. Operation or necropsy may reveal a contusion or wound of the scalp and fracture of the bones; the dura is intact and the brain appears normal, but a deep, clearly circumscribed haematoma is found.

3) Primary Head Injury and Haematoma Secondary to an Intracranial Space-Occupying Lesion. The primary head injury causes vascular disorders in the brain resulting in a haematoma within a tumour, or vascular malformation. Here is an example: The pilot of an airplane hit his chin against the frame of the windscreen when, due to a defect, the plane took off abruptly. After a brief loss of consciousness, he fully recovered and felt quite well for a few

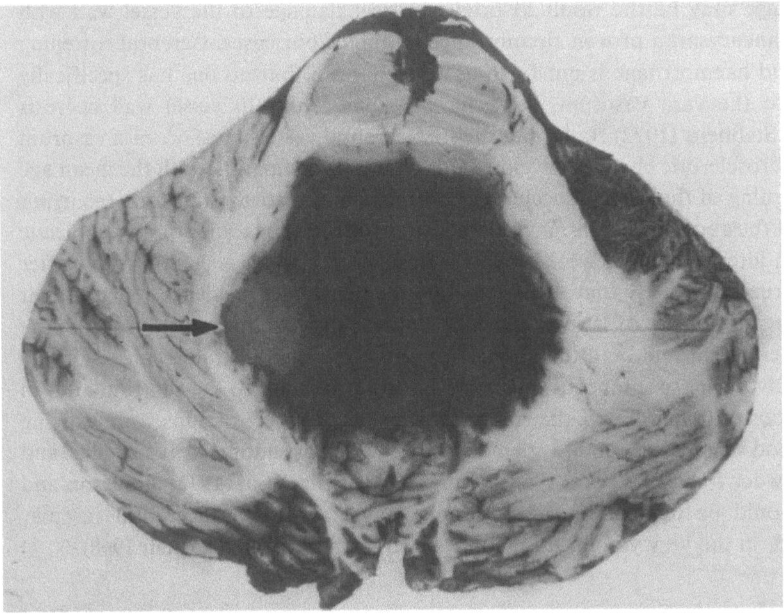

Fig. 1. Cerebellar medulloblastoma → in a young man, with large haematoma which developed after minor head injury

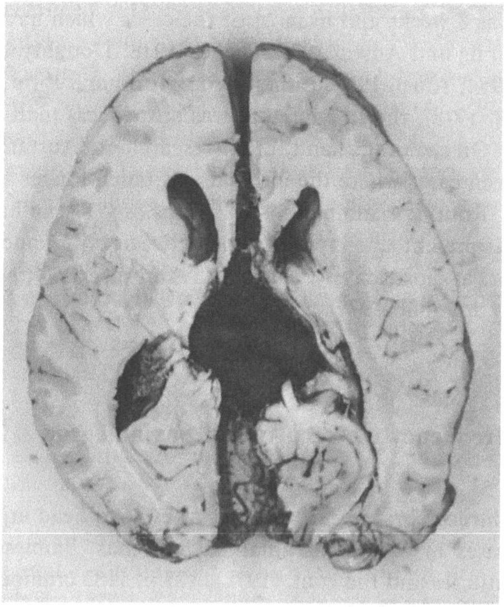

Fig. 2. Angioma of the choroid plexus in the pineal region with haematoma precipitated by a head injury

days. On the third day he complained of headeache, nausea, vomiting and disturbances of balance. Two days later tonsillar herniation developed and he died. Necropsy revealed a small tumour (medulloblastoma) and a large haematoma (Fig. 1).

Head injuries often set the stage for a clinical picture of ruptured angioma. In our statistics there were three cases of angioma of the choroid plexus whose clinical onset was marked by a head injury and which developed in two stages (Fig. 2).

4) Epileptic Seizures – Secondary Trauma with Subsequent Haematoma

2.9.4 Delayed Traumatic Apoplexy

R. Vara-Thorbeck, Granada

The average number of patients suffering from severe cranio-cerebral injuries who are admitted each year to my department of surgery in the University Hospital of Granada is 492, which represents 24.4% of all patients admitted.

From 1972 to 1978 I have operated on nine delayed traumatic intracerebral haematomas. The last three of these operations have been performed during the last 12 months.

Bollinger (1891) was the first to describe delayed traumatic apoplexy, and his study was based on four necropsy cases. Bollinger cited the following criteria for diagnosis: (1) the absence of pre-existing vascular disease; (2) a definite history of trauma; and (3) an asymptomatic interval and a subsequent apoplectiform episode.

In 1904, Bailey distinguished three types of traumatic apoplexy: a severe form coincident with the injury; a subacute form, where apoplexy develops days or weeks after the trauma; and a chronic form, that develops many months later.

Naffziger and Jones (1928) felt that the maximum time for traumatic haemorrhage to develop was 8 weeks and in most of the cases which have appeared in publications (Rosenhagen 1930; Craig and Adson 1936; Russell 1938; Doughty 1938; Symonds 1940; De Jong 1942; Jamieson 1954; Ameli 1957; Litner 1961; Morin and Pitts 1970; Barathan and Dennyson 1972; Brown et al. 1978), the free interval was always less than 120 days.

On the other hand, other researchers (Austarheim 1956; Hillbom and Anttinent 1957) have seen cases where the interval was much longer – in one case, 11 years.

Routine examinations by means of CT scan have made neurosurgical diagnosis much easier. At present, the lapse of time between injury and surgical treatment has been reduced to hours or, at most, days (Paxton and Ambrose 1974; Merino de Villasante and Taveras 1976; French and Dublin 1977).

Frequency of Occurrence: Sex and Age

Intracerebral haematomas as a result of head injury are infrequent. Krenkel (1970) recorded 80 cases in 612 intracranial haematomas. Jamieson (1972) found 63 in 11000 craniocerebral injuries and Pia et al. (1978), 127 in 5583 craniocerebral injuries. We have operated on 65 cases of a total of 2886 cases of severe craniocerebral injury.

However, if the severe traumatic intracerebral haematoma is relatively rare, delayed traumatic apoplexy is even more so. The majority of publications on the subject present between one and four cases. Baratham and Dennyson (1972) saw 21 cases of a total of 7866 patients with craniocerebral injuries. Over the last 7 years we treated and operated on nine patients with delayed apoplexy from a total of 2886 severe craniocerebral injuries.

The youngest patient was 14 years old and the oldest, 74; most of the patients were between 50 and 70. This is in line with the figures produced by Baratham and Dennyson (1972) (21 cases), but not with those of Morin and Pitts (1970) (24 cases), who reported that the highest incidence of haemorrhages occurred between the ages of 30 and 40. There was a clear preponderance of males over females (8 to 1).

Aetiology

It is obvious that the factor which directly causes the haemorrhage is a craniocerebral injury. There exists, nevertheless, some disagreement among authors as to the intensity of the causative trauma, though most of them are of the opinion that it is usually not very severe. In our cases injury was very slight in five (there was no initial loss of consciousness), while in three cases there was a moderate trauma (a fall on the stairs, of some three to five steps, producing a loss of consciousness lasting less than 60 min), and in one case the trauma was severe – the patient was run over by a car, losing consciousness for more than 6 h.

In the literature we find wide variations in the degree of importance given to the following which may be considered as predisposing factors: arterial hypertension, cerebral arteriosclerosis, cerebral atrophy, alcoholism and diabetes. Of our nine patients only three showed clearly predisposing features (Fig. 1).

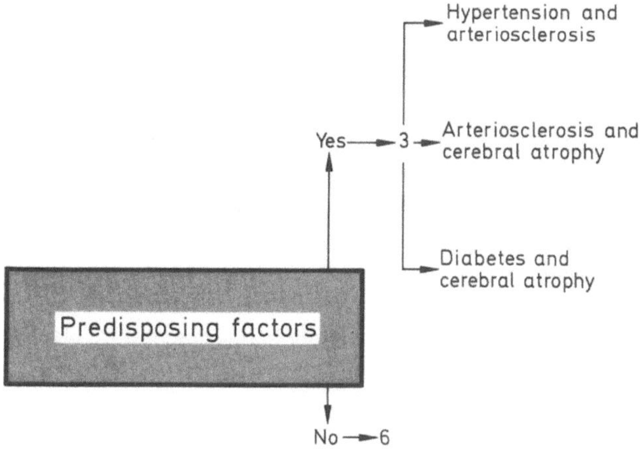

Fig. 1. Predisposing factors

Pathology

As regards the situation of the haematomas we found a marked preference for that side of the brain where the injury took place. Thus, in seven of our patients the delayed traumatic apoplexy occurred on the same side, and in two cases on the opposite side. (In one of the latter cases we found a small subdural haematoma on the same side as the original injury.)

Six haematomas were situated in the left cerebral hemisphere (four temporal, one parietal and one temporoparietal). Three were situated in the right hemisphere (two in the frontal lobe and one in the temporal lobe) (Fig. 2).

All the haematomas were subcortical, varying in depth and extent, but in no case did they reach the basal ganglia. Only two produced a slight laceration in the outer wall of the lateral ventricle.

The size of the haematoma varied between 5 – 6 cc and 40 – 60 cc; the volume was found to bear a direct relation to the lapse of time between injury and surgical treatment. The cavity was nearly filled with liquid blood, which could be evacuated easily, but at the base we always found clots which had to be aspirated.

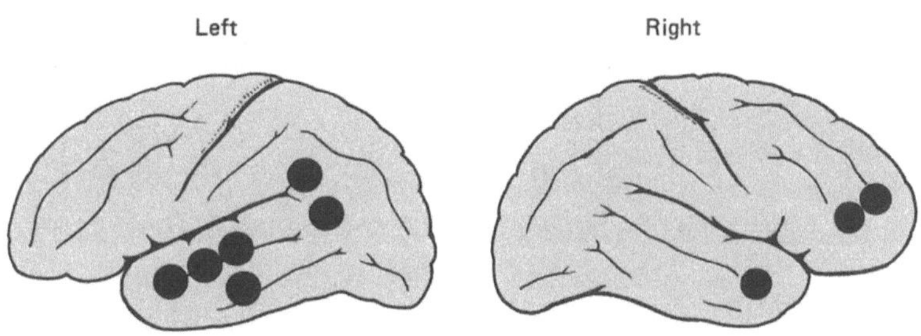

Fig. 2. Distribution of haematomas

Neurological Symptoms

As far as the neurological symptoms are concerned, the existence of an asymptomatic free interval can be said to be pathognomonic for the diagnosis of a delayed traumatic apoplexy.

In our cases the shortest interval was 1.5 h and the longest, 6 months. As can be seen in Table 1, this interval varied between 1 and 48 h in two cases, between 5 and 15 days in three cases, between 16 and 30 days in two others, between two and three months in one, and in one case the interval was 6 months.

The clinical signs and symptoms shown by our patients are seen in Fig. 3. The most frequent symptoms were disturbances of consciousness (but in no case was there deep coma), hemiparesis and hemiplegia. Only in one case did we observe a paralytic dilatation of one pupil. This was on the side opposite to that on which the intracerebral haematoma was situated and was due to the existence of a concomitant subdural haematoma on the same side.

Table 1. Interval between injury and onset of symptoms

Interval	Number of cases
1 – 48 h	2
5 – 15 days	2
16 – 30 days	2
2 – 3 months	1
6 months	1

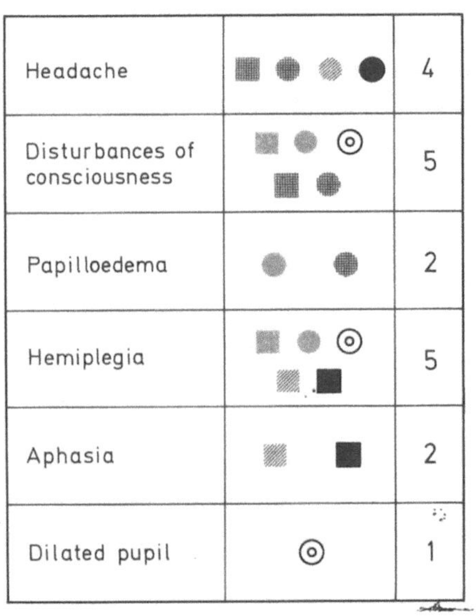

Fig. 3. Neurological signs and symptoms

Diagnosis

Diagnosis of the definite existence of the haematoma and its localization was carried out in all our patients by means of a carotid angiogram on one or both sides. Echo-encephalograms carried out on six patients proved positive in only one case (a middle-echo shift and complex echo haematoma). We applied computerized axial tomography in our three last patients, and the results were clearly positive in two cases and doubtful in one.

Treatment

All our patients underwent a surgical operation: In all cases we carried out a frontal, temporal or temporoparietal osteoplastic craniotomy. It was necessary to perform a double craniotomy in only one case (where there was a subdural haematoma on the same side as the original injury and an intracerebral "contre-coup" haematoma).

In general the cerebral cortex had a normal aspect, although in one case we found signs of a traumatic cerebral lesion. We located the haematoma and punctured it with a Cushing's needle. We then opened the cerebral cortex very slightly and aspirated the clots in the cavity. We did not see any vascular haemorrhage, so after covering the cavity walls with fibrin foam, we left a drainage tube and closed the dura mater.

Results

Three of our patients died in the immediate postoperative period (that is, within 12 days). Two of these were more than 70 years old, the other was 56. All had developed severe respiratory complications, which bore no apparent relation to the lapse of time between injury and surgical treatment. Two of our patients did not recover from their hemiplegia or aphasia. The remaining four patients recovered and were able to resume their normal lives.

2.9.4.1 Discussion

K. J. Zülch, Cologne: The type of lesion which is the so-called late apoplexy plays a certain role in legal medicine in Germany and opinion about it is not clear. Bollinger listed four points of importance: trauma in a legal sense, an interval, apoplectiform onset and no concurrent disease. However, confusion still exists.

Let me briefly recall a case of a 25-year-old racing car test-driver. During a test drive, he had a minor accident with a very slight blow to his head. There was no loss of consciousness and no confusion. Over the next days he had a slight headache. He had a check-up in a hospital and was sent for a 2-week rest. After 4 weeks he took up driving again. On the first drive with another test-driver beside him, he deviated the car always to the left so that at the end of the race, his colleague asked him to stop driving. The patient went home, after half an hour became confused and after an hour unconscious. He died the same night. At autopsy a great clot in the centrum semiovale was found, and the most interesting discovery was perivenous oedema with macrophages. There were all the signs of a lesion which must have been at least 2 weeks old and could correspond to the first trauma.

To summarize the requirements for defining the condition as a "late apoplexy": The patient should be below the age of arterial disease, i.e. he should be younger than 45, and he should have no vascular diseases or blood disorders. There must be a history of trauma, as well as an interval of at least 6 days, and pathological proof that there has been trauma to the brain substance.

J. Glowacki, Cracow: In the Department of Neurotraumatology of the Medical Academy in Cracow, among 140 cases of intracerebral haematomas there were 6 cases with "spontaneous haematomas" occurring some time after the head injury. The interval between the trauma and the operation was, in one case, 4 months; in one case, 1 year; in two cases, 3 years; in one case, 4 years; and in one case, 5 years. All patients were admitted to the department because of signs of increased intracranial pressure. All of them were subjected to angiography, and neither in this examination nor in the biopsy specimens taken at operation was there evidence of vascular malformation or tumour.

Question: The concept of late apoplexy just given may be all right for the pathologist. The term may be also acceptable if only young patients are concerned. What about the older group of patients with mild trauma and "late apoplexy"?

K. J. Zülch, Cologne: The problem with older people is more complicated, this is the age of vascular disease. It is therefore necessary to prove the correlation and not merely to assume that the late apoplexy is connected to the trauma.

H. W. Pia, Giessen: There are many factors which contribute to the bleeding: age, hypertension, minor trauma, coagulopathy, sometimes all at the same time.

K. J. Zülch, Cologne: Sure, but the insurance companies will say, hypertension is a disease, coagulopathy is a disease and each of them alone can be the cause of bleeding. This limits our opinion quite considerably.

K. Jellinger, Vienna: From the pathological point of view I cannot distinguish between the so-called spontaneous or post-traumatic lesions, with extremely few exceptions. A considerable number of traumatic or post-traumatic haematomas also occur in the lateral region of the putamen and claustrum between the grey and the white matter. We should not forget also that there may be a haemorrhage in the vicinity of the previous damage or necrosis with a secondary erosion from which the haemorrhage may occur. I think in these cases we can clearly accept the connexion. I am not so sure whether we can accept this connexion for haematomas occurring after considerably longer delay.

2.10 Haematomas of Unknown Aetiology

W. Luyendijk, Leiden

From the start of the neurosurgical department in Leiden in 1954 until and including 1977, 140 patients suffering from intracerebral haematoma were operated on.

A survey of the aetiology (Table 1; Fig. 1) shows that the number of cases which are finally classified as of unknown aetiology amounts to 49, being 35% of the total case material. Together with the familial cases it numbers 60, i.e. 43%. At the time of operation, more cases

Table 1. Survey of case material

	10	11 – 20	21 – 30	31 – 40	41 – 50	51 – 60	61 – 70	71 – 80	80 yrs	Total
Trauma	3	5	4	1	8	10	6	3	–	40
Tumour	–	2	2	2	–	4	2	–	–	12
Aneurysm AVA, etc.	–	5	4	4	1	5	1	1	–	21
Haemorrhagic diathesis	3	–	–	–	–	1	–	–	–	4
Unknown aetiology	2	3	3	3	11	15	9	3	–	49
Familial	–	–	–	–	3	8	–	–	–	11
Surgical compl.	–	1	1	–	–	–	1	–	–	3
Total	8	16	14	10	23	43	19	7	–	140

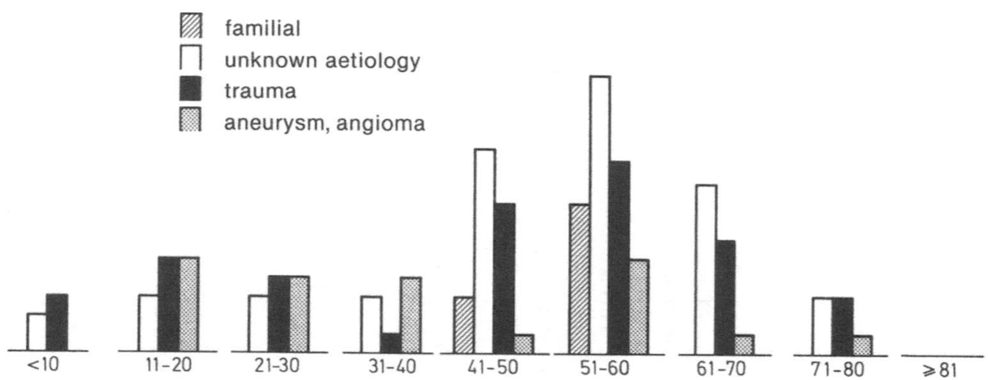

Fig. 1. Histogram showing the aetiological backgrounds of the intracerebral haematomas per decade of age

seem to belong to this category of unknown aetiology. However, pathological examination of the wall of the haematomas, and sometimes its macroscopical aspect, has revealed the presence of a tumour or vascular pathology which hitherto was not suggested by the history nor indicated by angiography or other pre-operative examinations. In this way 16 cases (11.4%) appeared to have an aetiology other than that expected, thus theoretically reducing the number of cases with unknown aetiology from 65 to 49.

According to the reports of the neuropathologist, eight patients suffered from a tumour: four malignant or semi-malignant gliomas, three metastases of a carcinoma and one giant cell sarcoma. In five of these cases this pathology was already suspected at the time of operation. In the other eight patients biopsy of the wall of the haematoma revealed vascular pathology, such as six small arteriovenous malformations and two haemangioblastomas. (Only in three cases were these anomalies suspected during the surgical intervention.)

However, the haematomas of unknown aetiology which occurred in 35% of the cases deserve further attention. Their incidence is remarkably high in the fifth, sixth and seventh decades of life (Fig. 2). When the familial cases are added, a striking preponderance is seen in the fifth and especially in the sixth decade. The sex ratio is 3 to 2, showing a majority of male patients.

The mortality in the group of the haematomas of unknown aetiology amounts to 43%, but is strikingly higher in the familial cases, i.e. 63%. As is indicated in the literature, the outcome in general is unfavourably influenced by increasing age and by a rapid development of signs and symptoms. If we consider the causative factors we have to realize that fundamentally, a haematoma is an extravasation which can only occur after rupture of the wall of a blood-vessel. Except in the case of a traumatic lesion, a pre-existing pathology must be consequently assumed. This seems to be likely in case of an aneurysm, an arteriovenous malformation and even a tumour. However, in cases of unknown aetiology it remains an open question whether even systematically performed small biopsies could provide us with adequate information. Even a careful search for small vascular anomalies by the usual methods of autopsy examination has not led to a complete solution of this problem (Odom et al. 1952; Nayrac et al. 1953; Van der Ark 1968).

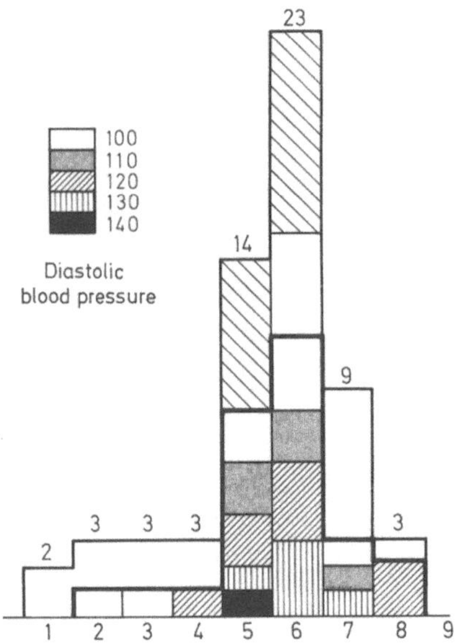

Fig. 2. Histogram of 49 intracerebral haematomas of unknown aetiology and 11 familial haematomas (coarsely striped), divided into decades of age. Cases with pre-existing arterial hypertension are surrounded by a thick line

On the other hand, Russell (1963) and Cole and Yates (1967) were able to demonstrate the existence of micro-aneurysms (as described by Charcot and Bouchard in 1868) with the help of low-voltage X-ray micro-angiography of brain sections after post-mortem perfusion with a contrast medium. They found the highest incidence in hypertensive patients 65 – 69 years of age.

In the group of haematomas of unknown origin the incidence of hypertension appears to be rather high. Hypertension is considered to have played a possible causative role only when it has been established for some time before the development of the haematoma, or when it was still present some time after the haematoma had been removed. Hypertension is assumed when the diastolic value is 100 mm Hg or more.

According to a governmental report concerning a large population research project in Holland, hypertension in the sense described has been found in 3.7% of males between the ages of 54 and 64, and in 4.0% of females in the same age group. However, the incidence of hypertension in haematomas of unknown aetiology is much higher. In the sixth decade it amounts to 67% (excluding the familial cases, it is 48%). In the whole group of 49 cases hypertension was found in 51% with a striking male preponderance of 37%.

From these figures it has to be concluded that arterial hypertension plays an important causative role in intracerebral haematomas of unknown aetiology.

As regards anticoagulants it appears from our case material that their influence is only very slight (Fig. 3). This conclusion agrees with a recent study by Wintzen (1979) regarding the incidence of intracranial haematomas among a large group of patients chronically treated with anticoagulants for all sorts of reasons.

In conclusion it is tempting to assume a vascular pathology as a fundamental factor developing in the fifth, sixth and seventh decade of life and then leading to intracerebral haematomas of unknown aetiology. A comparable situation is established in the group of familial haematomas and may underline this suggestion.

How far micro-aneurysms will develop on the basis of this vascular pathology and, after rupture, will initiate the development of intracerebral haematomas, remains an open question.

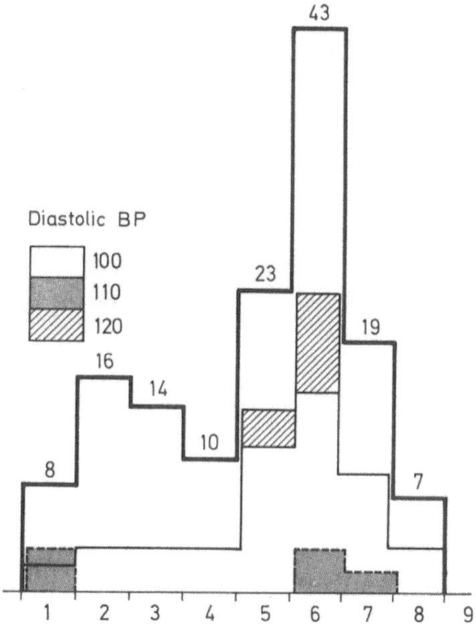

Fig. 3. Histogram of 140 surgically treated intracerebral haematomas divided into decades. The haematomas of unknown aetiology and familial cases (striped) are surrounded by a thin line. The dotted areas indicate the cases of haemorrhagic diathesis and those treated with anticoagulants

2.11 Stroke and ICH in Spontaneously Hypertensive Rats

W. Rascher, R. Dietz, H. Haebara, A. Schömig, D. Ganten, and F. Gross, Heidelberg

Cerebrovascular damage occurs in many forms of experimental hypertension in rats, and its incidence depends largely upon the speed and intensity of the increase in blood pressure and upon the absolute height of the blood pressure. This paper reports the results of pathophysiological and histological studies in the stroke-prone substrain of spontaneously hypertensive rats (spSH) which has a high incidence of cerebrovascular stroke (Okamoto et al. 1974). Such a strain of spSH has been bred for 4 years in our institution.

Of 185 spSH, 72 (39%) kept under normal conditions developed stroke within the first year of life. Among the cerebrovascular lesions, three different types can be distinguished: anaemic infarction (59%), cerebral haemorrhage (33%) (Fig. 1), and haemorrhagic infarction (8%).

Studies were undertaken to investigate the possibilities of either reducing or enhancing the blood pressure increase and influencing the development of cerebrovascular damage. Variations in the concentration of salt in the diet changed the course of blood pressure development. In 7 – 8-week-old spSH rats, a low-sodium diet (1 mmol/kg Na) induced an initial

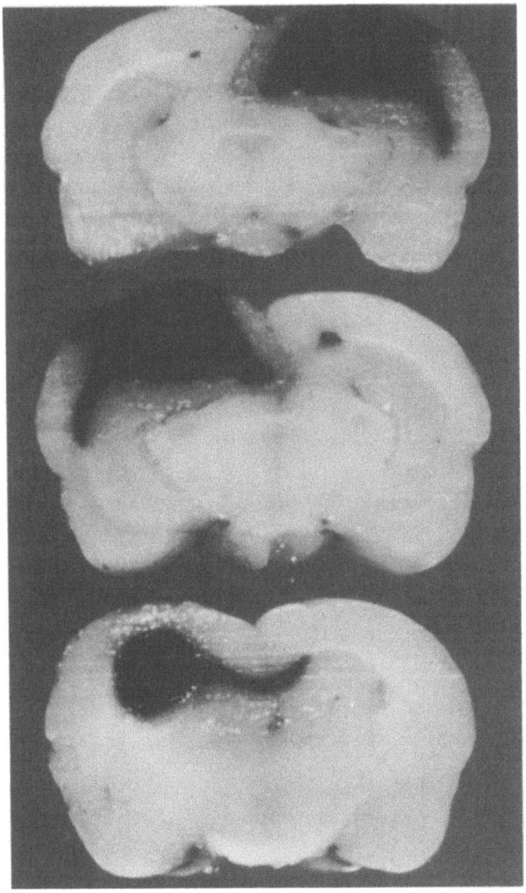

Fig. 1. Cerebral haemorrhage in spSH rats with perforation into the ventricles

reduction in blood pressure which was followed by a delayed and diminished increase, whereas a high sodium diet (1000 mmol/kg Na) accelerated the development of hypertension. In the latter group, symptoms of cerebrovascular lesions were seen in five of ten rats within 2 – 4 weeks after starting the administration of the high sodium diet. At the end of this experiment, the average blood pressure in the group on the low salt diet was significantly lower than that of the controls. In the same group, the plasma angiotensin II concentration was about 7 times normal, whereas it was slightly reduced in the rats on the high salt diet (Dietz et al. 1978).

To study the sensitivity of spSH rats to additional hypertensinogenic stimuli, various types of experimental renal hypertension were elicited. In 7 – 8-week-old spSH rats, a stenosis of one or both renal arteries (1-clip, 2-kidney; 2-clip, 2-kidney hypertension) or renal artery stenosis after unilateral nephrectomy (1-clip, 1-kidney hypertension) caused a rapid rise in blood pressure. Within 7 – 14 days, blood pressure in these rats increased to values that are otherwise found only at the age of 9 – 12 months (Dietz et al. 1978). Extensive vascular lesions occurred in all three types of renal hypertension. In rats with 1-clip, 2-kidney hypertension, the incidence of stroke was 61% and rose to 69%, if 1% saline was given as drinking fluid. For animals with 2-clip, 2-kidney hypertension, the incidence of cerebrovascular lesions was 72%, and 76% with 1% saline. The most severe and frequent lesions in the brain were observed in rats with 1-clip, 1-kidney hypertension. In these animals, the incidence of cerebrovascular lesions was 92%. The incidence increased to 96% with the addition of salt to the drinking fluid. The renin-angiotensin system was only stimulated in rats with 1-clip, 2-kidney hypertension.

In the brain of spSH rats, vascular lesions are mainly found in three zones (Fig. 2): most frequently in the area between the posterior and the terminal branch of the middle cerebral artery; second, in the area between the second and the third branch of the middle and anterior cerebral artery; and, finally, in the area between the first branch of the middle and the anterior cerebral arteries (Haebara et al. 1977). This distribution of lesions differs from that seen in man as a consequence of high blood pressure. In humans, cerebral haemorrhages as well as anaemic infarctions are more frequently found in the deeper parts of the hemisphere or in the brain stem and only rarely in the cortex or the subcortical parenchyma.

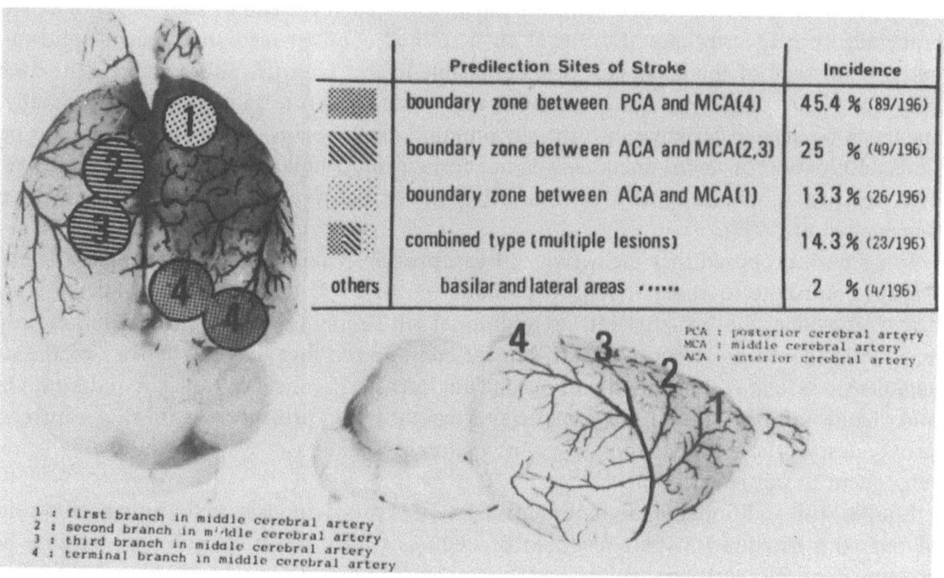

Fig. 2. Predilection sites of cerebrovascular lesions in spSH rats

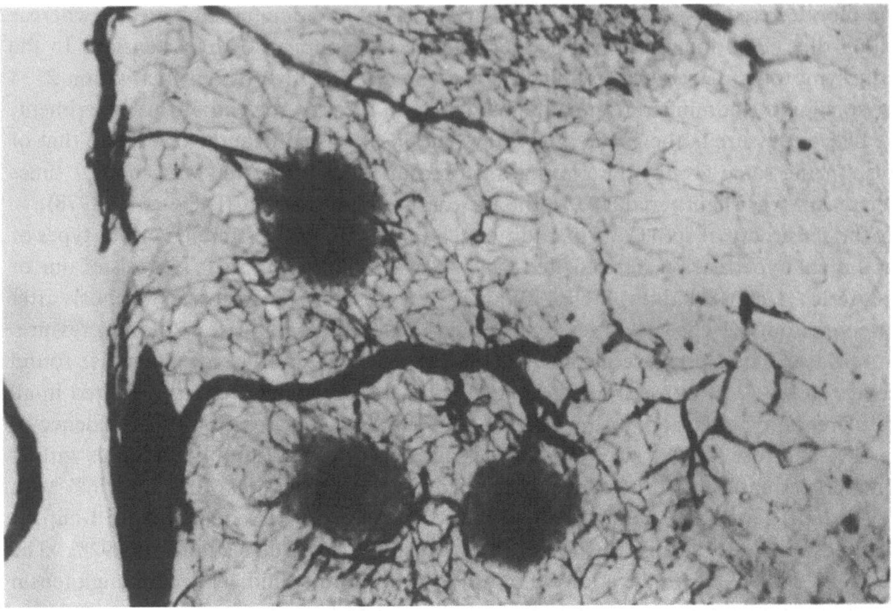

Fig. 3. Micro-aneurysms in brain vessels of spSH rats. The brain was perfused with X-ray contrast medium and dyestuff. Leakage of the dyestuff from the micro-aneurysm filled with contrast medium (dark centre) is indicated by the grey surrounding zone

Intracerebral haematomas are the consequence of the rupture of intracerebral arterioles or of small aneurysms that have been formed along them, subsequent to the development of high blood pressure. The micro-aneurysms are mostly situated at the end of small arteries and at the branching sites of arterioles. By means of a stained contrast medium it can be shown that initially, the wall of the aneurysm is impermeable to the dyestuff. Subsequently, the dyestuff leaks out of the contrast medium, indicating an increase in permeability (Fig. 3) and, finally, the aneurysm bursts and bleeding into the surrounding tissue occurs. In any other vascular bed, a similar formation of micro-aneurysms is not found, but cellular hyperplasia of the vessel wall with obstruction of the lumen, fibrinoid necrosis and perivascular infiltration are observed (Haebara et al. 1977).

It has been proposed that the activity of vasopressor systems, such as the renin-angiotensin system, contribute to vascular lesions (Brunner et al. 1973). From our experiments reported here, it is evident that in spSH rats an additional salt supply favours the rise in blood pressure and the incidence of cerebrovascular damage, despite the fact that the activity of the renin-angiotensin system is suppressed and plasma angiotensin II concentrations are reduced. On the other hand, salt restriction has a beneficial effect on blood pressure and on the occurrence of stroke, despite the fact that the activity of the renin-angiotensin system is markedly increased subsequent to salt restriction.

Studies with additional renal hypertension in spSH rats demonstrate the enhanced sensitivity of rats with hereditary hypertension to procedures which are also known to increase blood pressure in normotensive animals. The rapid increase in blood pressure after renal hypertension accelerated the occurrence and incidence of cerebrovascular lesions up to 61% – 92%.

In conclusion:

1) Cerebrovascular damage is more severe, the more rapidly increases in blood pressure occur.
2) The activity of the renin-angiotensin system does not contribute to vascular lesions.
3) The distribution of lesions in the brain of spSH rats differs from that seen in humans with high blood pressure.
4) Stroke-prone spontaneously hypertensive rats are highly susceptible to other hypertensinogenic factors such as high salt intake or renal artery stenosis.
5) Intracerebral haematomas are the consequence of the rupture of intracerebral arterioles or of micro-aneurysms that have formed along them, subsequent to the development of high blood pressure.

Acknowledgement

We are grateful to Professor Dr. Hackenthal for the determination of angiotensin II concentrations.

3 Epidemiology

3.1 Epidemiology of ICH in Europe

R. Lorenz, Giessen

If we are to speak about the epidemiology of intracerebral haemorrhage it means we must clarify the morbidity, mortality, distribution and age of this subgroup of cerebrovascular diseases (CVD). A number of difficulties exist in solving the inherent problems involved. CVD are not subjected to registration as infectious diseases are. So, in general, only national statistics of mortality are available, which can be compared on an international basis since the international classification of diagnosis (ICD of 1968) was introduced by the World Health Organization (WHO). The morbidity can be estimated only by analysing scientific literature. But as is well known, such data have to be handled carefully because they are based on certification of death where errors are often present and misinterpretations are possible.

The total mortality in West Germany (FRG) is between 0.9 and 1.2% yearly (Fig. 1), taking into consideration the data available between 1952 and 1971[1]. The number of deaths due to intracerebral haemorrhage and cerebrovascular diseases (ICD 430 – 436, 438) is between 10.8% and 13.3% (Fig. 2) of the total mortality, corresponding to a mortality rate of 131 – 150 per 100000 population. As compared with tumours of the central nervous system the corresponding rate per year is 1.6 and 3.0 per 100000 population (Fig. 3). Thus, the death rate from intracerebral haemorrhage and cerebrovascular diseases is around 100 times higher than that from neoplasms of the CNS. In respect to intracerebral haemorrhages only, one has to expect a mortality between 7087 and 7692, that is to say 0.9% – 1.0% of total mortality or nearly 12% of the group mortality (Table 1). Age-specific death rates show a strikingly accelerating rate with increasing age, the peak lies about the period from 65 to 80 years (Fig. 4). As regards the symptom of hypertension as a pathogenetic factor in intracerebral haemorrhage, one sees a significant preponderance of the subgroup of haematomas without hypertension (Fig. 5), but hypertension still figures as the one most important pathogenetic factor. It stands to reason that in the group of intracerebral haemorrhages, all cases with traumatic haematomas and haemorrhages originating from aneurysms and A-V malformations are excluded.

Unfortunately it was not possible for me to get similar exact data for all European countries. However, we are able to see the figures of Goldberg and Kurland (1972), cited by Kurtzke in 1976. Table 2 shows that the majority of countries have a mortality rate near 100 per 100000 with a variation between 48 (Belgium) and 153 (Finland). The FRG figures are high. The standardized death rate for the EEC (Fig. 6) was published by Garraway (1976), using WHO statistics of 1972. The quota of intracerebral haemorrhages ranges between 10% and 18% in the various countries.

Regarding the morbidity, one can only calculate crude rates. Considering the fact that in clinical studies the mortality rate lies between 80% and 85%, if conservatively treated, and between 24% – 50%, if operatively treated (Luyendijk 1972), one can estimate a morbidity rate of about 100 – 200 for Belgium and 300 – 600 for Finland per 100000 population.

---

1 Data kindly supplied by Statistisches Bundesamt, Wiesbaden, FRG

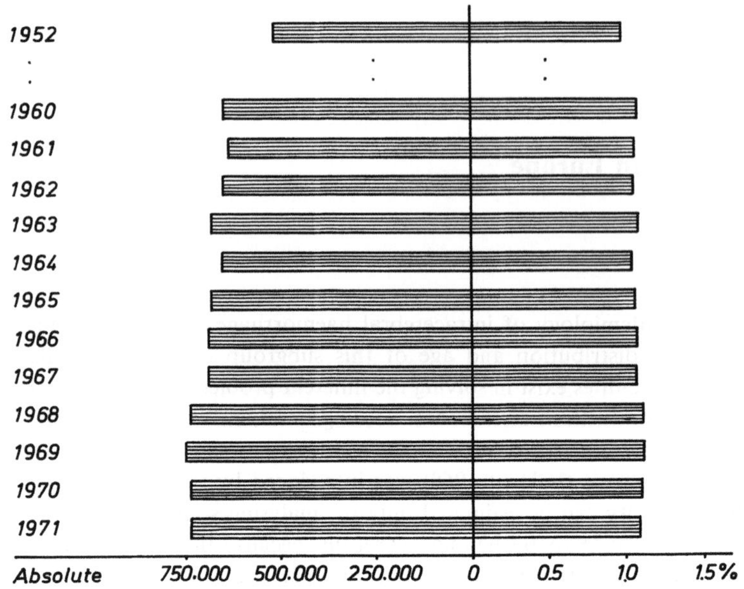

Fig. 1. Total mortality in West Germany

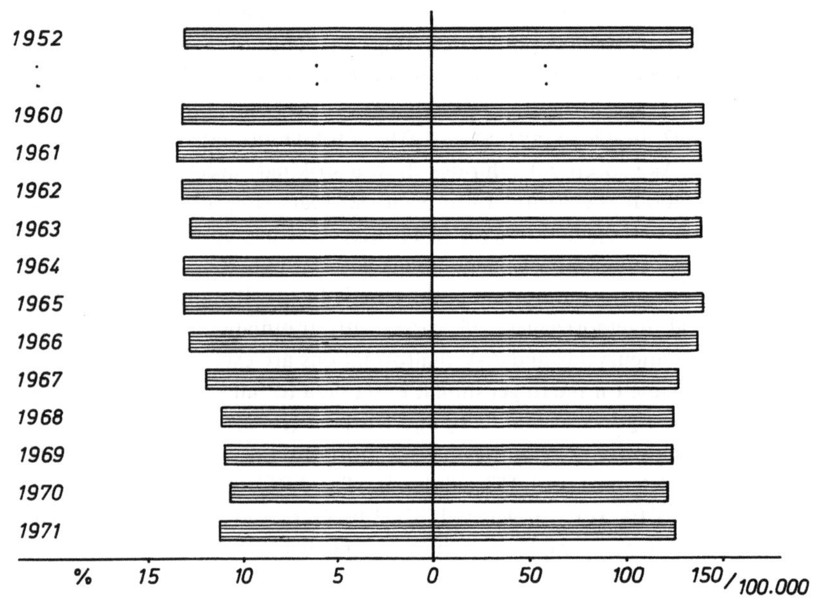

Fig. 2. Percentage of mortality and mortality rates per 100000 population due to intracerebral haemorrhage and cerebrovascular disease (ICD 430–436, 438) in West Germany

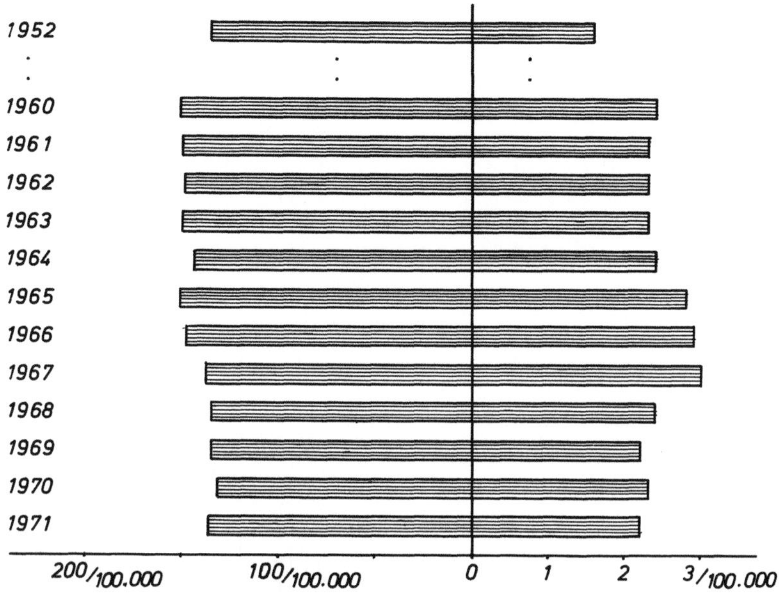

Fig. 3. Mortality rates per 100000 population due to intracerebral haemorrhage and cerebrovascular diseases (ICD 430 – 436, 438) compared with neoplasmas of the CNS (ICD 371)

Table 1. Mortality due to intracerebral haemorrhages (ICD 431) and its relation to total mortality

Year	Total ICH	% of Total Deaths
1969	7692	1.03
1970	7087	0.96
1971	7483	1.02

Thus, the morbidity and total mortality from intracerebral haemorrhage is much higher than published figures from neurological and neurosurgical units would suggest. For instance, in a given period of 25 years in our department 135 cases were treated. These considerations show the need for further careful work and are a challenge for co-operation between practioners and specialists in internal medicine, neurology, and neurosurgery.

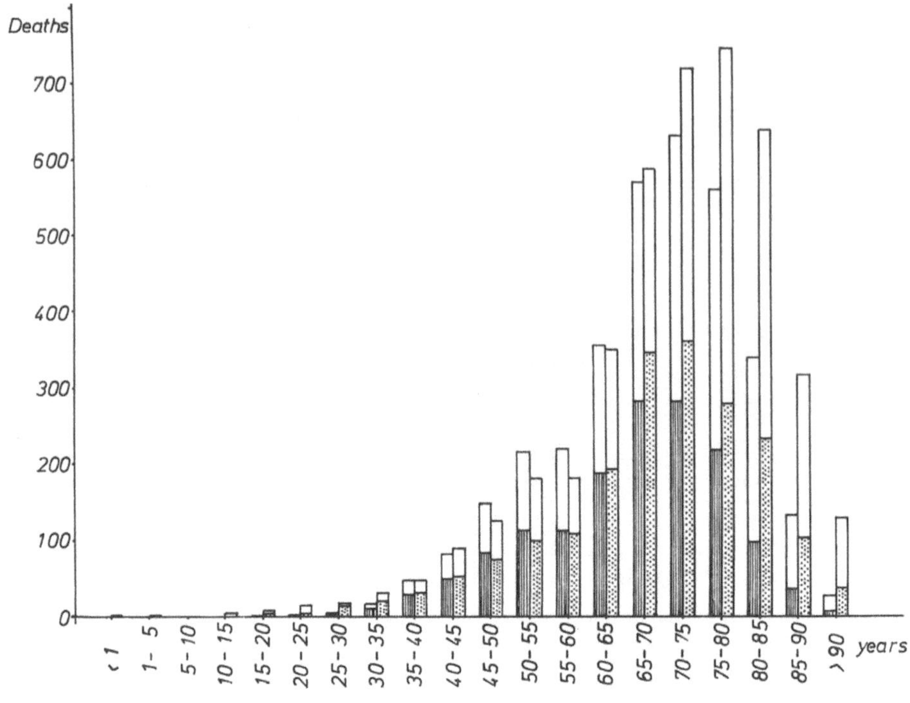

Fig. 4. Death rate due to intracerebral haemorrhage and their distribution according to sex and age. ▥ with (ICD 4310) and □ without (ICD 4319) hypertension. □ female rate

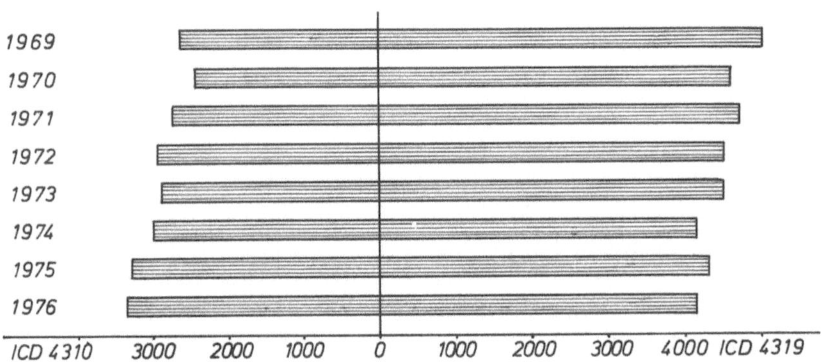

Fig. 5. Intracerebral haemorrhage with hypertension (ICD 4310) and without hypertension (ICD 4319)

Table 2. Mortality rate in various countries[a]

Country	Rate	Country	Rate
Norway	98	Italy	125
Sweden	104	Portugal	124
Finland	153	Israel (Jews)	115
Denmark	100	U.S. Africa (Whites)	101
Scotland	148	Iceland	106
England-Wales	116	Canada	97
Northern Ireland	123	United States (total)	100
Ireland	98	United States (Whites)	95
West Germany	142	United States (Non-whites)	165
France	99	Mexico	36
Belgium	48	Colombia	48
Netherlands	97	Uruguay	146
Switzerland	109	Chile	100
Austria	114	Australia	118
Czechoslovakia	86	New Zealand	102
Greece	75	Philippines	17
		Japan	209

[a] Cerebrovascular disease (CVD). Average annual age-adjusted (to U.S. 1950 population) mortality rates per 100000 population by country, mostly for 5 years within 1951 – 58 (Goldberg and Kurland 1972)

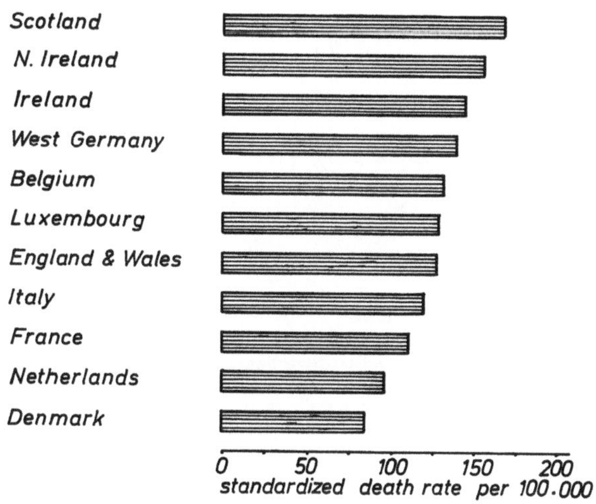

Fig. 6. Age-adjusted mortality from cerebrovascular disease in the EEC (C. M. Garraway 1976)

3.2 Epidemiology of Hypertensive ICH in Japan

H. Kanaya, Morioka

Diagnostic criteria for hypertensive intracerebral haemorrhage differ according to the researcher and have not been fixed. The author considered hypertensive intracerebral haemorrhage as a disease in a patient with a history of vascular hypertension before the stroke and with no cause of cerebrovascular diseases other than vascular hypertension. In Japan, the most common cause of death is cerebrovascular disease, the actual number of deaths from this source being 170000 annually. The high death rate among those afflicted with cerebrovascular disease is mainly due to hypertensive intracerebral haemorrhage and cerebral infarction. In this paper, the annual trends in death rate for hypertensive intracerebral haemorrhage in Japan are discussed and compared with the death rate from cerebral infarction (Vital Statistics; see references).

Death Rate for Cerebrovascular Diseases in Various Countries

These results were compared with the age-adjusted death rate based on the age structure of the Japanese population for 1970 using the World Health Statistics Annual 1970 and 1971 (Fig. 1). The death rate for cerebrovascular diseases per 100000 of the population in Japan is much higher than in other countries; it is more than double of that in Germany. The death rate for hypertensive intracerebral haemorrhage in Japan is also much higher than in other countries.

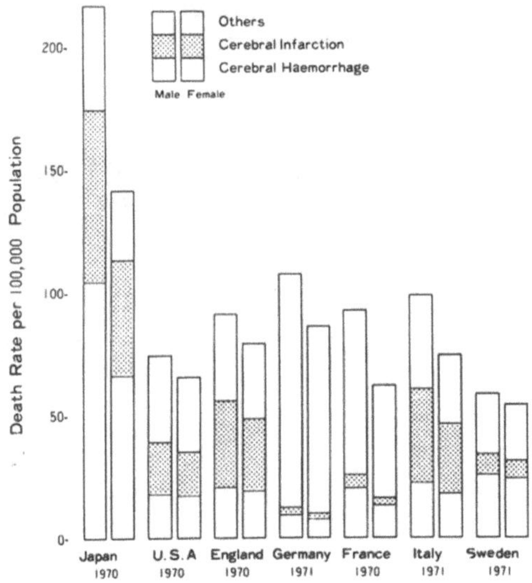

Fig. 1. Age adjusted death rate from cerebrovascular disease in some countries (per 100000 population)

Death Rate for Hypertensive Intracerebral Haemorrhage

Figure 2 shows the annual trends in cerebrovascular diseases in Japan from 1951 to 1976. These data were prepared on the basis of the population structure for 1965 using Vital Statistics in Japan. The death rate for cerebrovascular disease per 100000 of the population reached a maximum of 133.5 in 1965 and thereafter decreased sharply to 89.0 in 1976. The death rate for cerebral haemorrhage was 113.2 in 1951. It decreased sharply from 1965 and reached 33.3 in 1976. However, the death rate for cerebral infarction gradually increased and reached about the same level as that for cerebral haemorrhage in 1976.

The age-adjusted death rates by sex, for hypertensive intracerebral haemorrhage are shown in Fig. 3. In all years, males showed a higher death rate than females. There was no difference between males and females in the incidence of cerebral infarction.

Annual trends in the death rate from cerebral haemorrhage according to sex and age are shown in Fig. 4. In males, the death rate per 100000 of the population increased with age. Cerebral haemorrhage in those 50 years old or over decreased remarkably from 1968. The same decrease was also seen in females.

Death Rate for Hypertensive Intracerebral Haemorrhage in Autopsy Cases

The above-mentioned death rate for cerebrovascular diseases was prepared from doctors' death certificates which do not necessarily indicate the correct diagnosis. Therefore, annual trends in hypertensive intracerebral haemorrhage and cerebral infarction were investigated using the Annual of Pathological Autopsy Cases in Japan published by the Japanese Pathological Society. Figure 5 shows the frequency of cerebral haemorrhage and cerebral infarction cases among total autopsy cases from 1970 to 1975. This frequency was about 5% before 1973, but from 1973 it fell to about 3%.

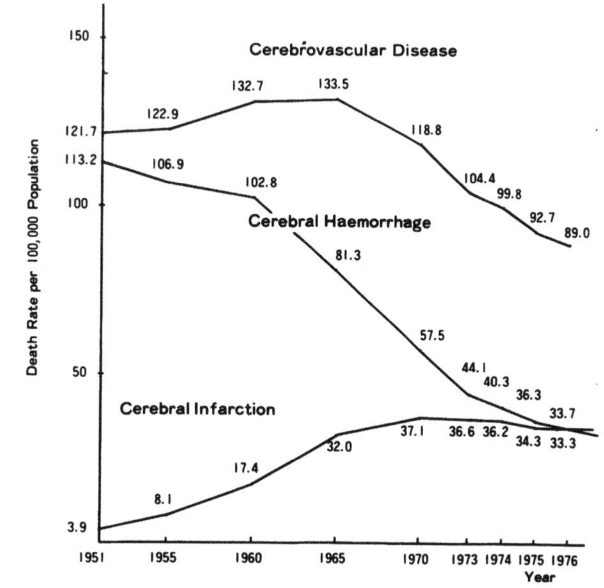

Fig. 2. Trends between 1951 and 1976 in age-adjusted death rate from cerebrovascular disease in Japan (per 100000 population)

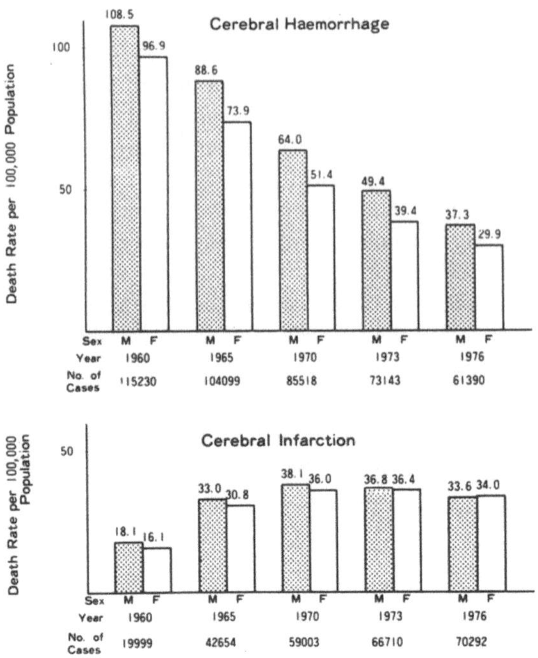

Fig. 3. Age-adjusted death rate from cerebral haemorrhage and cerebral infarction by sex in Japan (1960 – 1976) (per 100000 population)

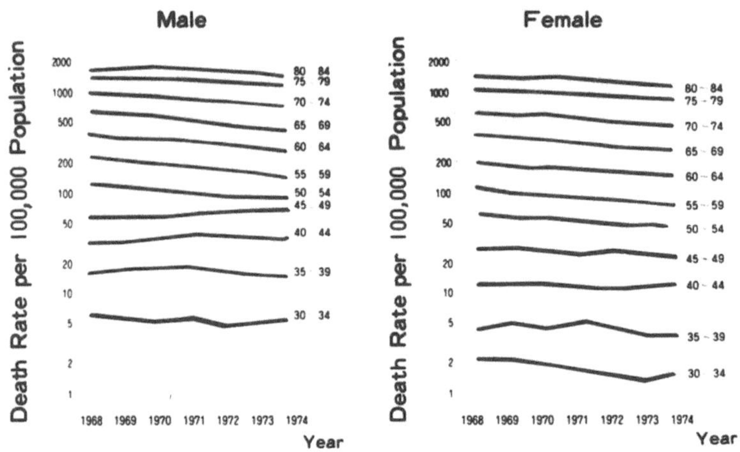

Fig. 4. Trends between 1968 and 1974 in death rate from cerebral haemorrhage by age and sex in Japan (per 100000 population)

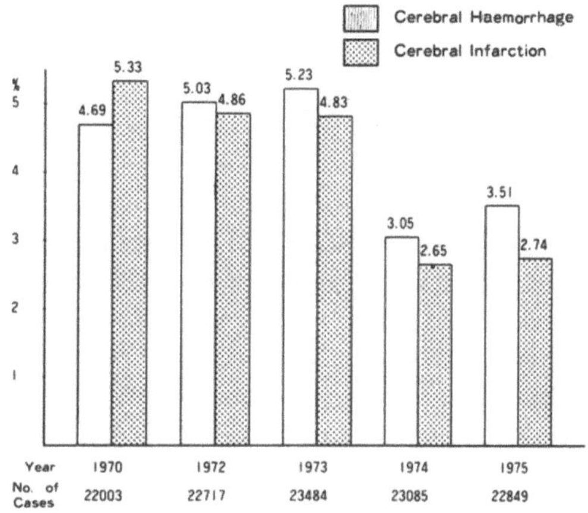

Fig. 5. Trends between 1970 and 1975 in frequency of cerebral haemorrhage and infarction in autopsy cases in Japan

Discussion

Recent conditions concerning cerebrovascular diseases in Japan have been described above. Cerebrovascular diseases have been decreasing every year and the age-adjusted death rate for cerebral haemorrhages was reduced by more than half in 1965. The main reason for this is the decrease in the death rate for cerebral haemorrhage in both men and women 50 years of age or over.

The reasons for the decrease in the death rate for hypertensive intracerebral haemorrhage since 1965 are not clear. The composition of the usual Japanese diet has changed fairly rapidly since World War II. As shown in Fig. 6, the increase in consumption of milk and milk products, meat and poultry, eggs, fat, oils and fruits is most remarkable, while consumption of rice is decreasing slowly. Takahashi (1978) reported that the traditional Japanese diet usually consisted of rice, miso soup made of bean paste, salted pickles and some fish or vegetables. These changes in the habitual diet may bear some relation to the morbidity of cerebrovascular diseases. Increase of cerebral infarction and decrease of cerebral haemorrhage seem to be related to the westernization of Japanese diet, as represented by an increase in consumption of meat, milk and eggs.

The cause for the decrease in hypertensive intracerebral haemorrhage in recent years in Japan is not clear, but it appears to be because preventive measures such as dietary improvements, blood pressure control and heating in cold regions have spread widely among Japanese in the last 10 years due to high economic growth.

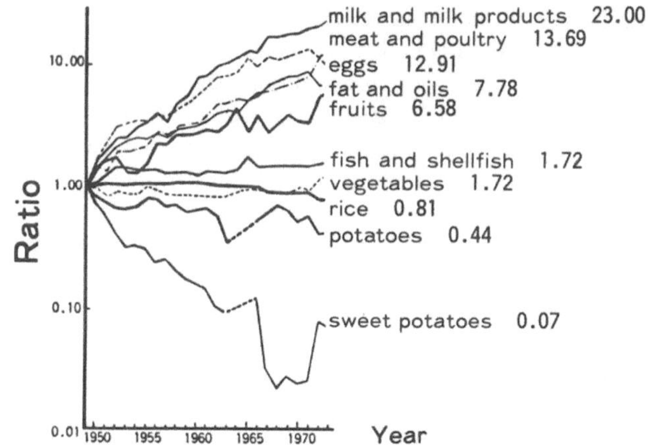

Fig. 6. Trends of food intake in Japanese people (1949 – 1973)

3.3 ICH and their Aetiology in India

R. D. Nagpal, Bombay

Epidemiology involves the study of the distribution of a disease in a population and the study of those factors which influence this distribution. It concerns variations in disease frequency related to such factors as time and place, and also the study of certain individual characteristics of those affected by the disease such as age, sex, race, socio-economic class and individual habits such as smoking and diet. No study has been done or is being done in India which tackles the epidemiology of spontaneous intracerebral haematomas, nor is there any form of national stroke registry. An attempt over the past 6 months to obtain this information, at least for the urban population, failed miserably. The questionnaire sent to the leading medical centres was either never returned or, when sent back, the figures were pitiably small. No information is available about the prevalence in the rural population which comprises 80% – 90% of India's population. In urban areas the problem is further compounded by a large floating population, making long-term follow-up futile and meaningless. Some information is available from an ongoing study of strokes in the young, under the auspices of the Indian Council of Medical Research. This information is shown in Table 1 (Dalal 1979). Haemorrhagic disease as the cause of stroke is seen to vary from 5.9% to 37.9%. These figures include intracerebral haemorrhages from aneurysms and arteriovenous malformations. It is not known how many of these were spontaneous intracerebral haematomas unrelated to arteriovenous malformations and aneurysms. The 102 patients under the age of 40 with a recent stroke, studied by Dalal 1979, showed an 8.8% incidence of spontaneous intracerebral haematomas. In southern India the incidence of stroke was determined as 56 per 100000 and 88 per 100000 in Vellore and Madras, respectively. These figures are very low when compared to the figures of 154 and 156 per 100000 for Carlisle, England and Rochester, Minnesota, United States, respectively. As already mentioned, even in these figures the incidence of spontaneous intracerebral haemorrhage is not separately available.

Faced with this problem of a paucity of information, I present data from 109 patients with spontaneous intracerebral haematomas treated at the Neurosurgical Department of the King Edward Memorial Hospital, Bombay, from 1957 to 1977. These 109 patients constitute 0.1% of total hospital admissions and 1.13% of the neurosurgical admissions over the same period (Table 2). Of these 109 patients, 66 had hypertension as the cause of haemorrhage, 2 had thrombocytopenia, 1 leukaemia and, in the remaining 40, the cause of the haemorrhage was unknown. Of the 109 patients, 74 were males and 39 were females, giving a male-to-female ratio of nearly 2:1. Concerning age distribution, the highest incidence was in the fifth and sixth decades, i.e. 30 and 28 cases, respectively (Fig. 1). Autopsies were performed in 48 of the 60 who died. The site of the haematoma in these 48 is shown in Fig. 2. In the remaining group of 61 patients which includes those still alive and those that died but where no autopsy was possible, the location of the haematoma was based on radiological and/or surgical findings (Table 3).

The mortality in the hypertensive group was high. Of this group, 45 patients (comprising 68.1%) died and the fate of another four is unknown.

More interesting is the group of 40 patients in whom the cause of haemorrhage could not be elucidated. In none of these was a possible causative factor such as hypertension, aneurysm, arteriovenous malformation, trauma or a bleeding disorder detected. The largest number of patients are seen to be in the third, fourth and sixth decades. The male-to-female ratio is 2:1, and 12 of these 40 patients died, with the greatest mortality being in the third and sixth decades.

Table 1. Incidence of acute cerebrovascular lesions in hospital populations in different urban areas of India[a]

Location	Authors	Year of study	Total	Ischaemic diseases		Miscellaneous	Haemorrhagic disease
				Cerebral thrombosis	Cerebral embolism		
Patiala	(Gupta et al. 1965)	1957–1960	260	185 (71.1%)	19 (7.3%)	31 (11.8%)	25 (9.6%)
Delhi	(Padmavati et al. 1963)	1954–1959	453	231 (50.9%)	29 (6.4%)	90 (20.7%)	103 (22.7%)
Agra	(Dube & Omar 1965)	1943–1962	480	374 (77.9%)	23 (4.8%)	9 (1.6%)	75 (15.6%)
Lucknow	(Misra et al. 1967)	1961–1965	454	339 (74.6%)	36 (7.9%)	16 (3.5%)	63 (13.6%)
Bombay	(Bharucha & Umerji 1962)	1959–1960	926	635 (68.3%)	20 (2.2%)	114 (12.3%)	157 (17.2%)
Bombay[b]	(Dalal et al. 1965, 1968)	1963 (7 months)	127	66 (52.1%)	26 (20.4%)	13 (10.2%)	22 (17.3%)
Hyderabad	(Naik et al. 1966)	1961–1963	866	640 (73.9%)	14 (1.6%)	52 (6.2%)	160 (18.5%)
Bangalore	(Krishna & Teja 1965)	1958–1964	189	79 (41.8%)	2 (1.0%)	88 (46.5%)	20 (10.6%)
Jamshedpur	(Khan & Rao 1951)	1947–1950	116	62 (53.4%)	6 (5.2%)	4 (33.4%)	44 (37.9%)
Vellore[b]	(Abraham & Daniel 1972)	1967–1972	850	607 (71.4%)[c]	48 (5.6%)	145 (17.1%)	50 (5.9%)

[a] In majority of retrospective studies the analysis is based on hospital records containing non-standardized information. Verification of diagnosis by angiography or necropsy is rarely possible

[b] Prospective studies

[c] 546 cerebral thrombosis, plus 61 internal carotid artery thrombosis

Table 2. Aetiology of intracerebral haemorrhage

Cause	No. of cases
Hypertensive	66
Non-hypertensive, unknown	40
Non-hypertensive, known	
Thrombocytopenia	2
Leukaemia	1
Total	109

Mortality rate of the ICH (A 85, i.e. ICD 430–438, WHO) per 1000 deaths

1968		1978		
Country	Total	Total	Male	Female
Austria	169.7	156.1	126.8	183.4
Belgium	94.7	132.0	109.6	156.6
Bulgaria	149.3	216.0	188.0	249.0
Czechoslovakia	103.7	161.5	133.7	192.7
Denmark	125.4	92.8	82.0	105.5
Finland	128.6	–	–	–
France	128.9	138.9	115.7	163.9
Germany (East)	–	63.7	52.4	73.2
Germany (West)	182.5	139.7	114.3	164.7
Great Britain	159.6	–		
England & Wales	–	126.1	95.8	156.5
Scotland	–	148.7	114.7	183.4
N. Ireland	–	143.4	110.8	179.4
Greece	95.3	165.8	133.4	200.5
Hungary	141.5	146.9	126.1	169.2
Iceland	80.1	107.2	90.3	129.5
Ireland	137.9	134.6	108.5	165.8
Italy	136.4	–	–	–
Luxembourg	174.5	116.2	103.8	130.5
Netherlands	93.3	108.1	87.3	134.6
Norway	156.3	142.0	116.7	172.3
Poland	35.9	–	–	–
Portugal	154.4	–	–	–
Romania	116.4	142.8	122.3	164.3
Spain	125.9	–	–	–
Sweden	128.1	108.6	88.5	133.0
Switzerland	119.7	120.0	97.6	145.2
Yugoslavia	65.8	108.2	93.3	124.3
Australia	117.8	140.7	102.7	188.4
New Zealand	106.3	128.8	94.4	170.8
South Africa	95.8	–	–	–
Canada	78.0	–	–	–
Chile	60.0	76.6	62.7	93.6
Colombia	29.6	56.9	47.2	68.3
Costa Rica	27.5	54.9	48.8	62.8
Dominican Republic	8.8	31.9	29.4	34.8
Ecuador	17.2	–	–	–
El Salvador	10.9	22.3	20.5	24.6
Guatemala	7.5	8.1	7.9	8.2
Honduras	–	24.5	22.6	26.8
Mexico	21.9	–	–	–
Nicaragua	17.9	–	–	–
Panama	46.4	–	–	–
Paraguay	24.6	69.2	63.1	75.9
United States	103.6	102.5	80.0	130.3
Uruguay	101.6	124.3	99.0	156.1
Venezuela	24.2	49.1	42.9	56.8
Egypt	–	5.5	6.2	4.7
Jordan	12.1	–	–	–
Syria	–	20.9	21.7	19.8
Kuwait	–	44.4	42.1	48.0
Israel	71.7	131.3	111.8	154.9
Iran	–	21.0	21.4	20.4

Table 4. Autopsy findings

Sex/age	
1. M/52	Haemorrhage 0.5 × 0.5 cm in the pons with left calcarine infarct
2. M/50	Right 7 × 5 × 4 cm haemorrhage in the basal ganglia. Temporal lobe herniation, pontine haemorrhage, calcarine infarct
3. M/30	Subarachnoid haemorrhage. Small punctate haemorrhages all over in connexion with small vessels. Subendocardial, mucosal and alveolar haemorrhages
4. F/28	Left ventricular hypertrophy + marked atherosclerosis. 8 × 6 × 5 cm haemorrhage in left putamen. Left cerebellar haemorrhage
5. M/55	Left parietal haematoma 5 × 4 × 4 cm. Partial skull autopsy only
6. M/14	Haemorrhage involving right putamen, g. pallidus and thalamus arterial or venous infarct
7. M/52	Severe atherosclerosis. 7 × 6 × 6 cm haematoma involving int. capsule, putamen, thalamus and ventricle, (R) calcarine infarction and brain stem haemorrhage
8. M/41	Right haemorrhage in basal ganglia with intraventricular spread. Massive cerebral oedema. No fracture
9. F/18	Right large haematoma destroying int. capsule and lenticular nuclei, intraventricular spread
10. M/38	Right internal capsular haemorrhage
11. M/22	Right external capsular clot, 10 × 8 × 6 cm, with secondary brain stem haemorrhage

Of the 12 who died, 10 were males and two were females. One of these 12 patients was discharged after evacuation of an intramedullary haematoma. He expired 3 months later at home, and thus no autopsy was possible. The autopsy material of the remaining 11 patients, initially classified as spontaneous intracerebral haemorrhage of unknown aetiology, was restudied carefully, and pertinent autopsy findings are given in Table 4. This re-examination showed a definitive cause overlooked at the earlier examination in six cases. Case 4 showed marked left ventricular hypertrophy and atherosclerosis, but had no hypertension when alive. Case 7 showed severe atherosclerosis of all the major cerebral vessels, again raising doubts about possible hypertension going undetected during his brief period in the hospital. Case 5 has to be excluded from the unknown category as only a partial skull autopsy was possible. In case 3, evidence of a bleeding diathesis was detected in the form of multiple haemorrhages in the subendocardium, intestinal mucosa and alveoli of the lungs. Case 6, after careful review of the slides, was diagnosed as a haemorrhagic infarct of venous or arterial origin. Case 8 may be said to have a traumatic clot, as there was history of a trivial fall. However, the clinical findings of a large head and advanced papilloedema spoke against a traumatic aetiology. In cases 1, 2, 9, 10 and 11, even this careful restudy failed to reveal the cause of haemorrhage.

It is this group of 40 patients, consisting mainly of those in their second and third decades, predominantly males without any detectable cause of haemorrhage, that has proved puzzling.

3.4 WHO Statistics of Mortality in ICH

J. Iizuka, Bonn

The following data were kindly supplied by the WHO Offices, Geneva.

It is obvious that these statistics must be cautiously interpreted because of the multiplicity of medical, social, political and administrative factors which influence the accumulation of data and differ from country to country.

Mortality rate of the ICH (A 85, i.e. ICD 430 – 438, WHO) per 1000 deaths

1968		1978		
Country	Total	Total	Male	Female
Austria	169.7	156.1	126.8	183.4
Belgium	94.7	132.0	109.6	156.6
Bulgaria	149.3	216.0	188.0	249.0
Czechoslovakia	103.7	161.5	133.7	192.7
Denmark	125.4	92.8	82.0	105.5
Finland	128.6	–	–	–
France	128.9	138.9	115.7	163.9
Germany (East)	–	63.7	52.4	73.2
Germany (West)	182.5	139.7	114.3	164.7
Great Britain	159.6	–		
England & Wales	–	126.1	95.8	156.5
Scotland	–	148.7	114.7	183.4
N. Ireland	–	143.4	110.8	179.4
Greece	95.3	165.8	133.4	200.5
Hungary	141.5	146.9	126.1	169.2
Iceland	80.1	107.2	90.3	129.5
Ireland	137.9	134.6	108.5	165.8
Italy	136.4	–	–	–
Luxembourg	174.5	116.2	103.8	130.5
Netherlands	93.3	108.1	87.3	134.6
Norway	156.3	142.0	116.7	172.3
Poland	35.9	–	–	–
Portugal	154.4	–	–	–
Romania	116.4	142.8	122.3	164.3
Spain	125.9	–	–	–
Sweden	128.1	108.6	88.5	133.0
Switzerland	119.7	120.0	97.6	145.2
Yugoslavia	65.8	108.2	93.3	124.3
Australia	117.8	140.7	102.7	188.4
New Zealand	106.3	128.8	94.4	170.8
South Africa	95.8	–	–	–
Canada	78.0	–	–	–
Chile	60.0	76.6	62.7	93.6
Colombia	29.6	56.9	47.2	68.3
Costa Rica	27.5	54.9	48.8	62.8
Dominican Republic	8.8	31.9	29.4	34.8
Ecuador	17.2	–	–	–
El Salvador	10.9	22.3	20.5	24.6
Guatemala	7.5	8.1	7.9	8.2
Honduras	–	24.5	22.6	26.8
Mexico	21.9	–	–	–
Nicaragua	17.9	–	–	–
Panama	46.4	–	–	–
Paraguay	24.6	69.2	63.1	75.9
United States	103.6	102.5	80.0	130.3
Uruguay	101.6	124.3	99.0	156.1
Venezuela	24.2	49.1	42.9	56.8
Egypt	–	5.5	6.2	4.7
Jordan	12.1	–	–	–
Syria	–	20.9	21.7	19.8
Kuwait	–	44.4	42.1	48.0
Israel	71.7	131.3	111.8	154.9
Iran	–	21.0	21.4	20.4

1968		1978		
Country	Total	Total	Male	Female
Ceylon	24.2	–	–	–
Thailand	4.5	10.5	11.5	9.2
Philippines	7.2	–	–	–
Formosa	64.9	–	–	–
Japan	171.9	247.1	235.6	260.5

4 Clinical Pathology

4.1 Cerebral Blood Flow in ICH (Is Outcome Determined by Irreversible Haemodynamic Factors?)

J. Overgaard, Odense

Introduction

Intracerebral haematoma exerts a complex influence on brain function. As a space-occupying lesion it may provoke intracranial pressure rises beyond the brain's autoregulatory capacity and by this effect alone reduce cerebral blood flow. As local perfusion pressure may vary and at least is unpredictable, regional cerebral blood flow is probably regulated by mechanisms which are even more difficult to define than the normal functional metabolic linkage (Kawakami et al. 1974; Sussman et al. 1974). In hypertensives the normal autoregulatory range of blood pressure variation is shifted to the right, i.e. the lower level of perfusion pressure compatible with the maintained cerebral blood flow has a higher value than in the normotensive (Skinhøj and Strandgaard 1973). In theory this effect of chronic elevated blood pressure would endanger such a patient's brain function more than normotensives with a proportionate spontaneous intracerebral haematoma.

In either condition an increased tissue perfusion should follow evacuation of the intracranial mass lesion if reduction of local tissue perfusion pressure plays the major role in flow depression. Prompt clinical improvement should result from surgery if blood pressure is not allowed to decrease. Other mechanisms may, however, be responsible as the beneficial effect of haematoma evacuation is often equivocal (McKissock et al. 1961).

Some of the problems encountered with these patients will be discussed in detail on the basis of haemodynamic investigations in a patient whose intracerebral haematoma was located in the left subcortical parietal region.

Case History

This 54-year-old woman had headache for some years and arterial hypertension, but was generally regarded as a neurotic. For 3 days she had intermittent hemiparaesthesia which was suddenly superseded by a right hemiplegia and aphasia. She was transferred to the neurosurgical department because the diagnosis of a middle cerebral artery occlusion was considered. On admission she was awake, but mental spontaneity was reduced and she could not talk. The visual fields suggested a right homonymous hemianopia. She had slight papilloedema and vascular changes compatible with hypertension, as well as a flaccid right-sided hemiplegia. Plantar reflexes bilateral extensive and blood pressure was 210/110 mm Hg.

Pre-Operative Haemodynamic Study

Under local analgesia a catheter was placed in the left internal carotid artery. A Seletz cannula was inserted into the frontal horn through a precoronal burr-hole, and a catheter was placed in the bulb of the jugular vein. Blood pressure and intracranial pressure were monitored through the respective catheters. Blood gases were analysed from samples obtained from the carotid and jugular vessels.

CBF was studied by the intracarotid Xenon-133 method (Lassen and Ingvar 1972). Washout was followed by 35 scintillation detectors placed over the left side of the head. Regional cerebral blood flow is presented as the rCBF init, and mean hemispheric flow is expressed as CBF init and CBF_{10}. Carotid angiograms and ventriculography were performed immediately after the study.

Results

The haemodynamic values obtained by the study are presented in Table 1. Flow was severely reduced despite maintained cerebral perfusion pressure in all runs. Evacuation of 15 ml ventricular fluid increased the perfusion pressure by 43% and CBF init by 39%, demonstrating impaired autoregulation. The corresponding regional flow changes are shown in Figs. 1 and 2 which reveal that all cortical areas are involved. The location of the haematoma is projected to the overlying cortical regions in Fig. 3. This area is not especially underperfused; the regional flows are well elevated over the hemispheric mean perfusion. The lowest regional flow values are located semicircular and anterior to the haematoma area. Mental effort increases flow in the haematoma area (Fig. 4). The oxygen uptake is low, but this is primarily because of low flow as the arteriovenous oxygen difference is only slightly reduced.

Operation

Immediately after this study the haematoma was evacuated. The approach was a craniotomy in the left parietal region. The dura was widely opened. The parietal cortex was pale, but only slightly protruding. Through a linear cortical incision the haematoma was found 2 cm under the cortex. It consisted of 100 ml of coagulated blood. It had dissected the white matter, almost reaching the ventricular ependyma.

Clinical Course

No dramatic improvement resulted from operation as she was still awake but mentaly inactive. Within the next week she could utter a few simple words in response to questions. The hemianopia and hemiplegia was unchanged. Systolic blood pressure was rather stable, i.e. 150 – 190 mm Hg. Drainage of ventricular fluid recovered about 400 ml/24 h. Intermittent ICP monitoring showed intraventricular pressure slightly elevated, i.e. 11 – 21 mm Hg. A control study was performed on the 7th postoperative day. At this time it was not possible to obtain blood samples from the internal jugular vein.

Postoperative Haemodynamic Study

This was conducted in exactly the same way as the pre-operative investigation. Autoregulation was assessed by induced elevation of the blood pressure. Mental activity was stimulated by the application of a painful stimulus to the right index finger. After the study a left carotid angiogram was done as well as a ventriculogram.

Table 1. Pre-operative haemodynamic study

	MABP	MIVP	CPP	$PaCO_2$	mhCBF init	$mhCBF_{10}$	$(A\text{-}V)O_2diff$	$CMRO_2$
Rest I	140	47	93	35	24.7 ± 3.9	25	6.90	1.73
Calculation	148	51	97	35	23.6 ± 4.3	27	7.05	1.90
Rest II	152	52	100	37	22.7 ± 3.4	23	6.57	1.51
Evacuation of 15 ml CSF (immediate)	150	7	143	38	34.8 ± 5.7	32	5.66	1.79
Evacuation of 15 ml CSF (19 min)	142	11	131	35	33.3 ± 5.5	32	5.86	1.87
Healthy controls				39	65.2 ± 9.8	55		
Units	MABP, MIVP, CPP: mmHg. $CMRO_2$: ml/100 g/min.			$PaCO_2$: torr.	$(A\text{-}V)O_2$diff.: (Sat. AO_2-Sat. VO_2) × 1.39 × Hb/100			

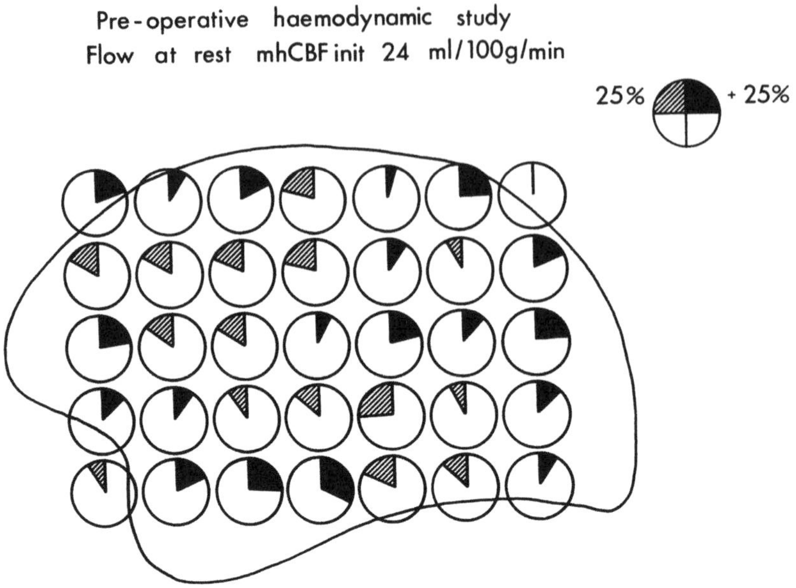

Fig. 1. Regional distribution of CBF init. A regional flow 25% above hemispheric mean (24) equals 30 ml/100 g/min. A regional flow 25% lower than hemispheric mean equals 18 ml/100 mg/min

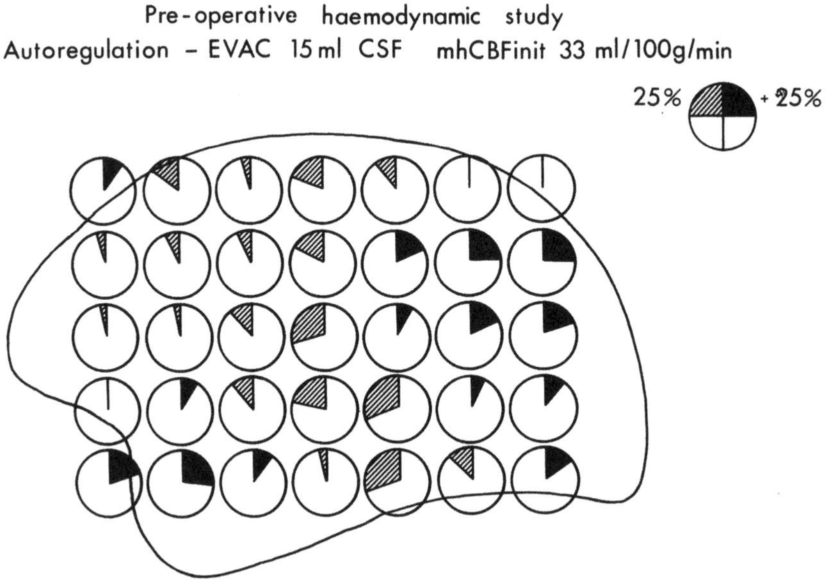

Fig. 2. Regional distribution of CBF init. A regional flow 25% above hemispheric mean (33) equals 41 ml/100 g/min. A regional flow 25% lower than hemispheric mean equals 25 ml/100 g/min

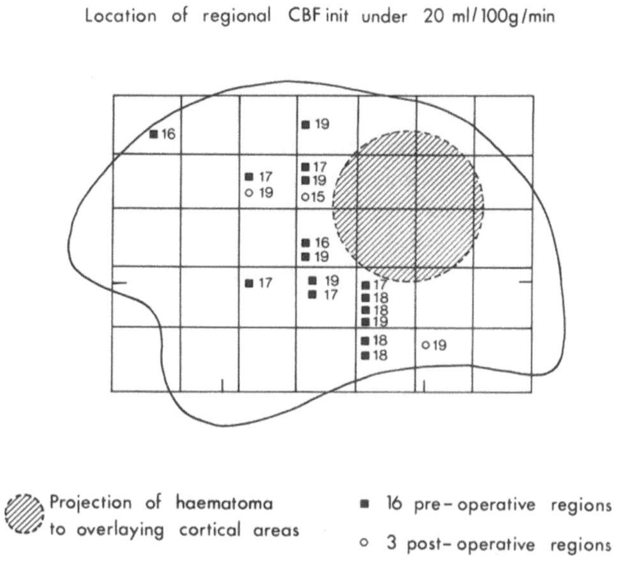

Fig. 3. The 16 pre-operative flow values were located in nine regions. Evacuation of 15 ml CSF increased regional flow to over 20 ml/100 g/min in seven of the nine regions. Only in two regions did flow then exceed 30 ml/100 g/min. The postoperative study disclosed that only three of the nine regions had a flow over 30 ml/100 g/min 1 week after haematoma evacuation

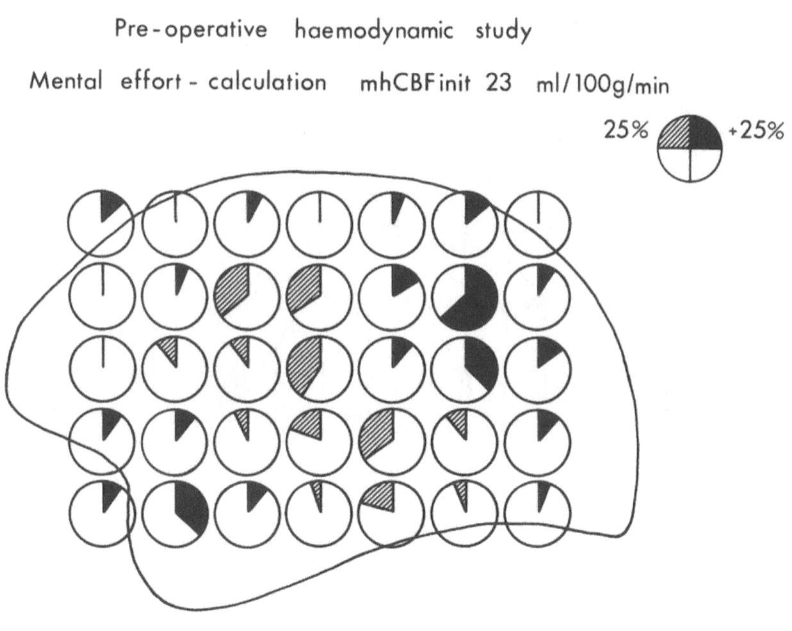

Fig. 4. The mental effort consisted in looking upon a tabula with simple arithmetic problems. As the patient could not speak it is not known if the patient did solve the problems. Regional flow was however redistributed in favour of the parietal cortex. A regional flow 25% above hemispheric mean (23) equals 29 ml/100 g/min. A regional flow 25% under hemispheric mean equals 17 ml/100 g/min

Results

The basic haemodynamic values are shown in Table 2. Mean hemispheric blood flow was very close to the pre-operative values. There was no regional hyperaemia. During the autoregulation test the perfusion pressure increased 35% and the mean hemispheric CBF increased 14%, which indicates a slightly impaired vasomotor adaptation to pressure changes. The regional flow distribution is presented in Figs. 5 and 6. The carotid angiogram showed normal arterial pattern, but the vessel diameter was very narrow throughout. The ventriculogram revealed moderately dilated ventricles, and pre-operative shifts had disappeared.

Table 2. Postoperative haemodynamic study

	MABP	MIVP	CPP	$PaCO_2$	mhCBF init	$mhCBF_{10}$
Rest	94	14	80	36	26.9 ± 3.8	29
Induced arterial hypertension	122	14	108	35	30.6 ± 4.4	31
Stimulation with pain	98	14	84	35	24.6 ± 3.6	29

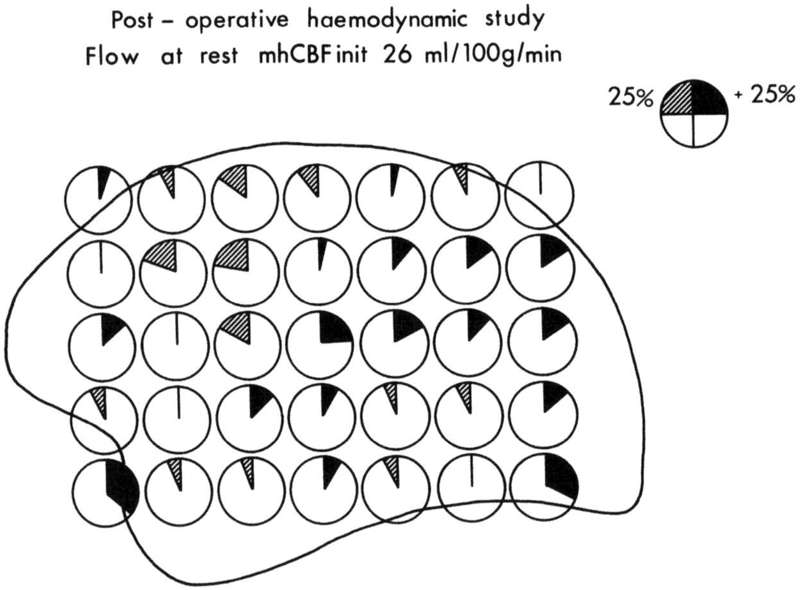

Fig. 5. Postoperative study at day 7. Regional distribution is still in favour of the parieto-temporal regions. A regional flow value over 25% of the hemispheric mean (26) equals 32 ml/100 g/min. A regional flow 25% under the hemispheric mean equals 20 ml/100 g/min

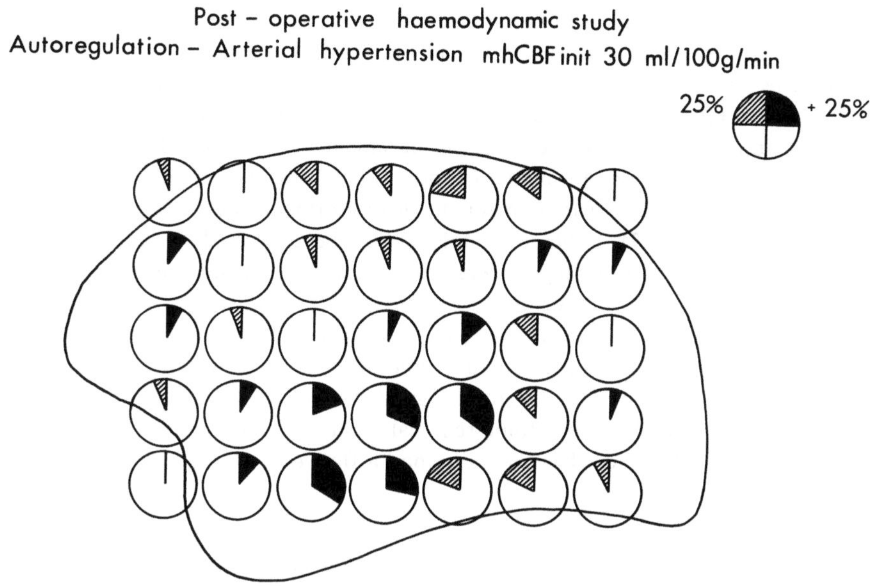

Fig. 6. Postoperative study at day 7. Autoregulation is especially impaired in the temporal lobe area (compare with Fig. 5). A regional flow 25% above the hemispheric mean (30) equals 37 ml/100 g/min. A regional flow 25% under hemispheric mean equals 23 ml/100 g/min

Discussion

Spontaneous intracerebral haematoma is followed by a reduction of hemispheric cerebral blood flow regardless of the location of the haematoma – deep, central or lateral, subcortical. The blood flow reduction is not correlated to the timing of investigation after the haemorrhage. The mean hemispheric blood flow is, however, related to the level of consciousness and inversely related to the size of the haematoma, as revealed on angiograms (Jaffe et al. 1970; Paulson 1971; Kawakami et al. 1974). Mean flow is often reduced to levels around 25 – 30 ml/100 g/min in comatose patients and 35 – 40 ml/100 g/min in awake patients. Hyperaemic areas located to the clinically relevant region or remote from it seem to occur in less than half of the studied hemispheres (Jaffe et al. 1970; Kawakami et al. 1974).

It has been suggested but not proven that "transhemispheric depression", or diaschisis, constitutes a part of the haemodynamic consequence following intracerebral haematoma (Skinhøy 1965; Slater et al. 1977). Flow-reduction in the contralateral hamisphere is not a peak phenomenon occurring in the first few hours after onset, but is "a process that increases during the first week" (Slater et al. 1977). If these results obtained in stroke patients with cerebral infarcts are valid for developments in cerebral haematoma also, delay in operating would exert an unfavourable influence upon the clinical outcome.

An analysis of this study of regional cerebral blood flow in a patient with a 100-ml intracerebral haematoma in the left parietal region confirms the experiences quoted. It is surprising, however, that ipsilateral flow values were so low. Although autoregulation was impaired, the effect of increased perfusion pressure was only slight, and regional flow never reached the normal range. The multidetector system disclosed that the distribution of regional flow was inverted; flow especially in the frontal areas was more reduced than in the parietal cortex.

This severely pathological flow pattern was not explained by an effect of high intracranial pressure as it persisted after the ICP had been reduced (Fig. 2). The frontal lobe may be regarded as remote to the location of the haematoma. It is well known that regional hyperaemia does occur in remote areas. In clinical studies this finding has been regarded as an effect of increased intracranial pressure causing displacement of the brain (Eudo, Larsen and Lassen 1977). Neither hyperaemia nor increased intracranial pressure were present after evacuation of CSF. A haemodynamic explanation for the inverted flow contours (Fieschi et al. 1968, Ingvar 1976; Eudo et al. 1977) is therefore not likely. The depressed frontal lobe flow may have another cause and it is perhaps relevant to regard the phenomenon as a consequence of insufficient information – transmission failure or diaschisis within the diseased hemisphere.

The calculated flow values were low, but only a few regions had a perfusion under 20 ml/100 g/min. Before CSF evacuation they amounted to 15% which decreased to 1.5% after evacuation. In both situations the total flow distribution is far away from the dispersion in healthy controls (Fig. 7). Haematoma removal was not as effective as CSF evacuation because the 7th-day study disclosed that no region had a flow over 39 ml/100 g/min.

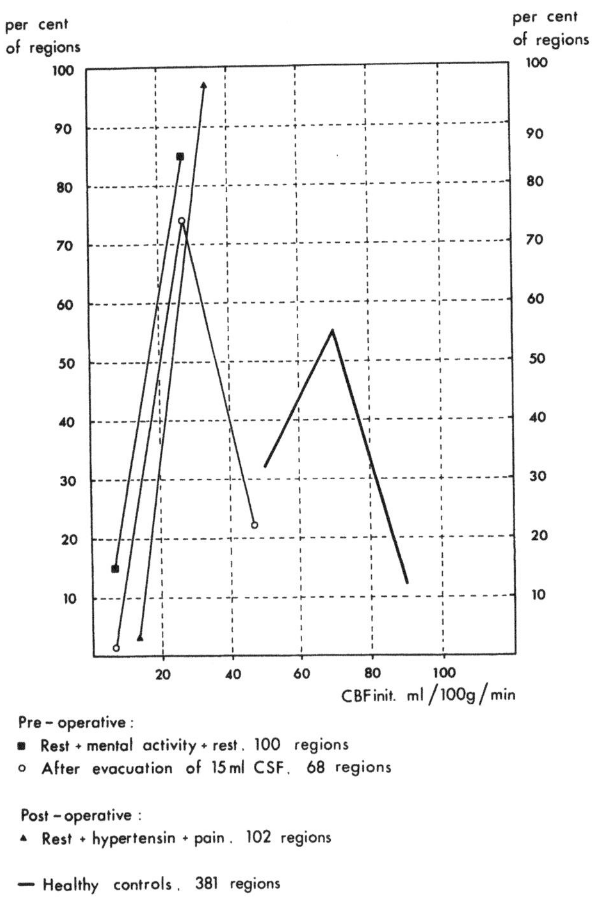

Fig. 7. Simplified histogram constructed as follows: All the pre- and postoperative regional flow values were-assigned to classes of flow intervals: 0 – 19, 20 – 39, 40 – 59, 60 – 79, 80 – 99 and 100 – 119 ml/100 g/min. (*X-axis*). The relative incidence of flow classes is expressed as percentage (*Y-axis*). The control values were obtained from studies of 9 healthy persons

Improvement of clinical deficits did not result from evacuation of CSF or haematoma. The explanation for this disappointing effect of treatment may be related to the occurrence of regional ischaemia. The concept of ischaemia has within the last few years been elucidated by experimental studies. Failing tissue perfusion with regard to functional demands may be called functional ischaemia. The exact flow values or a threshold below which demands exceeds supply is not known for the human brain. Extrapolating from the normal flow distribution it may be suggested that a regional flow lower than 40 ml/100 g/min will not allow undisturbed function in conscious man (see Fig. 7).

Electro-encephalographic homeostasis is disturbed when flow is reduced to 20 – 16 ml/100 g/min (Boysen 1973). In animal experiments it has been shown that evoked cortical electrical responses were undisturbed as long as cortical perfusion was kept between 20 and 12 ml/100 g/min. A 50% reduction of the response occurred at a cortical flow of 16 ml/100 g/min. It may be suggested that this failure of transmission of signals may constitute the basis for the diaschisis phenomenon (Branston et al. 1974).

At this level of tissue perfusion morphology is still intact. The first step in disintegration may be connected with the release of potassium, which was found to occur when local flow falls between 11 and 7 ml/100 g/min (Astrup et al. 1977). If these flow values are maintained for 2 – 3 h it has been shown that microscopic infarction develops (Morawetz et al. 1979). Local flow of that magnitude is probably always associated with clinical deficits, but is not invariably permanent, as reversal of hemiplegia in animals has been observed when the duration of these low perfusion rates was less than 60 min. It was also disclosed that there was no difference in the vulnerability of white and grey matter to ischaemia (Morawetz et al. 1979).

Analysing the experimental findings it is clear that some of the details obtained in the presented case study are features that perhaps explain the bad prognosis. First a total of 16 regions had flow values lower than 20 ml/100 g/min. A few were close to the threshold values for information transmission failure (Fig. 3), and these regions were located in a ring-shaped zone outside and anterior to the haematoma area. It may be assumed that flow at that low level had persisted for many hours, leading to disturbances of the thalamocortical transmission lines. In turn, the reduced information reduced function and metabolism, which especially affected the frontal lobe regions. As coupling of function and metabolism still worked, the perfusion of those areas was regulated down to basal metabolic demands. Evacuation of CSF was not followed by a substantial improvement in flow distribution nor of clinical deficits. In the "ischaemic" ring-shaped zone only two regions out of nine increased the flow above 30 ml/100 g/min. At the postoperative study one week later no further flow increase had occurred. The clinical experience of reversing severe neurological deficits by induced elevation of perfusion pressure could not be repeated in this patient (Symon 1978).

It is tempting to suggest that functional prognosis is determined primarily by the presence of flow lower than 20 ml/100 g/min in a few – or perhaps only one – cortical regions! This condition may be tolerated within a time scale of less than 1 h. If regional flow is kept above that level functional prognosis should improve.

Clinical Conclusion

As a guideline for surgery on intracerebral haematomas located within the telencephalic subcortical white matter physiological investigations support the hypothesis that haematoma evacuation should follow within 60 min to secure optimal outcome. When this interval cannot be observed the lesion may induce a severe depression of hemispheric or global brain function, which persists in spite of haematoma evacuation. Therapeutic measures have hitherto not been recommended for this secondary effect on intracerebral haematoma.

4.2 Intracranial Pressure in ICH

J. W. F. Beks, Groningen

One of the early attempts to give an explanation of intracranial dynamics was embodied in the Monro-Kellie doctrine. The core of this doctrine is still valid, i.e. that the total volume of the intracranial content is constant, but their conclusion, i.e. that the volume of the different components could not change, is wrong. Obviously they could not appreciate that there is a free communication between the vascular bed of the brain and the extracranial veins, and they obviously did not know about the CSF, which is rather surprising, considering that Monro's father discovered the foramen which bears his name (Lundberg 1975).

The ability of the intracranial blood and the CSF to pass out of and into the cranial cavity, is the main mechanism responsible for what we now call "spatial compensation" (Langfitt 1969), a process in which the blood passes out into the sinuses mainly through the bridging veins.

Clinical and experimental data suggest that swelling of the brain may cause obstruction of these extracranial veins and, consequently, congestion and further swelling of the brain tissue. This mechanism is supposed to be involved in the production of acute increases in intracranial pressure (ICP).

The CSF may be displaced from the cranial cavity in two ways. Increments of the intracranial contents can be rapidly compensated for by displacement of CSF into the spinal subarachnoid space, provided that there is an open communication between the cranial and spinal compartments. A slower compensation can be achieved by ordinary CSF absorption, which is directly correlated to ICP.

The capacity for spatial compensation will be reduced if any of these pathways is blocked, e.g. by blood in the subarachnoid space. Any intracranial expanding lesion, whether it is a tumour or abscess, a haematoma or a swollen infarct, will produce a distortion or a shift of the brain. This shift leads in turn to secondary, vascular sequelae in other vital structures.

Deformity may develop very quickly in association with a rapidly expanding lesion, but it tends to be maximal when the lesion is expanding very slowly (Miller and Adams 1972).

As shift and distortion contribute to the spatial compensation, they can occur in the absence of any significantly raised ICP. The pattern of inevitable deformity depends not only on the rate of enlargement, but also on the site of the expanding lesion. As the lesion expands, so also does the hemisphere. The surface of the brain is pressed against the unyielding dura, gyri are flattened, sulci are narrowed and CSF is displaced from the subarachnoid space. The lateral ventricle on the side of the lesion and the third ventricle become reduced in size, and there is a lateral shift of the midline structures, away from the lesion. The next stage is the development of internal herniation, viz. displacement of brain tissue from one intracranial compartment to another. The morphology, pathogenesis and clinical aspects of brain stem herniation were discussed by Pia (1956).

If the volume-pressure relationship is one of the cornerstones in intracranial dynamics, the interrelation between the cerebral blood flow and ICP is an other one. I would like to stress the reciprocal character of this interrelation. On the one hand, variations of the vasomotor tone of the cerebral resistance vessels may cause variations of the ICP by letting in more or less of the systemic arterial blood pressure into distensible vessels of the cerebral vascular bed.

On the other hand, variations of ICP may cause changes of the cerebral perfusion pressure and cerebral blood flow. Consequently, a rise in ICP may elicit an auto-regulation response i.e. a reduction of peripheral resistance by dilatation of the cerebral vessels, which may cause a further rise in ICP and so on. If the intracranial buffering capacity is compromised, this chain reaction is likely to cause rapid elevation of the ICP (Miller and Adams 1972). However, the pressure-volume relationship and the interplay between the ICP and the dynamics of the intracranial blood and CSF are of particular importance for the understanding of certain phenomena in cerebro-vascular accidents.

Increased ICP is common as a result of intracerebral haemorrhage which produces a space-occupying mass with its resultant reactive brain swelling, sometimes aggravated by ventricular obstruction. However, it was only when continuous recording of the ICP was introduced into clinical practice by P. Janny and later by N. Lundberg, that it became possible to study in detail the ICP variations in cerebro-vascular accidents and to evaluate their clinical significance. As far as I know, apart from the reports of Janny (1976, 1978) no studies on the ICP in cerebral haemorrhage have been published. Our series includes 21 consecutive cases of massive "spontaneous" intracerebral haematoma. The patients are classified in four groups according to their neurological condition, using the classification of Van den Ark and Kahn (1968):

	Number
Group 1: Neurologically normal	1
Group 2: Focal neurological signs	5
Group 3: Dulled conscious response and localized neurological signs	7
Group 4: Comatose	8
	21

The haematomas originated from:

1) Angiomas	5
2) Aneurysms	4
3) Hypertension and arteriosclerosis	8
4) Tumours	4
	21

The correlation between the neurological status and the cause of the haemorrhage was:

	Angiomas	Aneurysms	Hypertension	Tumours
Group 1	–	–	–	1
Group 2	3	–	2	0
Group 3	1	2	3	1
Group 4	1	2	3	2
	5	4	8	4

In these cases we used an epidural pressure transducer for continuous monitoring. In the majority of the cases (15) we saw an increased ICP (above 20 mmHg) in the first 24 h.

	Number	ICP	Died
Group 1	1	1	0
Group 2	5	2	0
Group 3	7	6	3
Group 4	8	6	6
	21	15	9

Patients in group 4, who were in a very bad clinical condition, had an increased ICP, i.e. over 60 mmHg. In none of these patients was there any reaction of the intracranial pressure to intravenous osmotic diuretics. All these patients died. In patients in a better clinical condition, the ICP decreased gradually in the first 4–5 days after the ictus. All the different causes of intracranial haemorrhage were associated with increased ICP.

	Number	Increased ICP	Died
Angiomas	5	1	0
Aneurysms	4	3	1
Hypertension	8	7	6
Tumours	4	4	2
	21	15	9

The location of the haemorrhage was

	Frontal	Temporal	Capsular	Parieto-occipital
Angiomas	2	2	–	1
Aneurysms	2	2	–	–
Hypertension	–	2	6	–
Tumours	2	1	–	1
	6	7	6	2

Like Ransohoff et al. (1970), we had very consistent indications for operation. The following categories were considered unsuitable for surgical treatment:

1) Patients who had symptoms of severe secondary brain stem compression.
2) Patients who had rapid progressive deterioration.
3) Patients who stabilized on a non-surgical regime.

It is our opinion that one should try, by all means, to reduce the increased intracranial pressure, to prevent further brain damage and to decide whether the patient's clinical condition is due to a severe destructive or irreversible lesion rather than to pure cerebral compression. The risk of a rebleed, after lowering the ICP, should be accepted.

4.2.1 Discussion

J. Zierski (Giessen): The number of ICP measurements among our patients with lobar haematomas is too small to permit definite conclusions, but our recent observations suggest that they are of considerable value for detection of rebleeding, particularly in patients with temporal haematomas who run the highest risk of decompensation. The situation of these patients is similar to those with traumatic temporal lobe contusion. Some of them will recover without operation, but others will require it. ICP measurement will help to differentiate between these two groups of patients. Parietal and occipital lobe haematomas do not usually require ICP monitoring.

Case report

A 45-year-old patient with spontaneous intracerebral haematoma became decerebrate during CT examination (Fig. 1). He was immediately operated on, the haematoma was removed and

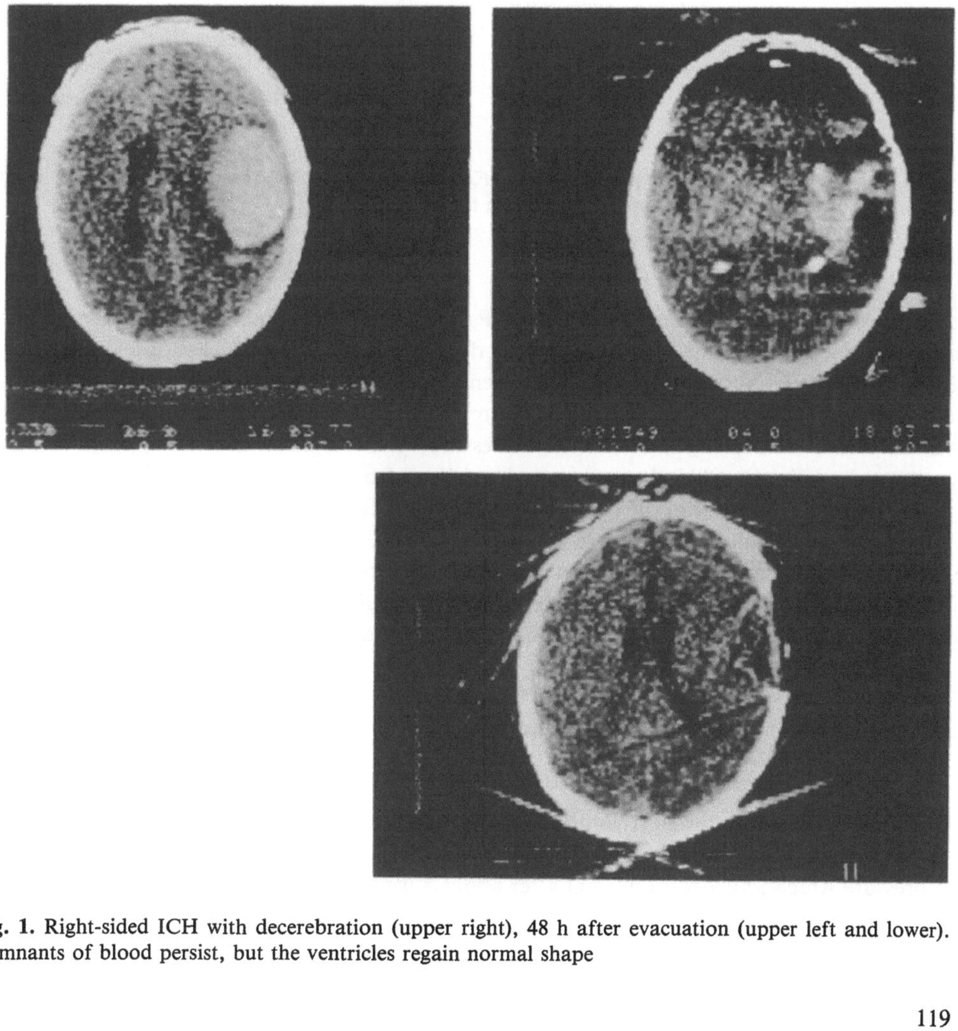

Fig. 1. Right-sided ICH with decerebration (upper right), 48 h after evacuation (upper left and lower). Remnants of blood persist, but the ventricles regain normal shape

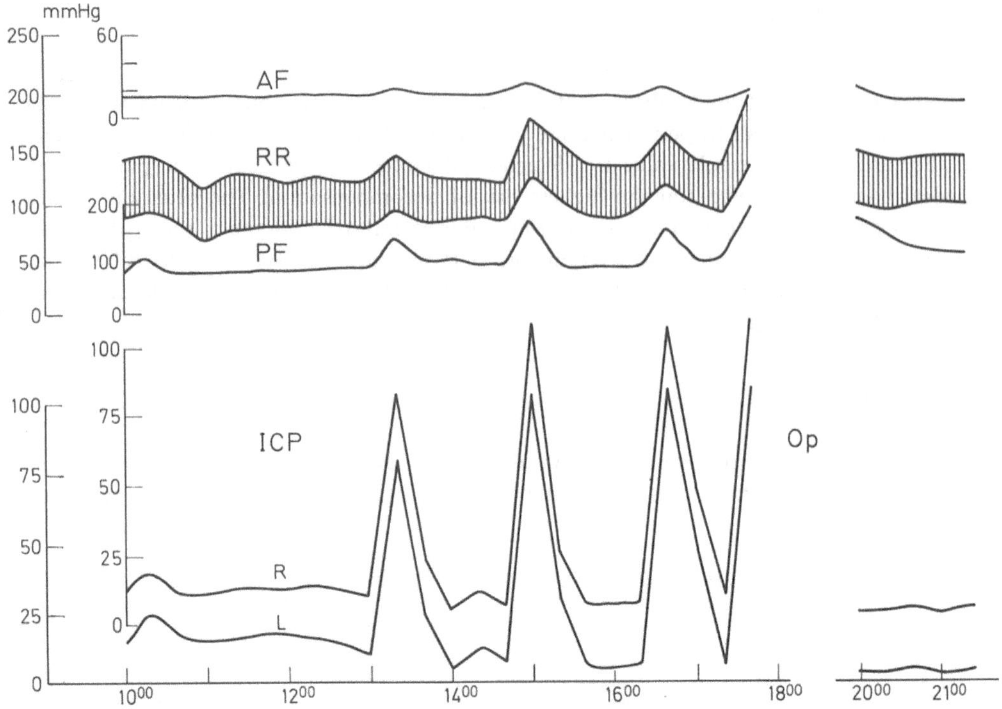

Fig. 2. Pressure tracing at the time of rebleeding. *AF,* respiratory rate; *RR,* blood pressure; *PF,* heart rate; *ICP,* mean intracranial pressure on the left and on the right side

bilateral subdural ICP measured (Phillips ICP Transducer). Decerebrate rigidity ceased a few hours after operation and in the following days his ICP remained slightly elevated up to 15 – 17 mmHg without pathological waves. Ten days later bleeding recurred. The curve (Fig. 2) shows the tracing of ICP, on R and L sides, respiration rate, blood pressure and pulse rate at the moment of rebleeding. The first high pressure wave was accompanied by a synchronous increase of respiration, blood pressure and pulse, and by transient slight dilatation of the R pupil, without any change in the level of consciousness. The ICP returned to the previous level. After the second high pressure wave the patient became more drowsy and with the third, he suddenly became comatose. Fresh haematoma was found and the bleeding vessel clipped. Postoperatively the pressure returned to normal. The patient made a very slow recovery, but unfortunately died 1 month later from pulmonary embolism.

Question: In cases in which the extremely high ICP does not responding to therapy, why didn't you try to lower pressure by evacuation of the clot?

J. Beks, Groningen:
Janny (1978) stated that even if you remove the clot, the pressure after the operation becomes elevated again. There was only a slight difference in the course, and our patients had an increase of pressure which returned to normal after about 3 weeks.

4.3 Sequential Changes in Tissue Surrounding ICH

J. Suzuki and T. Ebina, Sendai

Introduction

When haematomas form after an intracerebral haemorrhage, there is transient, physical injury to the brain due to the mass of the haematoma itself, and this determines the degree of consequent cerebral deficit. However, progressive injury to normal brain tissue surrounding the haematoma can also be brought about at the same time by secondary changes, such as brain oedema, degeneration and necrosis, which can often be seen at the time of extirpation of an intracerebral haematoma if some time has elapsed since the haemorrhage. Consequently, such secondary brain injury can be avoided by extirpating the haematoma before secondary changes in the tissue surrounding the haematoma have occurred. For lateral-type hypertensive intracerebral haematomas, we have been advocating early operation in which a trans-Sylvian approach is used for early removal of the haematoma. We have had good results with both mortality and morbidity (Suzuki and Sato 1972, 1976).

However, there have been few reports concerned with when and how the changes in the tissue surrounding the haematoma occur in the acute stage after intracerebral haemorrhage. To understand such changes, we have made continuous observations of the histological changes in the tissue surrounding haematomas, by using stereotactic operations to produce a haematoma in the lateral internal capsule of adult dogs.

Furthermore, to determine whether the changes in the tissue surrounding the haematoma are caused by the physical pressure of the haematoma or by factors within the haematoma itself, oil-wax has been injected into the same site as the haematoma and a comparative study made of the subsequent changes in the oil-wax and haematoma cases.

Experimental Method

Production of the Putaminal-type Intracerebral Haematoma and Preparation of the Specimen

Twenty-five adult, mongrel dogs weighing 7 – 13 kg were used. They were anaesthetized with pentobarbital and placed in the apparatus for stereotactic operations. A 0.4-mm diameter needle was placed from above into the lateral region of the internal capsule, 30 mm anterior, 13 mm lateral and 13 mm rostral to the midpoint of the line connecting the external auditory canals. Autologous blood (2 ml) was injected using the body blood pressure of the femoral artery, thereby producing a putaminal-type intracerebral haematoma. At various intervals after production of the haematoma the dogs were killed by an injection of calcium chloride (two dogs at 30 min, two at 3 h, three at 6 h, two at 12 h, three at 18 h, six at 24 h, three at 30 h, two at 36 h and two at 48 h). The brain was immediately excised and fixed in 10% formalin solution. Despite the fact that equal volumes of blood had been injected into the same site, it was seen after fixation that the haematomas were not always uniform, because of the secondary effects of the blood injection. There were some large haematomas, and some haematomas were located outside the lateral internal capsule. In these experiments, only those brains were used which had haematomas of roughly uniform size, located in the lateral portion of the internal capsule.

Histological samples were obtained from one dog each at 30 min and 3, 6, 12, 18, 24, 30, 36I and 48 h by making a frontal section passing through the chiasmal region and staining with haematoxylin-eosin and elastica-Masson. Histological investigations were made in each sample on the tissue surrounding the haematoma to assess the progressive changes.

Injection of Oil-Wax into the Lateral Portion of the Internal Capsule in Dogs and Preparation of Specimens

A 50% fixative paraffin and 50% olive oil mixture was heated and dissolved and cooled to normal temperature. In a mixture of oil and wax in these proportions the material can pass through a 0.4-mm diameter needle at around 35 °C, but solidifies at around 20 °C.

Fifteen adult mongrel dogs weighing 7 – 15 kg were used. They were anaesthetized with pentobarbitol and placed in the apparatus for stereotactic operation. An injection needle (0.4-mm diameter) which had been warmed to 40 °C was inserted into the lateral region of the internal capsule. Liquid oil-wax (2 ml) warmed to 35 °C was injected by hand over a period of 2 – 3 min. To prevent reflux of the oil-wax after removal of the needle from the site into which it had been inserted, the needle was left in a fixed position for about 10 min after injection. The dogs were killed by intravenous injection of calcium chloride 30 min and 3, 6, 12, 24, 36 and 48 h after the oil-wax injection. The brain was immediately removed and fixed in 10% formalin solution. After fixation, the surface of the brain was inspected and all specimens that had oil-wax at sites other than the lateral portion of the internal capsule and all those showing signs of secondary haemorrhage resulting from the injection were excluded from the study. Histological samples were prepared from seven animals, one each at 30 min and 3, 6, 12, 24, 36 and 48 h after the oil-wax injection. The samples were prepared as in the haematoma group from frontal sections passing through the chiasma using haematoxylin-eosin and elastica-Masson staining. The histological appearances in the brain tissue surrounding the oil-wax region were observed and compared with those in the haematoma samples.

Results

Progressive Histological Changes in Brain Tissue Surrounding the Haematoma

In the brain tissue removed 30 min after haematoma production, a clear border between the haematoma and the brain tissue was evident and strip-like areas of status spongiosus were found (Fig. 1).

Three hours after haematoma production, the boundary between the haematoma and the brain tissue was clear, but the width of the surrounding layer of status spongiosus had enlarged, and there was infiltration of fluid into the substance of the brain and into the perivascular area.

Six hours after haematoma production, red blood cells of the haematoma were found to have infiltrated heavily into the surrounding brain tissue. In that area, tissue was destroyed and necrosis had begun (Fig. 2). (Areas in which such changes are found are subsequently referred to as the necrotic zones.) Immediately external to that portion a layer of perivascular bleeding with spherical and ring-like haemorrhages was seen in the vicinity of capillaries, particularly venous capillaries (Fig. 3). (Areas in which such changes are found are subsequently referred to as perivascular bleeding zones.) Moreover, a zone external to that was found to show status spongiosus (Fig. 4). The border between the necrotic and the perivascular bleeding zones was distinct.

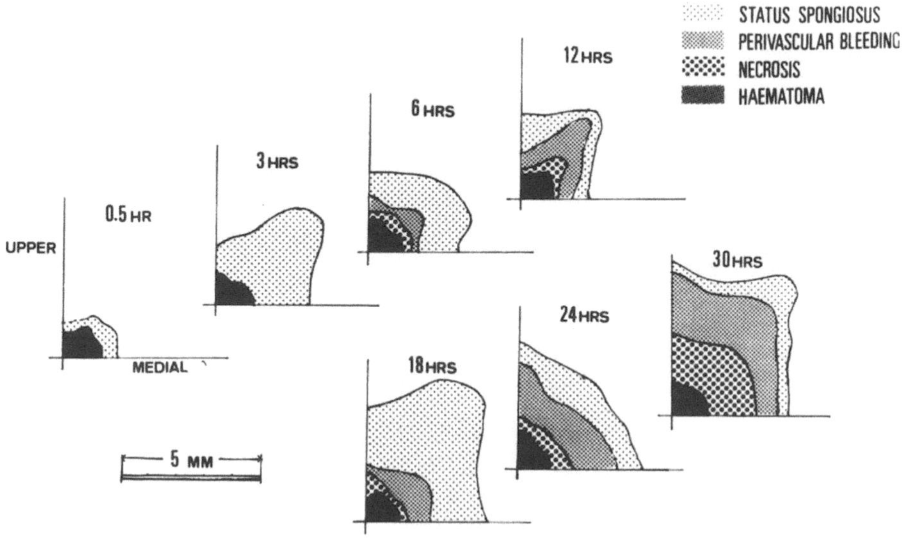

Fig. 1. Microscopical changes in the brain tissue around the haematoma after injection. The charge in status spongiosus was found in brain tissue 30 min after haematoma production. Changes in the status spongiosus, the perivascular bleeding and the necrosis were found in brain tissue 6 h after haematoma production, and the extent of these changes was found to increase with time

Twelve hours after haematoma production, external to the border between the haematoma and surrounding tissue, the three layers – necrotic, perivascular bleeding and status spongiosus – were still identifiable and the extent of each had increased.

In the sections taken 18, 24, 30, 36 and 48 h after haematoma production, the extent of all three zones was found to increase with time. The border between the necrotic zone and the perivascular bleeding zone was found to become indistinct because of multiple perivascular haemorrhages.

Progressive Histological Changes in Brain Tissue Surrounding the Oil-Wax

Thirty minutes after the oil-wax injection, the border between the oil-wax surrounding brain tissue was clear and no necrosis was apparent. The status spongiosus changes found 30 min after haematoma production were not seen in the surrounding brain tissue (Fig. 5).

Three hours after oil-wax injection, the border between the oil-wax and surrounding tissue was well defined, but slight status spongiosus was found in the brain tissue near the border. Compared with the haematoma cases, the changes were slight and not extensive. The infiltration of fluid into the brain and the perivascular area which was seen in the haematoma cases was not found.

Six and 12 h after oil-wax injection, the status spongiosus zone, which had appeared after 3 h, increased in severity with time. After 12 h slight perivascular bleeding was found at several places in the brain tissue at the border.

Twenty-four hours after oil-wax injection (Fig. 6), the status spongiosus zone grew wider, the brain tissue near the border with the oil-wax showed slight perivascular bleeding and one portion of the haemorrhage showed fusion and necrotic changes. Nevertheless, the changes were extremely mild in comparison with those in the animals with haematoma.

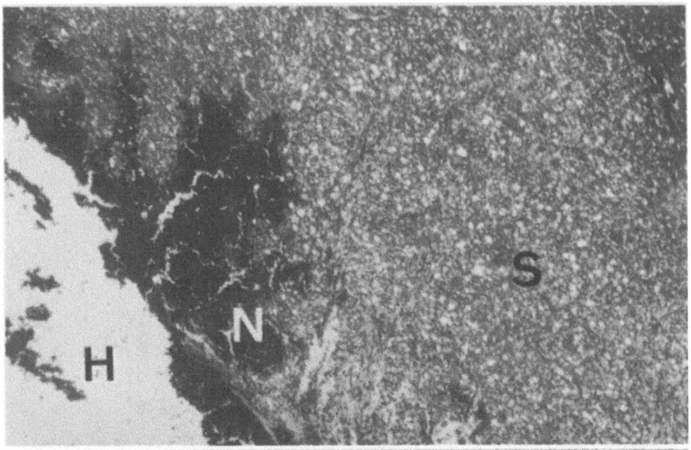

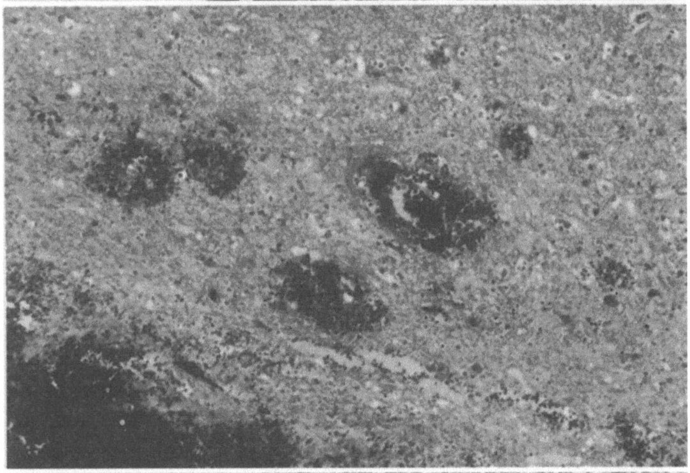
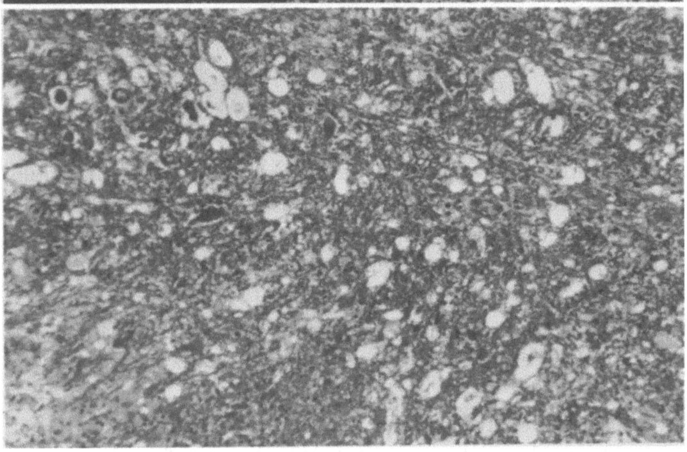

Fig. 2. Necrotic change (6 h after haematoma production). Red cells of the haematoma were found to have infiltrated markedly into the surrounding brain tissue so that tissue in that area was destroyed and necrosis had begun. *H,* haematoma; *N,* necrosis; *S,* status spongiosus. ×60

Fig. 3. Perivascular bleeding change (12 h after haematoma production). Perivascular bleeding with spherical and ring-like haemorrhages. ×150

Fig. 4. Change of status spongiosus (30 h after haematoma production). ×150

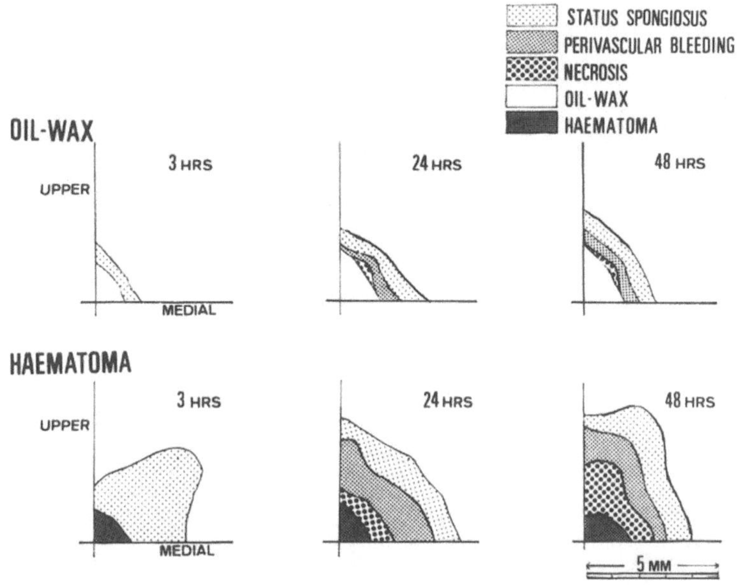

Fig. 5. Microscopical changes in brain tissue around the oil-wax and the haematoma. The changes in the brain tissue around the oil-wax were slight and much less in extent compared with the haematoma cases

Thirty-six hours after oil-wax injection, no marked differences from the 24-h specimens were noted in the brain tissue, but the degree of perivascular bleeding had worsened slightly.

Forty-eight hours after oil-wax injection, the status spongiosus layer had increased in size, the perivascular bleeding was more marked, and the necrosis of the border region between the oil-wax and brain tissue had advanced. Nevertheless, extensive necrotic and perivascular bleeding layers such as those seen in the haematoma group were not found.

Characteristics of Changes in Brain Tissue Surrounding the Haematoma according to the site

A tendency was found for the necrotic zone, perivascular bleeding zone and status spongiosus zone, which arose in the brain tissue around the haematoma and expanded peripherally with time, to progess more markedly in the superomedial, medial and superior directions (Fig. 7).

Discussion

Using stereotactic methods, intracerebral haematomas were produced in the lateral portion of the internal capsule in adult dogs and, using the same methods, oil-wax was injected into similar sites for comparative analysis of the subsequent changes in the surrounding brain tissue.

In the brain tissue surrounding a haematoma, a status spongiosus zone had already appeared 30 min after haematoma production. Subsequently, three zones developed around the haematoma: a necrotic zone, a perivascular bleeding zone and a spongiose zone, all of which extended peripherally with time.

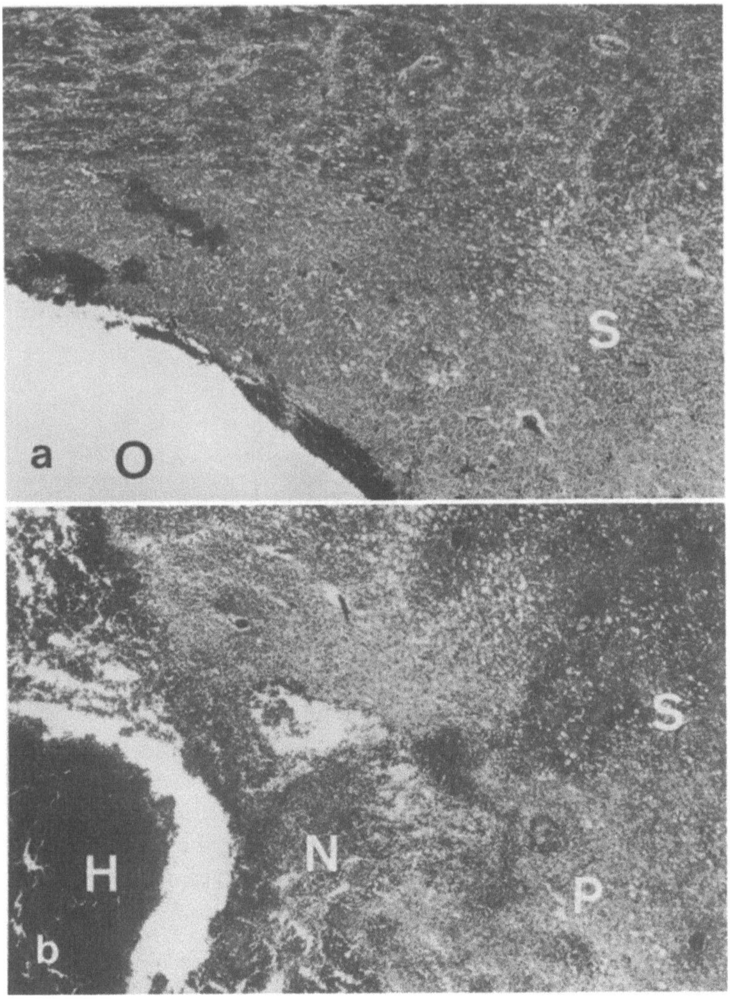

Fig. 6a, b. The changes in the brain tissue surrounding the oil-wax (*a*) and the haematoma (*b*) 24 h after injection. The changes surrounding the oil-wax were slight and much less in extent compared with the haematoma cases. *O,* oil-wax; *H,* haematoma; *N,* necrosis; *P,* perivascular bleeding; *S,* status spongiosus. ×60

Status spongiosus was found within 30 minutes of haematoma production, but after oil-wax injection only a mild status spongiosus was found after 3 h. This indicates that status spongiosus changes are not due solely to the physical insult of the haematoma on the surrounding brain tissue, but rather that plasma components from the haematoma infiltrate the surrounding brain tissue and accumulate in the intracellar spaces, leading to a pathological state similar to brain oedema. Of course, the physical insult alone gives rise to brain oedema in the surrounding tissue. That is to say, the mild status spongiosus changes which begin to appear 3 h after oil-wax injection are thought to be brought about by secondary changes in blood vessels due to the physical insult of the oil-wax. This means that the status spongiosus changes of the brain tissue surrounding the haematoma are caused by invasion of the surrounding tissue by plasma components from the haematoma immediately after the haematoma formation. From

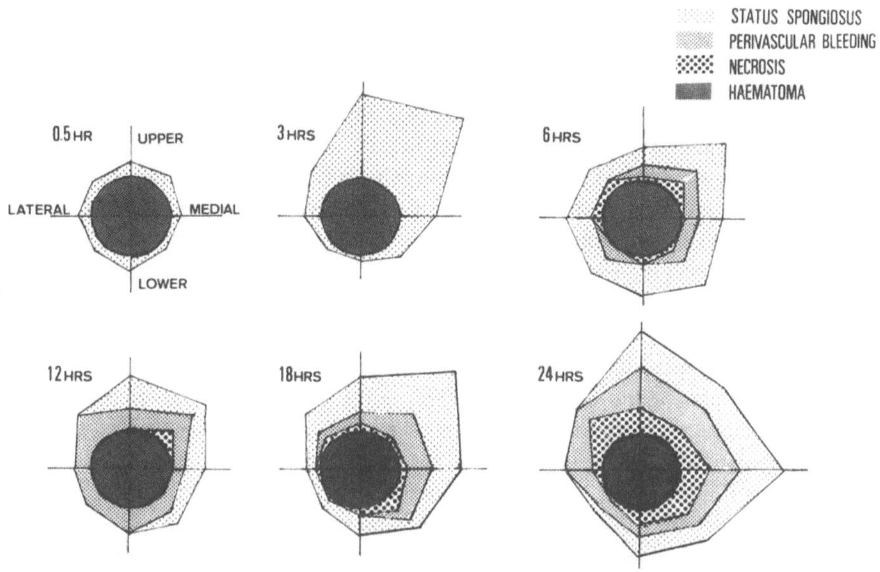

Fig. 7. Distribution of microscopical changes in brain tissue around the haematoma. A tendency was found for changes in the brain tissue around the haematoma to progress more in the superomedial, medial and superior directions

around 3 h thereafter, the influence of the haematoma on the blood vessels of the surrounding brain tissue is felt, and the pathological condition becomes worse.

The perivascular bleeding layer appeared after 6 h in both the haematoma and oil-wax cases and worsened with time. However, the degree of perivascular bleeding was far more pronounced in the haematoma cases. From this fact it is thought that in brain tissue which has received physical insult, the changes in the blood vessels which bring about perivascular extrusion of red blood cells appear after 6 h. The development of status spongiosus in the perivascular brain tissue depends little upon the influence of the rate of change in the vessel walls due to the physical pressure, but more upon the degree of such changes. This zone of perivascular bleeding is particularly marked near the haematoma or oil-wax and progresses with time. Furthermore, such bleeding is more marked in the superomedial and medial directions, which easily succumb to ischaemia, rather than in the lateral direction. Because of this it is thought that the changes in the vascular walls caused by perivascular bleeding are due to the circulatory insufficiency brought about the physical insult of the mass.

The necrotic zone, like the perivascular bleeding zone, appeared 6 h after haematoma production or oil-wax injection, but the causes were different. In the haematoma cases, the formation of the necrotic layer was due to two factors. The first is that the red blood cells from the haematoma directly infiltrate the surrounding brain tissue, causing its destruction. A marked necrotic layer is formed 6 h after haematoma production, and the red cells invade the surrounding brain tissue evenly, creating a clear boundary between the necrotic layer and the perivascular bleeding layer. The other factor is the necrotic layer formed by the fusion of many perivascular haemorrhages. This layer is found external to the necrotic layer and becomes more marked with time.

The boundary between the necrotic and perivascular bleeding layers is distinct until 12 h after the production of the haematoma, but thereafter it becomes gradually blurred. It is thus thought that the progressive enlargement of the necrotic layer is brought about by the direct infiltration of red blood cells into the tissue surrounding the haematoma until the 12th hour, after which the primary cause of necrosis is the fusion of numerous perivascular haemorrhages.

It is thus apparent that when an intracerebral haematoma occurs, secondary changes such as brain oedema, haemorrhage and necrosis, are rapidly brought about. Furthermore, these changes are not due merely to the physical impact of the haematoma on surrounding brain tissue, but are found to be greatly enhanced by the infiltration of plasma components from the haematoma into the brain tissue. With regard to the results of these experiments, it is thought that if extirpation of the haematoma is carried out at an early stage, before irreversible necrosis and perivascular bleeding has occurred, the secondary changes in the surrounding area will be minimized and a better result obtained. In these experiments, the secondary changes in the tissue surrounding the haematoma were particularly severe on the medial side, i.e. on the side towards the internal capsule. Thus, in cases of putaminal-type intracerebral haematoma it is important to extirpate the haematoma at an early stage to prevent secondary pathological changes in the internal capsule, and thus encourage a more favourable outcome.

With regard to clinical cases of hypertensive putaminal haematoma, we have previously published our results (1972) showing low morbidity and mortality rates using a trans-Sylvian approach for extirpating the haematoma at an early stage as this causes much less damage to the brain. As mentioned above, necrosis and perivascular bleeding, which are irreversible changes brought about by red cell invasion, are found 6 h after haematoma production in the surrounding tissue.

Consequently, in cases of hypertensive intracerebral haematoma, even if the primary destruction of brain tissue cannot be avoided because of the impact of the haematoma itself, the secondary, irreversible changes to surrounding brain tissue can be brought to a halt by haematoma extirpation within 6 h. Even in cases where more than 6 h have elapsed, secondary changes can be reduced provided that the original brain damage is minimized by prompt surgical extirpation. This means that early operations for hypertensive intracerebral haematoma are important both in terms of saving lives and obtaining a favourable functional outcome.

4.3.1 Discussion

K. J. Zülch (Cologne):
I think that by evacuation of the clot, if there is no rebleeding, you can prevent quite a bit of damage. But in hypertensive haematoma, within very few minutes, maybe half an hour, the destruction of the internal capsule and the region around it is already so extensive that I would discourage removing the haematoma. The neurological defects in these patients are far more extensive than those with other large infarcts.

4.4 Brain Abscess Following ICH

O. Busse, Giessen

Case Report

A 45-year-old male was subjected to laser recanalization of a urethral stricture. The operation was performed under epidural spinal anaesthesia. Four hours later, a left-sided hemiparesis suddenly developed and was followed by drowsiness and disorientation. Lumbar puncture revealed blood-stained CSF, and computerized tomography showed a haematoma in the region of the internal capsule with ventricular compression (Fig. 1a). His general condition and left-sided weakness improved gradually. He had mild pyrexia and slightly increased ESR, and the white cell count was 11000 – 22000. A repeat CT scan 1 week later showed progressing resorption of the haematoma (Fig. 1b). Four weeks after the cerebral incident sepsis developed, but the blood cultures were negative. The patient was treated with antibiotics. The hemiparesis

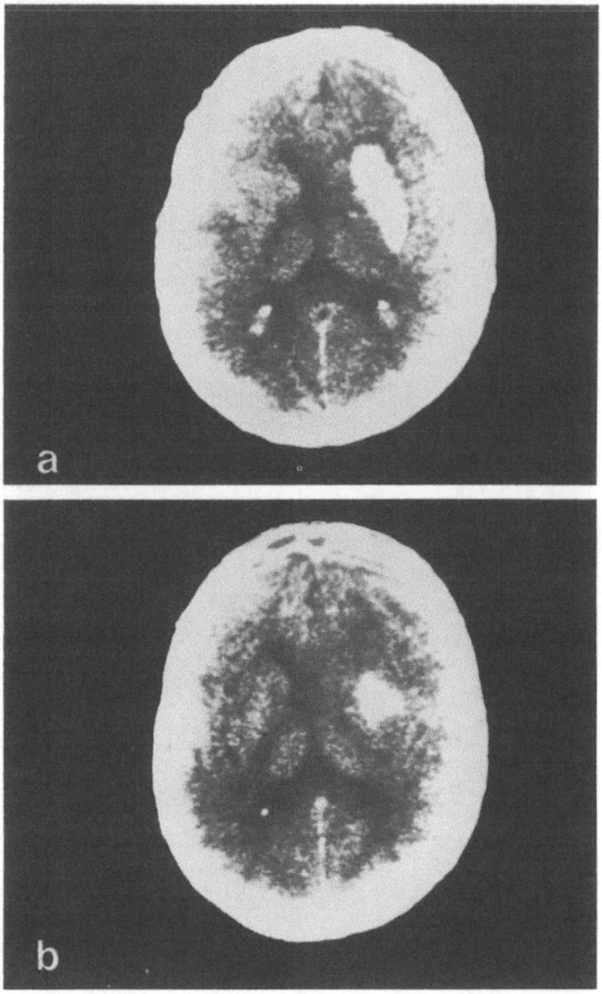

Fig. 1. a Haematoma of internal capsule with ventricular compression. **b** One week later good resorption of the haematoma

slowly improved, but he remained mentally slow and disorientated. Two months after the onset of the haemorrhage, cerebral angiography was performed and showed a space-occupying lesion in the area of the previous haemorrhage. Ring-like vascularization was shown in the angiogram. The CT scan showed an area of diminished density surrounded by a capsule with increased density, which enhanced after administration of contrast medium. It was thought that this indicated a brain abscess (Fig. 2). The abscess was punctured and 30 cc pus were recovered. The cultures were negative.

The pathogenesis of this brain abscess and its relation to the haemorrhage are difficult to interpret. Meningitis after lumbar puncture cannot be completely excluded. The haematoma cavity could have been a locus minoris resistentiae during the sepsis. The third possibility is a clinically silent bacteriaemia with bleeding occurring from a mycotic aneurysm, and subsequent formation of an abscess in the area.

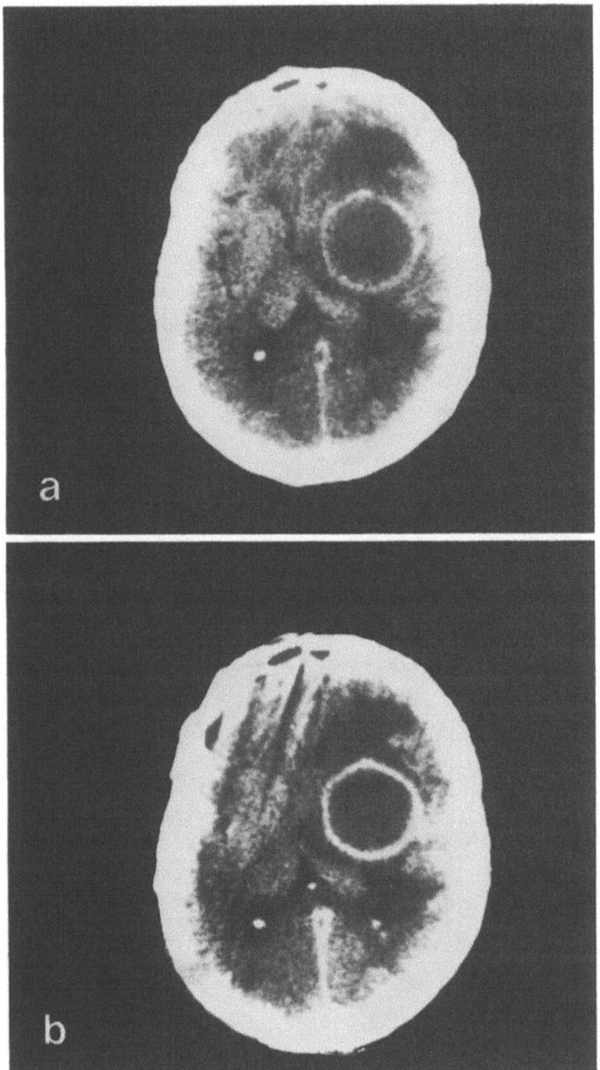

Fig. 2a, b. Brain abscess of the basal ganglia before **a** and after **b** contrast enhancement

5 Aetiological Aspects of Location

5.1 Pathology and Aetiology of Supratentorial Haemorrhage

K. Jellinger, Vienna

About 80% of all spontaneous intracerebral haemorrhages occur in the cerebral hemispheres and 20% in the brain stem and cerebellum (Fig. 1). The most frequent sites of intracerebral bleeds are in the basal ganglia and cerebral hemispheres and of these, 60% – 80% rupture into the ventricles (Mutlu et al. 1963; Yates 1976; Hurtig and Reivich 1977; Jellinger 1977). Haemorrhages into the basal ganglia account for 40% – 66% of all primary intracerebral bleeds and 5% – 7% of all cerebral vascular accidents (Huckman et al. 1970). Basal ganglia haemorrhage is a common, often catastrophic, occurrence accounting 40% of other non-hypertensive spontaneous bleeds which more often occur in the hemispheres (Fig. 1; Table 1). Evaluation of aetiological factors in a personal autopsy series and a sample of histologically examined neurosurgical cases (Table 1) demonstrates that in post-mortem material, about 70% of the basal ganglia haemorrhages are associated with hypertension (including eclampsia, etc.). Hemispheric haematomas most often result from vascular malformations, i.e. ruptured aneurysms (about 22%), angiomas (about 15%) and brain tumours (16%) rather than from hypertension (19%) and other vascular diseases or blood dyscrasias and coagulation disorders (9% – 10% each). For comparison, it is of interest to note that only one-third of the cerebellar and brain-stem haemorrhages were due to hypertension, while blood dyscrasias and angiomas were the second and third most important causes of cerebellar haematomas, and 50% of the brain stem bleeds were due to vascular malformations (Table 1). In biopsy material, the large majority of surgically treated lobar haemorrhages result from histologically proven vascular malformations of different sizes, while tumours and hypertension or other vascular diseases constituted the next most common recognizable causes. In almost 18% of this series no satisfactory cause for the haemorrhage could be identified.

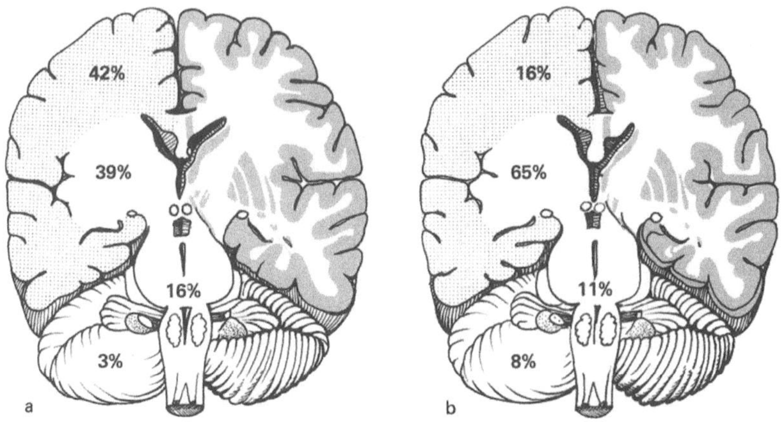

Fig. 1. a Sites of "spontaneous" non-hypertensive cerebral haemorrhages (mod. W. Schiefer 1972) and of **b** hypertensive cerebral haemorrhages (2050 cases; see Jellinger 1979)

Table 1. Aetiology and location of spontaneous intracerebral haematomas

Cause	Autopsy series (435 cases)				Biopsy series (112 cases)	
	Basal ganglia	Hemispheres	Cerebellum	Brain stem	Basal ganglia	Hemispheres
Hypertension	112	43	11	5	3	6
Aneurysm	5	59	1	–	–	3
Angioma	15	33	7	8	–	61
Tumours	5	37	3	1	–	12
Blood disease						
Coagul. disorders	4	19	9	1	–	2
Other vascular diseases [a]	6	21	1	–	–	6
Others, unknown	13	13	2	1	2	17
Total	160	225	34	16	5	107

[a] Phlebothrombosis, vasculititis, senile amyloid angiopathy

From post-mortem studies, the following predominant sites and extensions of supratentorial haemorrhages have been distinguished (Courville and Friedman 1942; Mutlu et al. 1963). These are summarized in Fig. 2 and have been confirmed by recent CT scans (Huk and Schiefer 1976; Dolinskas et al. 1977; Hier et al. 1977).

1) A lateral type affecting the putamen and its surroundings which accounts for one-fourth to one-third of all haematomas. This "typical" putaminal haemorrhage or "striatum apoplexy" may remain localized or extend into the internal capsule, lateral ventricle (Fig. 3) or to the white matter of the frontal, temporal and occipital lobes (Figs. 4, 6). In about 75% – 90% of the lethal cases it ruptures into the lateral ventricle (Freytag 1968; Jellinger 1972), while extension into the contralateral basal ganglia is rare.

2) The medial type arising in the thalamus or caudate nucleus occurring in about 10% which may destroy the hypothalamus and brain stem (Fig. 5), and in 90% – 97% ruptures into the ventricle. This type is frequently seen in both hypertension and deep AV malformations.

3) The quadrilateral type affecting the whole area of the basal ganglia, extending from the ventricle to the insula (Fig. 6) occurs in about 20% of all central haemorrhages.

4) The intermediary type of localized haematoma affecting either the striatum or the thalamus is present in about 20% each. It may or may not rupture into the ventricle (Fig. 7).

5) Haemorrhage into the hemispheric white matter and cerebral lobes accounts for about 16% of all hypertensive bleeds, but for 40% – 45% of other spontaneous non-hypertensive haemorrhages (Fig. 1).

The most frequent site of hypertensive haemorrhage is in the putamen, external capsule and claustrum, i.e. in the supply area of Charcot's lenticulostriate arteries which arise at a right angle from the main trunk of the middle cerebral artery. The predilection for hypertensive haemorrhages in this area has been related to vascular morphology and haemodynamic factors (see Zülch 1971; Jellinger 1972, 1977). In 75% – 87% of the cases, the bleed via the internal capsule ruptures into the dorsolateral corner of the lateral ventricle (Fig. 3). Less frequently the haemorrhage extends into the frontal white matter (about 30%), the temporal lobe (about 20%) or the parieto-occipital region (about 15%). Non-fatal putaminal haemorrhages later present as

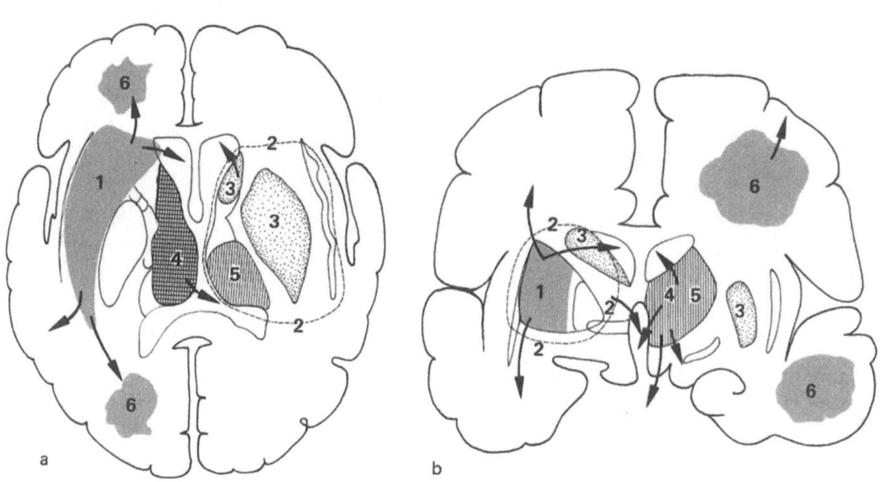

Fig. 2a, b. Predominant sites and extensions of hypertensive cerebral haemorrhages. **a** horizontal section and **b** coronal section. 1, striatum-claustrum haemorrhage; 2, quadrigeminal haemorrhage into total basal ganglia; 3, localized striatal haemorrhage; 4, 5, thalamic haemorrhage; 6, hemispheric and white matter haemorrhages

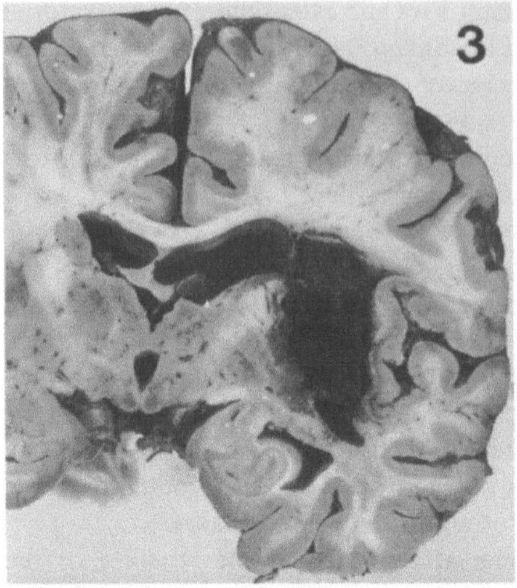
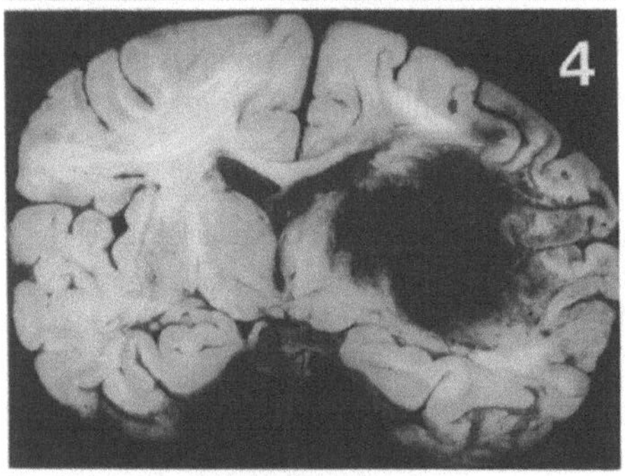
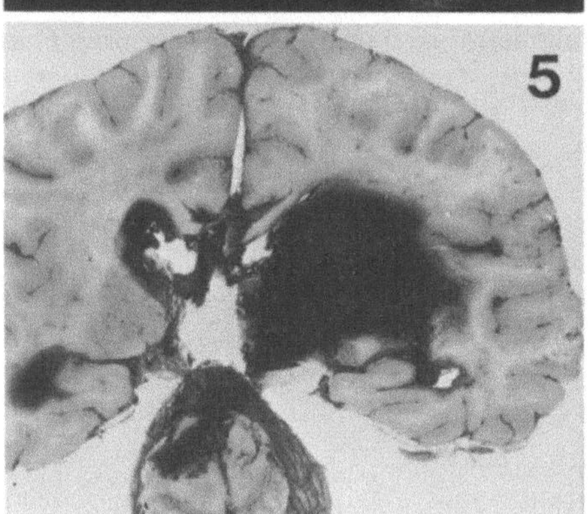
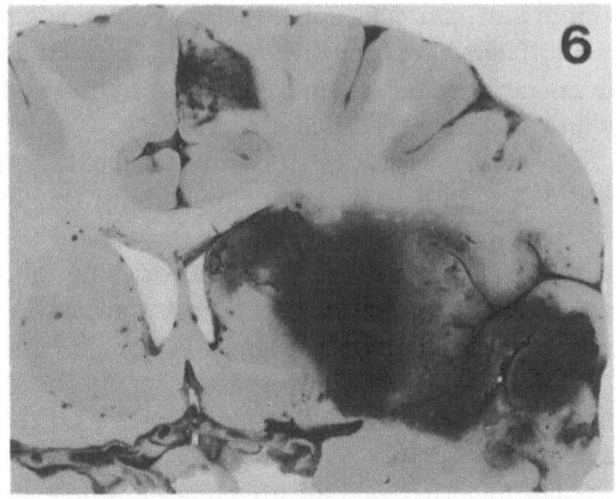
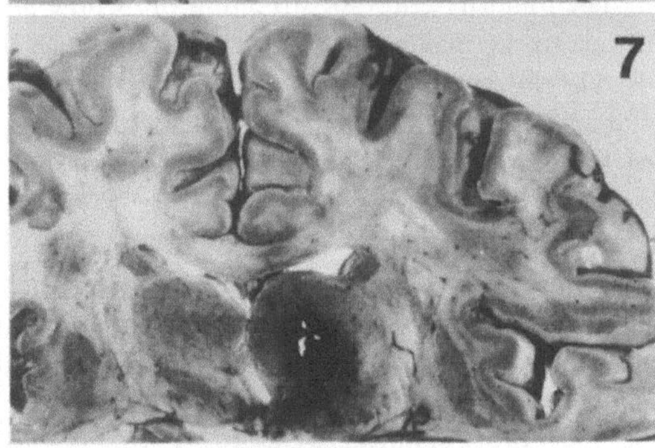
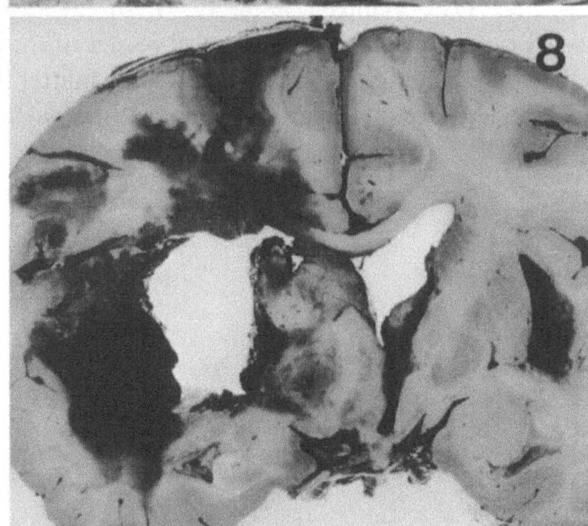

Fig. 3. Striatal haemorrhage extending through internal capsule to lateral ventricle
Fig. 4. Hypertensive striatal haemorrhage extending into insula
Fig. 5. Medial basal ganglionic haemorrhage with secondary brain stem haemorrhage
Fig. 6. Striatal haemorrhage extending into temporal lobe
Fig. 7. Small thalamic haemorrhage in hypertensive individual
Fig. 8. Massive basal ganglionic haemorrhage extending into frontal white matter with old contralateral lenticular haemorrhage

single or multilocular cavities which in 15% – 20% may show some traces of survived rupture into the ventricular system (Freytag 1968; Jellinger 1972). In about 15% – 20% of all recent fatal putaminal haemorrhages there are additional cystic cavities of an old contralateral lenticular "slit" haemorrhage (Fig. 8).

The medial type of ganglionic haemorrhage has much higher overall mortality owing to frequent intraventricular rupture or extension into the brain stem (Fazio et al. 1973). In addition, 30% – 50% of all supratentorial haemorrhages of all aetiologies are associated with secondary haemorrhage into the brain stem due to increased intracranial pressure (Freytag 1968; Jellinger 1977).

About 25% of the hypertensive supratentorial bleeds and more than half of the non-hypertensive supratentorial haemorrhages are located in the hemispheric lobes, the most frequent site being near the trigone of the lateral ventricle (30% – 40%) and the frontal lobe (about 25%), less often in the temporal and parietal lobes (15% – 20%). The cerebral hemispheres are most often affected by "atypical" haemorrhages arising from blood dyscrasias, vascular malformations or other vascular diseases. Hemispheric haemorrhages may remain circumscribed, and some of these would probably have escaped diagnosis before CT became available, while about 40% rupture into the ventricles, and 50% – 66% rupture into the subarachnoid space.

5.2 Haematomas in Hemispheric Lobes

J. Zierski, Giessen

Spontaneous intracerebral haematomas may occur in any region of the brain. However, for hypertensive haematomas and those due to cerebral atherosclerosis, the region of the basal ganglia is the site of predilection (Lazorthes 1956). We do not know exactly what factors are decisive in limiting the expansion of a haematoma to that region in some patients and why in others the bleeding expands into the white matter of the hemisphere, resulting in huge lobar clots.

The figures for the incidence of lobar distribution of haematomas vary considerably, depending on the method of study and classification used, but a relatively high incidence in the frontal and temporal lobes is obvious.

Giessen Series. Review of the Material

The aetiology of spontaneous intracerebral haematomas in our series of 135 cases, excluding haemorrhages caused by vascular malformations seen in angiography or at autopsy, is shown in Table 1. Of these haematomas, 52.5% occurred in patients with established arterial hypertension.

Patients with blood dyscrasia had haemorrhages of the dissecting type which spread into the white matter of the hemispheres and were not limited to one lobe.

In 5.3% of patients the cause of haematoma was a tumour. Only such patients were included in whom the pre-operative angiogram showed no tumour circulation and in whom tumour

Table 1. Aetiology of spontaneous intracerebral haematomas

	Number	%
Fixed arterial hypertension	71	52.5
Blood dyscrasia and anticoagulant therapy	14	10.4
Suspected micro-angioma	10	7.4
Tumour	7	5.3
Periarteritis nodosa	1	0.7
Other (cerebral atherosclerosis, venous thrombosis, unknown)	32	23.7
Total	135	

tissue was found by biopsy. Histologically, melanoma, oligodendroglioma, ependymoma, glioblastoma and chorion-epithelioma or seminoma were represented. In all these cases the haematoma was limited to one or two lobes.

In ten patients (7.4%) with lobar haematomas, micro-angioma was suspected. They had no hypertension, their average age was 43.5 and the malformation could not be demonstrated by angiography either before or after operation. The diagnosis of suspected micro-angioma was based, therefore, on operative findings and the exclusion of other possible lesions.

The distribution of haematomas is shown in Table 2. Of these, 63 were limited to one lobe with a clear preponderance in the frontal and temporal lobes. Forty-six haematomas spread in the white matter of two or three adjacent lobes. Frontoparietal haematomas correspond to the

Table 2. Location of haematomas

Frontal	20
Temporal	29
Parietal	8
Occipital	6
Frontotemporal	3
Frontoparietal	6
Temporoparietal	7
Parieto-occipital	20
Temporoparieto-occipital	6
Frontoparieto-occipital	4
Multiple	8
Isolated: basal ganglia, thalamus, ventricle, brain stem	14
Cerebellum	4
Total	135

Table 3. Spontaneous haematomas, lobar haematomas and involvement of deep structures

	Number	%
Ventricular rupture	46	34
Basal ganglia (putamen, caudate nucleus head and tail, internal capsule)	55	30.7
Thalamus	4	2.9
Brain stem	4	2.9

"suprasylvian" or "supra-insular location". Posteriorly situated multilobar haematomas correspond to the often used designation of "carrefour".

Of 135 cases, rupture of the haematoma into the ventricular system occurred in 34%. In 30.7% a lobar haematoma was in continuity with a haematoma occupying the putaminal region, head and tail of the caudate or internal capsule. In almost 3% of cases, lobar haematomas were combined with thalamic or brain stem haemorrhage (Table 3).

Summary

Lobar involvement cannot be attributed to any particular aetiological factor. Haematomas in patients with hypertension have some predilection for the temporal and frontal lobes. Single-lobe haematomas without involvement of deep structures are mostly of unknown, probably atherosclerotic origin or are caused by minute vascular malformations not demonstrable by routine tests. Intracerebral haematomas developing in combination with anticoagulant therapy show the greatest tendency to spread in the white matter and become multilobar. One should make the restriction that these observations are based on a rather selected group of patients who have been specifically referred for surgical treatment and may not be representative of those haemorrhages due to hypertension which are smaller in size and show a less dramatic clinical course.

Examples of lobar haematomas of different aetiology are given in Figs. 1–5.

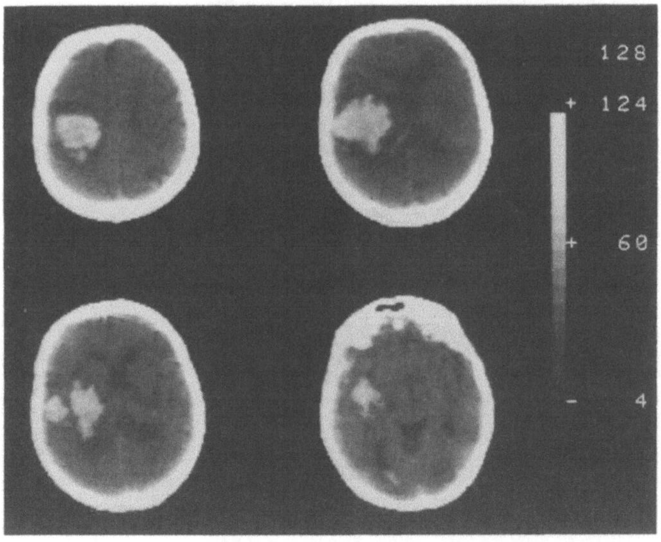

Fig. 1. Spontaneous intracerebral haematoma involving the internal capsule and spreading into the white substance of the temporal and parietal lobes

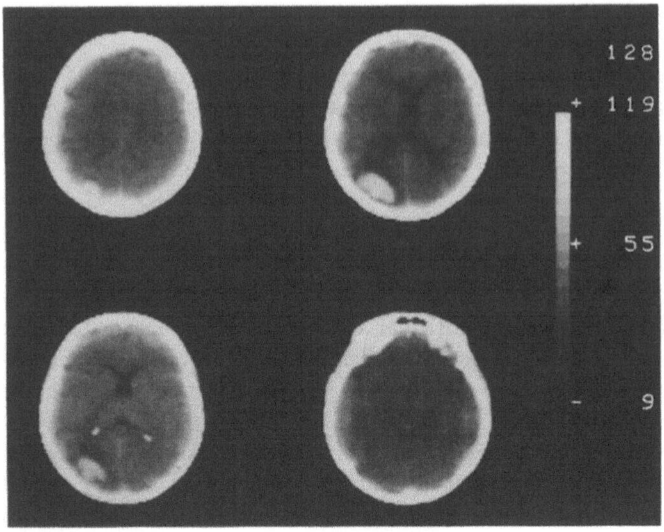

Fig. 2. Subcortical occipital monolobar haematoma of unknown aetiology

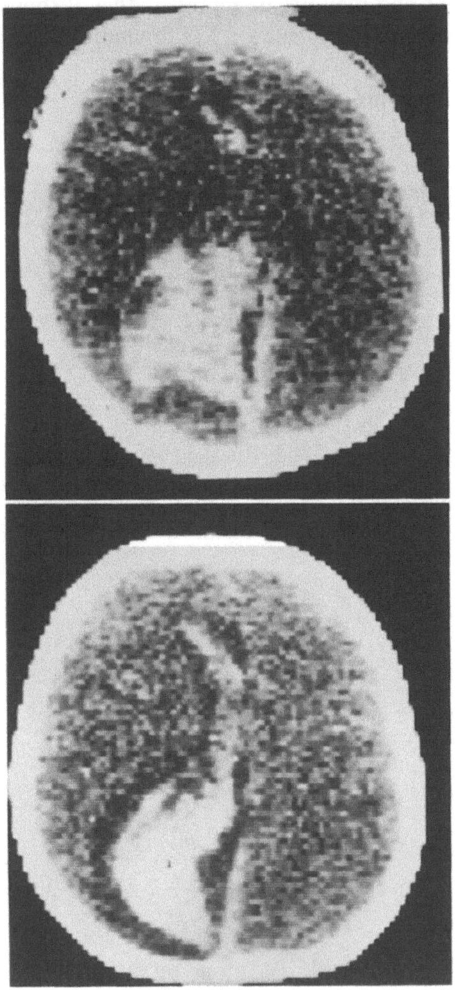

Fig. 3. Huge dissecting fronto-parieto-occipital haematoma in a patient who was receiving anticoagulant treatment

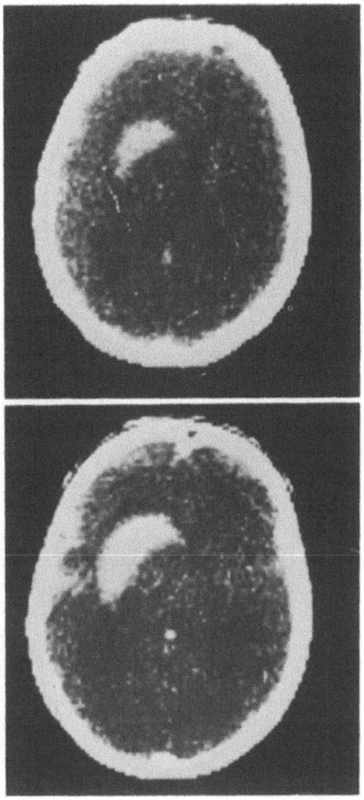

Fig. 4. Haematoma in the head of the caudate nucleus in a young patient. This haematoma was almost certainly caused by a small angioma

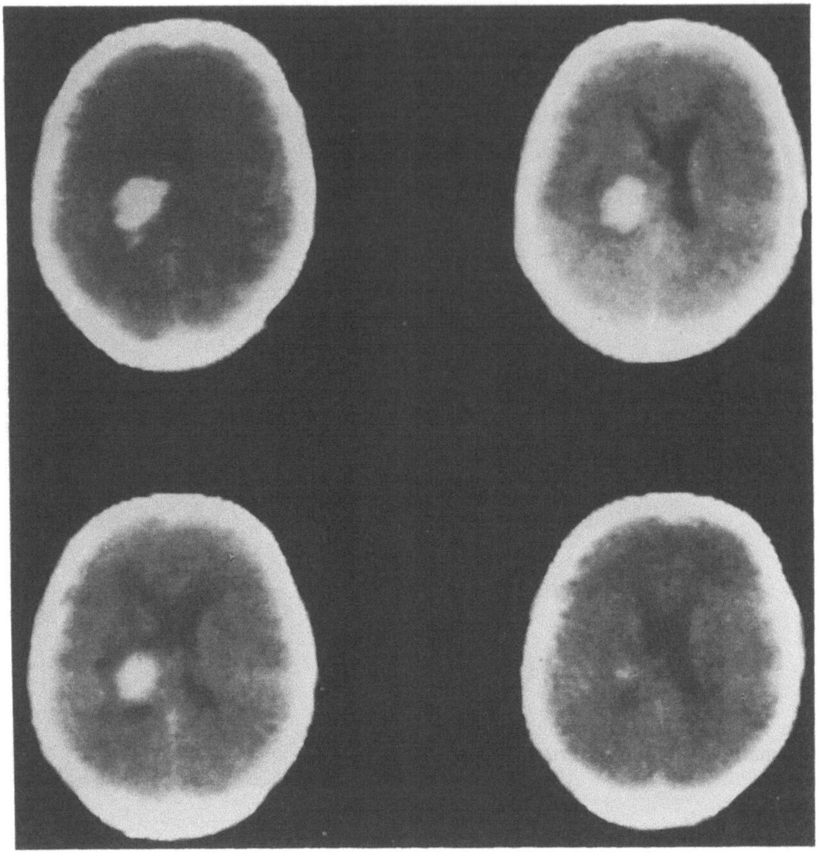

Fig. 5. Hypertensive paraventricular haematoma. Almost complete resorption after 35 days (right picture, lower row)

5.3 Intraventricular Haematoma and Haemorrhage

H. W. Pia, Giessen

Intraventricular haemorrhage, first described by Sanders (1881), was of little neurosurgical interest when I started my examinations in this field in 1960 (Pia 1953 – 1977). There had been reports about morphological findings and clinical case histories, in which attention had been drawn to various forms of haemorrhage, abnormal clinical symptoms and progress, to spontaneous recoveries and to a few cases treated successfully by operation.

In our first series of 54 cases in combination with 135 intracerebral haematomas (Pia 1966, 1968), we found an incidence of 6% with ICH caused by aneurysms, 24% with those of angiomas and 40% of those with haematomas of different aetiology.

Classification

We described a morphological classification based upon the various forms of intraventricular haemorrhage (Fig. 1). Total haematocephaly, or complete intraventricular tamponade, presents a filling of the entire ventricular system by blood clot. At autopsy a complete cast of the ventricle system is found (Fig. 2); there is no intraventricular CSF.

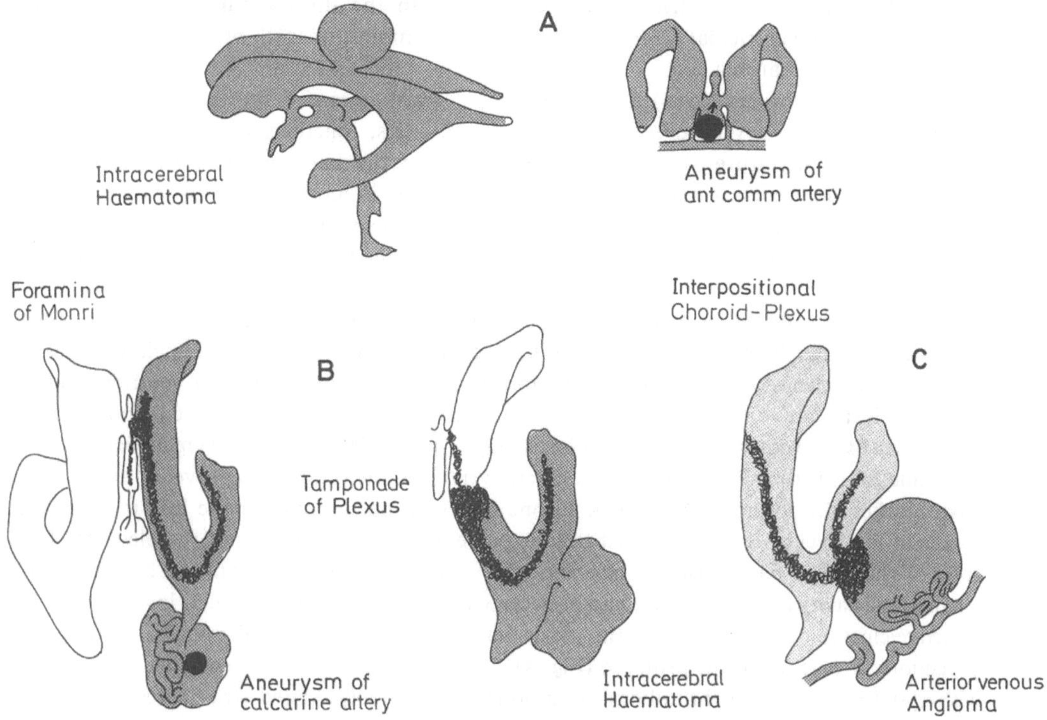

Fig. 1A–C. Morphological classification of intraventricular bleeding (Pia 1968). **A** Total ventricular tamponade (parenchymal haemorrhage with rupture into the ventricle or ruptured basal aneurysm), **B** Partial ventricular tamponade (ruptured angioma or parenchymal haemorrhage), **C** Blood-stained ventricular fluid (choroideal plexus closes the site of rupture)

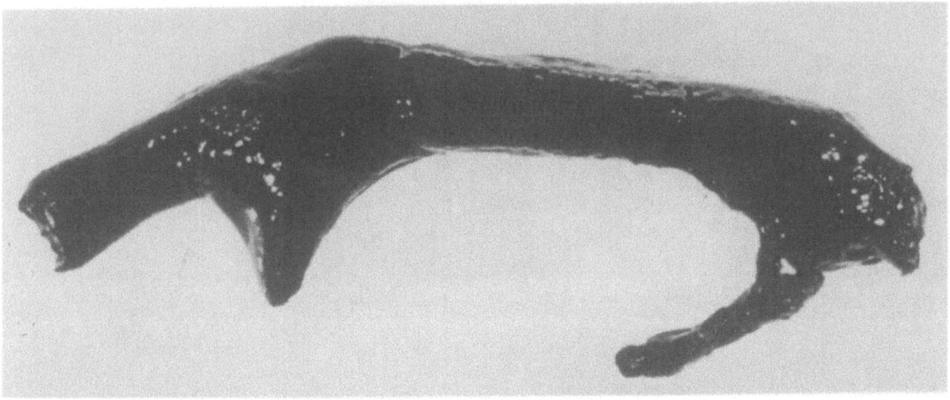

Fig. 2. Cast of the ventricle in total haematocephaly (Total ventricular tamponade)

In partial haematocephaly, or partial intraventricular tamponade, a collection of blood fills circumscribed portions of the ventricular system, usually one lateral ventricle and only rarely both. In addition, we have seen haematomas in circumscribed areas of one lateral ventricle, mainly in the posterior and inferior horn, at times extending to the trigone. Other types often encountered at autopsy are those with clots in the third ventricle, the aqueduct and fourth ventricle or in only one of these cavities. As in cases of total haematocephaly, the clots formed a cast of the part of the ventricle involved (Fig. 3). In the third group of intraventricular haemorrhage, the ventricular CSF contains a variable amount of fresh blood without showing any signs of a haematoma.

Janny and co-workers (1966) described as open haematomas a special form of localized haematoma, which they observed in eight personal cases, together, with eight similar cases reported in the literature. The bleeding originated in the basal ganglia, the haematomas extended into one ventricle and they were totally resorbed in most cases. This form of isolated intraventricular haematoma seems to be rare in hypertensive haemorrhage. It is a common finding in ruptured arteriovenous malformations of the head of the caudate nucleus or of the ventricle itself.

Up to the present time the causes and the pathogenic mechanism of these characteristic forms of intraventricular bleeding have scarcely been discussed. We found and concluded that the ventricular bottlenecks, the foramen of Monro, the outlets of the fourth ventricle and the choroid plexus are of greatest importance in the formation of generalized and localized ventricular haematomas. The choroid plexus plays a part in the closure of ventricular ruptures.

In nine cases with a complete clot in a lateral ventricle, the plexus was proved in two cases to have blocked the foramen of Monro. In one case of a haematoma of the inferior horn, the plexus at the level of the compressed trigone prevented further advance of the bleeding. In 27 cases of ventricular haemorrhage there were nine in which portions of the plexus bulged into the haematoma cavity and the rupture had been closed by this prolapse (see Fig. 1, lower right). The effective closure of the rupture by the plexus had been proved by the histological findings in a post-mortem case of plexus prolapse (Fig. 4). The plexus showed severe degenerative changes with cyst formation and thrombotic occlusions of the widely dilated stroma vessels, in other

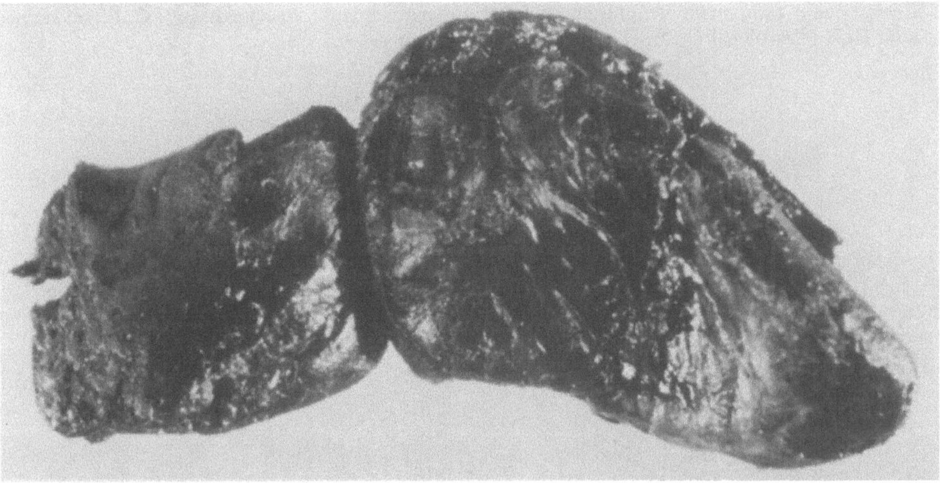

Fig. 3. Cast of a haematoma of a lateral ventricle in partial haematocephaly (Partial ventricular tamponade)

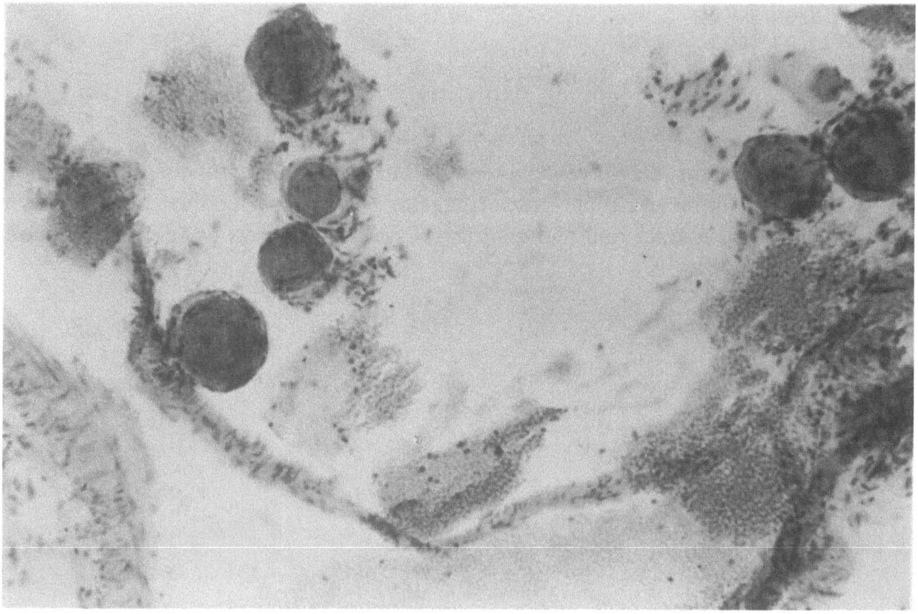

Fig. 4. Compressive lesion of choroid plexus in a case of plexus prolapse into an intracerebral haematoma, with closure of the ventricular rupture

Table 1. Intraventricular bleeding[a]

	Hypertension	Aneurysms	Angiomas	Various	Total
Total haematocephalus total ventricular tamponade	8	9	8	7	32
Partial haematocephalus partial ventricular tamponade	9	4	9	3	25
Ventricular haemorrhage	23	2	35	8	68
	40	15	52	18	125

[a] Neurosurgical University Clinic, Giessen, 1954 – 1972

words a picture of compression damage. A further protective mechanism is a local or generalized shift, with narrowing or displacement of the ventricular lumen.

Concerning the aetiology and distribution of the different types, we found that hypertensive, aneurysmal and angiomatous bleedings and those of other aetiology are combined with the three forms of intraventricular involvement (Table 1). Aneurysm cases show a tendency to total haematocephaly, whereas hypertensive ICH and angiomatous ICH mainly to intraventricular haemorrhage.

In our material neither the site of the ICH nor the age of the patient provided any reliable indication as to aetiology. This is particularly true for the concept that it is only capsular haemorrhages that show a special tendency to ventricular eruption.

The morphological and clinical findings of the pre-CT period may be helpful in reaching a correct classification and interpretation of intraventricular bleeding and the reasons why the ventricles are involved.

5.3.1 Discussion

C. Arseni and A. Gontea, Bucharest

The following situations may be encountered in intraventicular extravasations of blood:

1) Catastrophic intraventricular haemorrhage or ventricular flooding; bleeding throughout the entire subpial, subarachnoid and ventricular system, manifest by severe coma with fever,

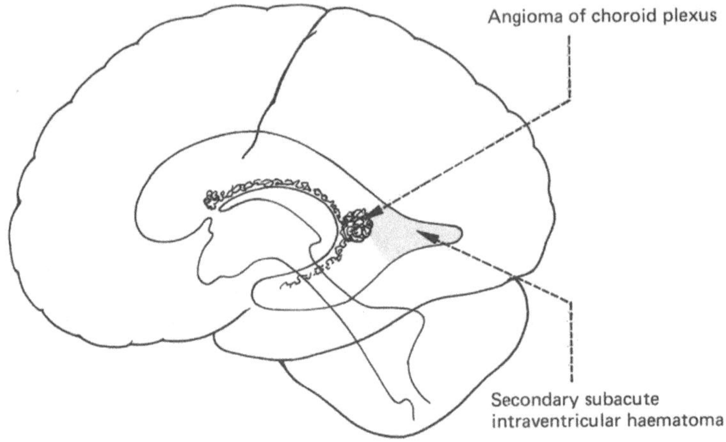

Fig. 1

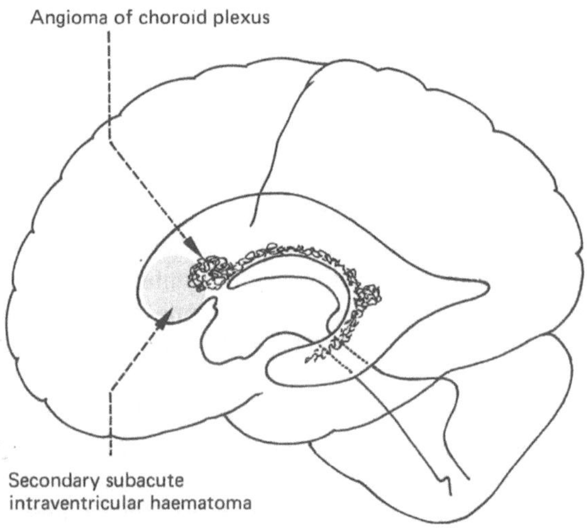

Fig. 2

decerebrate rigidity and bilateral extensor responses. Haemorrhage is produced by rupture of an aneurysm at the base of the brain and is encountered in elderly patients.

2) Common intraventricular haemorrhage, due to aneurysms in the basal nuclei and accompanied by coma, hemiplegia and intraventricular haemorrhage, affecting especially the older patients.

3) Acute and subacute secondary intraventricular haematoma (Figs. 1, 2) with or without loss of consciousness lasting hours or days and showing discrete neurological signs in young subjects. Haemorrhage is slight and even limited to one part of a ventricle, but it may recur. It is associated with angiomas and more rarely aneurysms of the choroid plexus vessels. Any young subject with repeated, moderate cerebral haemorrhage should be suspected of having an angioma of the choroid plexus. In nine cases the diagnosis of angioma of the choroid plexus was suggested by this presentation. Some had normal carotid and vertebral angiography.

4) Late secondary intraventricular haematoma (Fig. 3). In our series 3 of 13 cases of angioma of the choroid plexus evolved as an intraventricular haematoma in two stages.

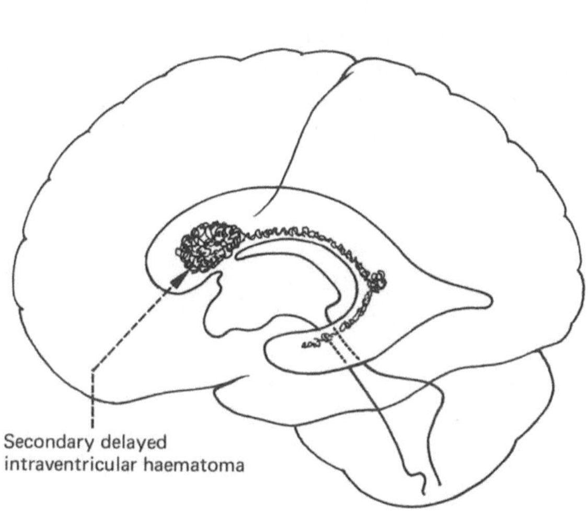

Fig. 3

5.4 Correlation Between Ventricular Haemorrhage and Chronic Cerebral Ischaemia in Adult Moya-Moya

J. Suzuki and N. Kodama, Sendai

Introduction

Ventricular haemorrhage is classified into two types: primary and secondary. In primary haemorrhage, the bleeding point is in the ventricle, while in secondary haemorrhage, it is outside the ventricle and subsequently the blood penetrates into the ventricle.

Five cases of secondary ventricular haemorrhage which appeared to be due to chronic ischaemia are presented. Correlations between chronic ischaemia and the ventricular haemorrhage are also discussed.

Case Reports

Case 1: A 25-year-old male had experienced febrile convulsions about twice a year in his childhood. He had a history of otitis media at the age of 10 and slight head injury at the age of 15. On 6 February 1975, he developed a sudden severe headache and vomiting without loss of consciousness. Lumbar puncture disclosed bloody CSF. He was admitted to our department on the 4th day after the onset, with the diagnosis of subarachnoid haemorrhage.

On admission, he was alert but complained of slight left frontal headache. The anteroposterior view of the left carotid angiogram revealed stenosis of the carotid bifurcation. The anterior cerebral artery was visualized, but the middle cerebral artery was scarcely visible and the poor Moya-Moya vessels were seen at the base of the brain (Fig. 1). The right carotid angiogram showed similar findings. The diagnosis of Moya-Moya disease was assumed and conservative therapy was adopted. Severe left headache and high fever of 38 °C continued in spite of the treatment. As his state of consciousness was deteriorating, continuous ventricular drainage (CVD) was instituted on 20 February. No CSF could be recovered by left ventricular puncture, but some old blood clot was. Right ventricular puncture revealed xanthochromic CSF. Conray ventriculography revealed a filling defect due to the blood clot in the left ventricle (Fig. 2). Consciousness was regained and headache disappeared after the ventricular drainage, which was discontinued a week later. The patient was discharged from hospital on 21 March (i.e. 7 weeks after the onset).

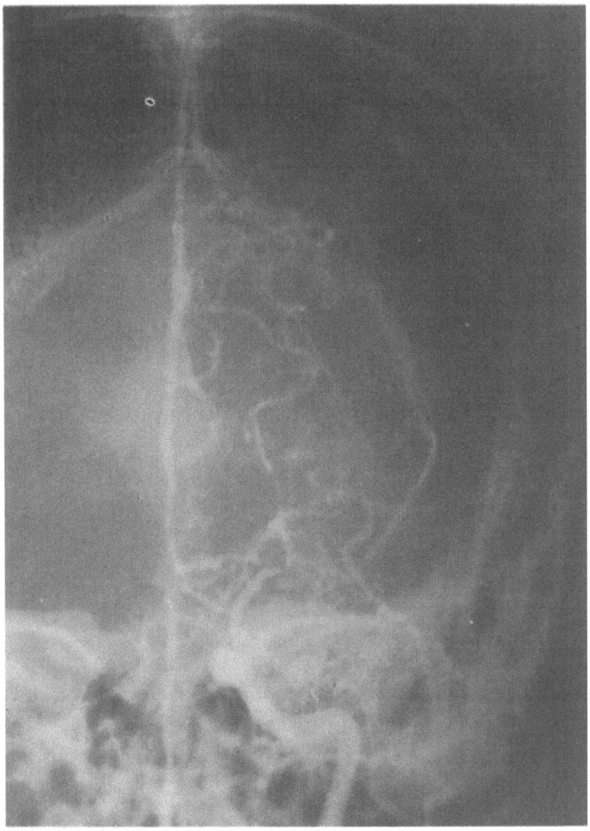

Fig. 1. Anteroposterior view of the left carotid angiogram on case 1. Stenosis at the carotid bifurcation and poor Moya-Moya vessels at the base of the brain are seen

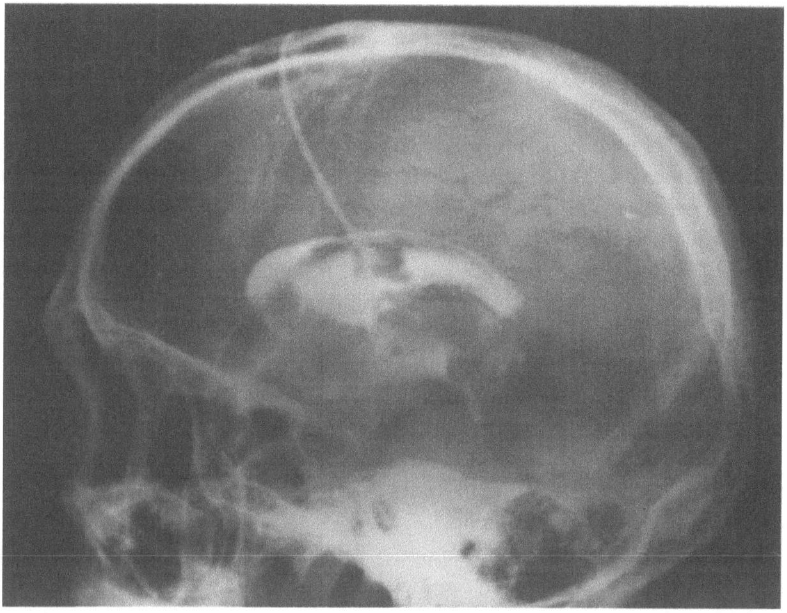

Fig. 2. Conray ventriculography on case 1. Filling defect due to blood clot is seen

Case 2: A 34-year-old female had a history of operation for sinusitis. She had suffered constantly from headache, which had sometimes been very severe during the last 5 years. On 17 September 1975, she developed a sudden severe headache and vomiting with disturbance of consciousness. On admission, she was semicomatose. Bilateral carotid angiography showed the typical indications of Moya-Moya disease. She became alert within 2 days of her admission. However, headache was still severe and a choked disc was found even 15 days after the onset. Continuous ventricular drainage was begun on 2 October. A brown blood clot was confirmed by right ventricular puncture, and conray ventriculography revealed a filling defect due to the blood clot. As her headache had improved, the drain was taken out after 1 week and the patient returned home on 31 October.

Case 3: A 41-year-old male developed a sudden severe headache accompanied by loss of consciousness on 20 December 1975. He was alert the next day, but the severe headache continued. Spinal tap disclosed bloody CSF. Neurological examinations revealed a slight left hemiparesis and sensory disturbance, and bilateral carotid angiography showed Moya-Moya vessels at the base of the brain. As the severe headache persisted, continuous ventricular drainage was set up. A filling defect due to blood clot in the right ventricle was found by conray ventriculography. Headache and slight left hemiparesis lessened with ventricular drainage, and the patient returned home on 4 February.

Case 4: A 40-year-old male had a tonsillectomy at the age of 35, hypertension was noticed at the age of 37. Around this time he lost consciousness for about 20 min after a bout of drinking. On 22 October 1975, he developed sudden temporal pain accompanied by vomiting and the headache persisted. On 26 October, he was seized by a sudden severe occipital headache and was admitted to our clinic. He was alert and showed no abnormal neurological findings. CSF taken on 27 October was xanthochromic. The left carotid angiogram revealed no abnormalities.

On the AP view of the right carotid angiogram, the right middle cerebral artery was found to be obstructed at the carotid bifurcation. Collateral pathways to the middle striate artery were formed via the perforating arteries which arose from the A.1 portion of the anterior cerebral artery. Because of these collateral pathways, the middle cerebral artery was poorly shown. As these collateral pathways were widened and tortuous, they must have been formed over a long period of time (Fig. 3). Right ventricular puncture confirmed the blood clot, and left ventricular puncture revealed pinkish CSF. Conray ventriculography showed the filling defect in the right ventricle. Continuous ventricular drainage lessened the headache, but the drainage could not be taken out because of the high CSF pressure. A ventriculo-peritoneal shunt was performed, and the patient was discharged from the hospital with a slight memory disturbance.

Case 5: A 16-year-old female had suffered from otitis media at the age of 14 and tonsillitis at 16. She had often complained of slight headache since July 1975, but had received no special medication.

On 14 December 1975, she suddenly developed repeated vomiting during sleep followed by a convulsion which lasted for 10 min. After recovering consciousness within an hour, she complained of a severe headache.

On admission, she was alert and had a stiff neck. The plantar reflex was extensor on the left, and a left carotid angiogram revealed no abnormalities. The AP view of the right carotid

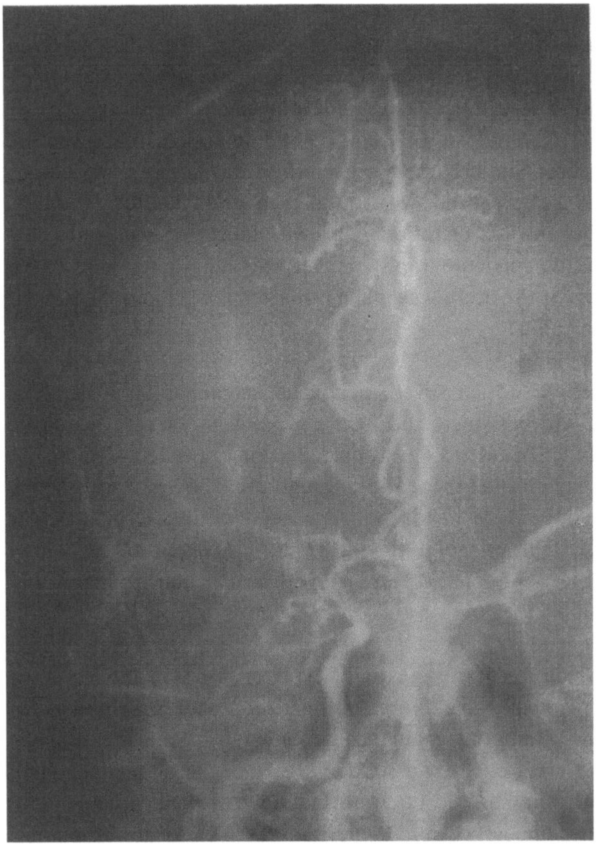

Fig. 3. Anteroposterior view of the right carotid angiogram on case 4, showing obstruction of the middle cerebral artery at its proximal portion. The middle cerebral artery is poorly visualized via the collateral pathway arising from the A_1 portion

angiogram revealed stenosis of the middle cerebral artery at the carotid bifurcation. A fine network of vessels which suggested collateral pathways was seen around the orbitofrontal artery. In the lateral view of the right carotid angiogram the ascending arteries and the angular artery were seen, but their diameters were almost half those of the opposite arteries.

On the basis of our former experiences, ventricular haemorrhage was suspected. A blood clot was aspirated by right ventricular puncture. The headache lessened with continuous ventricular drainage, and she was discharged from hospital on 24th January.

Discussion

It has usually been considered that ventricular haemorrhage is caused by rupture of an aneurysm or AV malformation, cerebral haemorrhage due to hypertension, bleeding from tumours and haemorrhagic diseases such as leukaemia, purpura, etc. However, our five cases of ventricular haemorrhage (Table 1) were not caused by the above-mentioned diseases. Three cases (1, 2 and 3) of five were instances of adult Moya-Moya disease (Kudo 1967; Nishimoto and Takeuchi 1968; Suzuki and Takahu 1968; Suzuki and Kodama 1971; Kodama and Suzuki 1974, 1978; Krayenbühl 1975; Meriwether et al. 1976). This disease has many unsolved problems. Its causes are not yet clarified, and there is still no agreement about the physiopathological interpretation.

However, the basic course of this disease is confirmed: As the bilateral stenotic change starting from the carotid bifurcation progresses, the main cerebral arteries gradually disappear and then a fine network of vessels appears at the base of the brain to compensate for the main cerebral arteries which are no longer shown on the carotid angiogram. It cannot be disputed that chronic ischaemia exists in this disease. The above-mentioned three cases showed no particular lesion that might have caused the ventricular haemorrhage, either by laboratory tests, carotid angiography, conray ventriculography or other examinations. Therefore, it seems to be most reasonable that some relationship exists between the ventricular haemorrhage and the pathological changes in the vessels of brain tissue in Moya-Moya disease.

In the other two cases (4 and 5) carotid angiography revealed stenosis and occlusion of the M1 portion of the middle cerebral artery and well-developed collateral pathways which were considered to have been formed over a long period of time. The ventricular haemorrhage was found on the same side. Carotid angiography of the opposite side and vertebral angiography showed no abnormalities liable to cause ventricular haemorrhage. The ventricular haemorrhage

Table 1. Summary of cases of ventricular haemorrhage

Case no.	Sex	Age	Symptoms	Carotid angiography	Conray ventriculogram
1	M	25	Headache, vomiting	Moya-Moya disease	Filling defect due to blood clot
2	F	33	Consciousness disturbance, nausea	Moya-Moya disease	Filling defect due to blood clot
3	M	41	Headache, consciousness disturbance, left hemiparesis	Moya-Moya disease	Filling defect due to blood clot
4	M	40	Headache, vomiting	Right MCA occlusion	Filling defect in the right ventricle
5	F	16	Convulsion, headache	Left MCA stenosis	Filling defect in the left ventricle

in these two cases may also be caused by stenotic and obstructive changes of the middle cerebral artery.

We have already reported on the three cases of Moya-Moya disease associated with aneurysm at the peripheral portion of the posterior choroidal artery (Kodama and Suzuki 1978). Each aneurysm was located in the brain tissue around the superolateral border of the lateral ventricle. These aneurysm shadows look different from the ordinary saccular aneurysms arising from the circle of Willis. Furthermore, three of them had disappeared completely on follow-up angiograms.

From these facts, we assume that these aneurysm shadows are not true aneurysms but pseudo-aneurysms which indicate the site of the bleeding point in the brain tissue. The course of these pseudo-aneurysms may perhaps be explained in the following way. Initially a small artery may rupture near the lateral ventricle so that the blood penetrates into it, but the small blood clot or, in other words, the pseudo-aneurysm, remains. The blood, which has penetrated into the lateral ventricle, circulates into the subarachnoid space. Therefore, the symptoms and signs may be misinterpreted as the result of a subarachnoid haemorrhage. Later, the blood clot is completely absorbed and disappears (Fig. 4).

It has been generally believed that the symptomatic recognition of Moya-Moya disease in adults is due to subarachnoid haemorrhage (Kanisasa et al. 1972; Lee and Cheung 1973), and the cause of the haemorrhage has been regarded as the rupture of the dilated Moya-Moya vessels in the subarachnoid space. There is no clear supporting evidence for this assumption. Our three cases already reported suggest that one of the mechanisms producing the symptoms may be the ventricular haemorrhage which follows the bleeding in the brain tissue. This concept was confirmed by ventricular puncture in cases 1, 2 and 3. The findings revealed by CT scans in recent cases and the fact that there have been several patients with intracerebral haematoma and ventricular haemorrhage among those Moya-Moya cases studied at autopsy also indicated the same conclusion (Vuia et al. 1970; Mirayama et al. 1974).

The fact that lateralized neurological symptoms and signs are not conspicuous in these five cases may indicate that the ventricular haemorrhage does not cause extensive damage to the brain tissue. Therefore, the exact bleeding point may be assumed to be at the superolateral border of the lateral ventricle, where pseudo-aneurysms were shown to exist (Kodama and Suzuki 1978).

According to the study of the vascular architecture by Softex, the arterial distribution around this region is scanty, because the central artery does not branch when it comes near to the

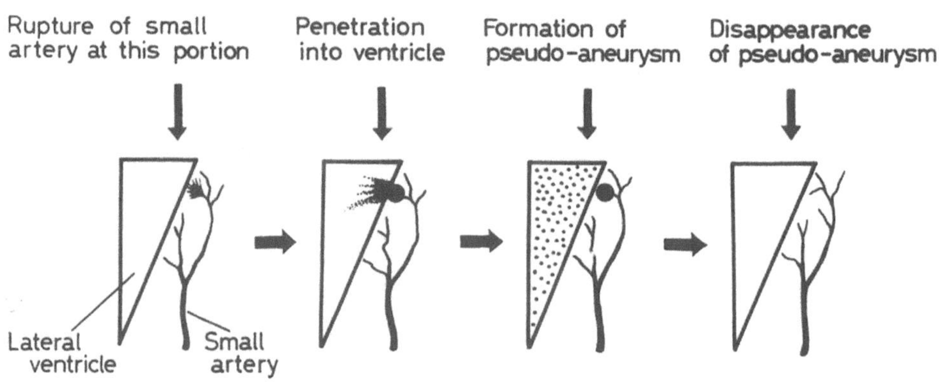

Fig. 4. Mechanism of the ventricular haemorrhage in Moya-Moya disease

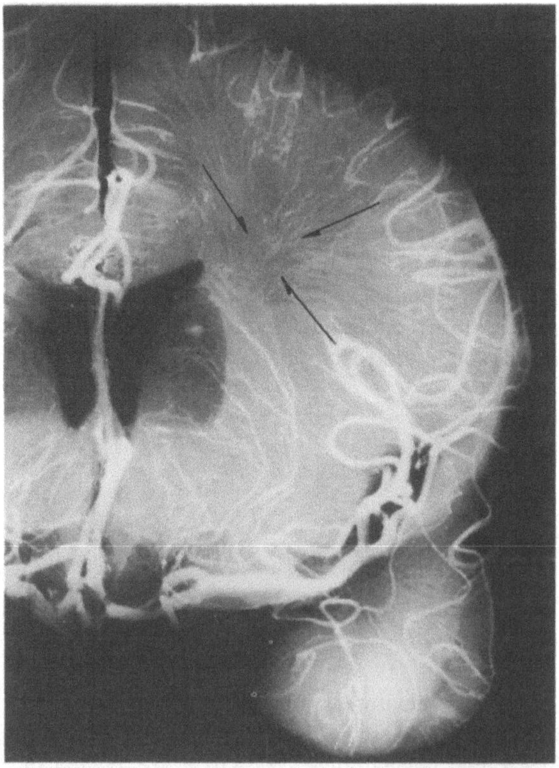

Fig. 5. Micro-angiogram of the human brain specimen. Vascularization at the superolateral border of the lateral ventricle is scanty (arrows)

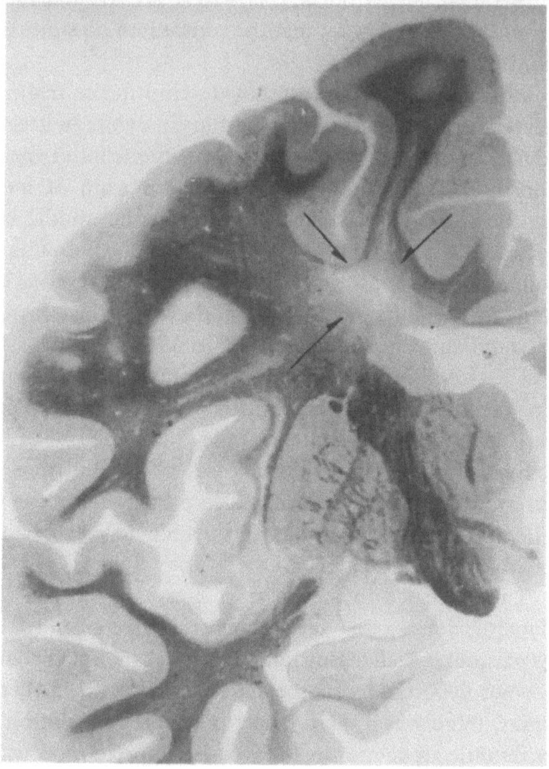

Fig. 6. Brain of a 23-year-old female suffering from aortic arch syndrome. Small focus of infarction at the superolateral border of the lateral ventricle (arrows) is shown

ventricular wall, and because the number of the capillaries is half that of the cerebral cortex (Kodama and Suzuki 1974) (Fig. 5). On account of the characteristic vascular architecture and the pattern of the blood supply, the deep portion of the white matter will be more affected than the cortex with its richer capillary supply and better blood flow, if any disturbance of blood flow exists on the proximal artery.

Figure 6 shows the brain of a 23-year-old female who suffered from aortic arch syndrome, in which there is chronic ischaemia due to progressive occlusion of the carotid artery. The changes of infarction are seen around the superolateral border of the lateral ventricle. From these facts, it naturally would be supposed that the focus of infarction occurred around the superolateral border of the lateral ventricle due to the chronic ischaemia in our five cases. However, it is not yet clear how the bleeding occurs. Either a haemorrhagic infarction might occur, or the small arterial wall in this focus might rupture on account of the change of arterial or venous pressure.

5.5 Cerebellar Haematomas

S. Kunze and W. Schiefer, Erlangen

Cerebellar haematomas may occur at any age. However, all larger statistical reports show a preference for the sixth and seventh decades. Data about the incidence of this lesion vary. Of all intracranial haematomas, 5% – 10% are located in the cerebellum. This corresponds to the proportion of the brain that the cerebellum occupies in relationship to the entire contents of the skull.

Most cerebellar haematomas develop in the region of the dentate nucleus. However, these haematomas seldom remain within the white matter. As a rule, the blood clot perforates the fourth ventricle or breaks into the subarachnoid space (Schiefer 1972). The demonstration by Dinsdale (1964) shows the close relationship of most cerebellar haematomas to the fourth ventricle (Fig. 1). The black region in the middle is affected most often, while the hatched section is less commonly the site of such haematomas. Only 3 of 53 cerebellar haematomas were found in the vermis, according to Dinsdale (1964). Thirty were located in the left hemisphere and only 19 in the right. This preference for the left side has also been observed by other authors (Hyland and Levy 1954; Rey-Bellet 1960).

The lateral projection shows the previously mentioned preferred localization in the region of the dentate nucleus (Fig. 2). The artery of the dentate nucleus, a branch of the superior cerebellar artery, is thought to play the same role in cases of hypertensive haemorrhages as the lenticulostriate arteries do in cases of haemorrhage into the basal ganglia. Branches of the inferior cerebellar artery may also participate in the blood supply of the dentate nucleus (Fig. 3). However, it is usually impossible to identify the actual source of the haematoma at operation or autopsy.

The preferred incidence at a later stage in life emphasizes the important role of arterial hypertension in the development of cerebellar haematomas. In a survey of such cases by McKissock, Richardson and Walsh (1960), Dinsdale (1964) and Norris, Eisen and Branch (1969), hypertension is the aetiological factor in three-quarters of the cases (Table 1). In nine cases, there was a disturbance in blood coagulation or the patient was undergoing treatment with anticoagulants. In some cases, hypertension was also present.

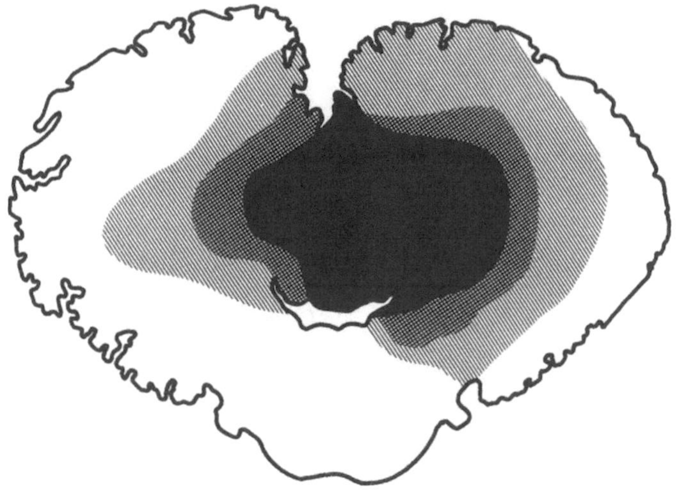

Fig. 1. Extension of cerebellar haematomas with relationship to the fourth ventricle and subarachnoid space. Black area represents greatest frequency of haemorrhage, cross-hatching shows moderate involvement (Dinsdale 1964)

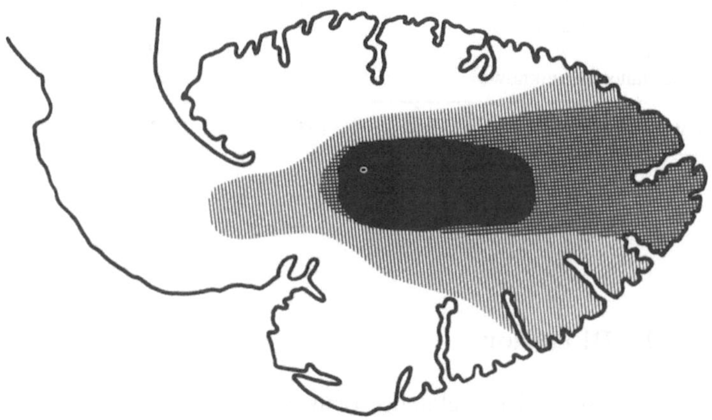

Fig. 2. The lateral projection shows the preferred localization in the region of the dentate nucleus (Dinsdale 1964)

In ten cases, an angioma or an aneurysm was found to be the cause of the haematoma and in two cases reported by Norris et al. (1969), metastatic tumours were the source of the haematoma. In the remaining seven cases, different causes such as micro-angiomas, acute infections or diabetes were mentioned. In some cases no cause could be found for the blood clot.

In summary, it may be said that the same aetiological factors play a role in cases of cerebellar haematomas as for cerebral haemorrhage. The hypertensive haemorrhages are usually found in the region of the dentate nucleus. Haematomas due to other causes are located in the vermis or else very lateral in the cerebellar hemisphere.

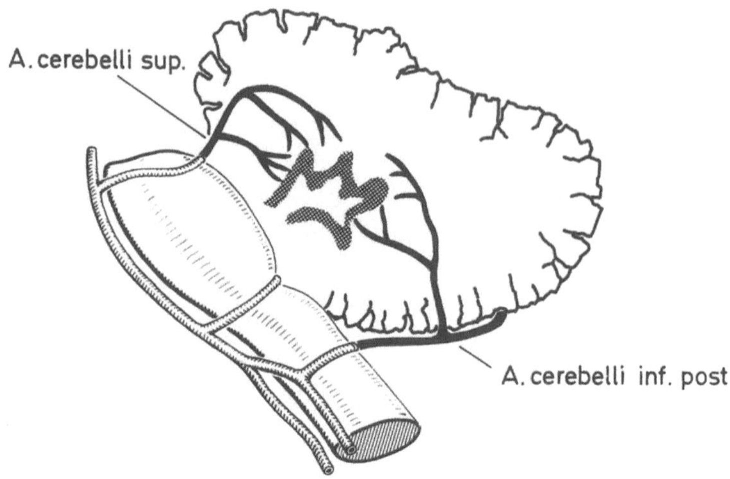

Fig. 3. Blood supply of the dentate nucleus

Table 1. Aetiology of cerebellar haematomas

Hypertension	77	73.3%
Bleeding disorder or anticoagulants	9	8.6%
Angioma, aneurysm	10	9.5%
Tumour	2	1.9%
Miscellaneous, unknown	7	6.7%
Total	105	100%

5.5.1 Discussion

L. Calliauw and I. Dehaene, Bruges

Intracerebellar haematomas of post-traumatic origin and haematomas due to a ruptured aneurysm or to an angioma, are excluded from this discussion.

The other spontaneous intracerebellar haematomas are commonly called "hypertensive" haematomas, as arterial hypertension seems to be the most common associated factor. Some authors believe that as many as 70% of all spontaneous intracerebellar haematomas are due to arterial hypertension (Brennen and Bergland 1977; Fisher et al. 1965; Freeman et al. 1973; Ott et al. 1974; Richardson 1972; Sano et al. 1964; Yoshida et al. 1978). However, in the large post-mortem series of Cole and Yates (1967), 100 cases were normotensive and 100 were hypertensive, according to their criteria of hypertension.

In our own series of 12 cases, there was only one case where a history of significant arterial hypertension was obtained. We have performed a post-mortem examination on each of the eight patients who died.

Case Reports

With Post-Mortem Examination

A 45-year-old male showed marked nephrosclerosis, possibly indicating unrecognized, and therefore untreated, hypertension.

One patient, a 77-year-old male, had arteriolosclerosis.

One patient had a blood dyscrasia, resulting in a chronic evolution with multiple haemorrhages.

In three patients there was a serious, but undiagnosed, infection. The most relevant example is that of a boy of 10 years. He was apparently in good health until one day at school, he had an acute onset of headache, followed quickly by deep coma. He was brought to our department, but died soon after admission. The post-mortem examination revealed an intracerebellar haematoma and also a severe purulent pericarditis and a purulent bronchopneumonia of earlier date than the onset of the haemorrhage. The two other patients also had a severe untreated infection (one chronic hepatitis with acute pancreatitis and one severe bronchopneumonia).

In these three patients there were no signs of intracerebral septic emboli or of intracerebral infection. Presumably the septic state produced a coagulopathy.

Only in two cases was there no demonstrable cause for the lesion and the history was not relevant.

With Operative Verification

Of four operated cases, three lacked any obvious predisposing factor for their haemorrhage. Of these three, one was the patient with the marked hypertension already mentioned.

Location

Two small haematomas were located in the dentate nucleus. The case of blood dyscrasia, and two of the three cases with infection, had multiple older haemorrhages in different parts of the brain. The other cases had large haematomas, mostly unilateral, sometimes ruptured into the fourth ventricle, without any precise origin of the bleeding. It is known that a micro-angioma can be destroyed by the haematoma.

Conclusion

Spontaneous haematomas in the cerebellum result from fragility of the blood vessels. This can be due to arteriolosclerosis, micro-angioma, infections, coagulopathy and hypertension. The presence of raised blood pressure is an additional factor. In our series, arterial hypertension was not the most frequent cause of the haemorrhage.

5.6 Spontaneous Brain Stem (Pontine) Haematomas

K. Sano and C. Ochiai, Tokyo

Spontaneous or primary brain stem haemorrhage excludes those haemorrhages associated with trauma, tumours, blood dyscrasia, aneurysms, clearly demonstrated arteriovenous malformations and Duret haemorrhage. Therefore, this paper deals with hypertensive or possibly hypertensive haemorrhage and haemorrhage caused by cryptic vascular malformations. These haemorrhages occur in various parts of the brain stem, but almost exclusively in the pons, although the haemorrhage may extend to the midbrain or to the diencephalon.

Pontine haemorrhages were reported to account for 6% of all intracranial spontaneous haemorrhages in autopsy material (Dinsdale 1964). In the era of computed tomography (CT), however, this percentage will probably decrease, because non-fatal haemorrhages in other sites will be increasingly disclosed. In one of our affiliated community hospitals, Aizu Central Hospital, pontine haemorrhages were found in 3% of all hypertensive haemorrhages in the CT.

From 1975 to 1978, 25 cases of spontaneous pontine haemorrhage (23 males and 2 females) were encountered in our clinic and our associated hospitals. Of these 25 cases, 23 were in patients over the age of 40 and among these, ten were known to have had hypertension prior to the haemorrhage. In the other 13 patients the blood pressure prior to the haemorrhage was unknown. There were two patients between the ages of 30 and 40; one had malignant hypertension, and the other had a small vascular malformation in the pons.

The latter case, a 32-year-old male, felt discomfort in the head during sleep and was found on waking to have a left-sided hemiparesis and hemihypaesthesia. Nausea and vomiting then appeared, accompanied by diplopia. He was fully conscious during the whole course of his illness. Positive contrast ventriculography revealed a small mass protruding from the floor of the fourth ventricle (Fig. 1). Operation was performed in the end of the 3rd week and a small subendymal haematoma, 1 cm in diameter, was removed. Histological examination showed a small arteriovenous malformation (Fig. 2). This patient is now well and working, 4 years after operation.

A similar case in 1970 (therefore not included in the present series) involved a 33-year-old male. He had right-sided hemiparesis and hemihypaesthesia and gradually developed difficulty in swallowing, dysarthria, left facial palsy and nystagmus. Operation was performed 6 weeks later and a small pontine haematoma was removed. However, he had a massive gastro-intestinal haemorrhage 3 days later and died. Autopsy disclosed a pontine haematoma (Fig. 3) caused by capillary telangiectasia (Fig. 4).

Therefore, in case of pontine haemorrhage without hypertension and below the age of 40, small, cryptic vascular malformations should be suspected as the cause.

Hypertensive pontine haemorrhage is reported to arise primarily from distal portions of the penetrating paramedian branches of the basilar artery and located at first near the junction of the basis pontis and the tegmentum (Dinsdale 1964). Nakajima et al. (1977) reported that these pontine vessels are similar to the lenticulostriate arteries in that the media is thin, the lumen is relatively large and the length from the basilar artery is relatively short.

Ooneda (1970) reported that vessels of this kind will receive greater tension to the wall from the blood pressure for the following reasons: $T = p \frac{r}{W}$ (Frank-Laplace). Here, T is the tension affecting the vessel wall, p is the intraluminal pressure, r is the inner radius, W is the

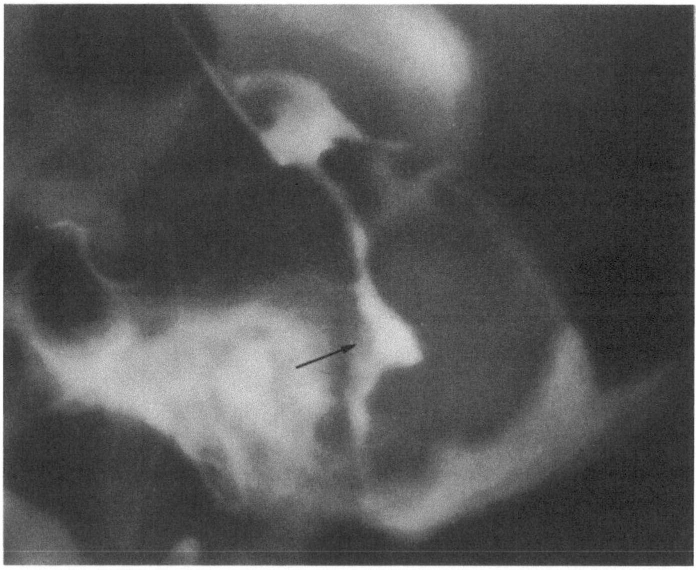

Fig. 1. Ventriculogram with small mass protruding from the floor of the fourth ventricle (arrows)

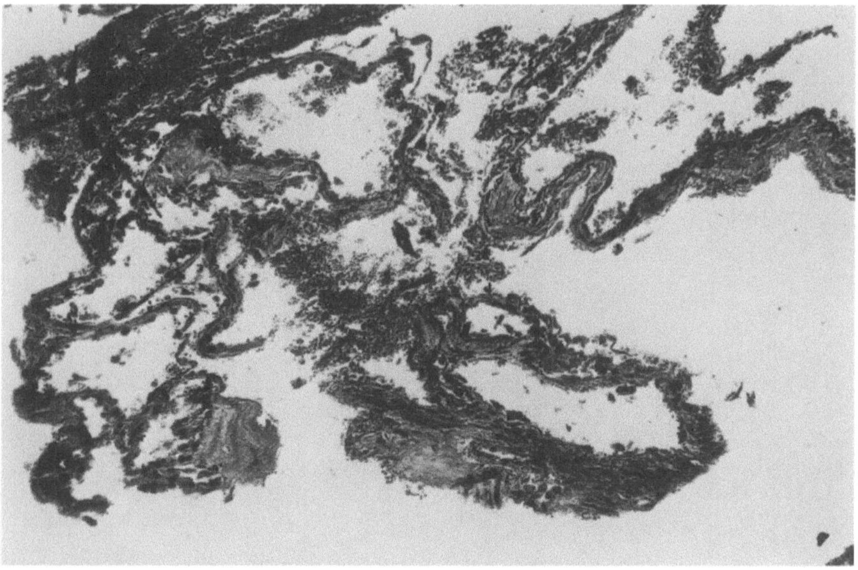

Fig. 2. Small arteriovenous malformation of the pons (see Fig. 1)

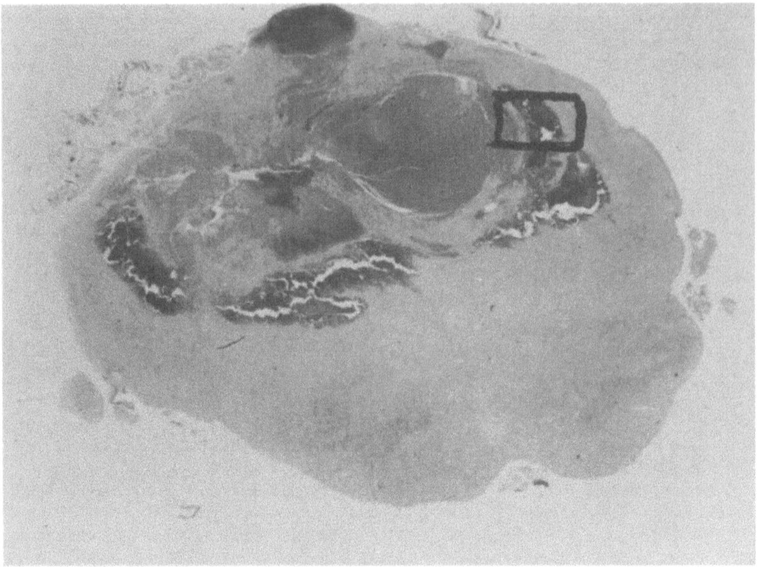

Fig. 3. Autopsy of the pons with pontine haematoma caused by a capillary telangiectasis

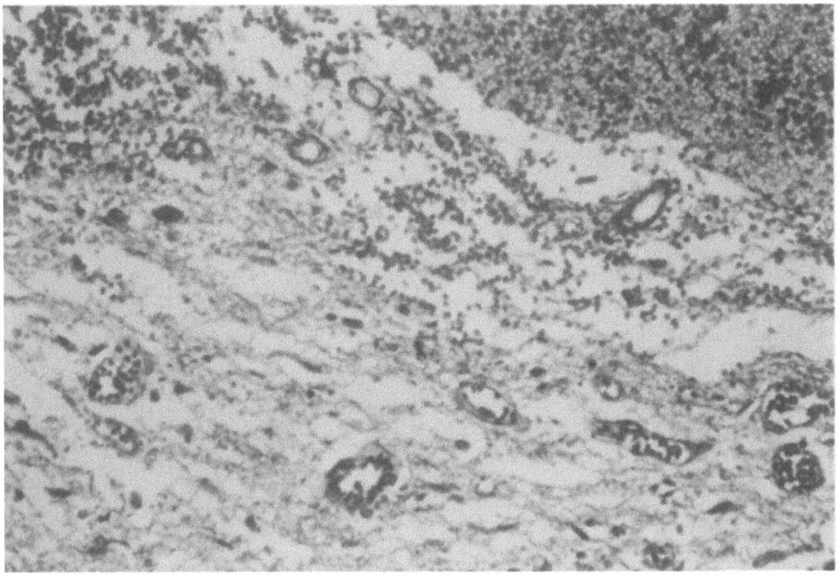

Fig. 4. Histological findings of a capillary telangiectasis (see Fig. 3)

thickness of the vessel wall. If r is large and W is thin and p is high, T must be large enough to distend the vessel wall and to cause angionecrosis, micro-aneurysms and, finally, rupture.

Besides, $\Delta P = \frac{8\eta l Q}{\pi r^4}$ (Hagen-Poiseuille).

Here, ΔP is the decrease of pressure at any length from the origin, η is viscosity of blood, l is the length of the vessel and Q is the quantity of blood. If r is large and l is relatively short, ΔP will be small and, therefore, hypertension (P) in the basilar artery will be kept in the distal portion of the perforating branches ($p = P - \Delta P$). Probably this explains why hypertensive haemorrhage in the brain stem occurs mostly in the pons.

According to Cole and Yates (1967a), the pons and the cerebellum are two sites of predilection for micro-aneurysms, outside of the cerebrum, although they are inclined to deny their causal relationship to hypertensive haemorrhage (1967b). Nakajima et al. (1977) and Fisher (1972) reported micro-aneurysms or bleeding globes surrounding pontine haematomas. Our micropaque injection studies also showed a micro-aneurysm-like globe surrounding the haematoma (Fig. 5).

Pontine haematomas rarely extend into the medulla, but may extend upward to the mesencephalon and the diencephalon (Dinsdale 1964). This is also true with our cases. The reason may probably be explained by the nerve fibre structures in the brain stem.

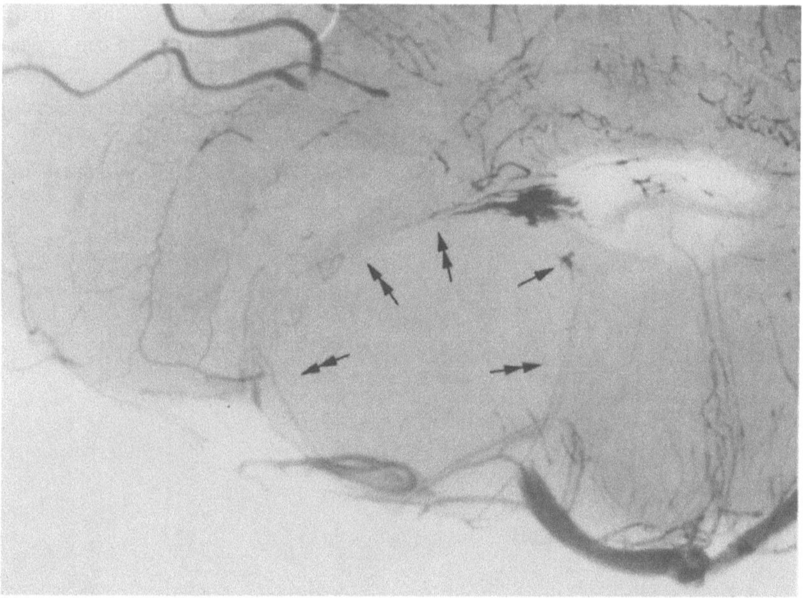

Fig. 5. Micropaque injection with a micro-aneurysm-like globe (single arrow) surrounding the haematoma (double arrows)

5.6.1 Primary Brain Stem Haematoma

C. Arseni and A. Gontea, Bucharest

Primary brain stem haematoma, a rarely diagnosed entity in the vascular pathology of the brain, raises problems in diagnosis and treatment.

Over the period 1935 – 1978 we dealt with three cases of primary brain stem, 25 of primary cerebellar and 336 of cerebral hemisphere haematoma. As regards the epidemiology, it appears that females predominate (2:1). All our patients were approximately 40 years old.

Hypertensive disease is of almost no importance in the causation of intrapontine haematoma. However, it is the main factor in 97% of patients with haemorrhage of the pons. In young subjects the haematoma is often secondary to a vascular malformation (we had five such cases; the youngest was aged 2.5 years).

Clinical Details

The first case was a male, age 43. Vertebral angiography was normal. On the basis of the patient's history and clinical picture a diagnosis of primary intraparenchymatous haematoma was made. The haematoma had a subacute course in two stages until operation. The haematoma was about 2 cm in diameter and 1 cm deep, situated in the lower part of the pons, that is in the upper part of the floor of the fourth ventricle. It was directed medially and yellow in appearance (Fig. 1). Through a 1.5 cm long and 1 cm deep midline incision, we came upon the haematoma. Most of it drained spontaneously, while the rest of it was removed by aspiration.

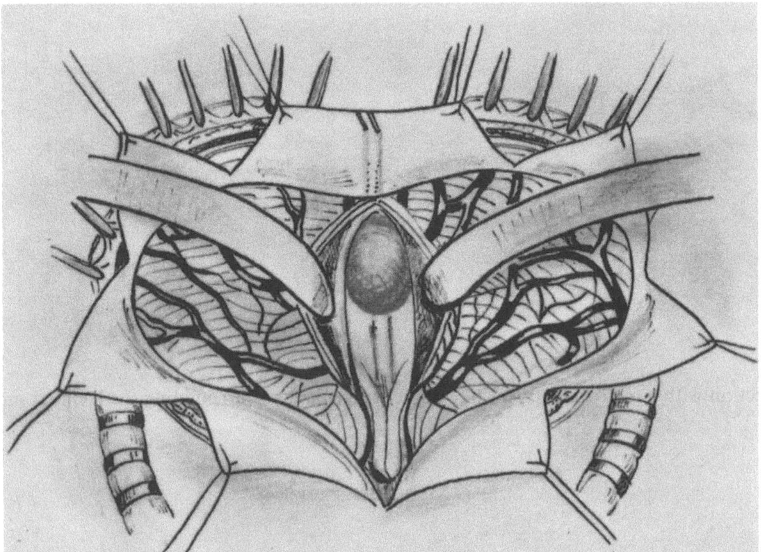

Fig. 1. Operative sketch in case 1, indicating an intrapontine haematoma in the upper half of the floor fourth ventricle

The second case was a 40-year-old female. On the basis of the history and clinical state consisting of onset of ictus, with two-stage subacute course and presence of a bulbar neurological syndrome, an intramedullary haematoma was suspected. Surgery was performed on the 3rd day after admission to hospital without the patient's being submitted to supplementary para-clinical examinations. Exploration of the floor of the fourth ventricle disclosed in its lower half, particularly on the left side, a violaceous-yellowish prominence with abreach in its centre spontaneously produced by the haematoma (Fig. 2). A left paramedian longitudinal incision, 1 cm long was made at that level to a depth of 1 cm, and a few clots (totalling 1 cc) were removed. The haematoma was about 1 cm in diameter.

The third case was a female, age 40. The diagnosis of tumour in the lower part of the brain stem was made on clinical grounds and after a slowly progressive course over about 3 weeks. At the operation we removed a round, 1.5 cm haematoma situated in the lower half of the fourth ventricle (extending up to the pyramidal decussation).

Discussion

There are very few reports in the literature on brain stem haematoma. Apart from our three cases, 14 cases of primary brain stem haematoma were reported. Most authors (Gros et al. 1948; Scoville and Poppen 1949; Dandy 1959; Tenuto and Cruz 1959; Paillas et al. 1963; Kempe 1964; Pouyanne et al. 1967; Koos et al. 1969; Obrador et al. 1970; Morin and Noterman 1971; Murphy 1972) have published one case each, two authors (Kowada et al. 1971; Papo et al. 1976) have published two cases each, while three cases were reported by us (Arseni). The first case was published by Dandy (1932). There were four cases of bulbopontine haematoma (Morin and Noterman 1971; Abrahams et al. 1971; Scott et al. 1973; Papo et al. 1976) and one of peduncular haematoma (Scoville and Poppen 1949), nine cases of haematoma in the pons (Gros et al. 1948; Tenuto and Cruz 1958; Dandy 1959; Paillas et al. 1963; Pouyanne et al. 1967;

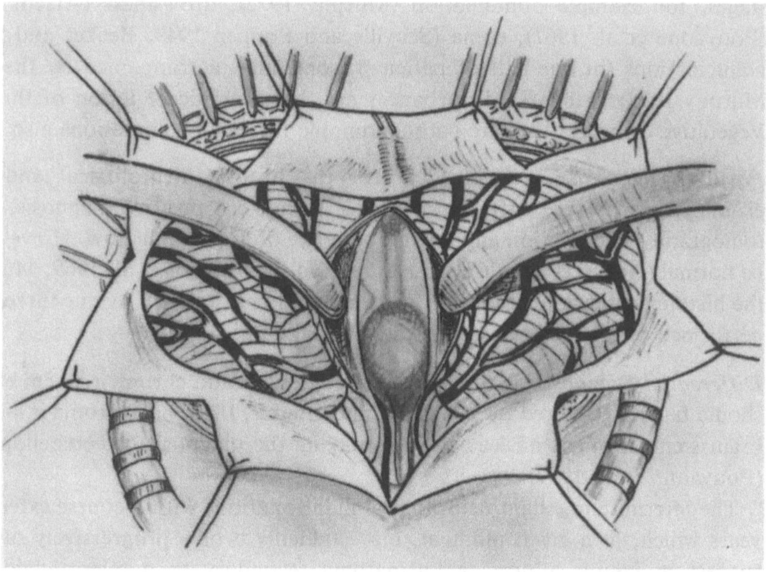

Fig. 2. Operative sketch in case 2, indicating an intrapontine haematoma in the lower half of the floor of the fourth ventricle

Koos et al. 1969; Murphy 1972; Kowada et al. 1971 – two cases) and three in the medulla oblongata (Kempe 1964; Arseni et al. 1967 – two cases).

Only one case was acute (Murphy 1972). The case reported by Becker and Silverberg (1978) was a haematoma secondary to an angioma demonstrated by a recurrence at 7 months when the patient was considered to have a small infarct; moreover, the case was not verified histologically.

Analysis of the history and neurological picture in our cases and in those published in the literature allowed us to draw the following conclusions:

1) The interval between the occurrence of the first neurological signs and the time of operation or death varied between 4 years (Dandy 1959), 3 years (Tenuto and Cruz 1958), 1.5 years (Scoville and Poppen 1949) and 1 year (Pouyanne et al. 1967), but in most cases the course was shorter than 3 months (Gros et al. 1948; Paillas et al. 1963; Kempe 1964; Arseni et al. 1967; Koos et al. 1969; Obrador et al. 1970; Kowada et al. 1971; Morin and Noterman 1971; Murphy 1972; Papo et al. 1976), and two cases were acute – 7 h (Becker and Silverberg 1978) or 1 day (Murphy 1972). The initial signs observed months or years before, reflected phenomena of vertebrobasilar insufficiency (in case of adult patients) or subclinical manifestations of micro-angiomas (in case of younger patients) rather than the formation of the haematoma. The time of formation of the haematoma corresponds to that of neurological signs which occur no later than 15–20 days after the blood extravasation. The course of the haematoma may be acute (3 days), subacute (below 2 weeks) or chronic. No matter what its form, the haematoma evolves progressively, in two stages, or it is static.

2) The clinical picture is polymorphous, which is characteristic of brain stem pathology. The variations in neurological manifestations depend on the brain stem segment involved, on the location (central or marginal) of the haematoma and on its volume.

It is not difficult to diagnose the site: There may be nuclear cranial nerve palsies, especially facial (16 of 16 cases), trigeminal and ocular paralyses (in one-half of the cases), hypo-acusis and disturbances of deglutition in a third of the cases. There may be pyramidal signs (14 of 17 cases), cerebellar disorders (one half of the cases) or alterations of consciousness in various stages, for example obnubilation (Murphy 1972), drowsiness (Arseni et al. 1967), stupor (Pouyanne et al. 1967), coma (Scoville and Poppen 1949; Becker and Silverberg 1978) and hallucinations (in one-half of patients), sometimes accompanied by fits (Arseni et al. 1967; Murphy 1972). All these disturbances are characteristic of lesion of the reticular substance. Vegetative disorders that are pathognomonic for brain stem lesions also may be found.

Positive Diagnosis: We consider that the history, neurological and cerebrospinal fluid examinations provide sufficient evidence to make a positive diagnosis. Certainly, computer tomography examination and angiography are of great value now. However, angiography may be normal (Arseni et al. 1967; Pouyanne et al. 1967; Koos et al. 1969; Murphy 1972), although the histological examination may show an angioma. In each of our three cases, operation was performed on the basis of exclusively clinical data.

Differential Diagnosis: If the course is progressive and chronic (Arseni et al. 1967), the lesion should be differentiated from a brain stem tumour. If the haematoma is localized laterally in the brain stem, it might mislead us into making the diagnosis of cerebellopontine angle tumour (Pouyanne et al. 1967).

The intermittent, slight neurological manifestations with a course extending over months or years which, at a given moment, may suddenly evolve progressively or in two stages might suggest in young subjects a haematoma secondary to a micro-angioma or, in adults, a metastasis. It should be emphasized that brain stem haematomas in children are most often secondary to an angioma. We had three such cases (the youngest child was $2\frac{1}{2}$ years old).

The slight and diffuse early symptoms might suggest a diagnosis of multiple sclerosis, but the mode of onset and the pattern of the symptoms should enable one to avoid this error.

The most difficult differentiation to make is between a haemorrhage in the brain stem and a haematoma in the same location. These lesions are still frequently mistaken for each other, and this is probably the main reason why so few communications exist in the literature concerning primary brain stem haematoma. The clinical picture of intrapontine haemorrhage commonly includes major disorders of consciousness (coma in two-thirds of cases), disorders in the respiratory rate, pinhole pupils, hyperthermia, motor disturbances such as tetraplegia, rapid deterioration and death. In the earlier history the patient has high arterial blood pressure, often malignant. Comparison of the clinical manifestations in brain stem haemorrhages with the most frequent signs in brain stem haematoma shows major differences. Hence, the differential diagnosis can and should be made correctly in all cases. The confusion is increased by the possible existence of blood in the CSF in cases of haematoma, as occurred in one of our cases. Another two cases were reported in the literature with descriptions of the CSF (Koos et al. 1969; Morin and Noterman 1971). The explanation of subarachnoid haemorrhage is a simple one, namely leakage of some blood from the haematoma to the surface. In almost all cases the nervous tissue between the haematoma and the subarachnoid space is very thin. Sometimes the site of leakage can be identified at operation.

For differentiation of haemorrhage from haematoma, one should constantly bear in mind the criteria we show in the following table.

Table 1. Differential diagnosis between haemorrhage and haematoma

Disease	Lesion	Onset	Course	Therapy
Haemorrhage	Diffuse laceration Malignant arterial hyper-tension (50%)	Ictal	Towards death or progressive remission	Exclusively conservative
Haematoma	Localized	Evolutive, often in two stages	As in intracranial expanding process	Exclusively surgical

We considered a case to be a primary haematoma whenever no determining cause such as trauma, tumour or vascular malformation was detectable, angiographically or surgically, and the pathological examination indicated a pure haematoma, as in our above-mentioned three cases. We consider that the first case of Pouyanne (1967) and the cases of Lewin (1934), Teilman (1953), Scott (1973) and Abrahams et al. (1971) cannot be included here because angiomas were found in pathological examination. The case reported by Becker and Silverberg (1978) should also be excluded because no pathological examination was performed. On the other hand there are cases reported as haemorrhage (Scoville 1949; Kawado et al. 1971) which in reality were haematomas (Myers et al. 1961), especially from haemorrhagic metastases (Arseni et al. 1971), multiple sclerosis (Scoville and Poppen 1949; Abrahams et al. 1971), or more frequently from vascular malformations (Levin 1934; Bergman 1950; Grotts 1950; Epstein 1951; Teilmann 1953; Lindheimer and Barrows 1962; Watanabe 1963; Pouyanne et al. 1967; Scott et al. 1973).

Conclusions

1) Primary brain stem haematoma is an entity which at present is well delimited pathologically, clinically and therapeutically, and is probably more frequent than would appear from the literature.
2) Primary brain stem haematoma occurs as a well-delimited blood extravasation which increases in volume progressively, being expansive in character, unlike primary brain stem haemorrhage which is diffuse, infiltrative, associated with necrosis in the vicinity and only seldom remits spontaneously.
3) Histological examination of the haematoma and of the membrane of the haematoma wall is essential to exclude secondary haematoma.
4) Three clinical forms of primary brain stem haematoma have been described: acute, subacute (with the progressive, stationary and two stage variants) and chronic (which is progressive). The onset is sudden, of moderate severity, with cerebellar and pyramidal symptoms, nuclear cranial nerve palsies (primarily facial) and a special type of alteration of consciousness. All these disturbances should be kept in mind whenever we are faced with a vascular accident, so that we may give the respective patient the correct diagnosis and treatment.
5) The aetiology of primary cerebellar haematoma is not yet elucidated. Various predisposing, favouring and occasional factors were presumed to act on the vascular wall, but very often these cannot be detected either. At any rate, there is no high arterial blood pressure.
6) The incidence of positive diagnosis of haematoma depends on the clinical examination and ancillary procedures, such as laboratory examination, CT and angiography.
7) Prognosis depends on the clinical form, promptness of diagnosis and the experience of the surgeon. In spite of the location of the lesion the prognosis is surprisingly good.
8) There is only one possible treatment: early removal of the haematoma, intensive care and appropriate rehabilitation.

6 Diagnosis

6.1 Angiography in ICH

6.1.1 Differential Diagnosis of ICH

R. Lorenz and A. Agnoli, Giessen

The indications and contra-indications for operative intervention in intracerebral haematomas are, in general, dependent on their pathogenesis. For this reason, pre-operative investigations, particularly contrast studies, have a very important part to play. Computer tomography has enriched the process of diagnosis in many ways (Terao et al. 1979). However, even today in individual cases the assessment and differential diagnosis can still be quite difficult.

On the basis of our own observations and misinterpretations, we would like to indicate some of the difficulties that can arise in making a differential diagnosis.

Actual Identification of Spontaneous Hypertonic Haemorrhages

Even a prominent AV malformation which has ruptured can be made invisible by the local pressure of the haematoma.

A 35-year-old patient (No. 271137931) was admitted in a decerebrate state 3 h after an apoplectic seizure. The blood pressure was in the hypertensive range. The angiogram revealed marked slowing of the circulation over the right hemisphere, and a large space-occupying lesion was seen in the parietal region with a small tangle of vessels and an early draining vein. A repeat angiogram, undertaken to confirm the findings, still showed nothing but the slowing of the circulation (arterial phase only apparent in the 7th second) and an avascular area in the parietal region (Fig. 1). The rapid evolution of the signs of pressure between the two angiograms had led by compression to a complete obliteration of the AV angioma. An immediate craniotomy allowed the evacuation of a haematoma of more than 200 ml and the removal of the AV angioma.

The bulbar symptoms regressed post-operatively and the patient recovered slowly. Over the year, during which he was followed up, he still showed some psychological disturbance and a left-sided hemiparesis.

Therefore, in cases which develop very acutely, the actual time at which the angiogram is done may decide if the correct diagnosis is made. Marked local and generalized rises of intracranial pressure in these patients can lead to compression of even a large AV angioma. The rise of the blood pressure can be interpreted, in the presence of signs of decerebration, as a reaction to this situation.

We recently had a similar experience in the case of a 13-year-old child (No. 180765571), who was taken ill suddenly, with a loss of consciousness rapidly progressing to a decerebrate state. Angiography merely showed signs of generalized raised intracranial pressure. The CT scan indicated thalamic and intraventricular haemorrhage, and an increase of density in the region of the draining veins raised the suspicion of an AV angioma. It was not possible to do anything further for the child. At autopsy a large AV angioma was confirmed.

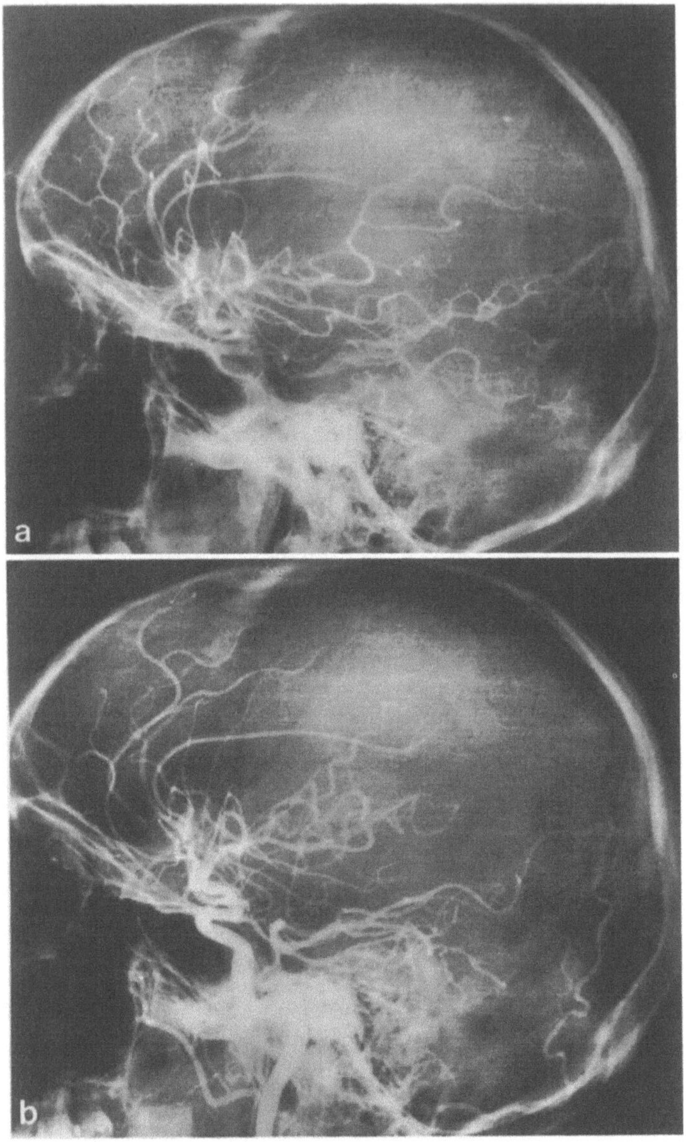

Fig. 1a, b. A marked local and generalized rise in intracranial pressure can lead to compression of a large AV angioma

Differentiation of "Micro-angiomas"

As compression of the vessels, either localized or generalized, makes even a large angioma invisible in the angiogram, in the presence of small angiomas whose compression is usually possible at an earlier stage, the angiographic demonstration of a "micro-angioma" is especially difficult. This has been pointed out by many authors during recent years. Laine et al. (1956) were probably the first to point out the possibility that so-called spontaneous intracerebral haematomas were due to rupture of micro-angiomas. Laine had reported in 1962 that a post-operative angiogram was absolutely essential, after the removal of a so-called spontaneous intracerebral haematoma, to exclude possibly vascular anomalies, which had escaped detection at the first investigation, on account of the local pressure.

A 40-year-old patient (No. 080938371) was admitted with raised blood pressure (230/140 mmHg), speech disturbances, right-sided hemiparesis, somnolence and mental slowing. The CT scan demonstrated a haematoma in the region of the left thalamus. In the first instance the angiogram only gave indirect evidence of a space-occupying lesion in the region of the basal ganglia. It was only in a control angiogram, 3 weeks after the haemorrhage, that the suspicion of a micro-angioma was raised. Later it was learnt from relatives and friends, that 20 years and 4 years earlier, the patient had suffered from a transient right hemiparesis. This information supported the diagnosis of micro-angioma, especially as according to the history, lower blood pressure values had previously been recorded.

In the above case it is evident that the resorption of the conservatively treated intrathalamic haematoma had made possible the demonstration of the micro-angioma. The hypertension must be regarded as reactive. The blood pressure subsequently returned to normal, after the resorption of the haematoma.

Differentiation from Tumours

A further important point in differential diagnosis of intracranial haemorrhages is distinguishing them from tumour.

A 15-year-old girl (No. 260659932) was admitted after a slowly progressive 4-month history, with extensive cranial nerve defects and spastic tetraparesis. The angiogram suggested an infratentorial space-occupying lesion, which in the ventriculogram was shown to be in the region of the floor of the fourth ventricle (Fig. 2). It was regarded as a brain stem tumour. Surprisingly, at operation there was a haematoma cavity, some 2 – 3 cm in diameter in the pons and medulla. No angioma was found on histological examination, although tumour was excluded. Four years later she is completing her professional training and shows merely a few cerebellar signs and a slight psychological syndrome.

Possibly, computer tomography might have enabled us to make a pre-operative diagnosis. Nevertheless, two further cases show the difficulties that can arise in distinguishing between intracranial and intratumoural bleeding, or in diagnosing a tumour when there is increased density in the CT scan.

A 21-year-old youth (No. 020657661) was taken ill with recurrent focal attacks in the left leg and left hand. When admitted 3 weeks later, he showed only mild mental disturbance and a slight accentuation of the reflexes in the left leg. The angiogram showed a right frontomedial space-occupying lesion, and the CT scan indicated a rounded lesion above and medial to the right lateral ventricle which showed practically no change after an injection of contrast (Fig. 3). A tentative diagnosis of a haemorrhage into a tumour was made and, as a differential diagnosis, a melanoma was considered. At operation a 2.5-cm haematoma cavity was found, just dorsal to the foramen of Monro, with small pathological vessels in the corpus callosum. A micro-angioma was confirmed histologically. The patient recovered rapidly and, at follow-up, showed no abnormalities.

As the shadow or increased density shown in the CT scan was not homogeneous, a tumour was initially thought of.

A further observation pointed in the same direction.

A 39-year-old man was taken ill suddenly, with giddiness and a sensation of numbness over the left half of the body. Later he developed ocular disturbances, which increased gradually, and other cranial nerves were affected. The angiogram showed a space-occupying lesion in the region of the midbrain and this was confirmed by ventriculography. The CT scan revealed an irregularly outlined area of increased density in the posterior part of the midbrain, i.e. the quadrigeminal region and pons, whose rounded shape and irregular borders suggested a metastasis (Fig. 4). At operation there was a haematoma cavity, 2.5 cm in diameter, whose wall contained pathological vessels. The patient recovered briefly, but died 14 days later from respiratory failure. At autopsy the haematoma in the pons was confirmed, and the micro-angioma was verified histologically.

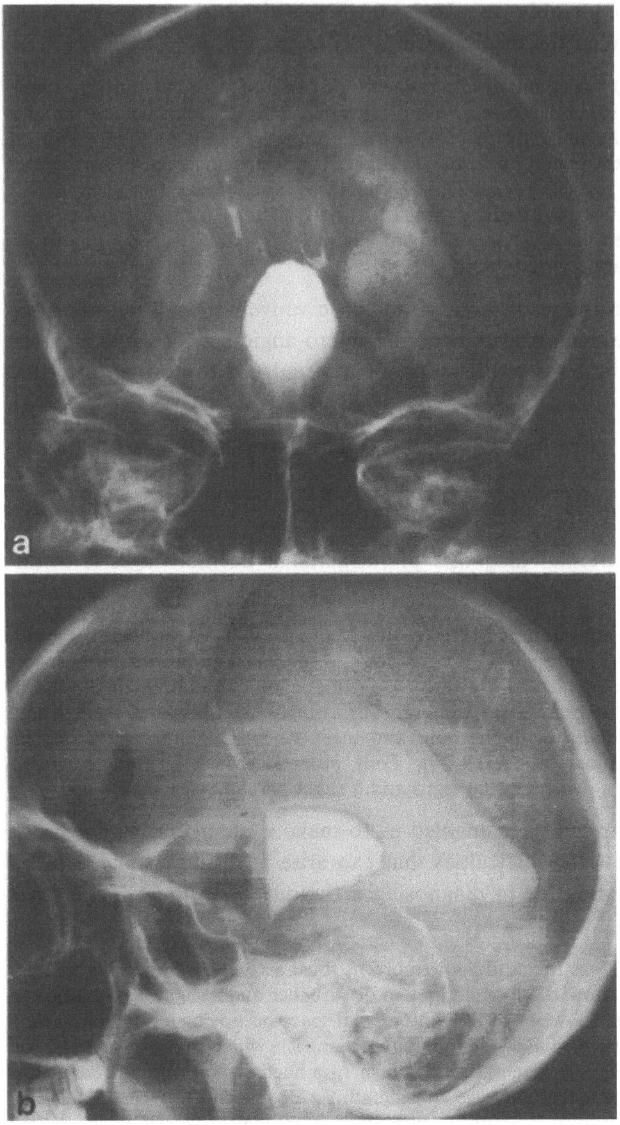

Fig. 2a, b. "Tumour" in the floor of the fourth ventricle, at operation shown to be a haematoma

An atypical location, a space-occupying lesion with rounded margins and a young patient would suggest the existence of a small haematoma from an angioma, in spite of a progressive course, with diffuse or irregular density in the CT scan.

Differentiation from So-called Arteriosclerotic Intracranial Haematoma

With advancing years the possibility is greater that we may be dealing with a so-called arteriosclerotic intracranial haemorrhage or, in the presence of vascular hypertension, that it is

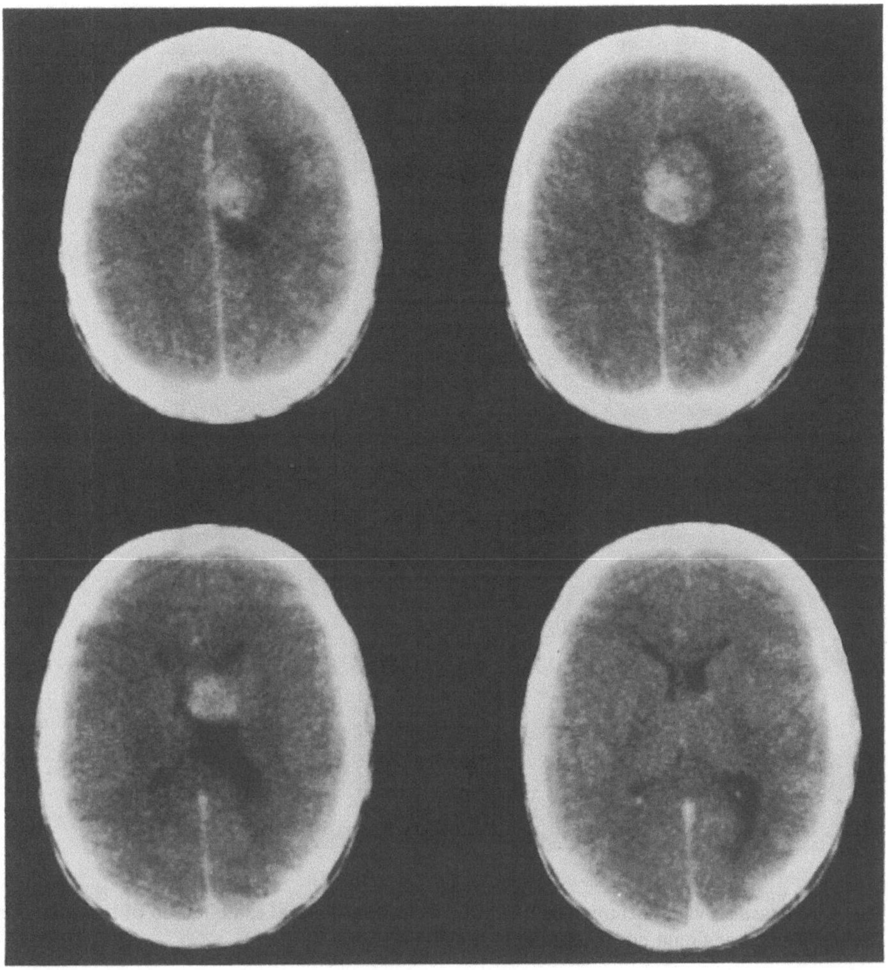

Fig. 3. "Intra-tumoral" haemorrhage, right frontomedial. Biopsy showed a spontaneous haemorrhage from a small angioma, which was not detectable in the angiogram

a haematoma resulting from this. As a rule, in these cases it is only the histological examination of the specimen that will allow an exact differentiation.

A 64-year-old man (No. 020803271) was admitted 17 days after an acute episode with headaches, giddiness and numbness, as well as constriction of the visual fields. The blood pressure was slightly raised. The angiogram showed a large space-occupying lesion in the left parieto-occipital region, and the air studies showed a downward displacement of the left lateral ventricle. At operation there was an intracranial haematoma with tamponade of the left posterior horn. An AV malformation was shown on histological examination. The post-operative angiogram gave no more evidence of the vascular malformation than did the pre-operative. The patient made a prompt recovery after the operation, although a homonymous hemianopia persisted.

In these patients the various contrast examinations were not able to establish the cause of the trouble, although the level of the blood pressure suggested that it was hypertensive in origin. Confirmation of the cause of the bleeding was only provided by the histological examination. The age and the slightly raised blood pressure (systolic 180 – 120, diastolic 110 – 70 mmHg) initially had made one think of a hypertensive haemorrhage.

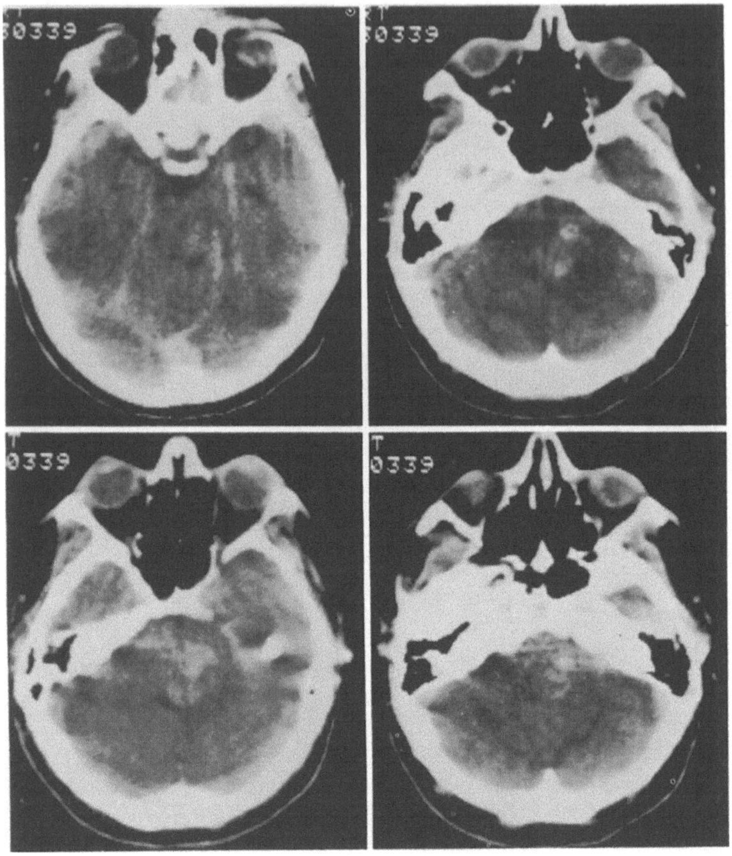

Fig. 4. "Metastasis with haemorrhage" in brain stem. Histological examination of the operation specimen showed a small angioma not detectable in the angiogram

Discussion and Summary

In spite of the improved diagnostic possibilities provided by magnification angiography and computerized tomography, the differential diagnosis of intracranial haemorrhages can be very difficult in individual cases. In many cases only the histological examination of biopsy or autopsy material will enable a conclusive diagnosis to be made. By paying attention to the age, the history, the site of the space-occupying lesion and the neurological findings and by painstaking analysis of the angiogram, the CT scan and, possibly, isotope scans, it will be possible in many cases to arrive at a correct provisional diagnosis, even pre-operatively (Luyendijk). At all events our observations show that even a progressive neurological picture over a long time and the irregular appearance of a space-occupying lesion of medium density in the scan, does not exclude the diagnosis of an intracranial haemorrhage. A consideration of the age, purely on its own, does not justify the conclusion that one is dealing with an arteriosclerotic or hypertensive intracranial haemorrhage. "Atypical" locations of haematomas strongly suggest the possibility of angiomatous haemorrhages. In many cases the actual time of the angiography is decisive for making the diagnosis; thus it is possible to be as much "too early" (compression of small angioma) as "too late" (compression even of a large angioma). A rise of the blood pressure, in terms of a "Cushing reaction", as a sequel to a rise of intracranial pressure must be distinguished from a true hypertension by a consideration of the history and course of the disease.

6.1.2 The Role of Angiography in the Neuroradiological Diagnosis of Intracerebral Haematomas*

L. Picard, J. Roland, J. Lepoire, and J. Montaut, Nancy

Introduction

Angiography was the most important neuroradiological investigation for the diagnosis of intracerebral haematomas before the era of computerized tomography.

Angiography was applied with the intention of providing answers to the following problems:

1) To reveal the presence of intracerebral haematoma. This haematoma could be diagnosed angiographically only indirectly. The diagnosis was based on such facts as the presence of an avascular space-occupying lesion, predilective site and clear clinical background. The margin for errors was large because a vascular space-occupying lesion could correspond equally well to a tumour. All neuroradiologists are well aware of the diagnostic problems posed by some intracerebral haematomas with the normal angiographic picture.
2) To determine whether the haematoma was "spontaneous" or whether it was secondary to the rupture of vascular malformation such as cerebral aneurysm or arteriovenous angioma. Over the years, it was shown that vascular malformations are a very frequent cause of intracerebral haematomas even in older people with arterial hypertension.
3) To define some physiopathological features of the space-occupying lesion such as possible existence of vascular spasm or delay of cerebral circulation connected with the presence of acute intracranial hypertension.

Since the advent of computerized tomography the diagnostic questions became modified in view of the fact that the existence of intracerebral haematoma could be demonstrated without any doubt by CT. Therefore, it was not astonishing that the question arose whether angiographic investigation is at all necessary. The aim of this report is to answer the question whether angiography is always necessary and if so in what circumstances.

This report is not based on upon statistical data. Some examples will be provided which seem sufficient to answer the question posed. If we exclude intracerebral post-traumatic haematomas which will not be analysed here, spontaneous intracerebral haematomas are usually secondary either to arterial hypertension in an arteriosclerotic patient or to vascular malformation, haemorrhage into cerebral infarct or tumour. It is worthwhile to analyse successively the different aetiologies to determine whether computerized tomography is able to provide sufficient information.

* In the CT pictures of this report the left side as seen by the reader corresponds to the right side of the cranium

Spontaneous Intracerebral Haematomas in Cases of Arterial Hypertension

Case 1: Mrs. B, aged 59, presented with diabetes, obesity, and severe arterial hypertension, treated irregularly for many years. On 15th October 1978, she developed acute left-sided hemiplegia with loss of consciousness and conjugate deviation of the head and the eyes to the right side. The CSF was blood – stained. Immediate computerized tomography (Fig. 1a, b) showed a deep intracerebral haematoma destroying the central grey nuclei. This form of haematoma is characteristic of spontaneous intracerebral haematomas in hypertensive patients. However, right-sided angiography performed immediately after admission (Fig. 1c) showed an aneurysm of the carotid siphon responsible for the haemorrhage.

This observation shows that the development of a spontaneous intracerebral haematoma in hypertensive patients may also be caused by vascular malformation. Computerized tomography is not in the position to reveal the aetiology of the haematoma – in this case the aneurysm – which could be demonstrated only by angiographic examination. We think, therefore, that there is an absolute necessity to perform complete angiographic examination as soon as the clinical condition of the patient permits.

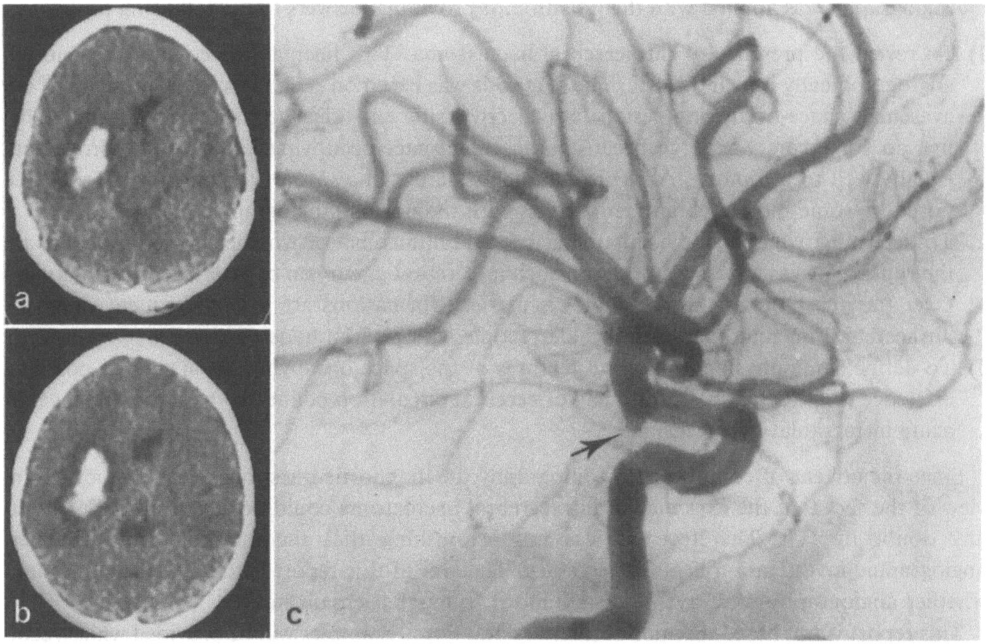

Fig. 1a – c. Spontaneous intracerebral haematoma in a patient with arterial hypertension, **a, b** Computerized tomography. Deep haematoma on the right side destroying the grey nuclei. Typical site of spontaneous intracerebral haematomas in hypertensive patients, **c** Carotid angiography. Lateral projection (subtraction). Small aneurysm (*arrow*) of the carotid siphon, the rupture of which was responsible for the intracerebral haematoma

The second case demonstrates the absolute necessity of performing an adequate and good quality angiography.

Case 2: A physician, 57 years old, presented with acute left-sided hemiplegia accompanied by an epileptic fit and severe headaches. There were no signs of subarachnoidal bleeding. Computer tomography showed right-sided central superficial haematoma with no signs of possible vascular malformation. Right-sided carotid angiography (Fig. 2) with enlargement and subtraction revealed a very small mycotic aneurysm responsible for the haemorrhage. This mycotic aneurysm, confirmed in pathological examination, presented therefore with acute signs without signs of infection.

The third case demonstrates that CT may be insufficient not only as far as the aneurysms are concerned, but also in cases of arteriovenous angiomas. A large arteriovenous angioma can be seen in computerized tomography usually because of the presence of calcifications and particularly because of the typical hyperdense zones with "vascular appearance" seen after the injection of contrast medium. However, in many cases, computerized tomography shows only the intracerebral haematoma, but no clues indicating the presence of an angioma.

Case 3: Mr. S., aged 55, presented with acute left-sided hemiparesis accompanied by headaches and vomiting. The CSF was blood – stained. Computerized tomography (Fig. 3a, b) showed a large haematoma in the right thalamus. Vertebral angiography on the right side showed that this haematoma was connected with a small arteriovenous angioma (Fig. 3c, d, e).

Analysis of these observations shows that computerized tomography is obviously insufficient for the diagnosis of vascular malformation such as aneurysms and even small angiomas. Taking into consideration the incidence of this malformation and patients with arterial hypertension it is necessary to perform routine angiographic examination in all cases, provided that there is no definite contra-indication.

Spontaneous Intracerebral Haematoma Due to Tumour

In these cases, CT may appear completely inadequate for diagnosis.

Case 4: Mr. P., aged 64, had a history which revealed arterial hypertension, myocardial infarct and gastric ulcer. He presented with acute subarachnoid bleeding and left-sided neurological deficit. Computerized tomography (Fig. 4) showed a large parietal haematoma on the right side. Right-sided carotid angiography showed pathological vessels characteristic of glioblastoma. The existence of this tumour could obviously not be demonstrated by computerized tomography alone.

Spontaneous Intracerebral Haematoma and Cerebral Infarct

The possibility of a large intracerebral haematoma discovered with computer tomography in patients who present with a vascular accident without subarachnoidal haemorrhage is well known. In some cases angiography proves that weare dealing with the alteration of a white infarct into a haemorrhagic infarct, as in the following case.

Case 5: Mrs. B., aged 44, presented with acute right-sided hemiplegia and aphasia. Computerized tomography showed a large deep frontotemporal left-sided haematoma with

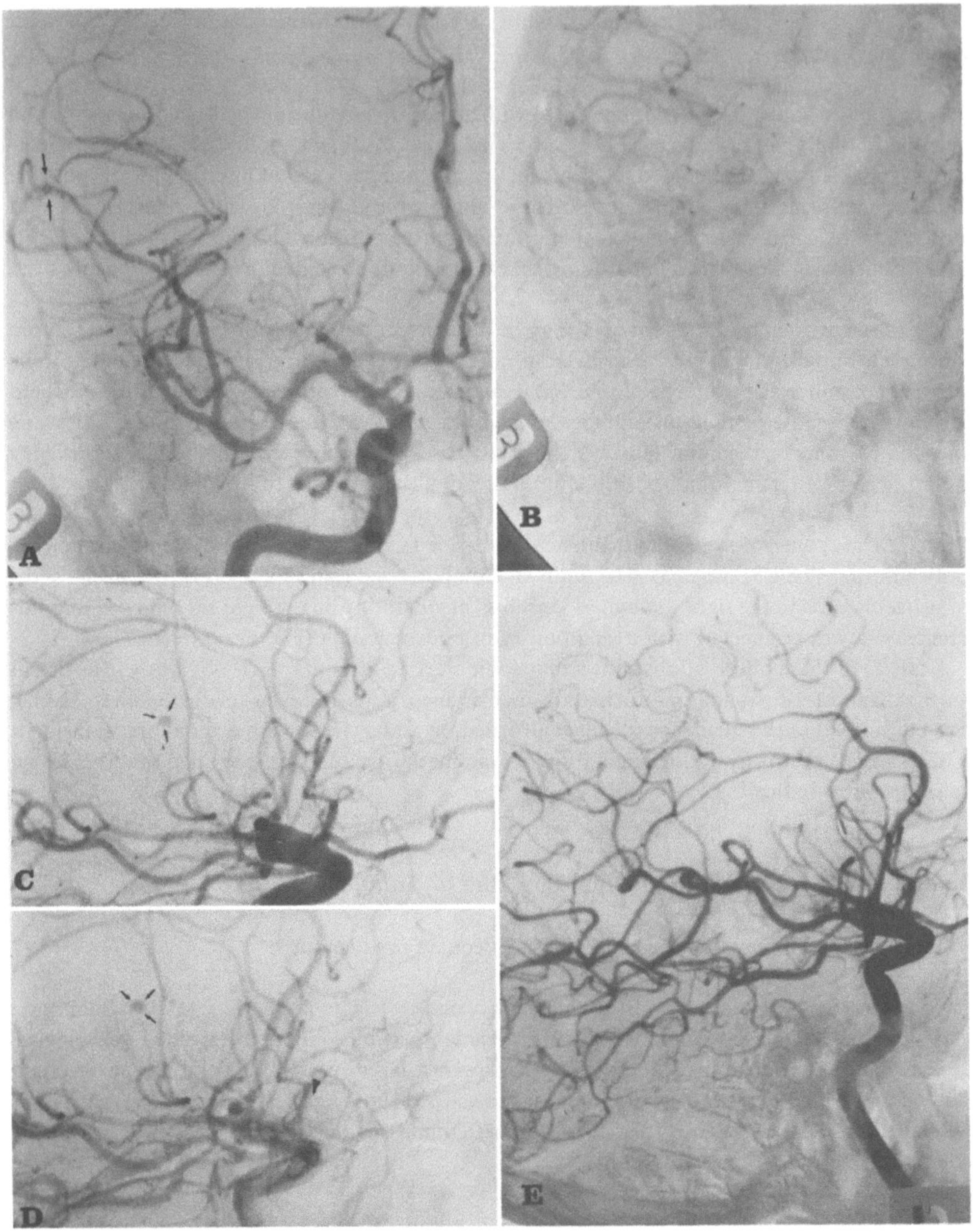

Fig. 2A – E. Intracerebral haematoma in the precentral region on the right side due to mycotic aneurysm. **A, B** Right-sided carotid angiography. **A – P** projection (enlargement and subtraction). There is a small distally located superficial aneurysm (*arrow*), **C, D** Right-sided carotid angiography. Lateral projection. The aneurysm (*arrow*) is located on a small supra-insular branch of the Rolandic artery, **E** Right-sided carotid angiography (postoperative). The malformation has been excised

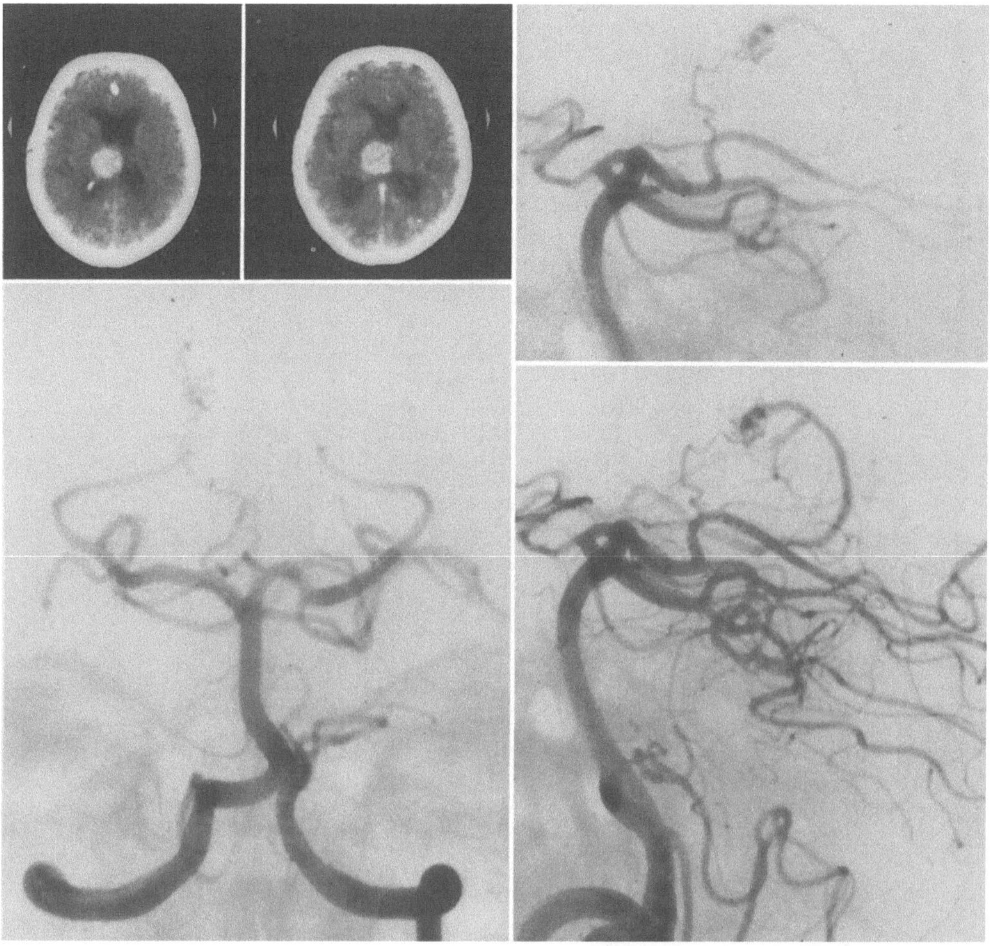

Fig. 3a – e. Thalamic haematoma due to rupture of the arteriovenous suprathalamic angioma on the right side. **a, b** Computerized tomography without contrast injection. Right-sided intrathalamic haematoma, **c** Vertebral angiography, A-P projection. Angiomatous vessel, paramedially, on the right side, **d, e** Vertebral angiography, A-P projection. Small arteriovenous angioma fed by the anterior thalamic branch of the posterior cerebral artery on the right side and draining through the posterior choroidal vein

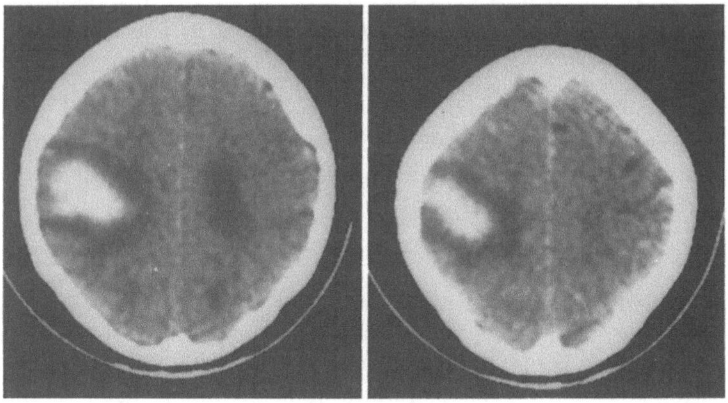

Fig. 4a, b. Haemorrhagic tumour in the right parietal region. **a, b** Computerized tomography without contrast medium. Large parietal haematoma on the right side surrounded by a hypodense zone which may correspond to oedema

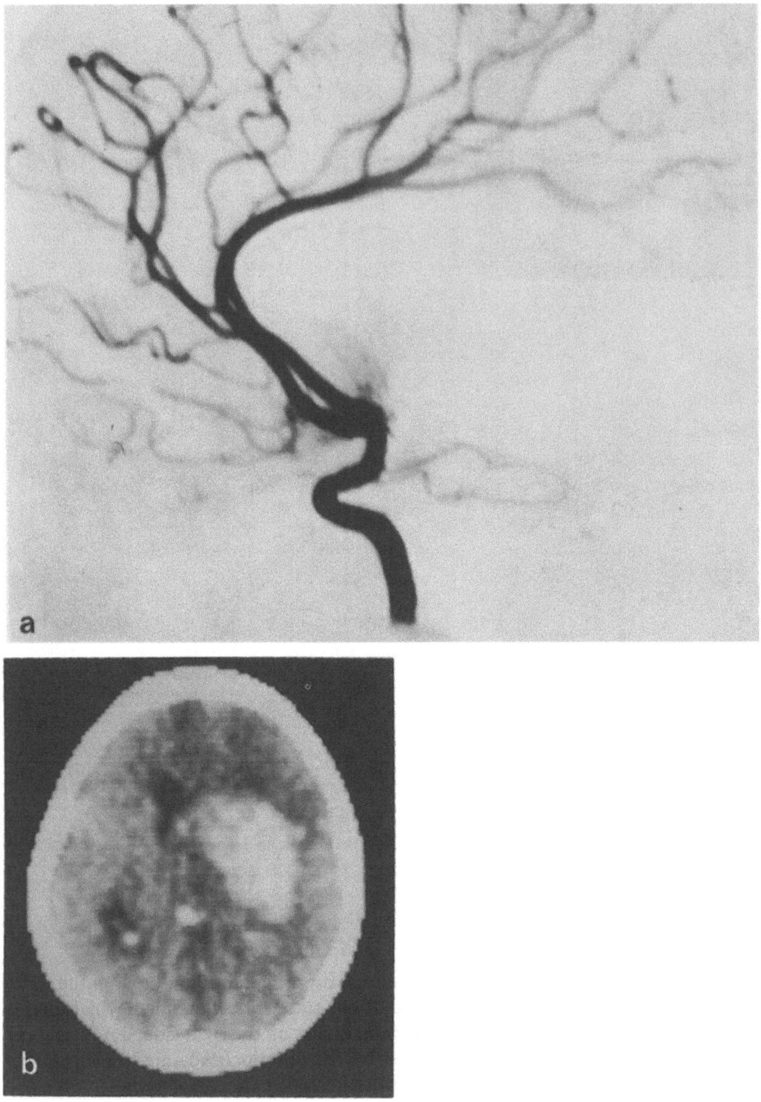

Fig. 5a, b. Intracerebral haematoma due to infarction. **a** Left-sided carotid angiography. Complete occlusion of the trunk of the left Sylvian artery at its origin, **b** Computerized tomography. Large intracerebral temporal haematoma on the left side destroying the central grey nuclei

intraventricular haemorrhage. Angiography revealed that this haematoma was secondary to the transformation of the infarction into a red infarct as a result of the occlusion of the middle cerebral artery (Fig. 5).

Conclusions

The physician is often asked to limit the diagnostic procedures because of economy and to perform only one examination which would permit the diagnosis and therapy. We have to ask ourselves whether such a demand is justified. Angiographic examination alone is obviously absolutely insufficient, not only because often it does not permit the diagnosis of the nature of the lesion, but also because there are difficulties in interpretation in certain sites particularly in cases of haematomas of the posterior fossa.

The cases described above show that computerized tomography is also often insufficient and does not permit a decision concerning treatment because of the inadequacy of information which is provided.

We think, therefore, that the neuroradiological investigations which are necessary in a patient suspected of having an intracerebral haematoma should include in the first instance computerized tomography. This investigation permits the diagnosis of the nature and the topography of the intracerebral haematoma. It has the enormous advantage of showing the possible accompanying oedema and also possible intraventricular spread of the bleeding. Computerized tomography reveals very small lesions, sometimes multiple, which are often completely missed by angiography. The second step is technically good angiographic examination using all the available possibilities to obtain the best information (selective angiography with catheterization, enlargement and subtraction). In some cases angiography may be avoided, usually with patients in whom this investigation is contra-indicated. Patients in whom operation is not contempleted because of advanced age or for other reasons, should not have angiography. The same is true for patients who present with malignant arterial hypertension. This should be treated first, before angiographic examination is performed. Also in some cases in which a haemorrhage occurs because of disturbances in blood coagulation (e.g. overdosage of anticoagulant treatment) computer tomography alone may be sufficient to diagnose intracerebral haematoma and to allow therapy to proceed.

6.1.3 Discussion

L. Picard, Nancy: I think that angiography is absolutely necessary in all cases where there is a possibility of treating the patient. The question is whether CT and angiography should both be done as in emergency.

H. W. Pia, Giessen: Every young patient with intracerebral haematoma should be studied by angiography. We have postponed angiography only in cases of absolute emergency and have removed the haematoma guided only by the CT findings. Such a patient will have an angiogram as soon as his condition permits.

B. Guidetti, Rome: With the establishment of CT scan our scheme has been changed. CT is performed immediately at the time of admission and repeated on successive days. Angiography is used only in those cases in which there exists the clinical doubt, although minimal, that the haemorrhage had been caused by the rupture of a vascular malformation.

6.2 Computerized Tomography (CT) in ICH

6.2.1 Diagnosis and Differential Diagnosis of Spontaneous ICH with CT Scan

E. Kazner, Munich, W. Lanksch, Munich, T. Grumme, Berlin,
and K. Kretzschmar, Mainz

Introduction

Computerized axial tomography is able for the first time to provide direct visualization of intracranial haemorrhages without risk or discomfort to the patient (Ambrose 1973; Baker et al. 1974; New et al. 1974; Scott et al. 1974; Kazner et al. 1975, 1978; Müller et al. 1975; Grumme et al. 1976; Kinkel and Jacobs 1976; Wüllenweber et al. 1976). The diagnosis of extravasated blood has become very easy by this new neurodiagnostic technique which is now indispensable in the management of patients with intracerebral haematomas and other space-occupying lesions. Even small haematomas of a few millimetres in diameter can be detected.

In many publications one can read that circulating blood normally cannot be seen in the CT scan because its absorption coefficient equals that of brain tissue. However, this is not the whole truth. Indeed, due to the partial-volume effect, blood even in the major vessels or sinuses usually does not differ significantly in density from the surrounding brain matter. But if circulating blood fills a larger area of a scanned slice, for instance in a big arteriovenous malformation, one can clearly see that blood has a considerably higher X-ray absorption than brain tissue. The example in Fig. 1 may serve as proof of this statement. It shows a giant aneurysm of the vein of Galen in an infant. The definitely hyperdense aneurysm area representing circulating blood is clearly visible before the administration of contrast medium. Such lesions would be more difficult to detect on plain CT scans in patients with low

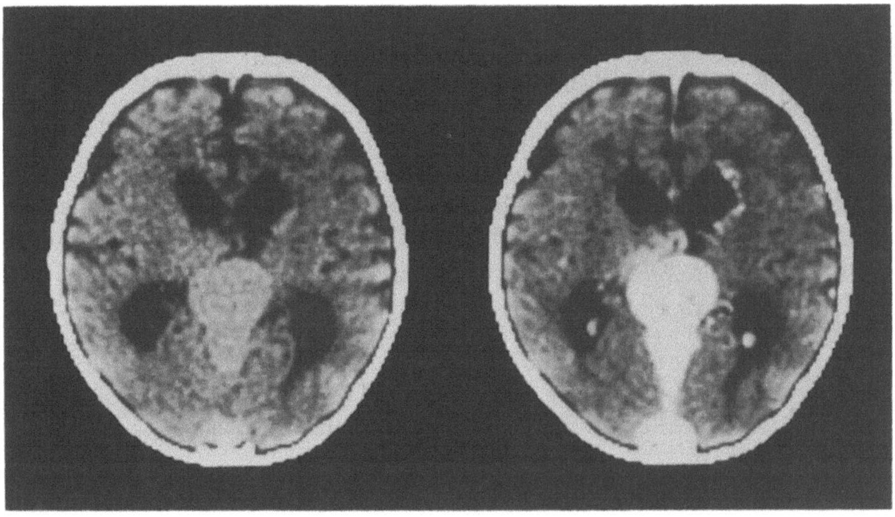

Fig. 1. Aneurysm of the vein of Galen in a 2-year-old child, demonstrating the high attenuation of circulating blood **a**. Significant increase in absorption after contrast enhancement **b**

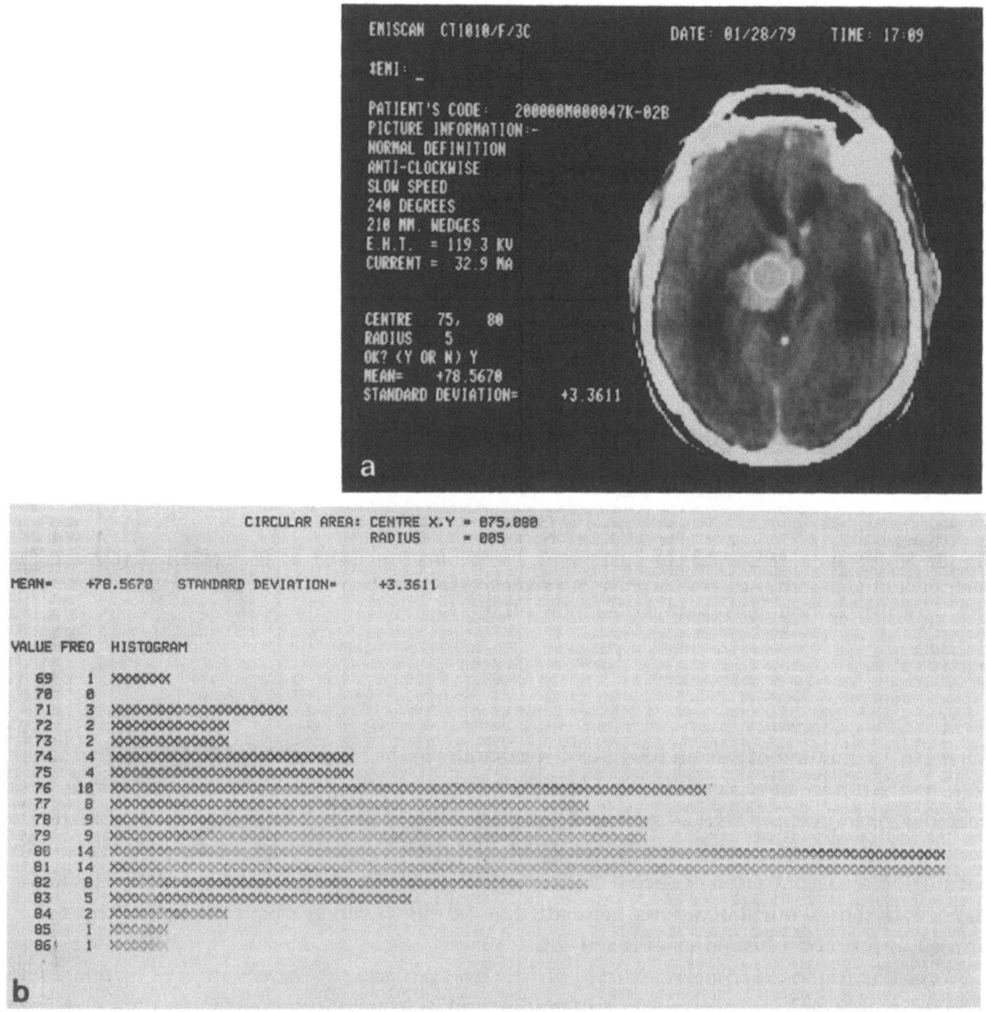

Fig. 2. a Attenuation measurement in the area of interest in a fresh blood clot (white circle). Mean absorption 78.6 Hounsfield units, **b** Histogram of the same blood clot as shown in Fig. 2a. The small standard deviation of 3.4 Hounsfield units points to a homogeneous haematoma

haemoglobin levels. In more severe anaemias a recent haemorrhage might not be distinguishable from surrounding brain tissue, since extravasated blood with a haemoglobin concentration of approximately 9 – 11 g % would have about the same attenuation as brain (New and Aronow 1976).

The attenuation of whole blood, haematocrit 45%, is 53 – 56 Hounsfield units, a value significantly higher than that of normal brain tissue, which is 30 – 38 Hounsfield units. Therefore, freshly extravasated blood within the brain, in the ventricles, in the subarachnoid spaces and the cisterns can immediately be recognized. Clot retraction following extravasation results in higher absorption values as the lower density serum is extruded, leaving a greater concentration of red blood cells (New and Aronow 1976). Thus, it becomes understandable that

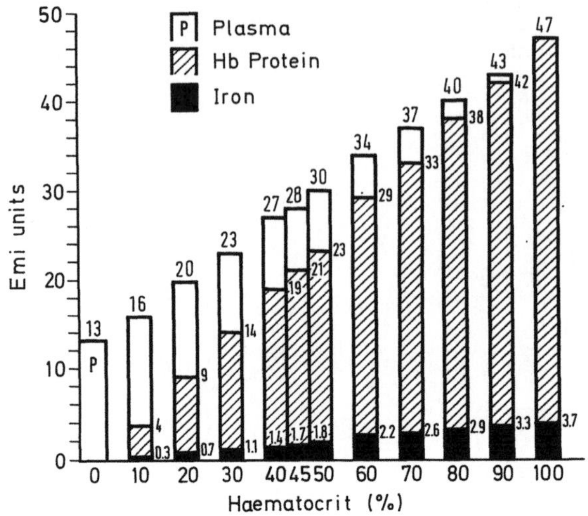

Fig. 3. Histogram showing the attenuation of whole blood at different haematocrit levels and the contributions of plasma, iron and haemoglobin to the total attenuation at each haematocrit level. One EMI unit = two Hounsfield units (New and Aronow 1976)

the mean attenuation of a fresh blood clot is generally in the range of 70 to 80 Hounsfield units. New and Aronow have demonstrated that a mean attenuation of 70 units corresponds to a haemoglobin content of 23 – 24 g % and one measuring 74 units, a haemoglobin concentration of 24 – 25 g %. An actual freshly retracted blood clot has a peak of 84 – 86 units. The haemoglobin concentration of such a clot reaches 26 – 28 g % and the haematocrit level is about 90%. With the aid of the computer these attenuation values can be calculated within seconds or printed in form of a histogram (Fig. 2a, b).

According to the experimental studies of New and Aronow, the attenuation of haemoglobin is based mainly on its protein constituent globin, and its iron content contributes only 7 – 8% of its total attenuation (Fig. 3).

Consecutive scans of intracerebral haemorrhages indicate that the absorption values rise in a very short period of time, corresponding to the formation of clot and clot retraction. In later stages the attenuation values decrease progressively.

Clinical Material

Our clinical experience with computed tomography in spontaneous intracerebral haematomas is based on 400 patients studied within the last 4 years in Berlin, Mainz and Munich. This group contains only patients with hypertensive haemorrhages, haemorrhages due to anticoagulant therapy or primary coagulopathy, verified micro-angiomas and spontaneous haematomas of unknown origin. Our definition of micro-angiomas is: "not visible in the angiogram".

An arterial hypertension was found in 45% of our cases; in 11% anticoagulative treatment or primary coagulopathy probably caused the haematoma. A micro-angioma was found in 5% of cases; in the remaining 39% the cause remained undetected. During the same period of time, 64 haematomas associated with an arteriovenous malformation and 126 intracerebral haematomas from aneurysms have been observed in addition, amounting to a total of 590 intracerebral haematomas.

The haematomas were found in the locations listed in Table 1. This distribution corresponds quite well to the reports in the neuropathologic literature. Haematomas within the basal ganglia, the thalamus, in the midbrain, the pons and the cerebellum amount to 58% of all spontaneous haematomas. Blood within the ventricles could be identified in 144 patients, or 36% of all cases, but in 57% of those haematomas within the basal ganglia and the thalamus. Frontal intracerebral haematomas, too, very often rupture into the ventricle (42%).

Fresh intracerebral haematomas are characterized as sharply delineated white areas (Fig. 4). After a few days the hyperdense haematoma is surrounded by a small zone of low density (Fig. 5). This low density is partly oedema or resolving haematoma, but most likely extruded serum. A finger-shaped oedema in the white matter develops only after several days at the

Table 1. Location of spontaneous intracerebral haematomas and frequency of intraventricular haemorrhage

Location	Number of patients	%	Intraventricular haemorrhage	%
Frontal	31	7.8	13	42
Temporal	50	12.5	2	4
Parietal	47	11.8	14	30
Occipital	31	7.8	5	16
Basal ganglia, thalamus	173	43.2	99	57
Midbrain, pons, cerebellum	59	14.7	6	10
Ventricular system	5	1.2	5	–
Multiple	4	1.0	–	–
Total	400		144	(36%)

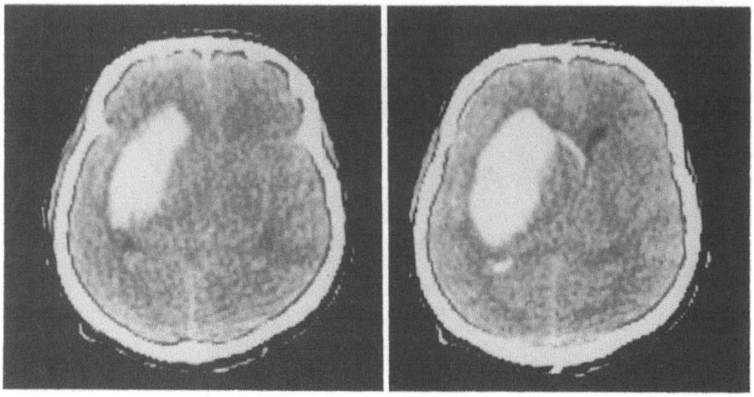

Fig. 4. Recent hypertensive haemorrhage in the left basal ganglia region, with penetration of blood into the left frontal horn

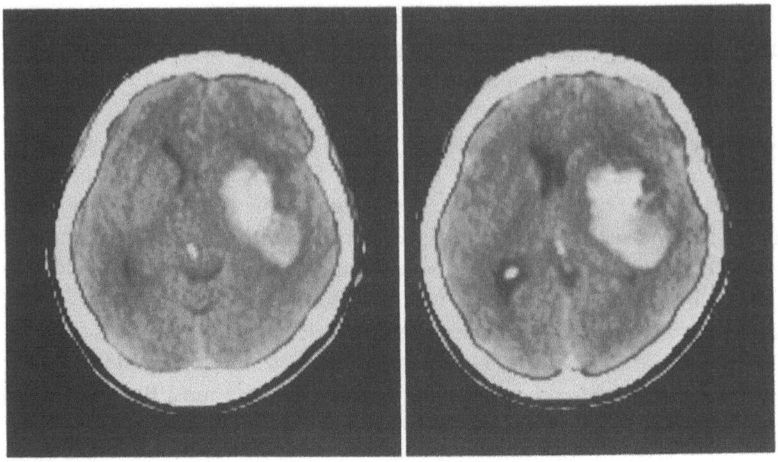

Fig. 5. Two-day-old hypertensive haemorrhage surrounded by a small area of low density

earliest (Fig. 6). A cockade-like or onion-like appearance of a haematoma suggests it has developed in several stages (Fig. 7).

Blood within the ventricles may exhibit different attenuation values. Clotted blood has the same absorption as within the brain parenchyma (Fig. 8). The attenuation of a CSF-blood mixture, frequently found in the occipital horns, is usually significantly lower; sometimes it equals that of brain tissue (Fig. 8a). Often a clear-cut border between CSF and the CSF/blood mixture is discernible. The accumulation of blood within the occipital horns is due to the sedimentation of blood cells in the supine position of the patient.

Ventricular penetration does not only occur with big intracerebral haematomas; even small globular haematomas may cause partial haematocephalus (Fig. 9). In a quarter of haematoma patients, there is blood in the subarachnoid space or the cisterns or both, mostly in combination with intraventricular blood.

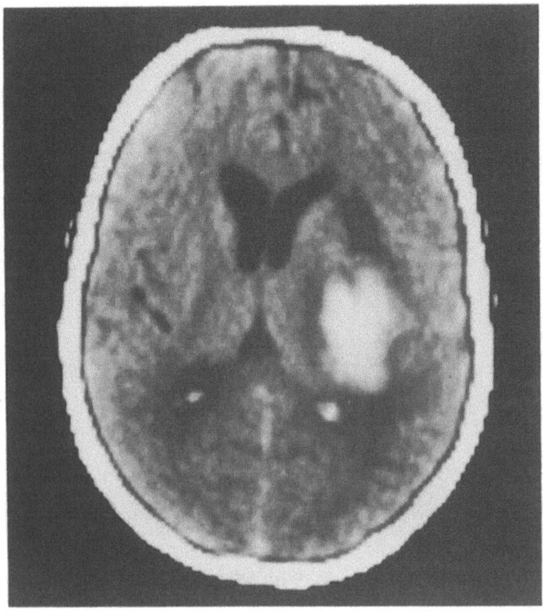

Fig. 6. Finger-shaped oedema in the white matter around a resolving intracerebral haematoma

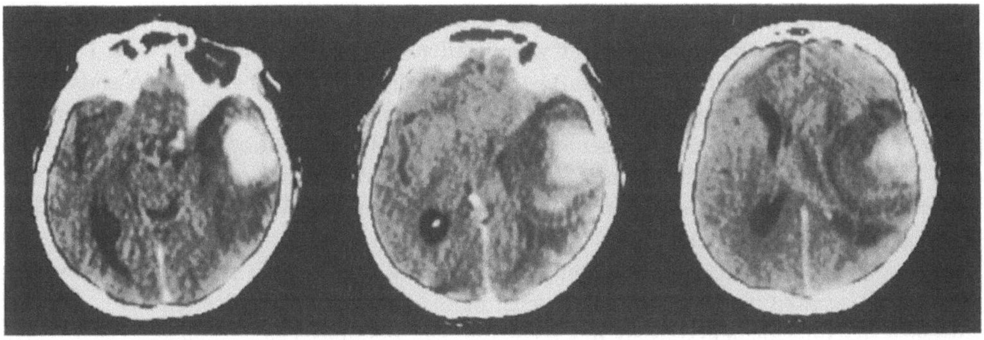

Fig. 7. Cockade-like aspect of an intracerebral haematoma, resulting from several haemorrhagic episodes

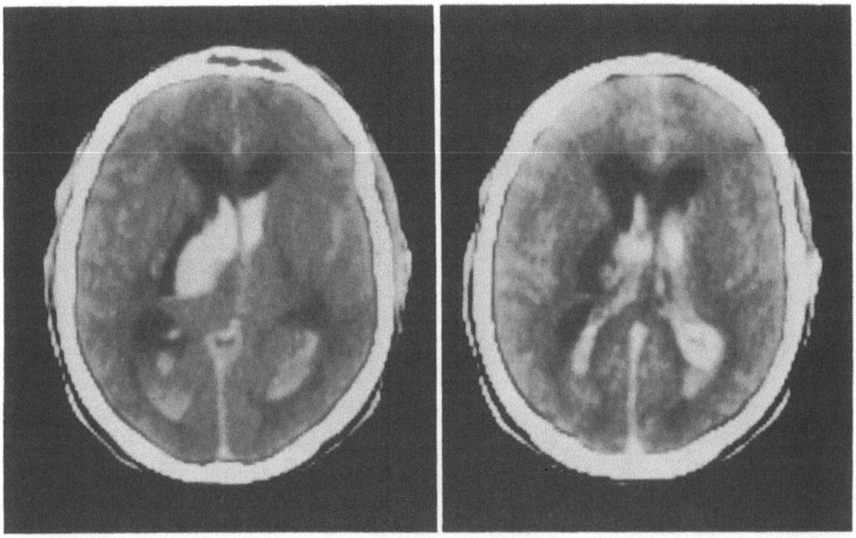

Fig. 8a, b. Intraventricular haemorrhage due to an AV malformation of the left choroid plexus. Clotted blood within the ventricles shows high attenuation values **a, b**. The attenuation values of the blood/CSF mixture within the occipital horns are significantly lower **a**

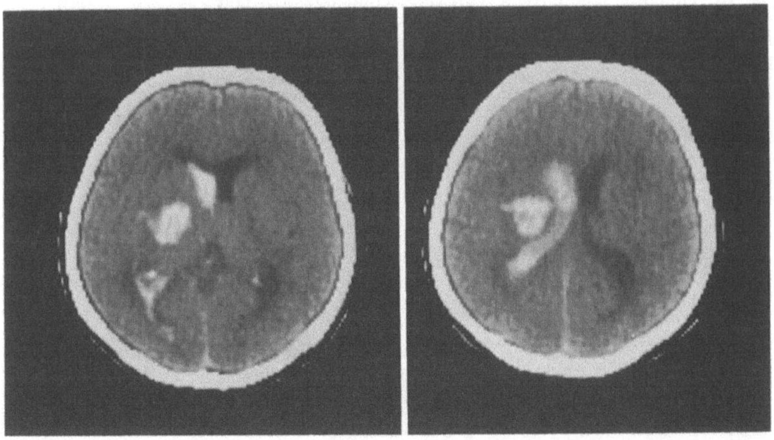

Fig. 9. Relatively small hypertensive haemorrhage with penetration into the ventricular system causing partial haematocephalus

The typical shape of a haematoma in the region of the basal ganglia is oval or oblong and is determined by the distribution of grey and white matter. In smaller haematomas the CT picture enables one to decide whether the lesion is located in the external capsule or the anterior or posterior limb of the internal capsule. In larger haematomas the exact origin cannot always be detected. The propagation of the haemorrhage follows the distribution of the white matter which obviously does not offer great resistance. The penetration into the white matter of the frontal or the parietal lobe follows the internal capsule. The penetration into the ventricular system occurs in a similar way.

In some cases, intracerebral haematomas seem to consist of several blood clots. However, this finding is caused by deep sulci which separate the spreading haemorrhage.

Isolated thalamic haematomas are much less frequent than basal ganglia haemorrhages (Fig. 10). Ventricular penetration occurs directly into the third ventricle with spread of the blood anteriorly and posteriorly. In one case we have seen a haematoma in the left cerebral peduncle extending to the thalamus. The cause remained undetected.

Pontine and cerebellar haematomas exhibit the typical shape and location as described by Dinsdale (Figs. 11, 12). In most cases of cerebellar haematoma the region of the dentate nucleus is involved.

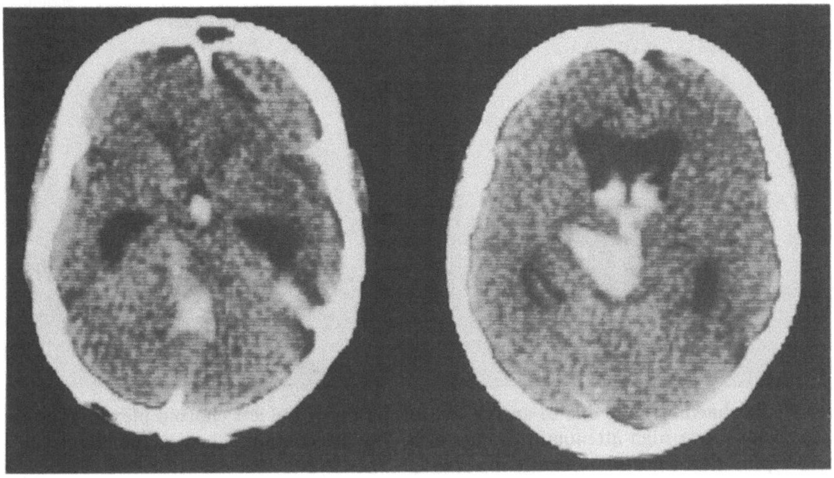

Fig. 10. Thalamic haematoma with ventricular haemorrhage

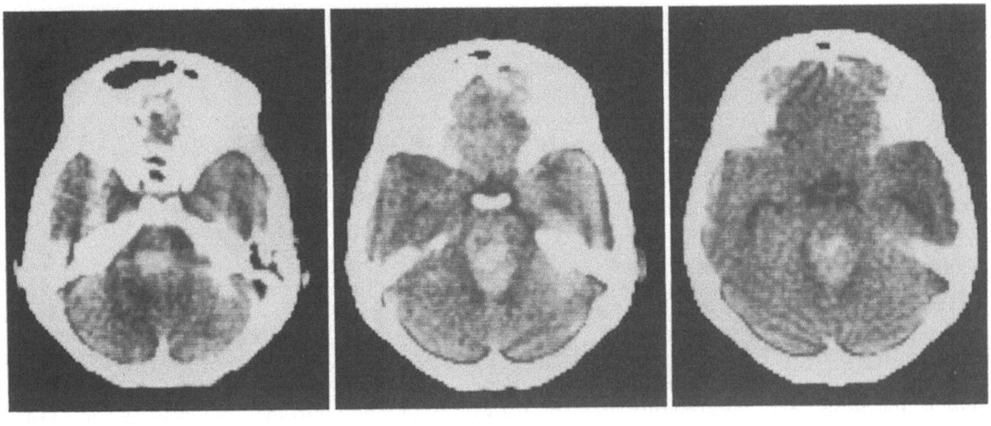

Fig. 11. Large pontine haematoma (operatively confirmed)

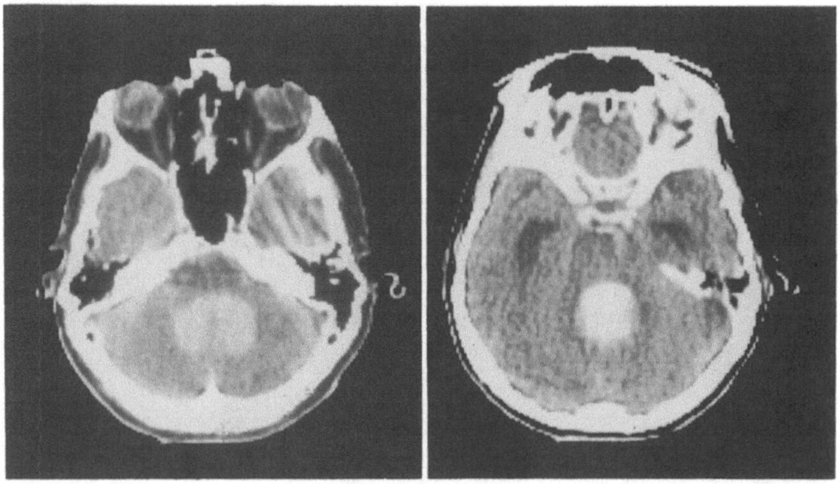

Fig. 12. Typical hypertensive cerebellar haemorrhage

Differential Diagnosis

When evaluating a CT scan which shows a hyperdense area typical of intracerebral haematoma as discussed already, some other diseases or conditions, apart from spontaneous hemorrhages, have to be considered in the differential diagnosis:

1) Intracerebral haematoma from an arteriovenous malformation;
2) Intracerebral haematoma from an aneurysm;
3) Haemorrhage into an arterial brain infarct;
4) Haemorrhage as a sequel to venous or sinus thrombosis;
5) "Chocolate cyst" (old unresorbed intracerebral haematoma);
6) Haemorrhage into a brain tumour (*glioma apoplecticum*);
7) Haemorrhage into an intracerebral metastasis;
8) Delayed or late post-traumatic intracerebral haematoma.

In haematomas near the cortex an AV malformation generally has to be considered. Figure 13 shows an example of a haematoma from a relatively small angioma of the right middle cerebral artery, with penetration of blood into the ventricles. In children, brain stem angiomas are not uncommon. Recurrent pontine symptoms point to the correct diagnosis. The CT scan shows a high density lesion.

Haematomas from aneurysms often show a very typical appearance in the CT scan. A haematoma in the frontal lobe or in the interhemispheric fissure between the frontal lobes is highly specific of an aneurysm of the anterior communicating artery. A haematoma arranged in the form of stairs is a characteristic finding in haemorrhages from an aneurysm of the pericallosal artery (Fig. 14). The typical shape is caused by the callosal cistern. Haematomas following the Sylvian fissure are typical findings in aneurysms of the carotid or the middle cerebral artery. The latter may also cause a circumscribed temporal haematoma, without evidence of blood in the subarachnoid space. Penetration of blood into the temporal horn is found with carotid aneurysms.

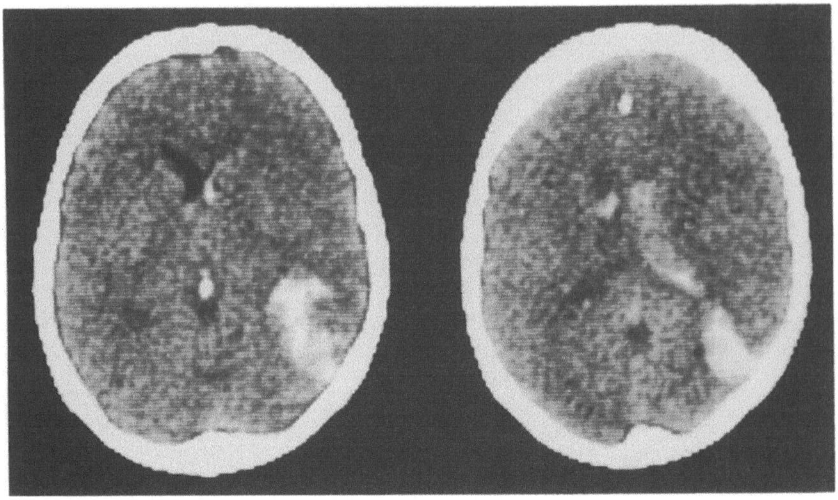

Fig. 13. Intracerebral haematoma in the right temporo-occipital region with ventricular haemorrhage due to an AV malformation of the right middle cerebral artery

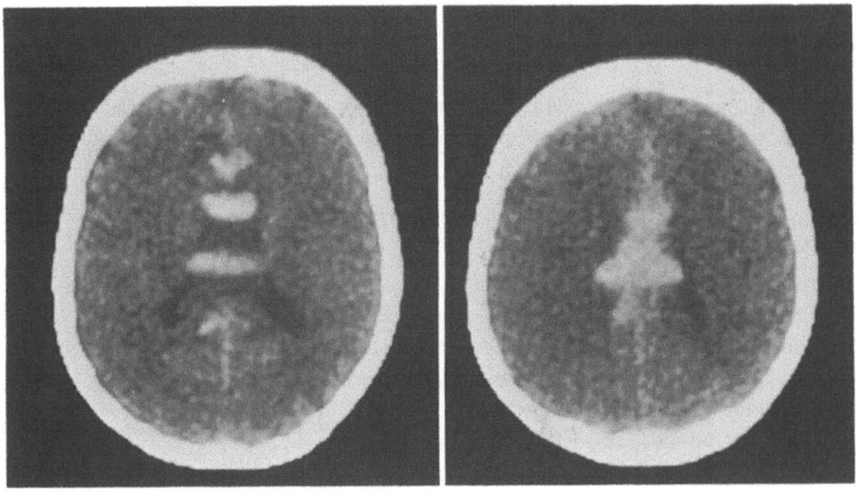

Fig. 14. Typical appearance of clotted blood within the callosal cistern from a ruptured aneurysm of the pericallosal artery

Haemorrhages into an infarcted area are quite rare. In the majority of our observations infarcts in the region of the posterior cerebral artery were involved. Up to the present, small petechial haemorrhages cannot be visualized in the CT scan. Haemorrhages in the parietal region near the midline, occasionally multiple and bilateral, may be found in patients with thrombosis of the superior sagittal sinus.

Old unresolved intracerebral haematomas are an unusual finding. The acute event may have occurred weeks or months ago. Nevertheless, the attenuation values often remain relatively high, similar to those of recent haematomas. At operation a cyst with a rough wall containing a chocolate-like creamy fluid will be found. Sometimes, remains of a micro-angioma are diagnosed microscopically in the cyst wall (Kazner et al. 1978).

Haemorrhage into a brain tumour or a metastasis is also a rare event. In 5–6% of our patients with glioblastomas, an intracerebral haematoma was present. Without using contrast enhancement the tumour can be missed (Fig. 15). Haemorrhages into cerebellar tumours in children are not unusual (Fig. 16). A haemorrhage into a pituitary adenoma is a rare event. In one patient, on the basis of the CT scan, we suggested the diagnosis of a cystic adenoma (Fig. 17), which turned out to be an old liquefied haematoma. Very typical are haematomas with metastases of malignant melanomas (Fig. 18). Occasionally, also in metastases of a renal hypernephroma, a haemorrhage will be observed. Metastases of a chorion carcinoma usually become manifest as intracerebral haematomas (Fig. 19).

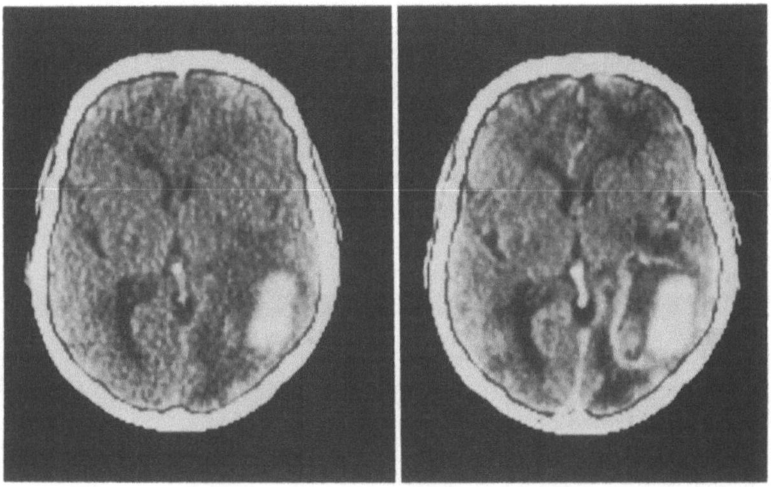

Fig. 15. Fresh haematoma within a glioblastoma. The tumour becomes visible only after contrast enhancement (right)

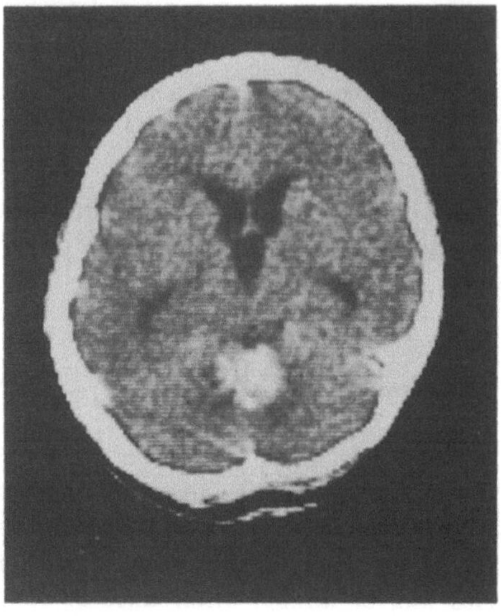

Fig. 16. Haemorrhage into a cerebellar astrocytoma in a 14-year-old child

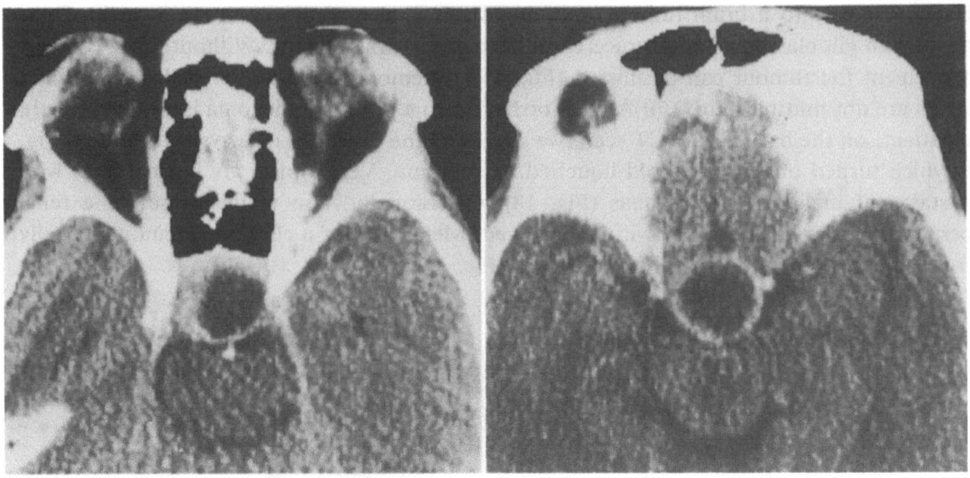

Fig. 17. Old liquefied haematoma (low absorption values!) within a pituitary adenoma. The small rim of vital tumour tissue takes up contrast material

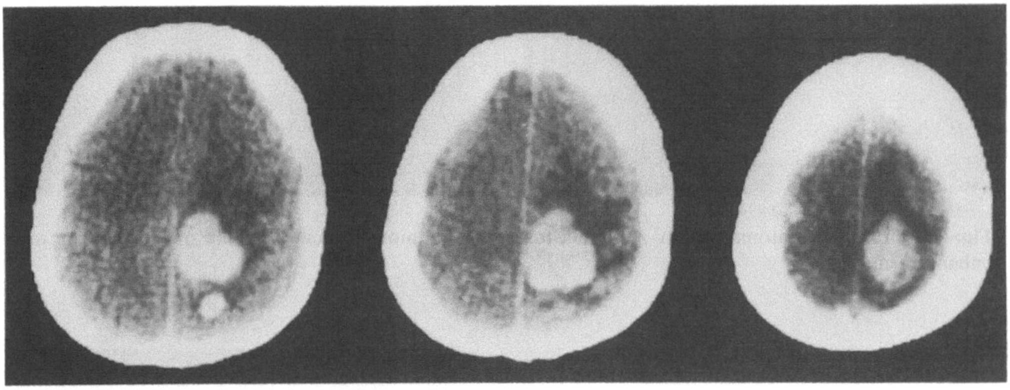

Fig. 18. Multiple metastases of a malignant melanoma with haemorrhage into the tumour tissue

Last, but not least, delayed and late post-traumatic intracerebral haematomas, as defined by von Monakow and Bollinger, have to be mentioned. We have recently reported on such observations (Lanksch et al. 1978).

Indication – Role of CT

Due to the excellent diagnostic possibilities offered by computerized tomography today, numerous patients with intracranial haematomas come to our notice in our clinical practice whom, before the introduction of CT, only a neuropathologist could have described with such accuracy. A CT scan is indicated in all patients with acute onset of neurological symptoms with or without disturbance of consciousness. CT should be performed before more

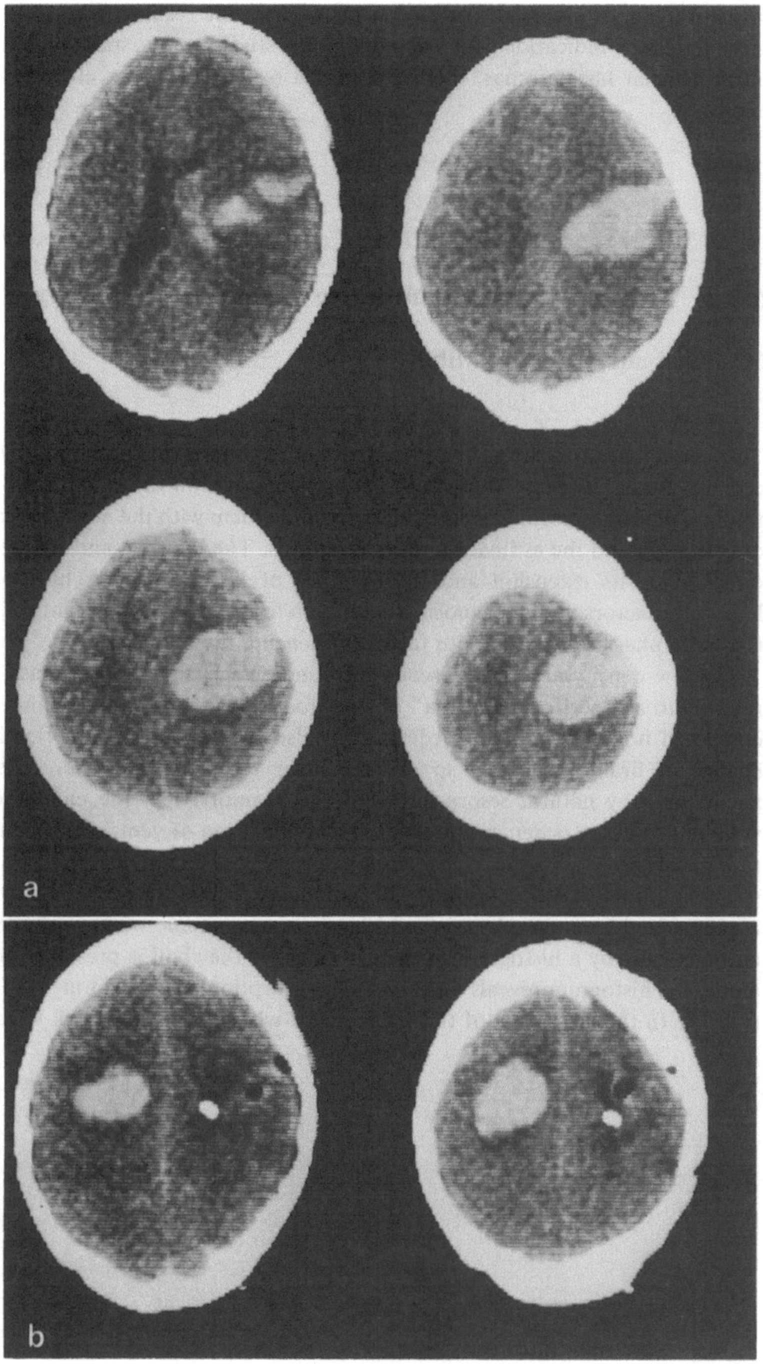

Fig. 19a, b. Recent intracerebral haematoma in the right parietal region in a 37-year-old woman due to metastasis of a chorion carcinoma (**a**). Nine days after the evacuation of the right haematoma, a second haemorrhage occurred, also due to a small metastasis not visible in the first CT scan (**b**)

invasive methods are used, because in many cases the result of the CT investigation allows a more precise indication for angiographic studies. In spontaneous intracerebral and intracerebellar haematomas, the CT scan can be used as an excellent guide for the operative approach.

6.2.2 Automatic and Quantitative Diagnosis of ICH by CT

M. Nagai and Y. Ueda, Mibu

There is no need to stress the usefulness of computerized tomography in the diagnosis of cerebrovascular disease. Many authors have reported on the classification of the types of CT findings in intracerebral haematoma, correlating them with the neurological grading, the timing of operation and the estimation of its prognosis. The location and the size of haematoma, the direction of its extension and the presence of intraventricular haemorrhage are the most important factors in the diagnosis. In addition to these, the significant role of perifocal oedema is also emphasized as a definite factor influencing the clinical course.

The low density area in CT scans surrounding the high density mass of the haematoma is referred to as "perifocal oedema" or "perifocal low density area". Since this area is probably composed not only of brain oedema, but also the residue of liquefied haematoma, necrotic change of brain tissue and so on, the latter term is preferable. After evacuation of the haematoma by natural resorption after the haemorrhage, the change of intracranial water volume, including oedema, liquefaction and dilatation of ventricle, becomes the main problem to be analysed.

The authors have developed an automatic, quantitative, diagnostic method utilizing computerized tomography, in which the intracranial water volume can be calculated automatically by a histogram of the CT value. If the skull is presumed to be filled with water alone, the histogram reveals a peak of the absorption coefficient at +5 Hounsfield Unit (HU) (Fig. 1). In the histogram of the CT value of whole brain, the peak is between 31 and 32 HU

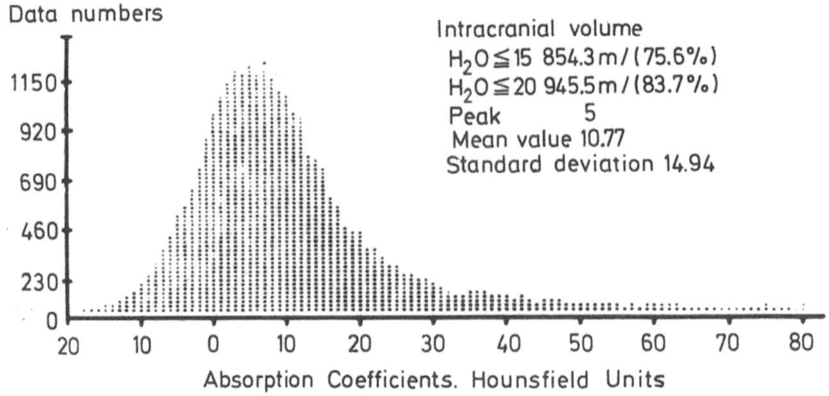

Fig. 1. Histogram of CT water value in skull

(Fig. 2). This number is almost constant in normal cases. When the intracranial water volume increases through any pathological processes, the peak of the histogram shifts to the lower value (Fig. 3). There is not only a shift of the peak, but a separation of the absorption coefficient into peaks also appears. One of them is the peak of water and the other is that of brain. In a case of severe hydrocephalus, for instance, the high peak of water and the low peak of brain are demonstrated in the histogram. The relative volume of the two peaks depends on the grade of hydrocephalus (Fig. 4). The absorption coefficients of bottom points between two peaks are in the range of 15 to 20 HU. From these results, the pixel of which absorption coefficient is under 15 HU should be regarded as the water component.

Proceeding to the next step, the separate calculation of CT value of each cerebral hemisphere can be carried out and drawn in histograms. Figure 5 shows the abstracted image of the left hemisphere drawn by similar technique of ROI (region of interest). The left half of Fig. 6 is a CT picture showing diffuse low density of the left hemisphere. The histograms of the whole brain, left and right hemispheres are illustrated on the right. In the diffuse low density of the left hemisphere, the peak of the histogram shifts to a lower value; meanwhile, that of the right hemisphere remains at 32 HU. Each histogram is shown separately in Fig. 7. The grade of the shift to the lower density is considered an important factor, related to the cerebral damage. In this case, which shows diffuse oedema of the left hemisphere due to acute obstruction of the left

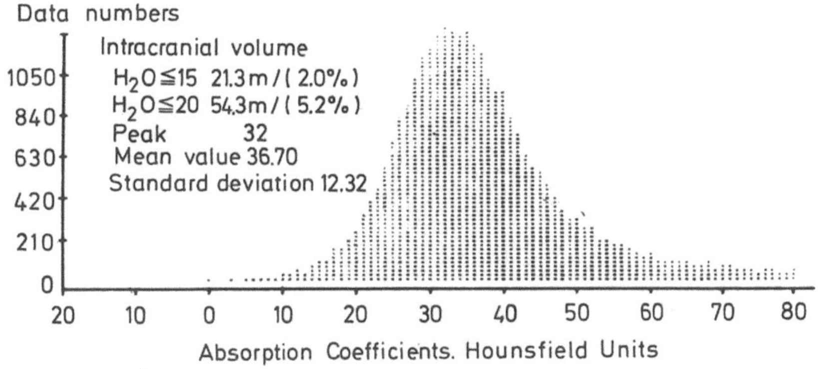

Fig. 2. Histogram of CT value of whole brain

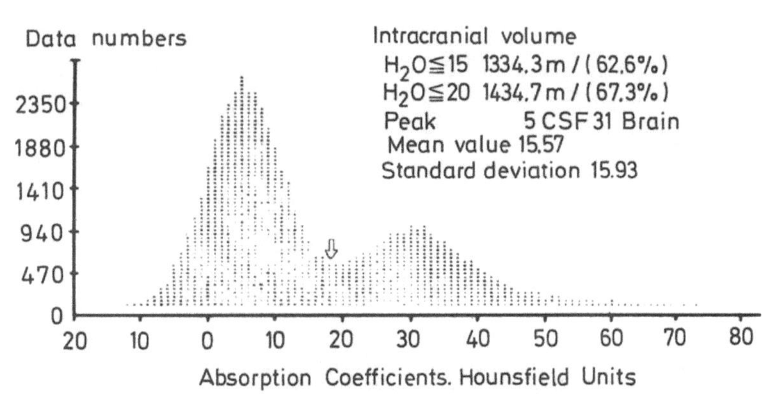

Fig. 3. Histogram of CT value of whole brain in severe hydrocephalus

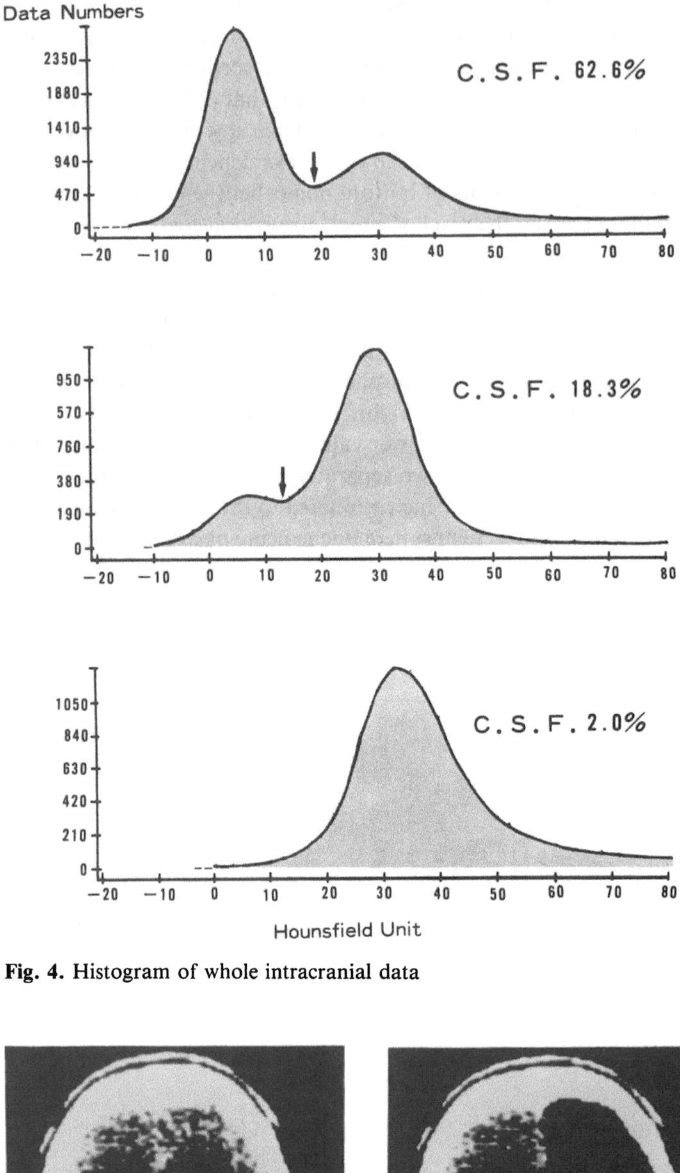

Fig. 4. Histogram of whole intracranial data

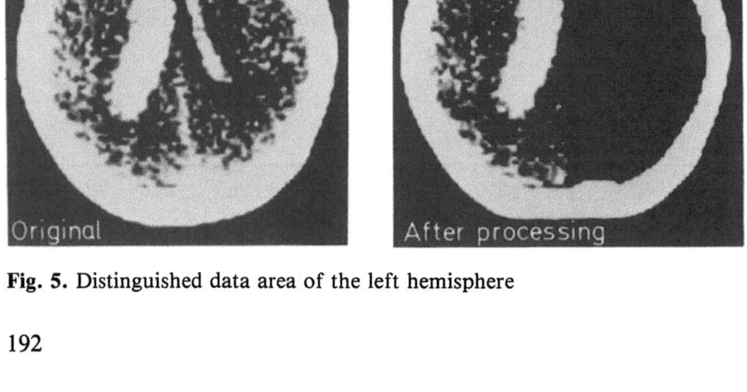

Fig. 5. Distinguished data area of the left hemisphere

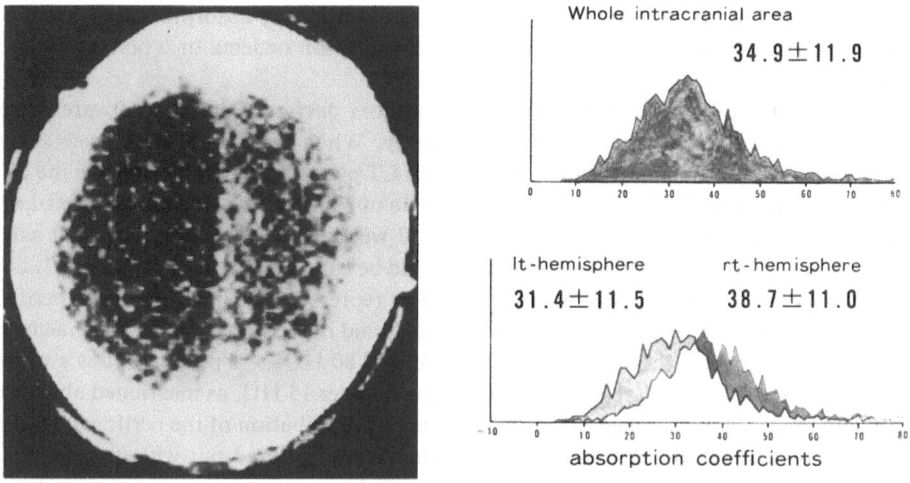

Fig. 6. Histogram of the separate hemispheres

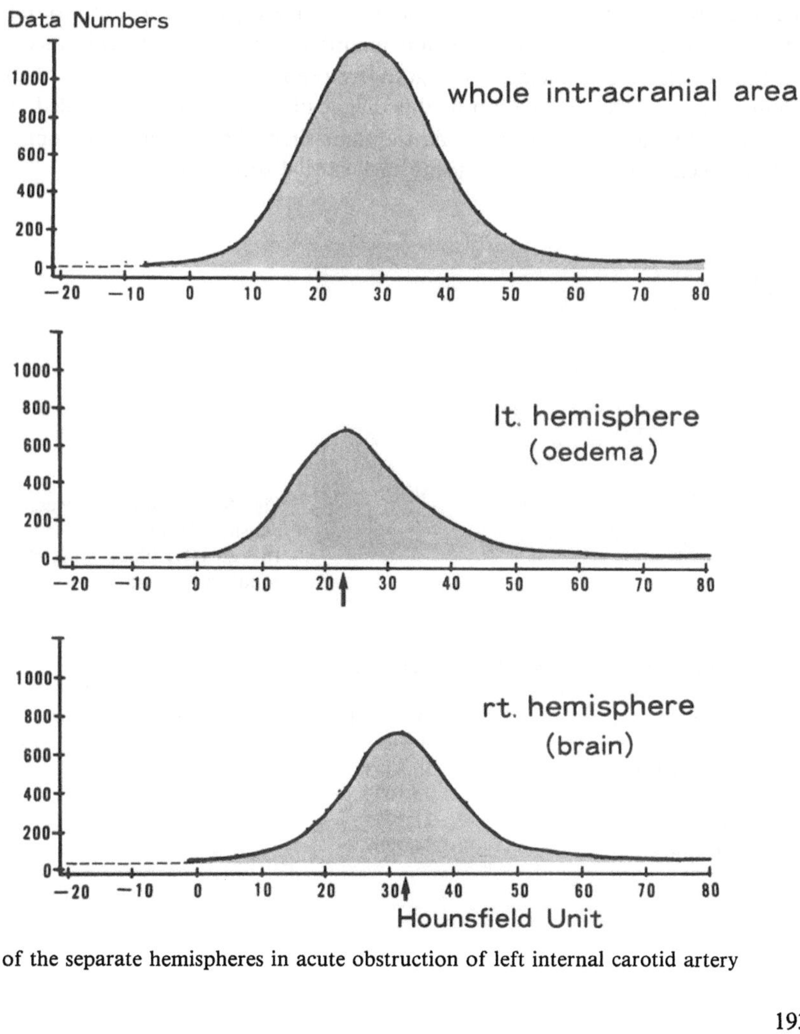

Fig. 7. Histogram of the separate hemispheres in acute obstruction of left internal carotid artery

internal carotid artery, the peak was at 23 HU. On average, an absorption coefficient between 16 and 26 HU could be regarded as a component of brain oedema or a perifocal low density area.

Using the basic data described above, the authors devised a special software programme visualizing the perifocal low density quantitatively. When two consecutive pixels between 16 and 26 HU are picked up and written in the file of CT pictures, they can be seen in the CT image as gray dots around the haematoma. The left side of Fig. 8 is the original picture of a case of intracerebral haematoma in a 64-year-old man, 2 weeks after the onset. The right side of the figure is the processed one. Such a procedure could be called "visualized processing". Since one pixel corresponds to 0.01 cm^3, the number of dots represents the quantity of the perifocal low density. This procedure is a kind of rearrangement, and in the same manner, the haematoma – the density of which is thought to be between 45 and 80 HU – is printed out as a white mass, and the water component (absorption coefficient is under 15 HU, as mentioned above) appears as a dark area in the CT image. At the same time, the distribution of the perifocal low density is clearly demonstrated in the picture. Each volume is also printed out with its mean value and standard deviation (Table 1). The three-dimensional sum of these numbers provides the real volume of each component. By means of this procedure, an intracerebral haematoma could be analysed, including its volume, the extent of perifocal low density and the size of the ventricles. The changes with time of each factor should be investigated in relation to the clinical course.

Preliminary attempts at the automatic quantitative diagnosis of the intracerebral haematoma and the associated pathological changes were reported mainly in terms of quantitative water volume analysis. The application of this diagnostic method in the detailed analysis of clinical cases should be developed further. At the same time, the capability of computed tomography could be extended still further by using such special software.

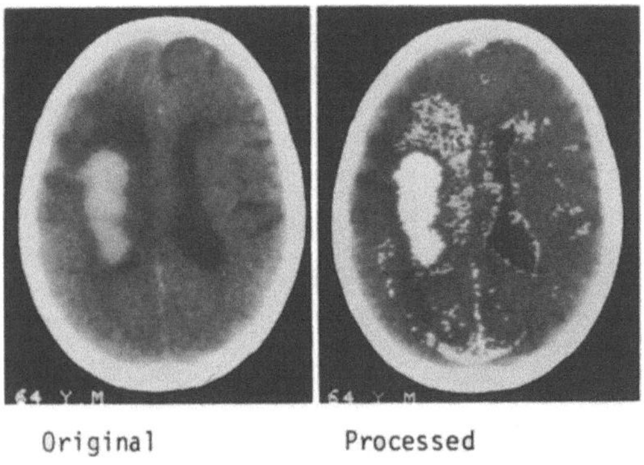

Fig. 8. Visualized processing of perifocal low density. White area, 45–80 HU; grey area, 16–26 HU; black area, ≤15 HU (one pixel is equal to 0.01 cm^3)

Table 1. Print-out of digital number of each volume

Data number	Mean value	Standard deviation
1 Slice brain 169.86	36.8783	13.7147
Ventricle 9.67	9.81075	4.18057
White matter and oedema 13.63	21.3771	2.73267
Haematoma 10.64	54.7707	6.41838

6.2.3 Intraventricular Haemorrhages in CT Scans

A. Laun, A. L. Agnoli, and L. Cristante, Giessen

Computerized tomography provided the possibility of early and easy recognition of small isolated or combined intraventricular haemorrhages (Dolinkas et al. Part I, II 1977; Pineda 1977). The number of cases is much higher than previously supposed (Tables 1, 2, 3). Further aid is provided by a new software evaluation system (Evaluscope; Siemens Co.). The aim of this study was to investigate whether the differential diagnosis between true intraventricular haematomas and haemorrhages is possible, to evaluate the rate of blood resorption and to provide some additional data and criteria for operative indications.

Experimental studies showed that the haemoglobin level in the blood and the concentration of calcium ions directly influence the absorption of X-rays and the density value measurement

Table 1. Intracranial haemorrhages [a]

	Number	%
Traumatic	286	4.9
Vascular malformations	148	3.5
Subarachnoid	23	0.5
Intracerebral	38	0.9
Subdural	48	1.1
	543	10.9

[a] 1975–1977

Tab. 2. Ventricular haemorrhages

	Intracranial haemorrhage	Intraventricular haemorrhage	%
AVM	148	12	8.3
Traumatic	286	14	4.9
Spontaneous	38	6	16.0

Table 3. Intraventricular haemorrhages [a]

	Number	%
Traumatic	14	35
Aneurysms	6	15
AVM	6	15
Spontaneous	6	15
Antifibrinolytic	2	5
Others	6	15
	40	100

[a] 1976–1978

(New and Aronow 1976). So far we have devoted little attention to these values. On the other hand, we found that blood cannot be recognized in the cerebrospinal fluid until the content is about 15%. In our cases the absorption values for water are ±0 units and for air (−)1000 units. Haemorrhages, on the 1st day, show absorption values between about 40 and 70 units.

As expected in serial measurements, the continuing decrease in the density of the haematoma was observed even if the visual difference was not recognizable. On the other hand, increase of density was observed in recurrent bleedings although the visual analysis of the picture showed, apart from the increase of the area of haemorrhage, no rise in density. This suggests that small, not clinically manifest, recurrent intraventricular and intracerebral bleedings can be recognized in computerized tomography. The histogram shows the frequence analysis of pixels with the same absorption values. In an acute haematoma the base of the histogram will be narrow. In repeated scans the shape of the histogram changes; it becomes wide and flat and has perhaps two or more peaks. This provides a good indication of the progress in the resorption of the haematoma.

In comparison with lobar intracerebral haemorrhages, intraventricular haemorrhages tend to be resorbed more quickly. However, these findings have to be confirmed in a larger number of patients. The main difficulty is connected with the exact repetition of identical serial scans, which is at present not possible without considerably more technical and financial assistance. This is also the reason why the planimetric measurement of the ventricular system for evaluation of progressive hydrocephalus remains inexact and time consuming.

Summary

Evaluation of density values in a histogram provides a better insight into the structure and resorption of intraventricular haemorrhages. It is still too early to say what help will be given in planning treatment. It is certain, however, that intraventricular haemorrhages and haematomas can be diagnosed more easily and that their number is much higher than previously supposed. The ease with which intraventricular bleeding can be recognized in computerized tomography should not overshadow the importance of the clinical condition of the patient, even if sometimes the demonstration of blood in the ventricular system encourages the use of drainage or the removal of a clot.

6.2.4 Brain Stem Haemorrhage

A. Laun and A. L. Agnoli, Giessen

Before the advent of computerized tomography, haematomas and haemorrhages in the brain stem were diagnosed on clinical grounds and only a small number could be diagnosed intra vitam. Dandy reported in 1932 about the first successful operative removal of pontine haematomas. Further cases were reported by Kempe (1964), Koos (1969), Obrador (1970), Arseni (1973, 1979) and Sano et al. (1979). Pneumo-encephalography and ventriculography provided only indirect evidence of pontine space-occupying lesions. Brain stem haematomas were therefore analysed usually from the pathological point of view of post-mortem findings

(Crompton 1971; Chodkiewicz 1973; Mitchell 1973; Vedrenne 1975; Budzilovich 1976). Angiographic findings in brain stem haematomas were described only in exceptional cases of small brain stem angiomas (Russo 1977; Sano 1979) or micro-angiomas (Lorenz and Agnoli, in press). Papo (1976) and Becker (1978) have shown that computerized tomography permits the demonstration of even very small haemorrhages in the brain stem.

Material

Of 12000 CT investigations performed in the Neuroradiological Department of the Neurosurgical Centre in Giessen in 1976–1979, there were 600 investigations performed in patients with cerebral cranial injuries. Brain stem haemorrhages were demonstrated in a total of 36 patients. Of this number, 28 had a craniocerebral injury (Table 1). Of 171 patients with subarachnoid haemorrhage seen during 3 years, brain stem haemorrhage was found in three cases of angioma and in one patient with cerebral aneurysm. Of 20 subdural haematomas that occurred in patients who received anticoagulant therapy, brain stem haemorrhage was found in one. Spontaneous haematomas were also found in two patients with uneventful past histories. Traumatic brain stem haemorrhages and their accompanying lesions are reviewed in Table 2.

Table 1. Aetiology of brain stem haemorrhage

Spontaneous	2
Spontaneous, accompanying subdural haematoma and cerebral aneurysm	1
Craniocerebral injury	28
Vascular malformation	
Arteriovenous angioma	2
Micro-angioma	1
Arterial hypertension	1
Coagulopathy	1
	36

Table 2. Traumatic brain stem haemorrhage (N = 28) and accompanying injuries

Solitary intracerebral haemorrhages	2
Multiple intracerebral haemorrhages	11
Subdural haematoma	4
Intraventricular bleeding	11 [a]
Infratentorial bleeding	3

[a] Intraventricular bleeding was connected, with the exception of two cases, with solitary or multiple intracerebral haemorrhages

Discussion

The reports on brain stem haemorrhages demonstrated by computerized tomography have been infrequent so far (Dublin 1977; French 1977). Becker reported in 1978 on a case of successfully operated brain stem haematoma diagnosed by computerized tomography. In this case there was neither angiographic nor histological evidence of tumour or vascular malformation.

In our series of 28 traumatic brain stem haemorrhages in only one case was a secondary bleeding, 4 days after the trauma, demonstrated. The investigation was performed immediately after admission and repeated 4 days later because of the development of a midbrain syndrome. Apart from the pontine haemorrhage there were bilateral, frontal, thin (0.6 cm) epidural haematomas which were evacuated. Six months after the injury the patient has only minimal neurological deficits (Fig. 1).

In all other cases of traumatic brain stem haemorrhages the haemorrhage could be demonstrated within the first 2 h after the injury (Rosaz and Laun 1980). They were combined with other intracranial or intracerebral lesions almost in every case (Table 2). The clinical diagnosis of pontine haemorrhage in this cases was not possible. Approximately 23% of patients with traumatic pontine haemorrhages survive the acute phase. One of the most important prognostic factors proved to be the early occlusion of the pontomesencephalic cisterns.

Computer tomographic demonstration of occluded pontomesencephalic cisterns within the first hours after the injury was almost invariably associated with a fatal outcome (Agnoli et al. 1979).

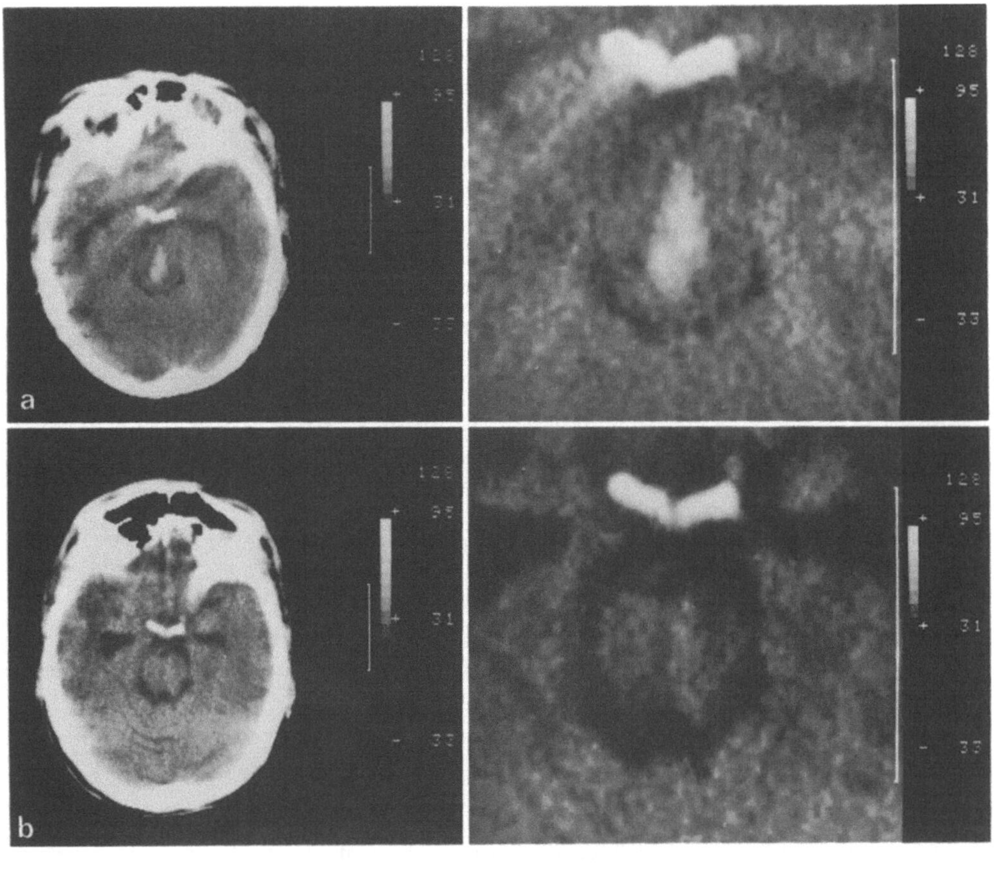

Fig. 1a, b. A 19-year-old male, with severe craniocerebral injury. **a** CT on the 4th day after the injury, tegmental haemorrhage. **b** 6 months later complete resorption of the haemorrhage, with normal configuration of the cisterns

Figure 2 shows the CT scan of a patient, with large arteriovenous angioma involving the midline structures and both occipital lobes, who died from spontaneous brain stem haemorrhage. Another patient with micro-angioma, confirmed on histological section, died 2 weeks after operative evacuation of an intrapontine haematoma.

The third case was a patient with spontaneous acute subdural haematoma in whom the postoperative angiography demonstrated an infraclinoid carotid artery aneurysm on the right side. Six months after the removal of the subdural haematoma the aneurysm was coated with muscle because occlusion with a clip was technically not possible. Six months after the coating an acute left-sided subdural haematoma developed. This was evacuated, but 21 h after the operation a large, fatal pontomesencephalic haemorrhage occurred. The only patient with brain stem haemorrhage due to arterial hypertension did not survive.

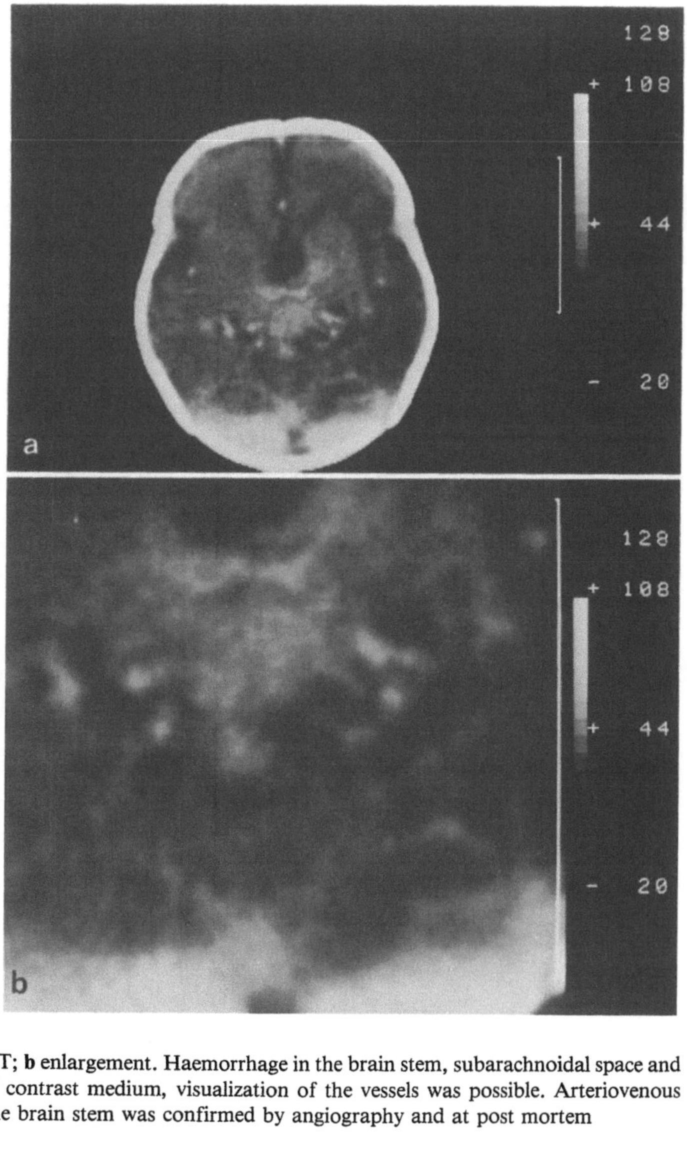

Fig. 2a, b. Female in a coma. **a** CT; **b** enlargement. Haemorrhage in the brain stem, subarachnoidal space and basal ganglia. After injection of contrast medium, visualization of the vessels was possible. Arteriovenous angioma with haemorrhage in the brain stem was confirmed by angiography and at post mortem

In both patients who survived the haemorrhage the resorption of blood occurred within 4 weeks (Fig. 3). This corresponds to the time of resorption reported for intracerebral haematomas (Messina 1975; Agnoli and Zierski 1980). The time of resorption is shorter when the extravasated blood is in contact with cerebrospinal fluid spaces (French and Dublin 1977; Laun et al. 1980).

It may be difficult to differentiate pontine haematoma from tumour of the brain stem (Duffner 1978); contrast enhanced CT is usually helpful in this respect (Fig. 4). It is indispensable to perform angiography to exclude a vascular malformation or tumour. The measurement of absorption values proved to be helpful in the diagnosis of brain stem haematomas (Laun and Rosaz 1980). The absorption values of these haematomas are approximately 40–60 HU. They can be demonstrated with appropriate software (HL programme).

The number of cases is too small to permit definite conclusions about the origin, therapy and prognosis of haemorrhages discovered by CT investigation. Primary haematomas caused by vascular malformations should be operated upon.

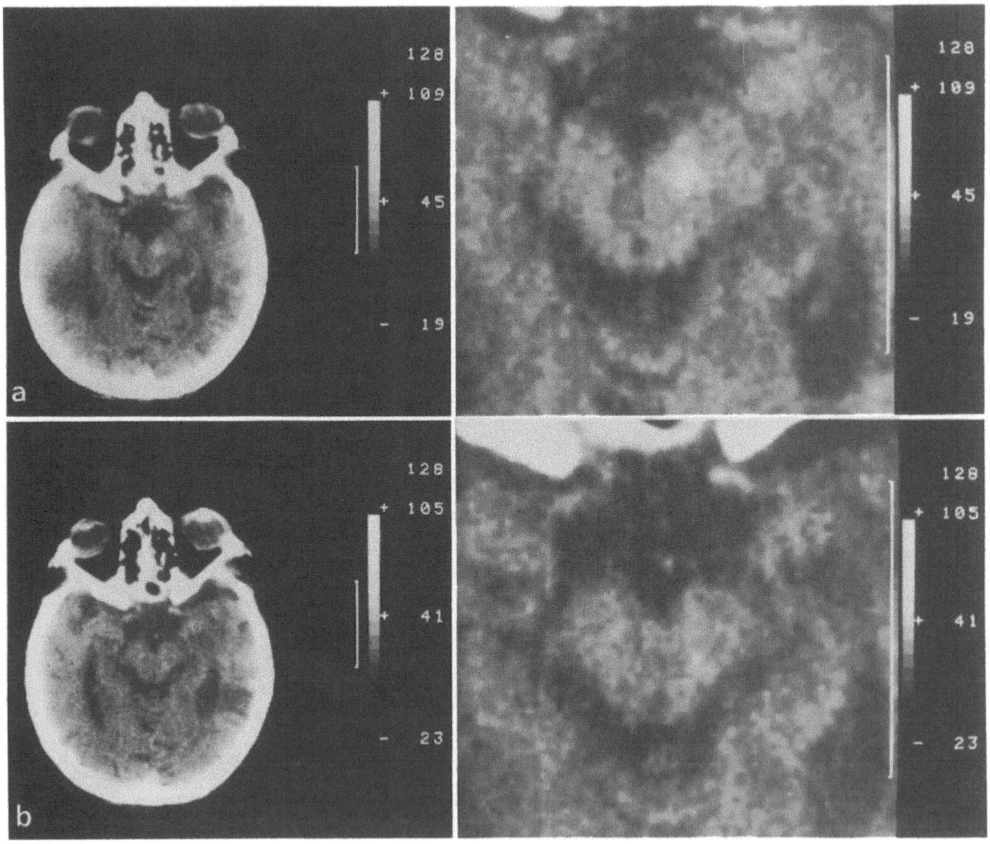

Fig. 3a, b. Haemorrhage in the brain stem in a female undergoing anticoagulant therapy. **a** Increased density in the right cerebral peduncle (haemorrhage); **b** 4 weeks later complete resorption. Minimal neurological deficits

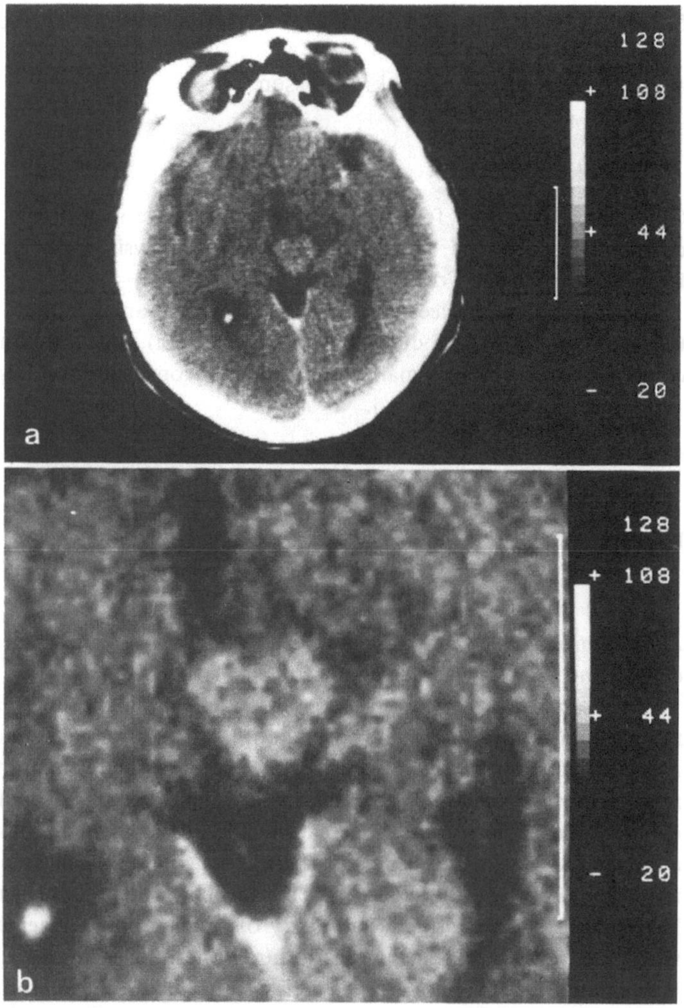

Fig. 4a, b. 42-year-old male. **a** CT after injection of contrast medium and **b** with enlargement. Increased density zone in mesencephalon on the right side. After injection of contrast medium enhancement suggested a tumour. Biopsy revealed a spongioblastoma, grade II

Summary

Craniocerebral juries are accompanied by haemorrhages in the brain stem in approximately 4% of cases. These haemorrhages were discovered as a rule within the first few hours after the injury and are probably primary in origin. Secondary haemorrhages seem to be exceptional. Brain stem haematomas in patients with arterial hypertension and vascular malformations are infrequent. For differential diagnosis it is absolutely necessary to perform CT after injection of contrast medium and complement the investigation by cerebral angiography. Our experience suggests that there is a quite number of brain stem haemorrhages which do not lead to death.

6.2.5. CT in Traumatic ICH – Measurement of Absorption Values

A. L. Agnoli and J. Zierski, Giessen

Our interest has been focussed on the quantitative measurement of absorption values and differential aspects of bleedings in CT. The analysis was performed with the aid of the Evaluscope (Siemens Co.).

The material was selected from 300 cases of cranial injury, which comprised extradural haematomas (25%), subdural haematomas (12%), intracerebral haemorrhages (21%) and combined forms (15%). Small traumatic contusions, subdural hygromas, gunshot injuries and scalp injuries are not included.

Results

Extradural Haematomas present in CT usually as a biconvex or lenticular zone of increased density and are very easily recognized (Fig. 1).

The mean absorption values were 70 – 75 U. The high upper values are probably related to the phenomenon of "computer overshoot" which is present under the bone. The planimetric measurements (at the area of the greatest extent of the haematoma) showed that there was no relation between the area measured and the clinical course. The differential diagnosis between epidural and acute subdural haematomas is difficult on the basis of density measurements, although on average the absorption values for acute subdural clots are lower. More important is the shape of the haematoma, particularly of its cerebral surface, the subdural haematomas having an irregular border. Planimetry of acute subdural haematomas showed that they are much less extensive that the extradural ones. The largest area counted for extradural haematoma was 5000 mm^2. The largest acute subdural haematoma had the area of 2000 mm^2. The situation is different with chronic and subchronic subdural haematomas. Measurement of the area affected by these haematomas showed values similar to those of epidural haematomas.

The average absorption values for *subdural haematomas* were 34 – 40 U. Those values were also recorded from areas close to the brain and to the bone. However, in the histogram, the largest number of pixels had absorption values ranging from 20 – 34 U.

Figure 2 shows different chronic subdural haematomas. It has to be remembered that subdural haematomas occasionally may be missed in CT. Fig. 3 shows a bilateral subdural haematoma. An increase of density is produced by an injection of contrast medium because of the enhancement of the haematoma capsule. The absorption values rise from 40 U. to 45 U. The absorption values for the highest number of pixels measured increase to 48 U.

Figure 4 demonstrates the stage of liquefaction of the clot. One part of the haematoma shows absorption values of 45 U. The majority of pixels have values of 42 U. The other part shows absorption values of 32 U., and the highest number of pixels has the value of 28 U.

In another example of bilateral subdural haematoma, considerable differences in absorption values were found. The absorption value for the largest number of pixels in the solid part of the haematoma was 42 U. and 43 U., respectively (Fig. 5). For the non-solid part of the haematoma the values were 20 U. (Fig. 5b).

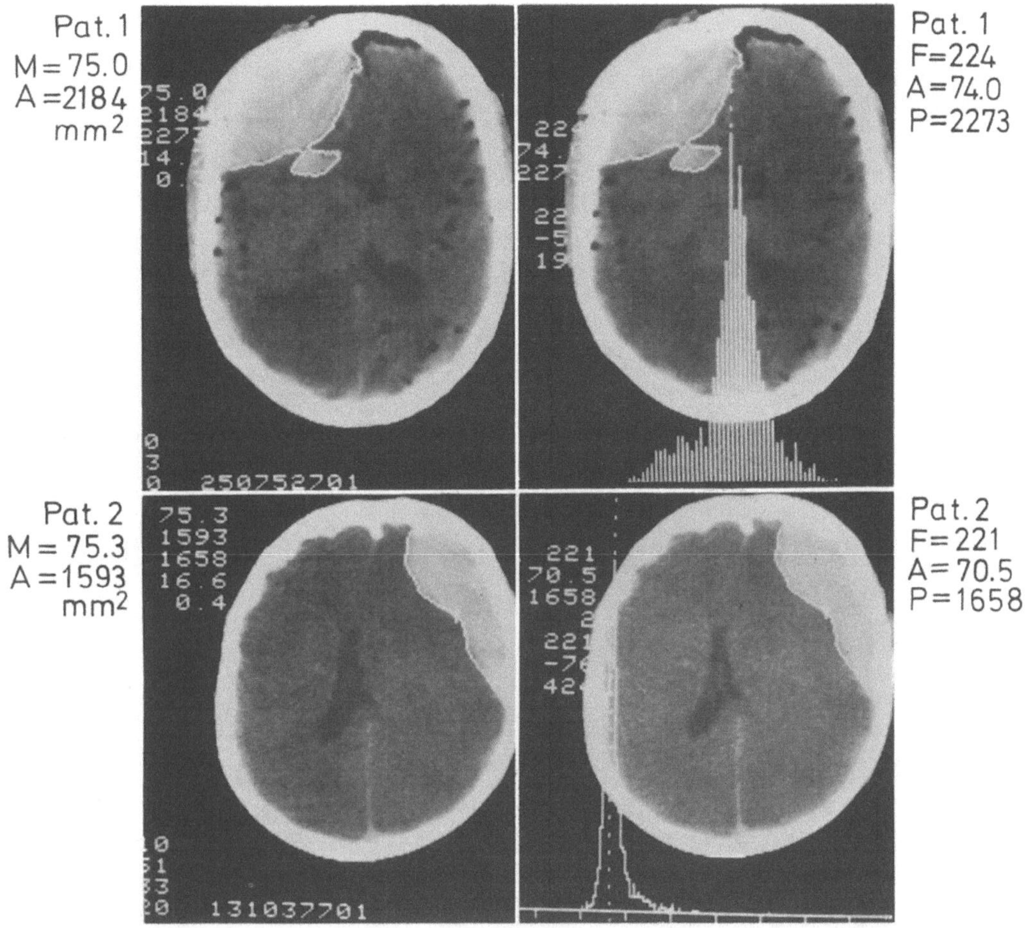

Fig. 1. Extradural haematomas. Mean absorption value (M) planimetry (A) and histogram with the number of pixels (P) counted

The measurement of absorption values in *traumatic intracerebral haematomas* shows a great scatter of values because surrounding oedema of variable extent is invariably present. The measurements were performed in cases examined between 1 and 24 h after the bleeding (immediate examination after haemorrhage may not show any changes in absorption values). The average values measured in our cases were 25 – 95 U., regardless of the size of haematoma. The highest number of pixels showed values from 20 to 45 U.

Resorption of blood can be followed in serial scans and documented by diminishing absorption values. The absorption values are already diminishing by the 3rd day after the injury. Figure 6 shows a decrease of average absorption values from 38 U. to 27 U., while Fig. 7 illustrates a decrease from 60 U. to 28 U. However, the rate of absorption is not always the same. Figure 8a shows two small intracerebral haematomas with average absorption values of 44 and 44 U., respectively. Six days later the density would appear to be less, but the absorption values remain unchanged. In another CT scan 10 days after the injury, one cannot differentiate between the two lesions. The average absorption values are 34 U.

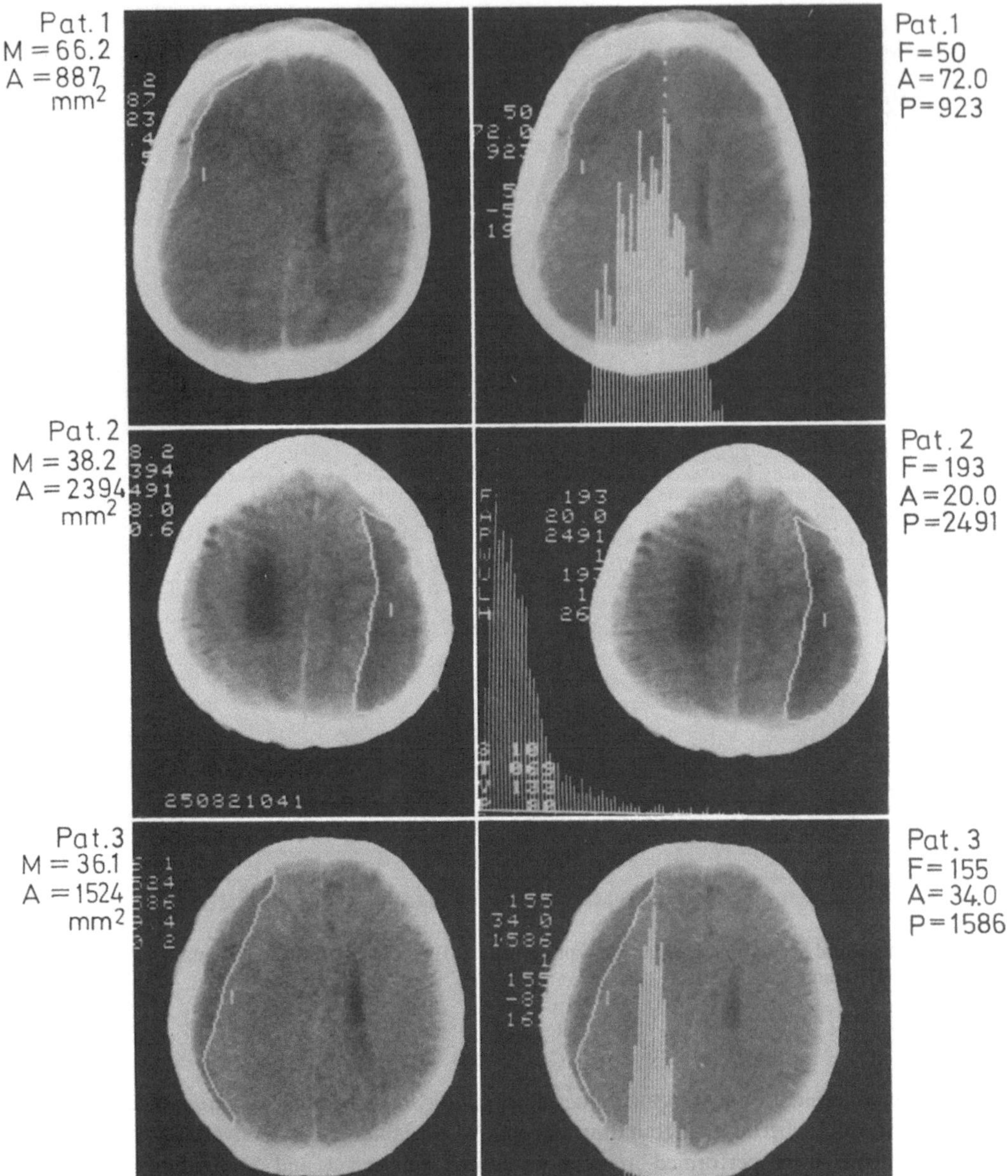

Fig. 2. Subdural haematomas

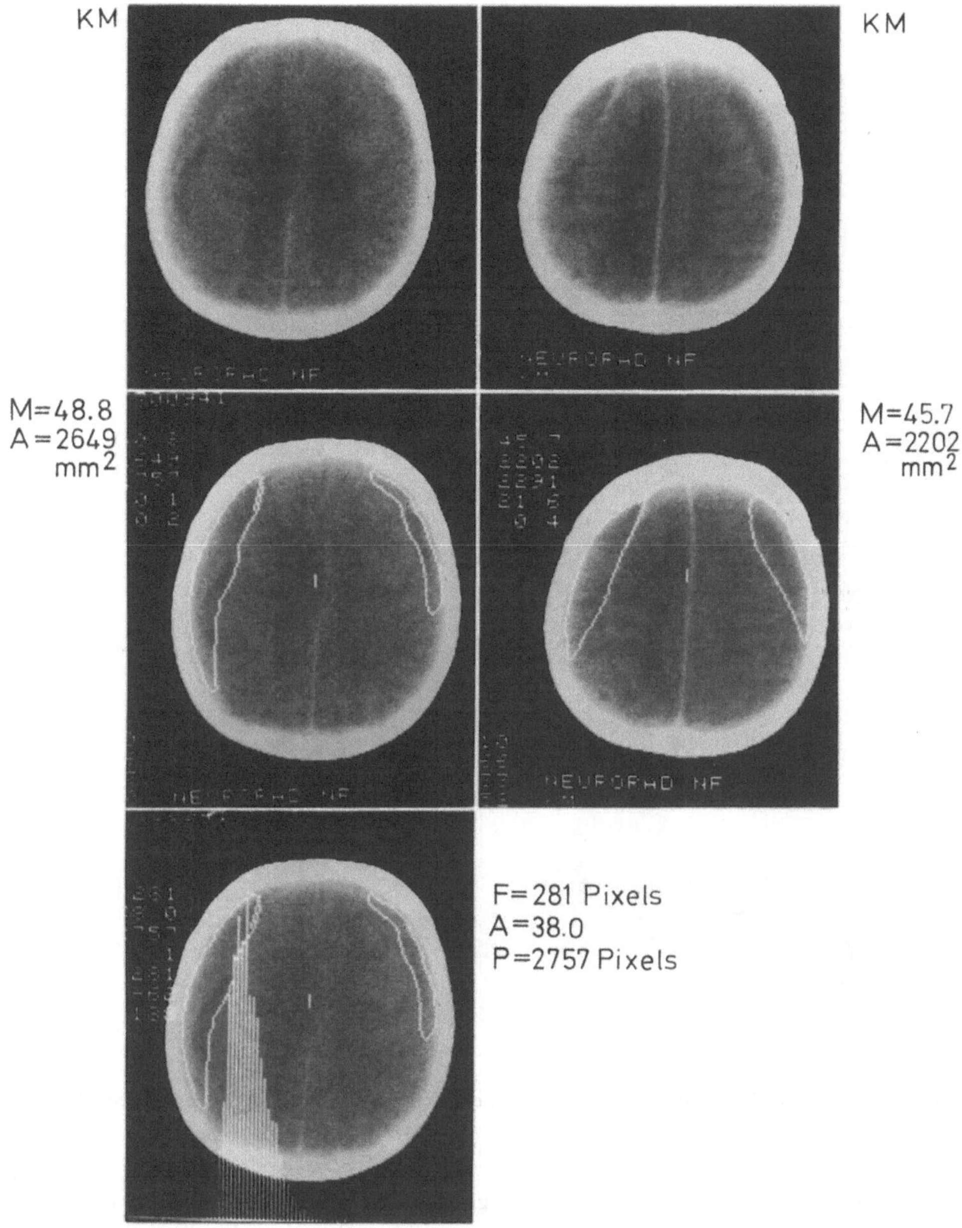

Fig. 3. Enhancement of haematoma capsule after injection of contrast medium

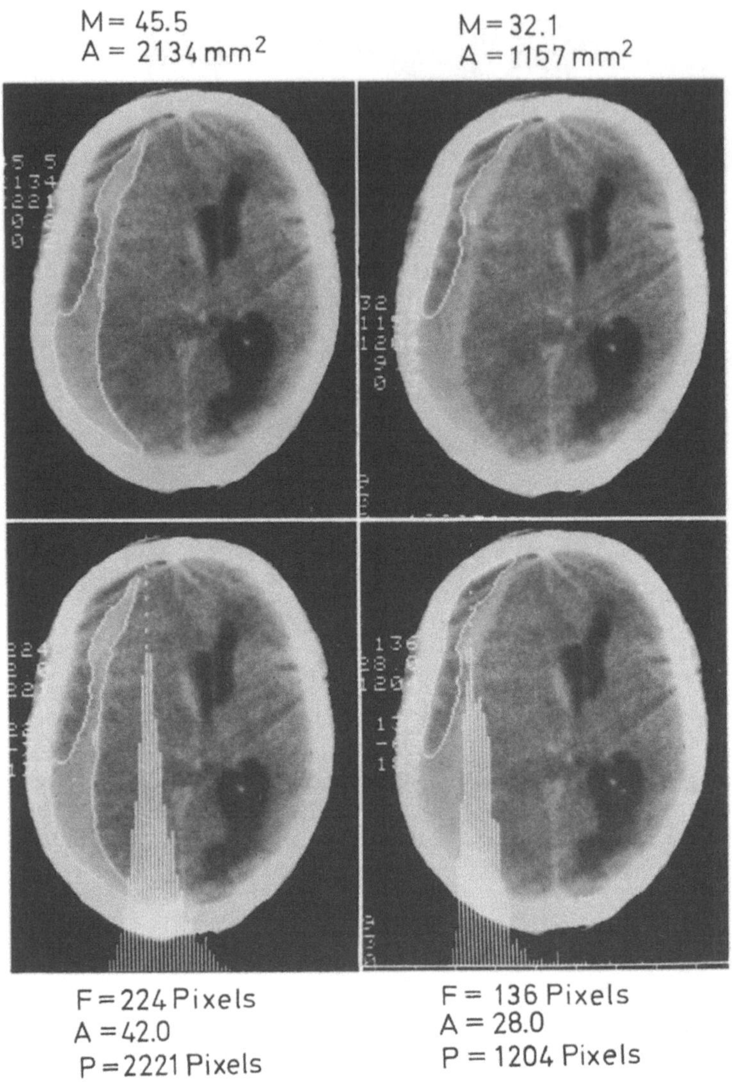

Fig. 4. Liquefaction of the clot in CT picture. Note the difference of absorption values between the layers of the haematoma

Figure 8b shows the same case with a histogram of the absorption values. If the highest number of pixels is taken into account it becomes evident that there has been a progressive reduction of values from 55 U. to 46 U. by the 6th day and 34 U. on the 10th day.

Intraventricular haemorrhages also tend to resorb very quickly. The reduction of absorption values from 39 U. to 27 U. was seen within 3 days (Fig. 9). Of ten cases with intraventricular bleeding, in three the blood was completely absorbed on the 3 day.

Great interest has been shown in measurement of ventricular size after an injury. In the development of ventricular enlargement within the first 4 weeks after the injury, the age of the patient, severity of trauma or type of lesion (subdural haematoma, intracerebral haematoma, contusion, etc.) do not seem to play any decisive role, i.e. the size of ventricle remained unchanged for over 3 weeks in a 70-year-old patient with subdural haematoma (Fig. 10) or

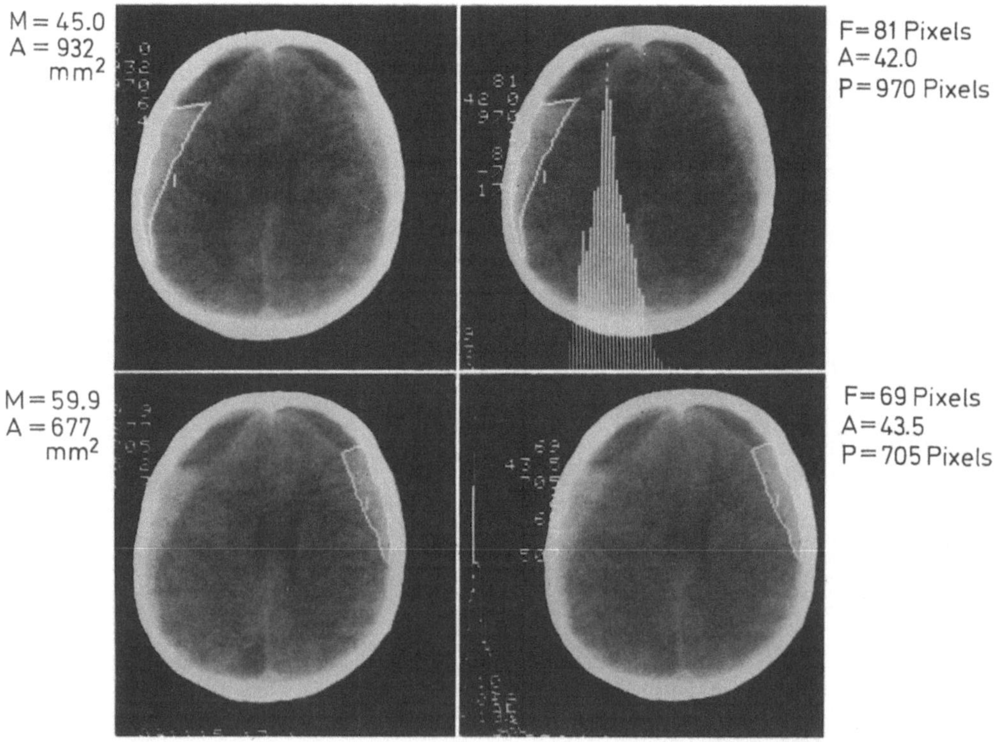

Fig. 5. a Solid parts. Differences of absorption values between solid and non-solid parts of subdural haematoma

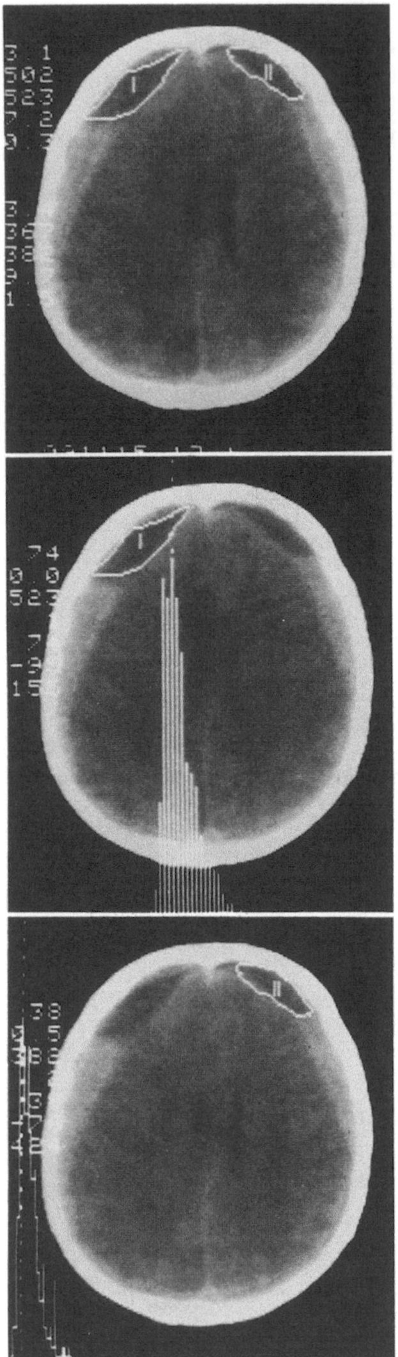

I : M=23.1
A =502mm²

II : M =33.4
A =367mm²

I : F=74 Pixels
A=20.0
P=523 Pixels

II : F=38 Pixels
A=20.5
P=382 Pixels

Fig. 5b. Non-solid parts

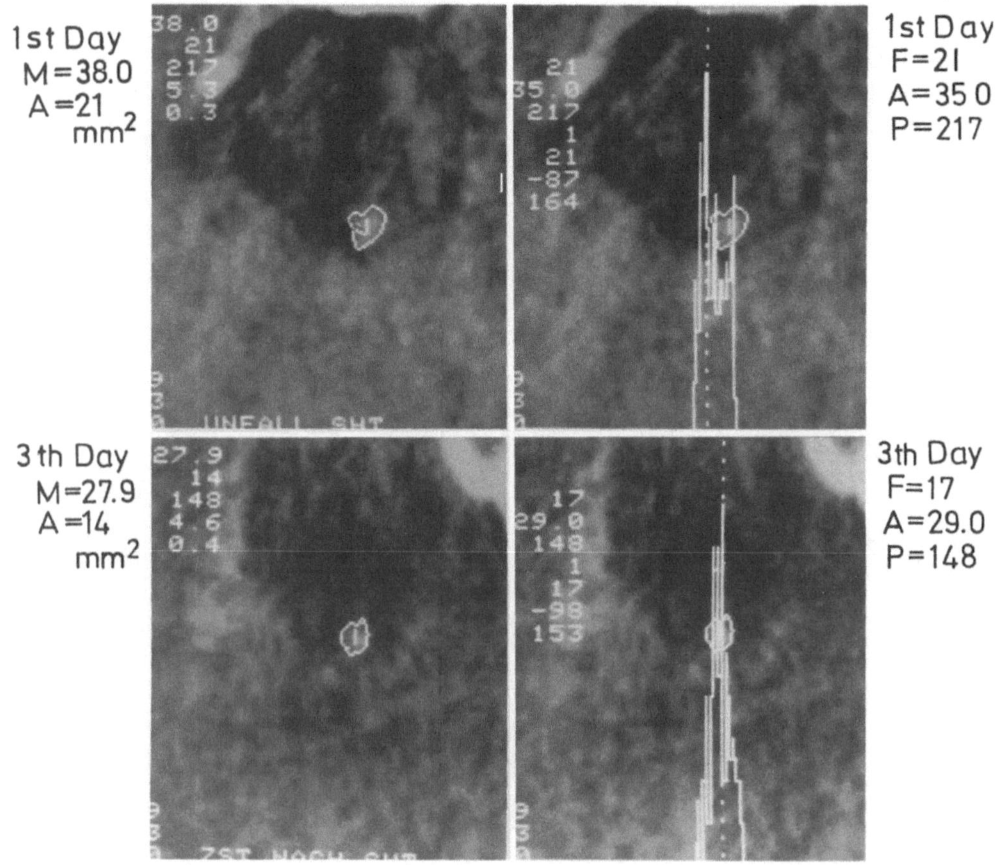

Fig. 6. Resorption of small intracerebral haematoma

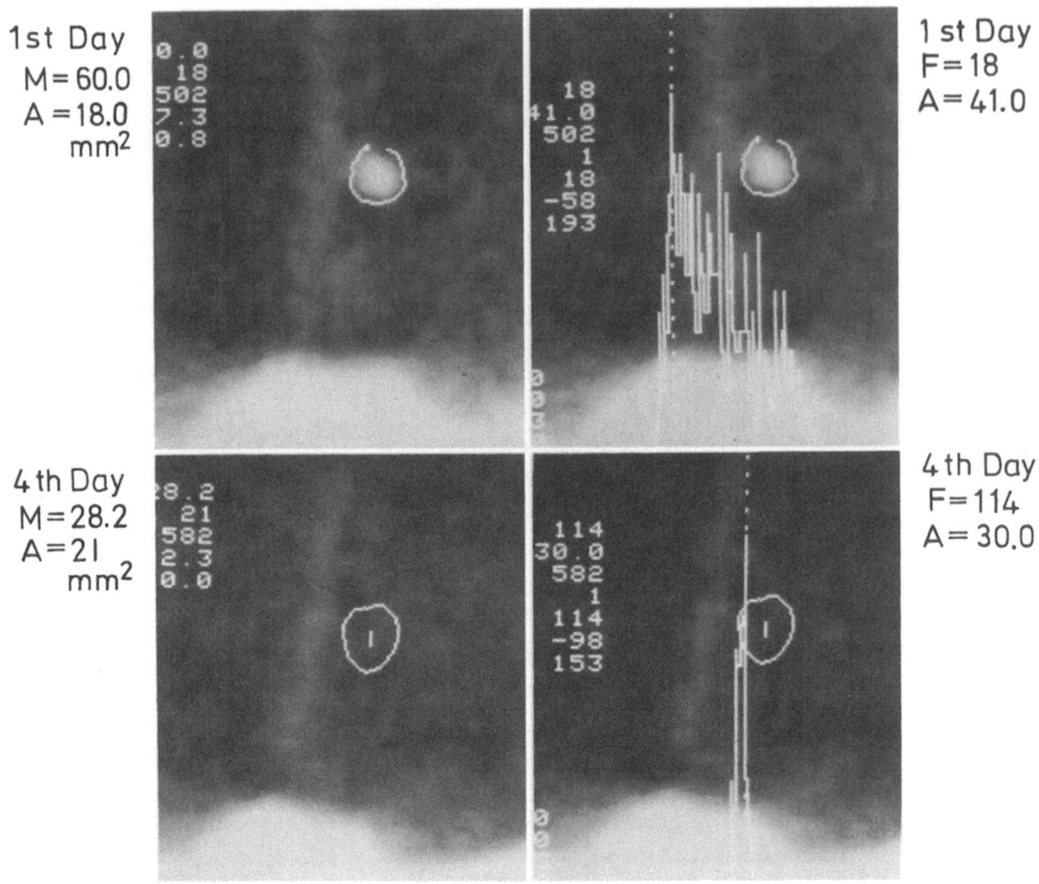

Fig. 7. Resorption of haematoma

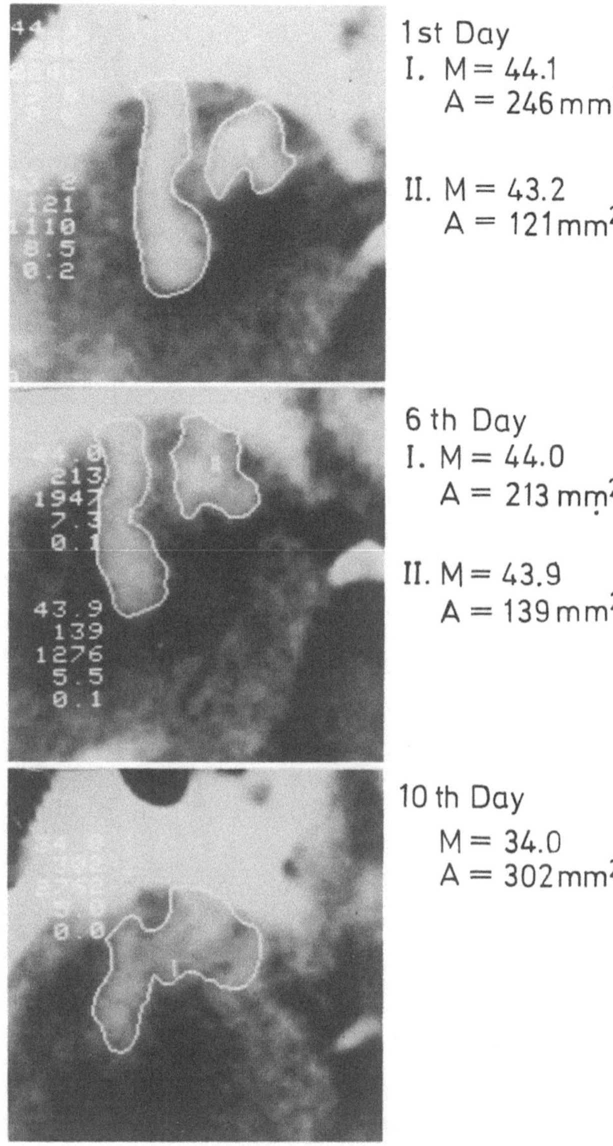

Fig. 8a. Resorption of haematoma. No change in absorption values 6 days after bleeding

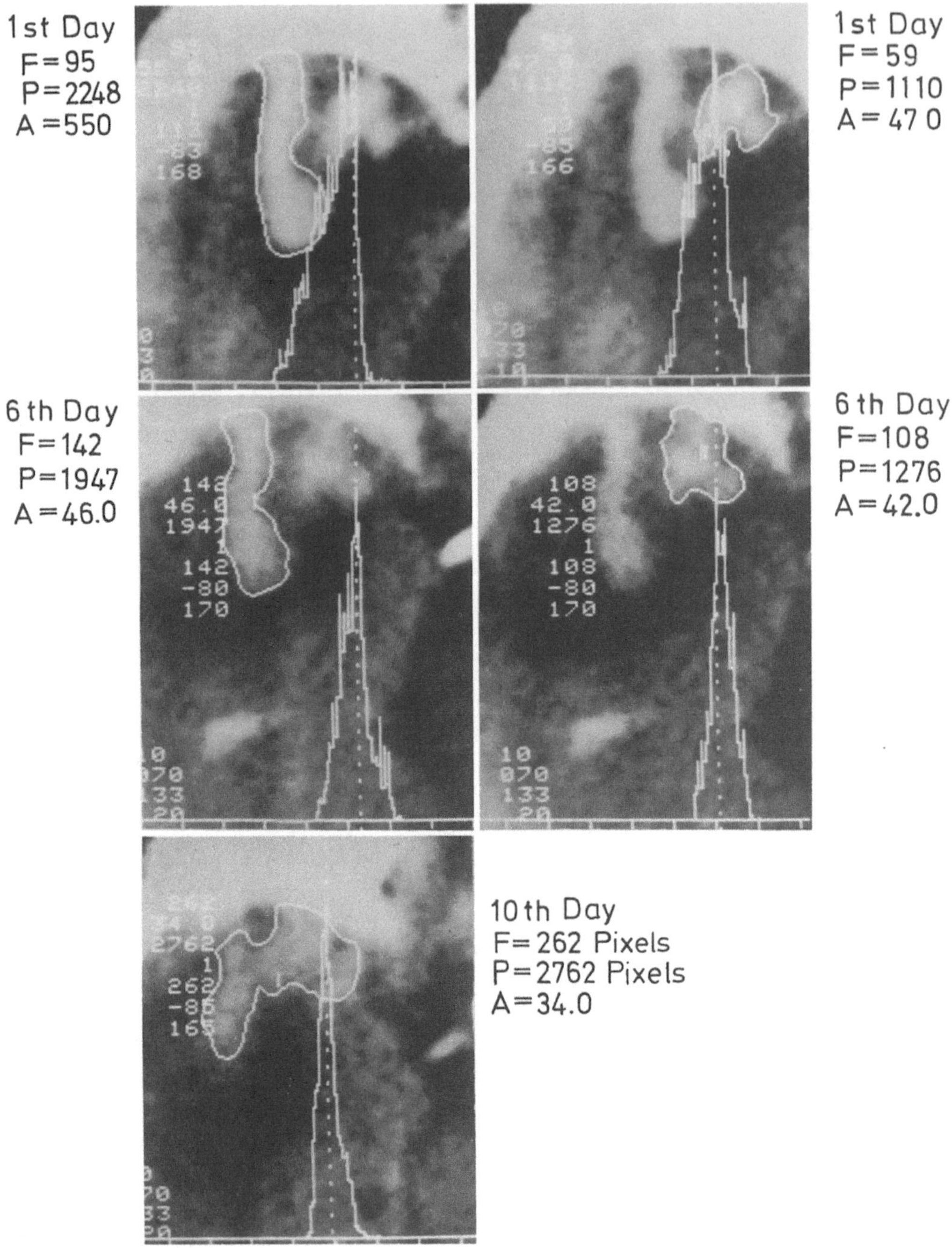

Fig. 8b. Resorption of haematoma. Note the change of the highest number of pixles between the 1st, 6th day and 10th day after bleeding

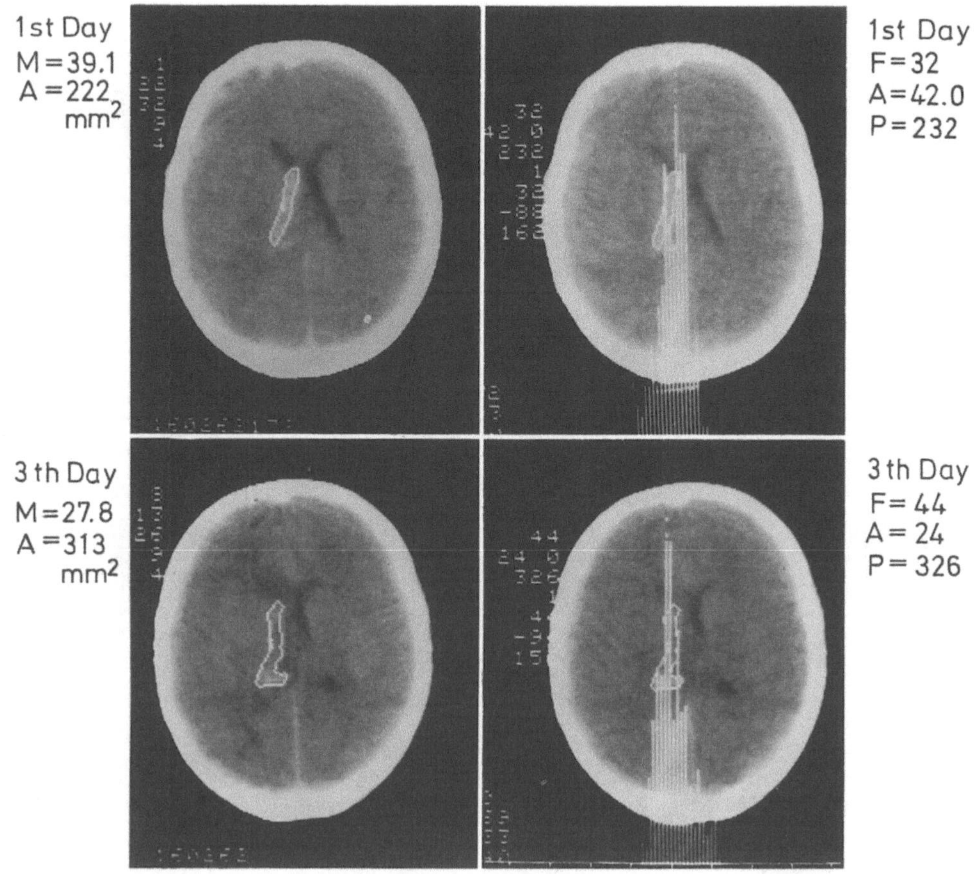

Fig. 9. Absorption of blood in the ventricle

could as well increase over the same period, as seen in an 80-year-old patient with subdural hygroma (Fig. 11).

Summary

In spite of difficulties connected with the exact reproduction of the same slice in CT in serial examinations, a considerable number of objective data can be gained about:

a) The extent of the lesion (planimetry);
b) The average absorption values and their change; and
c) the average absorption values of the largest number of pixels and their change (histograms).

Our preliminary observations suggest that for obtaining objective data concerning the resorption of blood and the structure of the haematoma, the elaboration of histograms and their evaluation is superior to the evaluation by mere measurement of absorption values. A further step will be the more exact analysis of pixels with low absorption values in order to define the zones of oedema.

We would recommend the development of appropriate software programmes for the analysis of the oedema zone surrounding the haematoma.

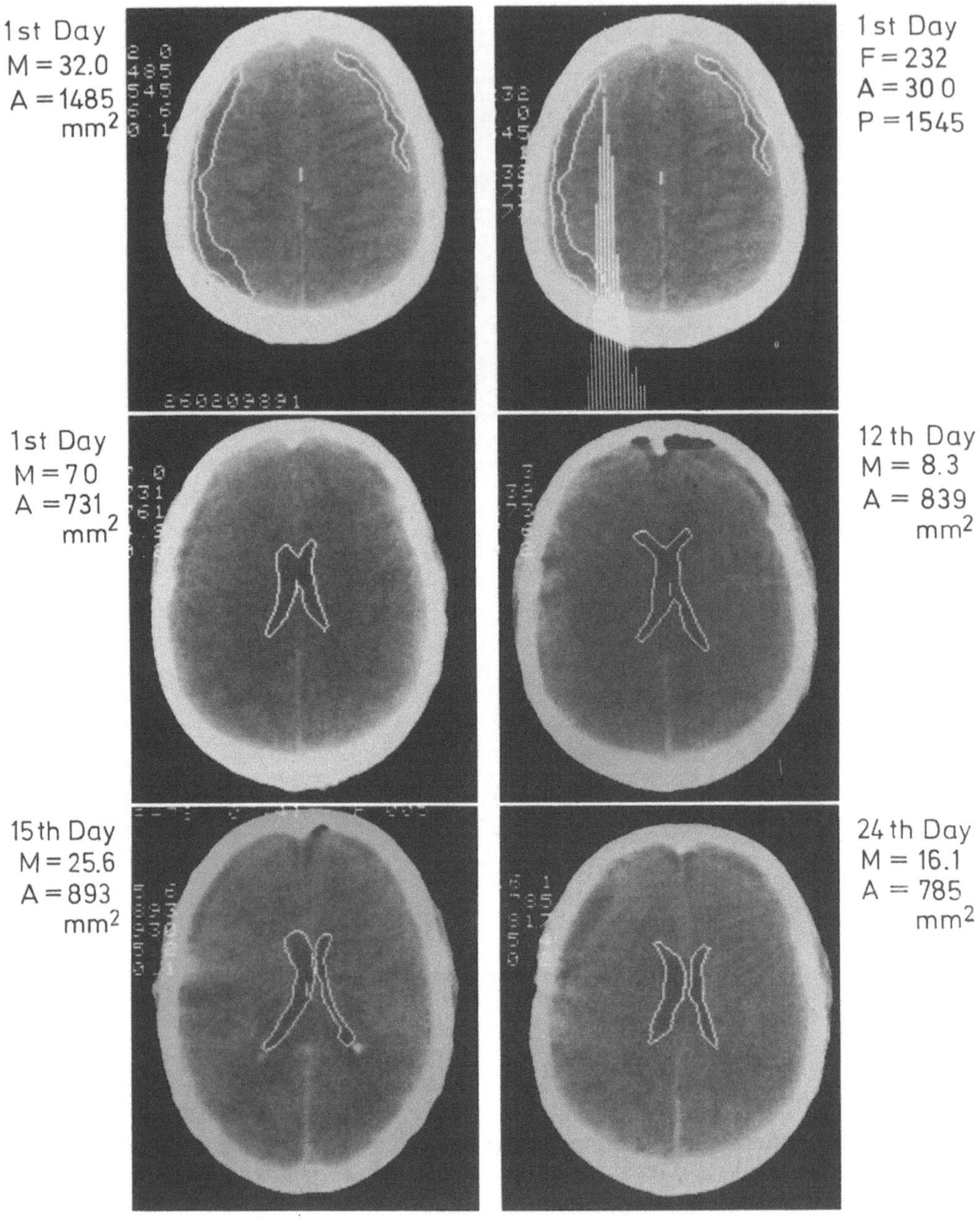

Fig. 10. Constant ventricular size in a patient with chronic subdural haematoma

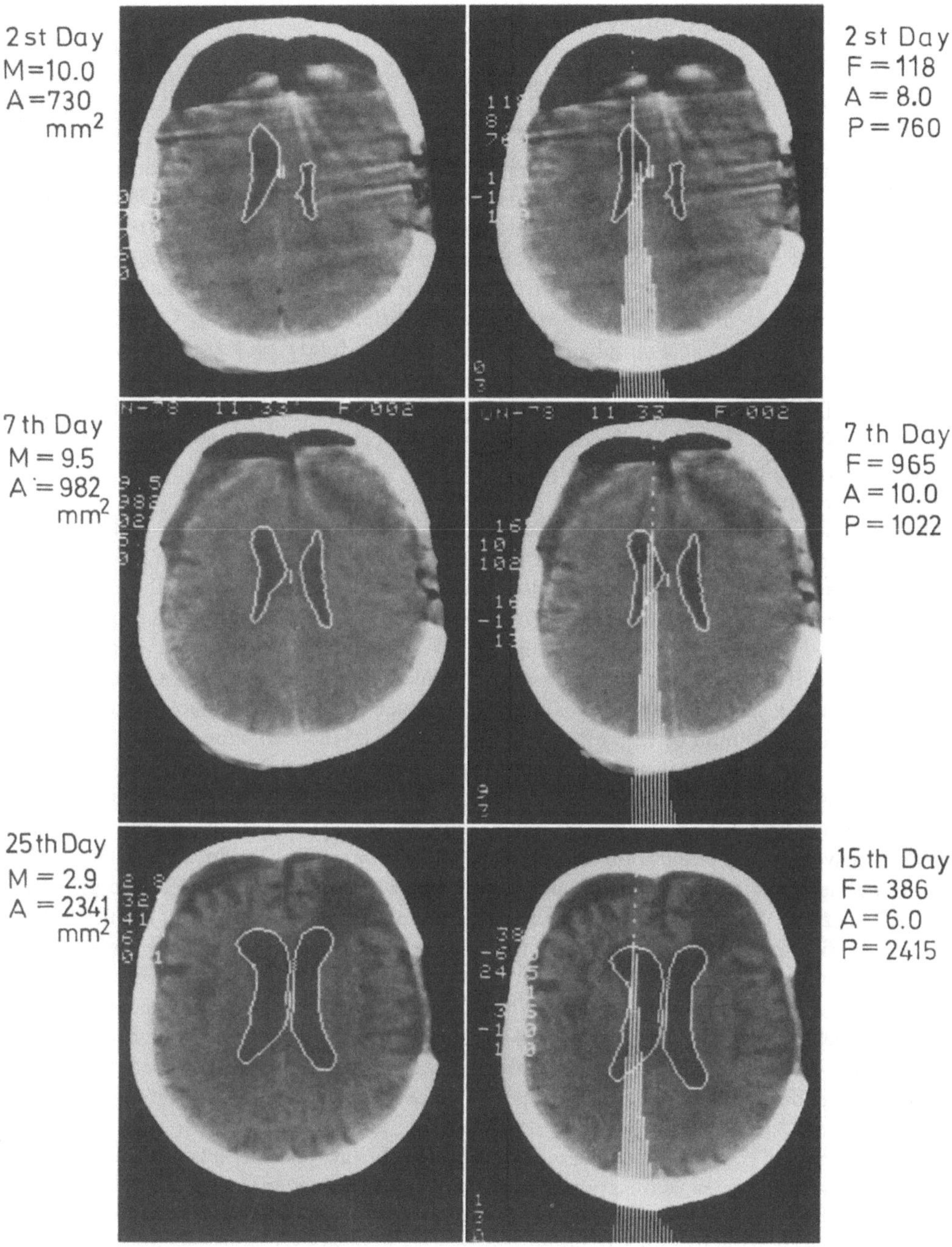

Fig. 11. Increasing ventricular size in a patient with subdural hygroma

6.2.6 Natural History and Follow-Up

T. Grumme, Berlin; K. Kretzschmar, Mainz, and W. Lanksch, Munich

Computed tomography (CT) is the first method to permit direct demonstration of space-occupying intracerebral haematomas. In addition, the procedure makes few demands on patients, most of whom are seriously ill. The introduction of CT has allowed us to study the natural course of spontaneous intracerebral haematomas. Older diagnostic methods provide limited information; the Echo-EG demonstrates regression of the midline shift and the EEG a return to normal brain wave activity, while brain scintiphotography shows a decrease in activity. Repeated carotid angiography is not permissible as a follow-up procedure and would, in many cases, merely document a reduction in the size of the mass lesion.

Our CT follow-up studies are based on results achieved by the CT study groups in Berlin, Mainz and Munich. Our own experience involves 103 cases of spontaneous intracerebral haemorrhage. Angiography was employed to exclude aneurysm and angioma as possible sources of bleeding.

Both the clinical condition of the patients and organizational considerations involving use of the scanner precluded adherence to a rigid schedule in performing follow-up studies. For this reason, we have chosen to present the results organized on a weekly basis up to the end of the 2nd month, and on a monthly basis thereafter. Some follow-ups consist of only a single study, either because the patients died or because they were transferred to other hospitals and later re-examined once in our clinic. An operation was performed in 25 cases, so these patients were no longer followed as cases of spontaneous untreated intracerebral haemorrhage. The period of follow-up was a maximum of 18 months after appearance of the haematoma.

Coagulated blood, which displaces and destroys brain tissue and which may penetrate the ventricles, has a significantly higher density than adjacent tissue. The signs of an intracranial space-occupying lesion are quite variable and depend on its position and size as well as on the presence of ventricular penetration and pre-existing brain atrophy. Perifocal oedema – or, rather, a zone of reduced density – is not evident immediately after the event. Two or three days later, a zone of reduced density may appear around the haematoma, which has not as yet changed in size or density. The nature of the hypodense zone is not entirely clear. Both resorption processes and development of oedema in lacerated tissue adjacent to the haemorrhage would seem to be present. When surgical intervention becomes necessary as a result of developing herniation, one finds evidence of both factors: localized brain oedema and collections of fluid resembling serum near the haematoma. However, one may encounter cases without a perifocal zone of reduced density. This occurs when brain tissue defects begin to appear.

The duration and course of the process of resorption may vary considerably as they appear in the CT scan. After a review of the available material, it is only possible to sketch out the natural course of this process. The size of the haematoma would seem to be a major factor. On the basis of our experience, we have found it convenient to classify intracerebral haematomas into two groups: those smaller than 1.5 – 2 cm in diameter and those larger. We shall first discuss the haematomas larger than 1.5 – 2 cm.

Neither the density nor the size of the intracerebral haematoma diminishes during the 1st week. Figure 1 shows a case of massive haematoma in the temporal lobe near the basal ganglia, with penetration of the ventricles. After a week, it appears that only the admixture of blood in the ventricles has diminished. A zone of slightly reduced density has appeared in the temporal region.

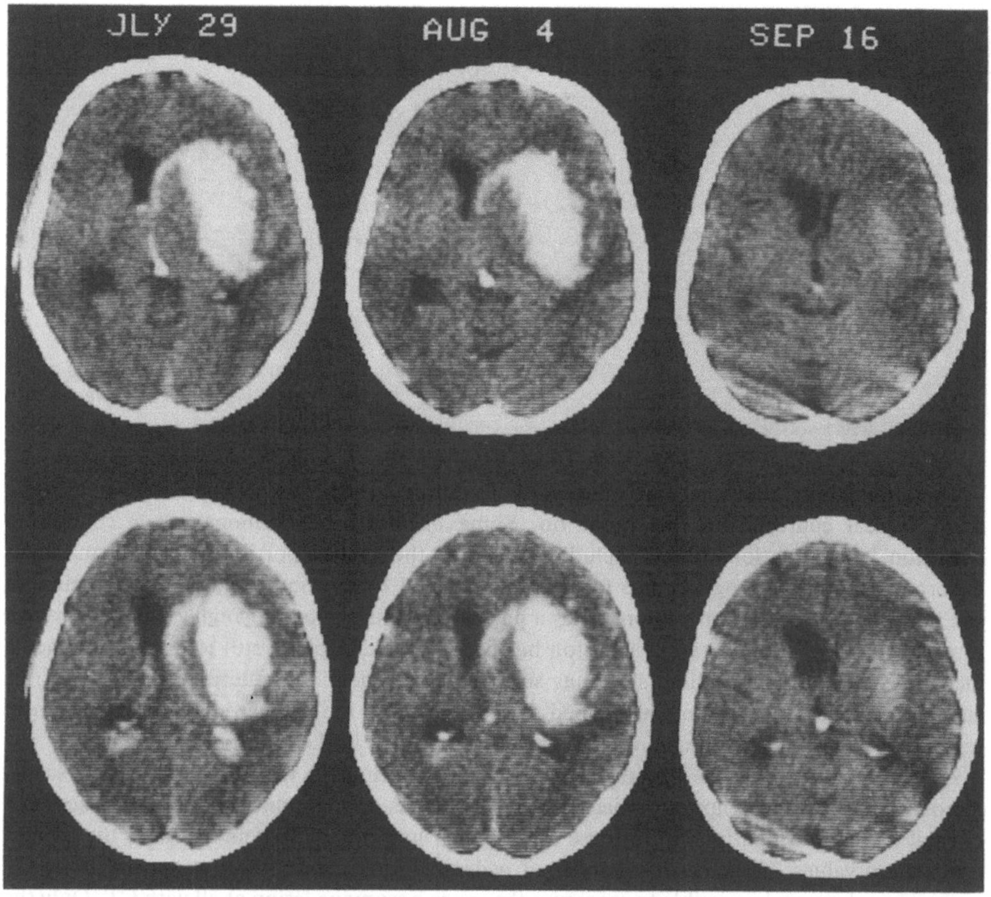

Fig. 1. Massive temporal intracerebral haematoma near the basal ganglia with penetration of the ventricles. Control investigations after 1 and 9 weeks

During the 2nd week, the density of the haematoma diminishes somewhat, with the central portions maintaining higher attenuation values, which would indicate that the haematoma decomposes from the periphery towards the centere. The border of the haematoma – usually a sharp, smooth contour – is no longer in evidence. Figure 2 shows a 12-day-old haemorrhage in the basal ganglia on the right side. The borders are not sharp and density is reduced in the periphery. In addition, there is a margin of reduced density around the haematoma. Since the attenuation values within the haematoma may vary considerably in this stage, measurement and graphic illustration of absolute values for the decrease in density provide little useful information. The highest attenuation values of fresh haemorrhages – about 84 Hounsfield units – are reduced to approximately 50 – 60 Hounsfield units during the 2nd week. The degree of midline shift does not change by the end of the 2nd week. The zone of reduced density may remain the same or increase slightly in size owing to the presence of localized oedema. The typical finger-shaped zones of oedema found in association with tumours are present in about 20% of haemorrhages in the temporal region or near the basal ganglia. To date, we have not found a single case of typical funnel-shaped oedema in spontaneous haemorrhage of the frontal region.

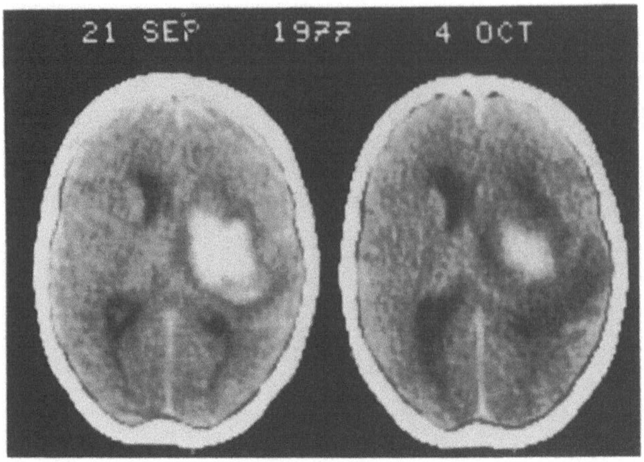

Fig. 2. Intracerebral haematoma of the basal ganglia. Control investigation after 13 days

The attenuation values become quite variable during the 3rd week. There seems to be no single typical course from this point on. Some haemorrhages demonstrate a continuing reduction in attenuation values, including those of the central portion of the haematoma. Resorption may have progressed so far that only a small zone of increased density remains, as can be seen in Fig. 3, which demonstrates a haemorrhage in the basal ganglia with penetration of the ventricles. In other cases the lesion has become smaller but is still evident as a zone of increased density. The midline shift has scarcely diminished. CT studies with i.v. contrast enhancement demonstrated a ring-shaped structure around the haematoma and the perifocal resorption zone. This phenomenon is the result of a defect in the blood-brain barrier.

As one might expect, the processes of resorption continue in the 4th week. In CT scans, almost all haemorrhages appear hyperdense in small areas. It is not uncommon to find zones of normal or reduced density within these areas which had originally demonstrated the highest attenuation values. If the perifocal zones of oedema and resorption do not appear in the CT scan, it may become impossible to recognize the space-occupying lesion at all with CT. Only the signs of displacement suggest the presence of a space-occupying lesion. If these signs are absent, one may come to the false conclusion that the intracerebral haemorrhage has resolved without

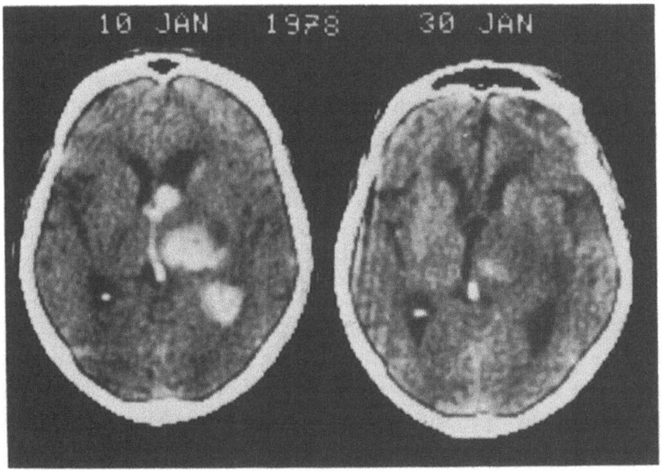

Fig. 3. Intracerebral haematoma of the basal ganglia. Control investigation after 20 days

sequelae. It is appropriate to mention that considerable problems in differential diagnosis may arise when patients are first examined with CT at this stage of their illness. This is generally true for all haemorrhages older than 10 days. CT studies made in the 4th week after haemorrhage may vary greatly. The haematoma is still slightly hyperdense, but there are also zones of reduced density in the area that had previously been hyperdense.

Hyperdense areas in the CT scan are exceptional in the 5th and 6th weeks. In general, the areas formerly occupied by haematoma appear as regions of normal or reduced density at this point. A midline shift is no longer present. There is a smooth transition from the perifocal zone of reduced density to the area formerly occupied by the – now completely transformed – haematoma. It is not certain that the incipient scar is present at this point.

The changes typical of the late stages of intracerebral haemorrhage may appear after 6 weeks, but often 8 – 9 weeks after the initial event. But very large haematomas may show, even after 9 weeks (Fig. 1), slight hyperdense and isodense areas; however, the haematoma has still not been resorbed. The appearance of the defects is extremely variable. The smallest defects appear as crescent-shaped areas of reduced density, while the larger defects may measure 3.5 × 4 cm and resemble cerebral infarction. The density of the defects attains values similar to that of the CSF. Distortion and dilatation of the ventricles on the affected side may often result, and midline structures may be displaced to the side of the lesion. Figure 4 shows an unoperated temporal lobe haemorrhage with a tissue defect 9 weeks after the event. Figure 5 illustrates a condition 9 weeks after haemorrhage near the basal ganglia.

In contrast to the larger haemorrhages, resorption seems to take place more quickly in the small haematomas less than 1.5 – 2 cm and a definite scar may be present after 4 weeks. In Fig. 6 the CT scan reveals no evidence of right cerebellar haemorrhage 4 weeks after the event. Even if no changes are evident in the CT scan, one may not conclude that the haemorrhage has healed without a scar. The lesion may be so small that it escapes detection as a result of the limited resolving power of the scanner.

Finally, a short discussion of the processes of resorption of intraventricular blood collections resulting from intracerebral haemorrhage is indicated. Decomposition of blood takes place more quickly in the ventricles than in brain tissue. At the end of the 1st week or beginning of the 2nd week, one usually finds isodense or slightly hyperdense zones in the posterior parts of the lateral ventricles. The extent of these changes depends on the extent of haemorrhage into the ventricles, while the location depends on the position of the patient. At the end of the 2nd

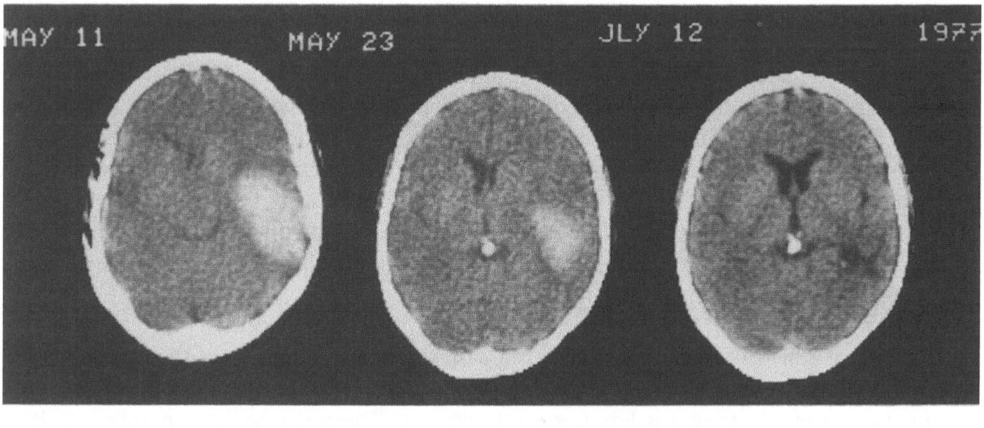

Fig. 4. Intracerebral haematoma, right temporal. Control investigations after 2 and 9 weeks

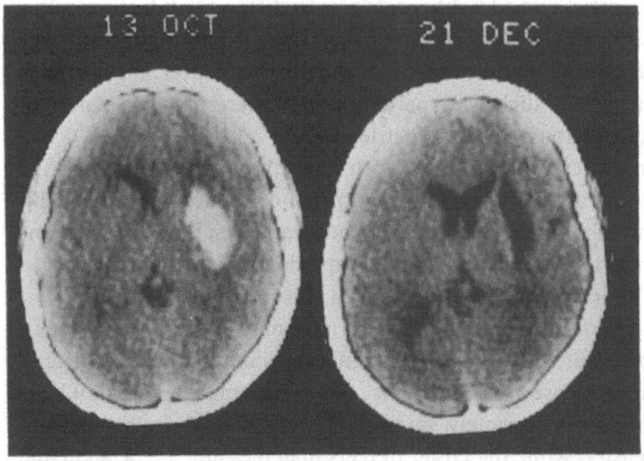

Fig. 5. Intracerebral haematoma near the basal ganglia. Control investigation after 9 weeks

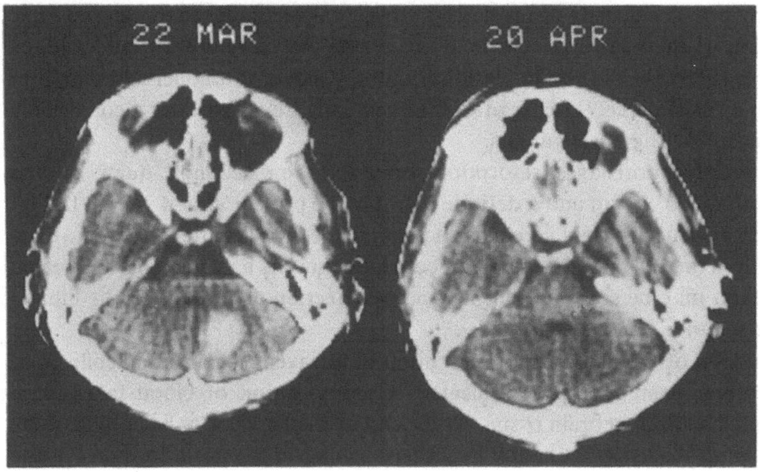

Fig. 6. Right intracerebellar haematoma. Control investigation after 4 weeks

week no blood clots are found in the ventricles, and the latter are often somewhat dilated. Rapid resorption may be explained by mixture of the blood and CSF.

In summary, we may draw the following conclusions about the natural history of spontaneous intracerebral haemorrhage, as it appears in the CT scan:

1) Speed of resorption depends on size of the haemorrhage. Haematomas smaller than 1.5 – 2 cm in diameter may heal with defects within 4 to 5 weeks. Larger haematomas require 6 – 7 weeks and usually 8 – 9 weeks. Blood in the ventricles is usually no longer demonstrable with CT after 14 – 20 days.
2) Regression of a midline shift does not parallel a reduction in size and density of the haematoma. Signs of a space-occupying lesion may still be present 5 weeks after haemorrhage. Regression of the midline shift is observed in the 3 week at the earliest. Occasional increases in the midline shift may be attributed to oedema.
3) A perifocal zone of reduced density appears on the 2nd or 3rd day, at the earliest, and is most probably a sign of a resorption process. In contrast to the situation found in brain tumours, cerebral oedema is less frequently present. These is usually a smooth transition from these perifocal zones of reduced density to the area of the developing tissue defect.

4) CT studies with i.v. contrast enhancement demonstrate in the 3rd or 4th week a ring-shaped structure around the haematoma and the perifocal resorption zone.
5) A defect is generally smaller than the original haematoma.
6) Normal CT scans following intracerebral haemorrhage should not be interpreted as evidence that the lesion has healed without a scar. Neuropathological evidence indicates that such conclusions on the basis of CT findings are not admissible.
7) Finally, one most conclude that intracerebral haemorrhage does not follow a single course in the CT scan. Size and location of the haemorrhage, penetration of the ventricles, perifocal oedema, extent of displacement of cerebral structures, pre-existing brain atrophy, age, general physical condition and previous illness may all cause great variation in these processes of haematoma transformation.

7 Conservative Treatment

7.1 The Immediate Care of Stroke

W. Dorndorf, Giessen

The immediate care of stroke includes general support measures and, in addition, special treatment. When the stroke is due to cerebral haemorrhage, special treatment consists mainly in the control of hypertension and in the reduction of intracranial pressure (Ramey et al. 1972; Toole et al. 1973; Meyer 1975; McDowell and Millikan 1978). General management including the following factors is important for both survival and the quality of survival:

Maintenance of patent airway
Maintenance of adequate lung ventilation
Appropriate therapy of cardiac dysfunction
Control of fluid balance, electrolytes and acid-base status
Maintenance of nutrition
Control of fever
Prevention of venous thrombosis
Coping with restlessness, nausea and singultus
Coping with seizures
Maintaining eye, oral and nasal hygiene and intact skin
Maintaining bladder and bowel function
Physical therapy

Many patients die, not directly from the effects of intracerebral haematoma, but from complications such as congestive heart failure, aspiration of gastric contents, pneumonia, fluid and electrolyte imbalance or pulmonary embolism. Preventing complications, therefore, is a valuable means of reducing mortality and morbidity, and of facilitating subsequent rehabilitation.

The acute stage of intracerebral haemorrhage is generally characterized by profoundly disturbed vital signs, as for instance by impairment of consciousness, elevated systemic blood pressure, respiratory and sometimes cardiac irregularities in association with a severe neurological deficit which usually makes its appearance abruptly. For professional management, these patients should be admitted to an intensive care unit in a neurological or neurosurgical department. After emergency treatment, i.e. respiratory care and initial management of intracranial hypertension, is instituted, followed by a physical examination and an attempt to obtain an accurate history about the patient, the necessary diagnostic procedures can be completed. Special attention has to be directed to respiratory pattern, to monitoring and support of vital functions, to continued evaluation of the neurological deficit and the management of any complication that may occur.

The first task of immediate care is the maintenance of an adequate airway and satisfactory pulmonary ventilation. Orotracheal intubation must be carried out if the attempt to clear the airway by suction is not successful. A nasogastric tube should be inserted to keep the stomach empty by aspiration. Regular measurement of paO_2, $paCO_2$ and pH are required to ascertain respiration and acid-base status. Tracheostomy becomes necessary if the airway control is unsatisfactory or if long-term respiratory assistance with a respirator is anticipated. Sterile aspiration techniques and adequate humidification of the airway must be guaranteed. In hypoxia, there is no objection to administering 1 – 2 litres oxygen per minute. Assisted or controlled ventilation may be indicated if CO_2 retention develops and results in respiratory acidosis. Another indication for controlled ventilation is an severe respiratory alkalosis. Immobility, insufficient coughing and aspiration favour the development of a segmental atelectasis which often precedes bronchopneumonia. Preventive measures are frequent turning, induced coughing and careful suction of tracheobronchial secretions. A recommended therapy is intermittent positive pressure breathing. Regular examination of the sputum, repeated chest examination and temperature control are necessary to detect an infection and commence appropriate antibiotic therapy.

Patients showing evidence of heart failure should be digitalized to improve cardiac output, to oxygenate the blood adequately and to prevent pulmonary congestion. Periodic measurement of the central venous pressure can be helpful in diagnosing impending congestive heart failure and in maintaining fluid balance.

In the first instance, nourishment of the patient takes place intravenously in the form of solutions of electrolytes, aminoacids and carbohydrates. The amount infused should approximately correspond to the urine output plus 1000 ml/24 h. Fever demands 750 ml more per degree centigrade. After 3 days, feeding by tube may be started to maintain the caloric requirements and avoid a negative nitrogen balance: 1500 calories per 24 h for the average patient. Fever over 39 °C should be reduced by administering appropriate medicaments. In most cases there is an infection of the respiratory or urinary tracts.

Many patients develop deep venous thrombosis of the paralyzed leg with subsequent pulmonary embolism in some cases. Early physical therapy, frequent change of position and elastic stockings may help in preventing the antecedent venous stasis.

Sedation, in the case of restlessness, is effected by the use of diazepam or, as an alternative, butyrophenon. Triflupromazine has proved effective against nausea and hiccup. Diazepam can be used against focal and generalized convulsions, and it can be combined with phenytoin and substituted by clonazepam (Rivotril) in the ratio of 10/1 mg.

In most patients, spontaneous intracerebral haemorrhage is caused by long-standing arterial hypertension which should be brought under control. When arterial pressure is excessively high and autoregulation is impaired or lost, cerebral blood volume increases, aggravating cerebral oedema and raising intracranial pressure. The elevated blood pressure should be lowered, but not so much as to impair cerebral blood flow. Only a reduction to about 160/90 mm Hg is advisable. The commonly used antihypertensive drugs such as reserpine, clonidine or hydralazine can be administered intramuscularly. Subsequent doses and the intervals of administration must be adjusted according to the effect on the blood pressure. When management is difficult, clonidine, hydralazine or methyldopa can be given intravenously and in emergency situations, diazoxide or sodium nitroprusside.

Intracranial hypertension in cerebral haemorrhage is usually caused by the combined effects of the mass lesion and the brain oedema (Katzman et al. 1977). Progressive enlargement of the haematoma and increasing brain oedema may be complicated by transtentorial herniation, a serious factor contributing to death in the acute stage. For reduction of increased intracranial pressure, intravenous infusions of hyperosmolar agents are used, such as mannitol or sorbitol. In general, they do not affect cerebral oedema, but reduce the fluid content of the normal brain, giving added space for the oedematous brain. Unfortunately, soon after the end of the infusion, intracranial pressure often returns to the previous level. On the other hand, possible rebound effects seem to be less of a problem using sorbitol and mannitol than with urea which was used formerly. Sorbitol is given in a concentration of 40%, mannitol in concentrations of 10% – 25%. Both of them produce an intense diuresis, so that dehydration, electrolyte imbalance and acidosis may occur. Therefore, fluid intake and output, electrolytes and acid-base status should be carefully controlled. Up to the onset of the activity of the applied hyperosmolar substances, induced hyperventilation may be indicated in the emergency treatment of elevated intracranial pressure. The resultant hypocapnia causes vasoconstriction and may diminish cerebral blood volume and reduce intracranial hypertension.

Glucocorticoids, such as dexamethasone, are used most effectively for reducing brain oedema associated with brain tumour. However, their value, if any, for patients suffering from stroke is not very impressive and opinion still differs about their effectiveness. The usual dose of dexamethasone is 24 – 28 mg daily. It is not clear whether very large doses – as high as 80 – 100 mg – are more effective. The administration of anti-ulcer medication is advisable. An open point is the value of aldosterone-antagonist spironolactone in the treatment of brain oedema associated with intracerebral haematoma; 4 × 200 mg daily is recommended.

The effect of fast-acting diuretics like frusemide on cerebrospinal fluid pressure is only mild at best. This indicates that such drugs should not be used alone in the treatment of brain oedema, but might be suitable in combination with slow-acting steroids.

There is still much to do in the immediate care of patients suffering from spontaneous intracerebral haematoma. However, prevention is better than cure. Thus, prevention of intracerebral haemorrhage by consistent treatment of the most important risk factor, hypertension, is a worthwhile task, considering the early, high mortality risk.

7.2 Conservative Therapy of Spontaneous ICH

H. Reisner, Vienna

Damage within the wall of the vessels or a pathological change in the content of a vessel is always a precursor of spontaneous cerebral haemorrhage. Disease in the wall of a vessel is most frequently arteriosclerosis, rarely it is hyalinosis; genuine hypertension leads more easily to haemorrhage than nephrogenic factors do (Davidoff 1958; Schiefer 1972; Reisner 1975).

Other rare vascular diseases (collagenosis, panangiitis nodosa and, exceptional nowadays, neurosyphilis) cause fewer cerebral haemorrhages, but more frequently interfere with the blood supply.

Haemorrhage in youth is usually caused by aneurysms or malformations within the vascular system. Haemorrhage from vascular tumours within the brain (glioblastoma multiforme) may show preliminary symptoms. Thus the haemorrhage does not occur as a first symptom in a completely healthy person (as in hypertensive intracerebral haemorrhage). One can also observe haemorrhage in spontaneous or iatrogenic disturbances of the coagulation mechanisms (e.g. in therapy with anticoagulants or antifibrinolytic drugs) (Klinger 1966). As a result of this, haemorrhage develops from pathological changes in the vessel walls or from disturbances of the coagulation mechanisms. Any treatment planned must depend on the particular cause. Acute haemorrhage needs conservative therapy with respect to both the pathological factors mentioned above. Disturbances of the blood coagulation mechanisms should be specifically treated in addition to acute medical, intensive care which is necessary. Diseases of the walls within the vascular system can sometimes be treated by surgical intervention, e.g. cases with vascular malformations or bleeding brain tumours (Krayenbühl 1965; Schiefer 1972).

Thus, conservative treatment is restricted except for prophylaxis and after treatment. Arteriosclerosis can rarely be influenced in any way. Collagenosis in the vascular system of the brain has a slightly better chance of treatment (immunosuppressive therapy); haemorrhages due to hypertension can be treated both by diet or medication. None of these measures is specific except in the treatment of neurosyphilis. One has to bear in mind that if the patient with haemorrhage survives (by conservative or neurosurgical treatment), the underlying illness is still not easy to treat and it sometimes progresses despite treatment.

Now that we have axial computer tomography, diagnosis of intracerebral haemorrhages has become much easier. Furthermore, one can also diagnose small intracerebral haemorrhages which may not always show typical clinical, diagnostic features. Sometimes in the CT scan one can see a cerebral haemorrhage which occurs clinically as a temporary disturbance of blood circulation within the brain (PRIND = prolonged reversible ischaemic neurological deficit) (Reisner 1961; Kazner et al. 1969; Grumme et al. 1976; Müller and Wiggly 1977; Pineda 1977; Walshe 1977; Reisner and Dal-Branco 1978).

Signs of intracranial pressure are not marked or may not be observed at all; clinical findings are represented by localizing neurological signs. These are merely small isolated haemorrhages which do not show any features on CSF examinations.

If cerebral haemorrhage is diagnosed the patient should be under intensive care, regardless of whether there is evidence of increased intracranial pressure. As a minimum the patient should at first be placed in a ward with facilities for intensive supervision and therapy. This should happen also with patients who are clinically not suspected of having a cerebral haemorrhage but in whom cerebral haemorrhage has been diagnosed in the CT scan.

Each small spontaneous intracerebral haemorrhage can have a progressive course and may ultimately break through into the fluid spaces. This group of patients does not require a full regime of intensive care.

One should use dehydrating agents, lower the blood pressure and, in addition, attend to cardiac and metabolic difficulties. Each patient, regardless of the location and size of the lesion, should be on strict bed rest combined with continuous clinical supervision including CSF examinations for a few weeks.

If the patient shows impairment of consciousness or is unconscious, a nasopharyngeal catheter, Mayo tubes or more likely intubation or tracheotomy should be employed; long-lasting unconsciousness sometimes needs nasal feeding. Antibiotic cover might be used with oxytetracycline, penicillin, oracillin, ampillicin, cephalexin or something similar. Intravenous infusions using 5% laevulose, isotonic NaCl or physiological Ringer's solution should be given, a minimum of 200 ml per day. Furthermore human albumin 2 × 50 ml, mannitol 2 – 3 × 100 ml/kg body wt., frusemide 2 × 1 – 2 ampoules of 20 mg. Dehydration depends on urinary secretion which should not be 500 – 700 ml less than the intake.

In cases of extrarenal insufficiency no mannitol, but rather sugar and lipoids should be given to avoid breakdown of protein.

The electrolyte balance is of great importance because of the substitution of potassium (KCl or potassium bicarbonate, Na^+ and Cl). Electrolyte solutions should be used combined with Elomel, etc.

When using aminoacids (aminosol) one has to consider the complications of possible malfunction of the kidneys, with increase of blood urea and urinary nitrogen.

Primarily renal malfunction requires mannitol, frusemide or dopamine. Acidosis needs sodium bicarbonate or Tutofusin, but not sodium lactate (danger: lactate acidosis).

In patients with hypertension, blood pressure should be lowered to 150–170 mm Hg [clonidine, continuous drip, reserpine 2.5 mg or leucinocaine-dihydroergotoxine (Panthesin-hydergin)]. Diabetic patients should receive appropriate treatment.

For cardiac treatment, digitalis glycoside combined with 0.125–0.25 mg strophanthine-K (Strophanthine, once or twice daily) should be given. Psychomotoric unsteadiness can be treated with lytic cocktail [one ampoule chlorpromazine (Largactil, Megaphen), promethazine (Phenergan, Atosil), dihydroergotoxine or three times daily one-third of one ampoule pethidine, chlorpromazine and promethazine].

Patients with long-lasting states of unconsciousness should be given parenteral feeding consisting of (a) Aminofusin, Aminosol-laevulose-Ethanol, Vitamins and 33% dextrose; (b) Intralipid 20% (2500 U. heparin) or (a) and (b) together as infusion. Feeding by stomach tube might be beneficial.

Treatment of brain oedema requires cortisone (48 mg dexamethason; 1st day, every 2 h 8 mg; 2nd day, 4 mg every 4 h; 3rd day, 8 mg every 4 h, followed by slow decrease of dosage). Cortisone therapy in oedema of the brain caused by traumatic haemorrhage seems to be more necessary than in cases of spontaneous intracerebral haemorrhage. The reason for this phenomenon might be primary shock in cases of traumatic haemorrhage. With clinical improvement all treatment should be gradually decreased.

In intracerebral haemorrhage one often observes paralysis of limbs (Reisner 1972); therefore, in these acute states one has to take care to prevent muscular contractions and stiff joints in the limbs involved. One should use specific positions for the patient in bed combined with careful passive movement of the involved joints. Special attention should be paid to joints of the fingers, hand and shoulder or ankle joint. If the general condition of the patient permits, physiotherapy might be of use; in cases of cerebral haemorrhage all these activities must be used with great caution, much more than in cases of cerebral insult due to disturbances of the cerebral circulation.

Active mobilization commonly starts after 4 weeks of illness. Further after-treatment demands physiotherapeutic rehabilitation, medication, diet, mental health and social activities. Special attention should be paid to factors of risk such as obesity, hypertension, diabetes and hyperlipoidaemia (Reisner 1975).

Summary

Conservative therapy in spontaneous intracerebral haemorrhages depends mainly on the state of consciousness of the patient. Patients with haemorrhages with only slight disturbances of consciousness need strict bed rest and dehydration and medication to lower the blood pressure, combined with cardiac help. All other cases need intensive care. Depending on the level of unconsciousness the patient has to be treated with intubation or tracheostomy. Besides specific therapy by infusion, dehydration and supervision of the electrolytes, one has to treat acidosis and renal insufficiency if they arise. If necessary, diabetes should also be treated. Cardiac help should not be ignored. Prophylactic antibiotics and use of the lytic cocktail (for sedation of psychomotor unsteadiness) are appropriate. In cases with long lasting unconsciousness parenteral feeding has to be used.

7.3 Rehabilitation After Acute ICH

K. A. Jochheim, Cologne

In May 1977, the White House Conference took place in Washington, D.C., bringing together 3700 disabled persons from throughout the United States. The summary of the final report has just been published. Among the major findings it is firmly emphasized that it is lack of co-ordination which prevents the disabled individual from getting the necessary service at the place and time needed. The problems arising from that gap, however, are not just individual problems, but they also affect the general planning of health and social services as well as their cost (Jochheim et al. 1977). Hoeck (1967) has outlined the need for co-ordinated efforts to rehabilitate stroke patients. According to his experience the main task is certainly the general assessment of the person to be rehabilitated which allows one to develop therapeutic aims as well as the planning and organization of the therapeutic work. Such assessment certainly has to recognize the present status as well as the long-term prognosis of the medical condition which includes the time schedule of the biomedical recovery as far as this is predictable. Such an assessment usually contains as a basis the immediate or permanent impairment remaining from the brain lesion, but there are additional factors to be mentioned which influence the therapeutic plan considerably. One major factor is the classification of disability resulting from functional limitations and from restrictions of activity. Functional limitations are defined as any obvious loss or reduction of the ability to carry out those individual functions that are expected of the person or parts of his body, and that are consequent upon impairment. Functional limitation is characterized by partial or total inability to perform specific mental, motor, sensory or other physical functions within the range and manner normally expected of the individual. Examples include disturbance of particular intellectual, behavioural, communication, posture, manipulative and other physical skills, as well as reduction of more generalized abilities such as endurance and tolerance. Restrictions of activity, however, mean any demonstrable loss or reduction of the ability to carry out such complicated or integrated activities as are expected of the person or the body and which are the result of functional limitations. Restriction of activity is characterized by inability or difficulty in performing voluntary activity customary to the individual and his whole body having regard to age, sex and normal social role. It relates to abilities that are generally accepted as essential components of everyday life; examples include disturbances of or inappropriate behaviour, in communication, in personal care such as continence and the ability to wash and feed oneself, in the performance of other activities in daily living and in locomotor activities such as the ability to walk. A list of two digit categories of disability was prepared for the World Health Organization by Philip Wood and co-workers (1979) (Table 1) and presents, if properly applied to any individual case, a comprehensive check-list, which enables the rehabilitation team to plan their treatment and management so as to minimize the handicap resulting from impairment and disability in the social contacts.

Figure 1 helps to explain the possibilities and limitations in overcoming disability in the main functional areas and the need for additional social activities to influence environmental factors. With this idea in mind the success of rehabilitation services could be orientated towards the goal of optimal re-integration into the different facets of social life. It is obvious that rehabilitation services in our present system of health care and social security are not meeting the challenge of disability resulting from stroke, in general, and from acute cerebral haemorrhage in particular. Rehabilitation facilities in close connexion with neurological and neurosurgical departments are still developed in only a few centres around the world. The tremendous increase of costs of

Table 1. Two-digit categories of disabilities

1	Behaviour disabilities
	Disabilities in autonomy (10 – 12)
10	Personal safety disability
11	Self-awareness disability
12	Severe behaviour disorder
	Disabilities in relations (13 – 16)
13	Family role disability
14	Social role disability
15	Occupational role disability
16	Other emotional disability
	Other behaviour disability (17 – 19)
17	Learning disability
18	Other education disability
19	Other behaviour disability
2	Communication disabilities
	Speaking disabilities (20 – 22)
20	Disability in understanding speech
21	Other disability in comprehension
22	Disability in talking
	Listening disabilities (23 – 24)
23	Disability in listening to speech
24	Other listening disability
	Seeing disabilities (25-27)
25	Disability in distant sight
26	Disability in near sight
27	Other disability in seeing
	Other communication disabilities (28 – 29)
28	Disability in writing
29	Other communication disability
	Physical disabilities:
	a) Activity restrictions
3	Personal care disabilities
	Excretion disabilities (30 – 32)
30	Controlled excretory difficulty
31	Uncontrolled incontinence
32	Other excretion disability
	Personal hygiene disabilities (33 – 34)
33	Bathing disability
34	Other personal hygiene disability
	Dressing disabilities (35 – 36)
35	Clothing disability
36	Other dressing disability
	Feeding and other personal care disabilities (37 – 39)
37	Disability in preliminaries to feeding
38	Other feeding disability
39	Other personal care disability
4	Locomotor disabilities
	Ambulation disabilities (40 – 45)
40	Walking disability
41	Traversing disability
42	Climbing stairs disability
43	Other climbing disability
44	Running disability
45	Other ambulation disability
	Confining disabilities (46 – 47)
46	Transfer disability
47	Transport disability
	Other locomotor disabilities (48 – 49)
48	Lifting disability
49	Other locomotor disability
5	Body disposition disabilities
	Domestic disability (50 – 51)
50	Subsistence disability
51	Household disability
	Body movement disabilities (52 – 57)
52	Retrieval disability
53	Reaching disability
54	Other disability in arm function
55	Kneeling disability
56	Crouching disability
57	Other body movement disability
	Other body disposition disabilities (58 – 59)
58	Postural disability
59	Other body disposition disability
6	Dexterity disabilities
	Daily activity disabilities (60 – 61)
60	Environmental modulation disability
61	Other daily activity disability

Table 1 (continued)

	Manual activity disabilities (62 – 66)
62	Fingering disability
63	Gripping disability
64	Holding disability
65	Handedness disability
66	Other manual activity disability
	Other dexterity disabilities (67 – 69)
67	Foot control disability
68	Other body control disability
69	Other dexterity disability
7	Situational disabilities and other activity restrictions
	Dependence and endurance disabilities (70 – 71)
70	Circumstantial dependence
71	Disability in endurance
	Environmental disabilities (72 – 77)
72	Disability in temperature tolerance
73	Disability in tolerance of other climatic features
74	Disability in tolerance of noise
75	Disability in tolerance of illumination
76	Disability in tolerance of work stresses
77	Disability in tolerance of other environmental factors
	Other activity restrictions (78 – 79)
78	Other situational disability
79	Other and unspecified activity restriction
	Physical disabilities:
	b) Functional limitations
8	Particular skill disabilities
9	Other functional limitations

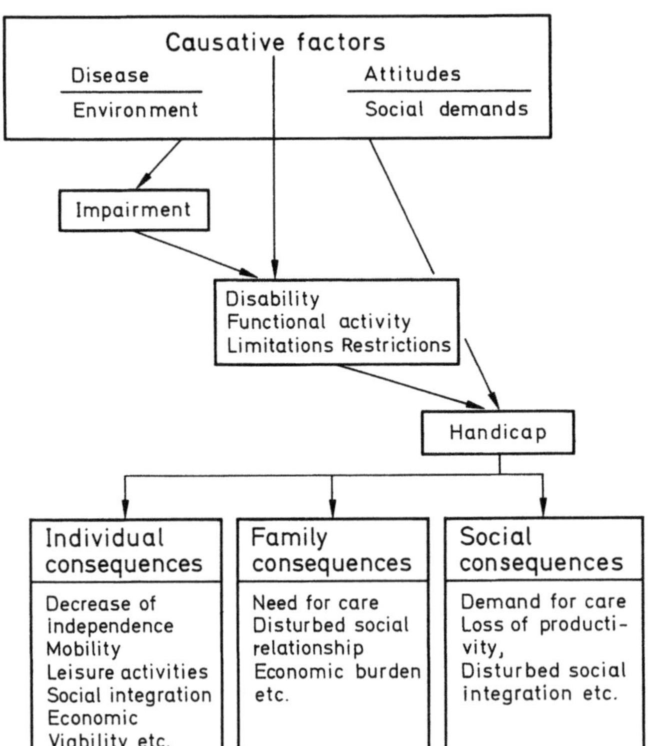

Fig. 1. Factors in causation and in rehabilitation after acute cerebral haemorrhage

hospital treatment in industrialized countries inevitably shortens the period in hospital, leaving the task of proper rehabilitation in the hands of well-meaning but frequently insufficiently skilled health workers and volunteers in the community. Modern medicine has overcome high death rates in many conditions, but now has to concentrate on proper rehabilitation to make a prolonged life acceptable for the patients. University and health system planners should consider re-organization of hospitals and outpatient services along the lines indicated.

7.3.1 Rehabilitation after Spontaneous ICH

O. Leitholf, Gailingen

In the last 3 years 49 patients with spontaneous intracerebral haematoma underwent rehabilitation in our clinic. Of these, 26 were under 45 years of age, and 28 were male. Up to the present, 33 of the patients came once, 13 twice, one four times and two patients came five times to us for treatment. Of these, 24 came in the 1st year and 16 between the 1st and 2nd year after the haemorrhage.

Forty of our patients had been operated on; in 28 of the patients the cause of the haemorrhage was unknown or undiscovered. Hypertension was the cause in 13 patients, decreased coagulability in six and, in two patients, haemorrhage was due to taking contraceptives.

In 12 cases the damage produced by the haemorrhage was situated in the left and, in six cases, in the right temporal region. In two other groups, each consisting of five patients, the haematoma was located in the right and left temporoparietal region. The other lesions were located evenly throughout the other regions. In one case the haemorrhage was infratentorial.

Immediately after the haemorrhage 35 of the patients had neurological disorders. Of these, two had a slight hemiparesis, ten a middle grade, and 23 a severe hemiparesis. After 2 years the picture had altered, for only three of the pareses could be defined as severe, while seven of the patients had a middle grade and eight had a slight paresis. In 12 there were no longer any symptoms.

In nine of the patients aphasia could be identified after the haemorrhage; this was still present after 2 years in eight patients, although in the majority of cases there were signs of improvement. In spite of this, one must say that the results of speech therapy were the least successful.

Psychopathological disturbances which were found in 32 of the patients after the haemorrhage were present in only 14 by the last examination, from which only middle grade or severe disturbances were recorded.

Fits occurred in the 1st year in 14 of the cases, during the 2nd year in another five and later in a further three patients. Of these 22 patients, eight had complete relief, six had only rare attacks and eight had them more frequently.

All types of treatment available were used on the patients. Each one had physiotherapy, 24 occupational therapy, and 34 had neuropsychological treatment which included speech therapy. Eight of the patients were assessed as to their fitness for work.

After 1 year ten patients were re-employed, after 2 years a further seven and after 5 years another four patients returned to work. Thus, there were altogether 21 patients who were capable of resuming work after the haemorrhage. Of these, 11 were working full-time and five part-time at their previous jobs. Four patients worked full-time and one patient part-time at another job. However, at the last assessment, 28 of the patients had not been able to return to work or were already receiving a pension.

In summary, one can say that of these 21 patients the majority were able to return to work *after* rehabilitation in our clinic although five patients had already been re-employed *before* admission to us. Eighteen patients had felt some improvement after the treatment, but were not yet ready to return to work. With ten patients no improvement could be achieved after rehabilitation, and they had to be regarded as incapable of work.

Of the 21 patients who were re-employed, the haemorrhage was situated on the right in 14 cases and on the left in seven. From a consideration of the history it would appear that in these patients who returned to work the cause of the haemorrhage was hypertension in three cases, decreased coagulability in three cases, and in two patients haemorrhage was associated with intake of contraceptives. It is striking to note that half of the patients with increased coagulability and both patients who took contraceptives were able to return to work.

Of these re-employed patients eight had no paresis after the haemorrhage. Among the other 13 who did have a paresis this had greatly improved. Six patients had been aphasic after the haemorrhage, which in one case had already recovered spontaneously before admission to us. In three cases the aphasia had improved after treatment, and in the other two it persisted unchanged. Of the 21 patients who returned to work 14 of them had psychiatric disorders. Ten of these who had severe deficiencies had shown some improvement, but in four cases the condition remained unchanged.

Of those patients who had returned to work eight complained of fits at their first examination, and at the last assessment three of these were free of attacks. Another six now had occasional fits, up to six times a year, and in one case there was no improvement and fits were still frequent.

I would now like to describe five patients, the first, three of whom were operated on:

A 24-year-old female experienced a spontaneous intracerebral haemorrhage, in the left temporoparietal region, 14 days after confinement. Post-operatively she had fits for 2 years which then ceased. She had dysphasia and was forgetful, but this showed no improvement with our treatment. The patient remained unable to work. The prognosis concerning the dysphasia must be regarded as poor after $4\frac{1}{2}$ years.

In another female patient with a right frontal spontaneous haemorrhage the cause was probably hypertension. Soon after the operation the left hemiparesis showed rapid signs of recovery. The neurological state was normal, though she was perhaps a little slow and showed signs of forgetfulness. This patient came to us 9 months after the haemorrhage. She was already capable of returning to her old job, and after her discharge she felt she had improved and was generally stabilized. Psychological testing showed no abnormalities.

A third patient came to us 6 months after her operation. In this case the haematoma was situated in the temporal basal ganglion and was extensive. As a result of two admissions to our clinic with a year between them, a great improvement was achieved subjectively as well as objectively. The patient, who at first was wheel-chair bound, was able to walk unaided at the time of her last discharge. The psychopathological picture was normal; she complained merely of occasional focal fits. The cause of the haemorrhage was unknown.

After these three quite different courses seen with operative treatment of spontaneous intracerebral haematomas, we now describe two patients whose haematoma was not operated on:

A 56-year-old man with hypertension suffered a large right temporal haemorrhage with perforation into the trigone. In spite of intensive treatment, his psychopathological disturbances and left-sided hemiparesis showed no improvement. The patient remained incapable of work.

In comparison, a young woman who came to us 15 months after a haemorrhage in the left internal capsule, was able to report a spontanous recovery of the paresis even before her admission. After the treatment she became mentally more balanced and stabilized. This patient had already resumed her former employment 3 months after the haemorrhage.

Because 21 of our patients with a spontaneous intracerebral haematoma were able to return to work either full-time or part-time, and another group of patients showed signs of improvement after a relatively short observation time and can be expected to return to work later on, one can look for more positive results than are normally expected from the rehabilitation of a spontaneous intracerebral haematoma, after operative or conservative treatment.

7.3.2 Discussion

H. Hacker, Frankfurt: We have been told that the number of stroke patients and especially those with intracerebral haematomas is enormous. We have also heard that intensive care should be established immediately, and probably for everyone. The costs of such a programme of management would be enormous. A compromise should be found – maybe intensive treatment for the patient with intracranial haemorrhage would be given only for a short time and then the patient would go back to his home-hospital. One should also ensure that rehabilitation takes place in the home surroundings as soon as possible because treatment in special rehabilitation centres is extremely expensive.

J. Gillingham, Edinburgh: In giving rehabilitation we must ensure that it is, in fact, effective. There is, at present, a study going on in Bristol (England), of the value of speech therapy using volunteers within the family who can do therapy in an intensive way. The early results seem to indicate that speech-therapy within the family is probably as effective as with trained speech therapists. We have to assess very carefully what is actually achieved by rehabilitation.

Another problem is surgery in the later stages, the aim of which is often to correct what has been caused by treatment at the earlier stages. It is important to provide good treatment initially so that there will be little necessity for late operations.

Rehabilitation centres on a national scale are not a realistic solution. In my opinion patients should return home as early as possible and the family must be involved in the rehabilitation process.

7.4 Initial Clinical Course and Prognostic Factors in ICH

F. Regli and D. Jeanmonod, Lausanne

Computerized tomography (CT scan) has become a most important tool in the diagnosis of intracerebral haematomas. This examination is approximately 90% accurate. Obviously the picture produced by the CT scan cannot distinguish between bleeding resulting from vessel rupture, tumoural necrosis or haemorrhagic infarction. In any event, to establish accurate criteria for the evaluation of treatment and prognosis of intracerebral haematomas it is mandatory to consider not only the results of the CT scan, but the whole range of clinical and paraclinical tests. In the following presentation the initial spontaneous course of intracerebral haematomas as well as the factors which determine their early and late prognosis will be described.

I. Initial Spontaneous Course of Intracerebral Haematomas

Intracerebral haematomas are typical examples of acute cerebrovascular accidents. They can occur without any prodromal symptoms and even when these are present, they are often vague and lack specificity. Their evolution is mostly progressive without fluctuations, but they can often show a striking reversibility of symptoms which can be attributed to compression factors and fibre dissection; both are reversible phenomena and do not cause permanent nerve fibre lesions. Previously, a distinction was made between massive destructive bleeding at the level of the basal ganglia and peripheral spreading of the bleeding with a more favourable course. Today, experience has shown that the clinical course of intracerebral haemorrhages is highly variable.

1) Acute Biphasic Course

The clinical incidence of this is at least 12%. It starts with focal neurological signs and the always-present diminution of consciousness, often accompanied by headache, vomiting and a meningeal syndrome, preceded by a non-specific prodromal phase. The early clinical course lasts between 1 hour and 2 days; this is followed by a period of 12 h to 19 days during which time a moderate-to-serious clinical neurological deficit is seen, but at the same time this is stabilized, as is the state of consciousness, generally without coma. Then after this plateau, one observes either a favourable clinical course with more or less serious neurological deficiencies, or a progressive deterioration over a 1- to 3-day period with increased focal hemispheric lesions and progressively clearer clinical signs of intracranial hypertension and brain stem compression. This type of clinical course, sometimes found in basal ganglia haematomas, is also typical of haemorrhages of the lobar white matter.

2) Variant of the Acute Biphasic Course

This second form is different from the first in that it appears suddenly but only the focal neurological signs are present. These are followed by a period of stabilization or a partial regression over a period of several days. After this period there is either an improvement or a worsening of the neurological symptoms, with a deterioration of the state of consciousness over a period of hours to weeks. This latter course frequently leads to deep coma and death. The incidence is difficult to evaluate. This pattern frequently indicates either a thalamic or a pontine haemorrhage.

3) Acute Triphasic Course

The incidence of this is difficult to evaluate. The initial symptoms correspond to those of the acute biphasic course, but they are followed by a phase of rapidly progressing neurological symptoms, especially of the hemispherical type. This phase is also followed by a rapid deterioration toward stupor, followed by coma similar to that already described in the first type. This type of clinical course has been described mostly in lateral putamino-capsular haemorrhages.

4) Hyperacute Course with Massive Flooding of the Ventricles and Severe Brain Damage

This clinical type presents with headache, flaccid hemiplegia and deep coma within 1 to 3 h and, occasionally, papilloedema. Frequently there are signs of ventricular tamponade. Of the deaths, 80% occur within 48 h, 60% within 24 h and some patients die within 2 h of the cerebrovascular accident.

The incidence is high, approximately 70%. This clinical course is classically described for a catastrophic haemorrhage of the basal ganglia and for a pontine haematoma.

5) Pseudotumoural Progressive Course (Slow Stroke)

The incidence is probably about 3%. After a prodromal episode there is a slow progression without remission of neurological symptoms, together with a decrease in the state of consciousness over a period of 7 to 14 days and sometimes longer. This slow, progressive phase can lead either to a regression of the symptoms with a favourable course, or to an increasing intracranial hypertension, with worsening of the hemispheric signs and finally compression of the brain stem. This form, which is sometimes found with lobar haemorrhages and occasionally with pontine haematomas, presents pitfalls for differential diagnosis.

6) Forms with Recurrence

Two types of recurrence may be distinguished; one is termed latent recurrent clinical course. In this case, there are repeated cerebrovascular accidents of greater or lesser importance, followed by a more or less complete return to normal; these correspond to small, recurring haemorrhages which are subsequently re-absorbed. The incidence of this type of clinical course is low and it is cited to illustrate the example of recurring intrapontine haemorrhages.

The second recurrent form is a frequently fatal superacute haemorrhage, which occurs a few days after the first haemorrhage. The incidence of this particular recurrent form is difficult to estimate. Certain authors consider it virtually non-existent; others state its frequency as between 3% and 8%. It would seem that the incidence increases to between 8% and 14% in postoperative cases where haemostasis has not been completely achieved. Spontaneously recurring cases are seen in cerebellar, but mostly in thalamic, haemorrhages.

7) Course with Extracerebral Complications

The clinical course is identical to that of the first form, except that about 2 weeks after the cerebrovascular accident, during a smooth recovery and in the presence of apparent clinical improvement, there is a sudden deterioration of pulmonary origin, and death frequently occurs within a few days. Pulmonary complications are by far the most frequent; predisposing factors are the age of the patient, pulmonary oedema, cardiac failure in the presence of hypertension, cardiorespiratory problems of central origin, bronchial congestion with abundant pulmonary secretions and coma which weakens the cough reflex.

8) Clinical Types of Cerebellar Haemorrhages

These four forms are similar to those already described.

a) Biphasic course. This form represents the highest incidence, i.e. 54%. The acute beginning is followed by a plateau period from 24 h to 8 – 10 days, during which a stabilization of the cerebellar symptoms occurs, with a normal or slightly lowered state of consciousness. It is during the 8 – 10 day period that one may observe a sudden and unpredictable decrease in consciousness with a rapidly progressive coma (5 h – 3 days) and death. The importance of rapid diagnosis is obvious.

b) Hyperacute course. This form has an incidence of 26%. Its course is rapid, with signs of brain stem compression and death often in 24 – 48 h.

c) Triphasic course. This form, the rarest, presents as an acute cerebrovascular accident followed by a phase of progressing cerebellar symptoms. Afterwards there is a progressive loss of consciousness which frequently leads to coma and death.

d) Chronic pseudotumoural course. The incidence is between 17% and 20%. Here the clinical course is slow and progressive, over a period of weeks or months, with an average of 3 weeks. There are purely cerebellar symptoms which sometimes progress episodically; the state of consciousness is normal. This often progresses to coma and death because of compression of the brain stem or pulmonary complications. This type of haematoma is frequently small and does not cause ventricular dilatation.

Explanation for the Deterioration in Intracerebral Haemorrhages

These varying clinical forms show the influence of the clinical picture, the pathogenesis and the pathology of this cerebral lesion. Many mechanisms can be the cause of deterioration in intracerebral haemorrhages. We can distinguish between early and late causes.

Early Causes of the Acute Deterioration by Massive Destructive Haemorrhages

Ischaemic necrosis caused by the elevated local pressure in the area of the haemorrhage, compressing the surrounding tissue.

Hyperacute intracranial hypertension.

Ventricular tamponade.

Fusion and spreading of the bleeding, due to pressure, toward the vital centres in the upper and lower part of the brain stem.

Late Causes of Deterioration by Peripherally Spreading Bleeding

These causes explain the progressive deterioration of the patient's condition which becomes apparent some 8 – 10 days after the acute onset.

Late cerebral oedema.

Osmotic phenomenon, in which an intracerebral blood clot progressively liquifies, so that at operation on about the 10th day, a reddish brown liquid, mixed with clotted blood adhering to the walls is found. The liquefaction probably results from an increase in the number of molecules through the breakdown of the large blood molecules. The liquid thus becomes hyperosmotic and attracts liquid from outside the haematoma, thus increasing its volume and making its action that of an intracerebral space-occupying lesion.

Hydrocephalus by partial compression or obstruction of the ventricular system by blood, or by obliteration of the re-absorption space by blood from subarachnoid haemorrhage.

Recurrent bleeding.

Extracerebral causes. The patient's condition may also deteriorate because of pulmonary complications, the first sign of which can be a decline in the state of consciousness and a slight deterioration in the neurological status.

II. Prognostic Elements

1. Initial clinical course
2. Site
3. Secondary extension
4. Intraventricular haemorrhage
5. Hydrocephalus
6. Volume
7. Causes
8. Rate of bleeding
9. Clinical factors
   Age
   Arterial hypertension
   Neurological findings

1) Type of Clinical Course

This aspect has already been discussed. It should be remembered that the clinical course of acute cerebellar haemorrhage shows an 80% mortality, whereas those with a chronic course have a mortality of only 40%.

2) Site of the Haematoma

This represents certainly one of the most important factors in prognosis. The mortality rate for lobar haematoma ranges from 9% to 22%, for putamino-capsular haemorrhage from 25% to 50%, for haemorrhage in the basal ganglia from 50% to 92%. The rates of adequate functional recovery are 50% for lobar haematoma, 33% for the putamino-capsular haemorrhage and only 14% for haemorrhage in the basal ganglia, respectively.

For cerebellar haemorrhages, the average mortality of 74% is high, but the rate of functional recovery is quite favourable at 66%. It is our opinion that it is extremely important today that with the help of the CT scan, we are better able to classify haematomas in the region of the basal ganglia. We can thus distinguish those haematomas which involve the basal ganglia globally from those localized at the level of the putamen or at the level of the caudate nucleus. In these latter sites there is a more favourable prognosis than in those lesions which involve all of the basal ganglia. It is also extremely important in clinical studies to give the precise location of haematomas, because their incidence varies in the different sites.

Thus, the putamen shows the highest incidence at 50.3% and the lobar haematomas have a 25.5% incidence, while for haematomas of the globus pallidus or in the whole basal ganglia the incidence is about 20%. Haematomas in the cerebellum or pons make up about 8% – 10% of the total.

3) Secondary Extension of an Intracerebral Haematoma

Approximately 74% of intracerebral haematomas extend beyond their primary location. The direction of this extension is related to the resistance of the white matter which surrounds the primary haematoma. This factor must be taken into consideration because, in fact, the prognosis for intracerebral haematomas always depends basically on the site of the primary haematoma itself. However, before the introduction of the CT scan it was sometimes difficult to differentiate a primary lobar haemorrhage from a secondary lobar haemorrhage following, for example, a haemorrhage originating in the region of the basal ganglia.

4) Intraventricular and Subarachnoid Haemorrhages

Blood is found in the ventricular system in 62% – 93% of hypertensive-type haemorrhages and in 75% of autopsies for spontaneous haemorrhages. The haemorrhage originates as follows: the incidence of ventricular bleeding is 97% in thalamic lesions, 71% – 87% in haemorrhages of the basal ganglia, 65% for pontine, 49% for cerebellar and 39% for lobar haemorrhages.

In total haematocephalus the blood obstructs all the ventricles and the mortality rate is 100%. With partial haematocephalus the ventricular haemorrhage involves only one lateral, or the third, ventricle; the mortality rate is 50%. With an isolated intraventricular haematoma the mortality rate is about 33%. Also with a bloody effusion into the ventricular system without a permanent collection of blood in the ventricles the mortality rate is about 33%.

It is rare for an intracerebral haematoma to extend through to the cortical surface, even in the case of lobar subcortical haematomas. Therefore, subarachnoid haemorrhage is most frequently caused by blood passing through the ventricular system as far as the foramina of Luschka and Magendie. This can occur in less than an hour. Subarachnoid haemorrhages do not influence the mortality rate of cerebral haematomas.

5) Hydrocephalus

This occurs either as a result of compression and displacement of the ventricles or ventricular occlusion by blood, or possibly by blood reaching and obstructing the subarachnoid spaces, thus preventing the subarachnoid re-absorption processes from taking place. This is a frequent occurrence in pontine and cerebellar haemorrhages, in which case there is compression of the medulla oblongata and a block of the fourth ventricle by clotted blood which can sometimes happen in a matter of seconds. It is also a frequent occurrence in thalamic and subependymal haemorrhages and those of the basal ganglia. It is obvious that a clot lodged anywhere and obstructing the ventricular fluid pathways will cause an acute hydrocephalus above that point, if obstruction is complete.

6) Volume of the Haematoma

The introduction of the CT scan has permitted the diagnosis of very small haematomas. These intracerebral haematomas, which from a clinical standpoint only present focal signs, would have been diagnosed as ischaemic softening before the advent of the CT scan. The discovery of these small haematomas has modified the frequency statistics for site and mortality. Thus, the incidence of thalamic haemorrhages has gone from between 15% and 18% to between 30% and 33% and haemorrhages in the head of the caudate nucleus from a lower incidence to an incidence between 30% and 33%.

7) Causes of Intracerebral Haematomas

The various causes of intracerebral haemorrhages other than the hypertensive form influence the prognosis not only by their intrinsic mortality, but also by their preferential location and their often multiple nature.

8) Rate of Bleeding

This can also influence the initial clinical symptoms. It often seems that the bleeding takes place over a period of 6 – 7 h. The rate of bleeding is directly proportional to the arterial hypertension and the decrease in cerebral tissue resistance in the area surrounding the haematoma. It is for this reason that a lacunar state or a diffuse cerebral atrophy could have a negative influence on the rate of bleeding. The rate of bleeding also depends as much on the location of the ruptured arterial wall as on the pathological state of the arteries themselves.

9) Clinical Factors

Age and Sex. The mortality rate increases over 60 years of age and reaches about 80% at more than 70 years. It would appear that the mortality rate is not influenced by the sex of the patients.

Arterial Hypertension. Hypertension can probably increase the rate of bleeding, increasing the pressure inside the haematoma, and therefore producing a rapid ischaemic necrosis in the area around the haemorrhage. It can also favour intracranial hypertension and increase cerebral oedema. It is striking that the mortality in normotensive operated patients was only 43%, while in hypertensive patients the mortality was 70%. It is also known that the mortality rate in patients with treated hypertension was substantially lower than that of patients who were not receiving treatment for their hypertension.

State of Consciousness and Neurological Examination. The state of consciousness is important in determining the prognosis as well as deciding the need for a surgical procedure. A persistent loss of consciousness leads to a mortality between 54% and 100%. A stupor leads to a mortality of about 70%; a drowsy state, a mortality rate of about 50%; and a normal level of consciousness, a mortality rate from 0% to 25%.

In a group of patients who survived an intracerebral haematoma, 30% of the patients were alert on admission, 20% in a coma and 50% were somnolent. In another group of patients who died after their haematoma 15% of the patients were somnolent and 85% comatose. It should be noted that with the exception of the brain stem signs, the neurological deficits are only slightly or not at all related to the prognosis, which means that the prognosis for hemiplegic patients who are alert is considerably better than for those patients who are somnolent with a normal neurological examination.

Closing Considerations

In the analysis of the initial clinical course of intracerebral haematomas as well as the search for prognostic factors two essential points must be considered when we are presented with patients suffering from intracerebral haematomas. It is only the detailed analysis of these factors which can show us the spontaneous course of the disease in each patient and in any event help us to choose between non-surgical or surgical treatment and to compare all the results of the different forms of treatment. It also helps us to decide the best moment to perform the surgical procedure.

7.5 Late Prognosis

H. Gänshirt and R. Keuler, Heidelberg

Late results after intracerebral haematomas naturally apply to only a small number of those cases which have suffered a cerebral haemorrhage. Regli and Jeanmonod (1979) found in an analysis of 77 publications that only one of five patients were still alive 1 month after a cerebral haemorrhage, and only two of 100 10 years later. Only one case in ten can be counted for the 5-year-late result. There is no doubt that these cases represent a select group with regard to age, gravity and location of the bleeding, the underlying causes and high-risk concomitant diseases.

The Minnesota study (Matsumoto et al. 1973) demonstrates the poor chances of short- and long-term survival in intracerebral haemorrhage. Comparisons with the survival time in intracerebral bleeding and in subarachnoid haemorrhage, cerebral embolism and thrombotic brain infarction show clearly that patients with cerebral haemorrhage have the poorest prospects of survival.

The 1971 Minnesota study (Whisnant et al. 1971) supplies additional information with regard to the slope of the long-term survival in thrombotic cerebral infarction and cerebral bleeding. On a short-term basis, infarction kills fewer patients than haemorrhage and the survival curve in cerebral infarction falls off much more slowly and steadily. On the other hand, patients with cerebral haemorrhage die of their condition mainly within the first weeks, after which the mortality curve is very much flatter than that in thrombotic infarction, because death occurs from recurrent bleeding in 5% of cases, but from recurrent infarction in 50% of cases. Myocardial infarction is to be expected in 8% of cerebral haemorrhages, but in 50% of brain infarctions. Fatal late complications are thus far rarer after cerebral haemorrhage than after cerebral infarction.

The site of the bleeding and any associated diseases doubtless have an influence on the long-term prognosis. Thus, patients surviving cerebellar haemorrhages have a very favourable prognosis, and prognosis for those with supratentorial lobe haematomas is more favourable than haematomas in the basal ganglia.

Results

The total number of brain haemorrhages admitted to our department within 10 years was 93. The intracerebral bleedings amount to 1% of inpatient admissions from 1969 to 1978 (Fig. 1).

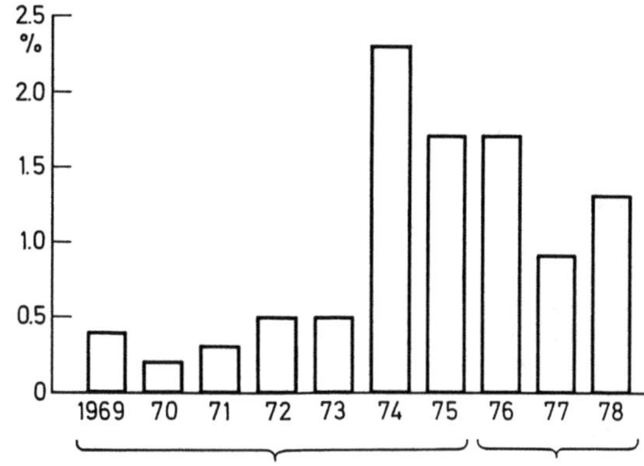

Fig. 1. Percentage in haematomas in total annual inpatient diagnoses

The number rose remarkably even before the era of computerized cranial tomography and has been 1.5% since 1974. The age peak is found in the sixth and seventh decades (Fig. 2). Males, with 53 cases predominate slightly over females (40 cases).

Of the patients with intracerebral haemorrhage, 41 (44%) died within the 1st week of the onset of the bleeding. On average, the 52 surviving cases (56%) were 12 years younger than those who died (Fig. 2).

Arterial hypertension was by far the most frequent cause of haemorrhage (Table 1). Patients with haemorrhages caused by trauma or angioma had a good prognosis for survival.

Significant associated diseases were frequent and were found in 38% of the survivors (Table 2), mainly diabetes mellitus and alcoholism. The concomitant disorders adversely affected those patients who were alive after the 1st week of the bleeding attack.

We did not observe a significant difference with regard to the late clinical result between cases treated surgically and those treated conservatively. Late mortalities were more frequent in the group treated conservatively, but the average age in the latter group was 16 years higher.

Three years after the haemorrhage, 28 patients of the initial 93 cases were alive (30%); 4 years after the bleeding there are 19 survivors (20%) and after 5 years, seven patients are alive (7.5%). The outcome is unknown in three cases (Fig. 3).

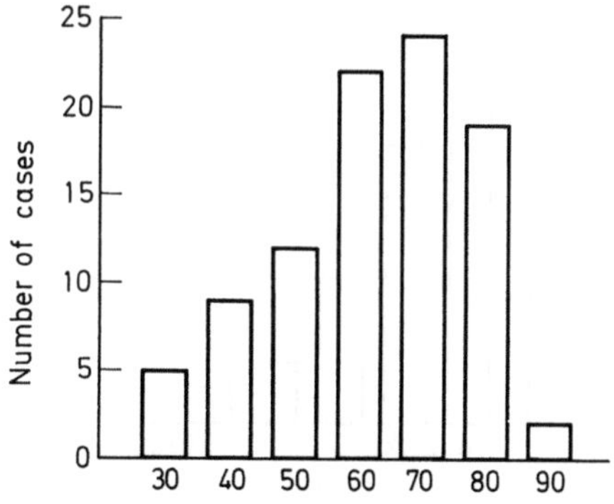

Fig. 2. Number of haematoma cases related to age. Mean age of group 57.7; mean age of survivors, 52.5; mean age of non-survivors, 64.3

Table 1. Underlying causes of haemorrhage

	n	%	Alive
Hypertension	52	55.9	26
Unknown	15	16.1	9
Trauma	7	7.5	6
Angioma	5	5.4	4
Aneurysm	5	5.4	2
Micro-angioma	2	2.2	1
Cerebral tumour	2	2.2	2
Anticoagulants	2	2.2	–
Cerebral venous thrombosis	2	2.2	2
Coagulopathy	1	1.1	–

Table 2. Associated diseases[a]

Diabetes mellitus	8×
Alcoholism	6×
Hyperlipidaemia	3×
Heart disease	2×
Renal failure	1×
	20× = 38%

[a] In 52 surviving patients only

If we look at the 28 cases with follow-up of 3, 4 and 5 years, 6, 7 and 5 cases, respectively, are normal or only slightly disabled, while 3, 5 and 2 cases, respectively, are severely disabled or totally dependent. The outcome for one case in each group is unknown. This means that two-thirds of the long-term survivors have a good prognosis and one-third a bad one as regards physical and mental recovery. The result is independent of whether the cases were initially treated surgically or conservatively.

Of the favourable cases six patients suffered from concomitant diseases and 13 cases did not, whereas of the invalid patients, seven had associated disorders and only two were free of them.

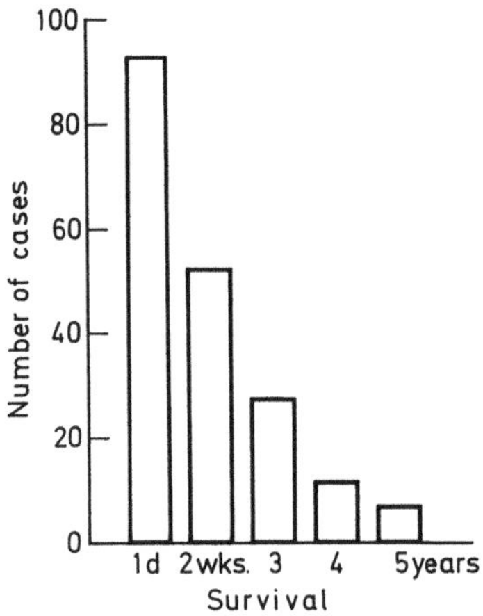

Fig. 3. Survival among 93 patients with haematoma

Haematomas have recurred in six of 93 cases (i.e. 6.45%).

There is no doubt that since the introduction of computerized cranial tomography more cases of intracerebral haematoma are being discovered, particularly those with minor haematomas, hitherto frequently taken for infarctions. In general these minor bleedings in the cerebral tissue have a good prognosis. It can therefore be supposed that in the near future more cases with a favourable late outcome will be seen.

Summary

The high mortality in cerebral haematomas means that only about 10% are alive after 5 years (in our study, the 5-year survival was 13%).

After 3, 4 and 5 years two-thirds of the surviving cases were clinically cured or only slightly disabled and one-third was severely disabled or required nursing care.

There was no difference in the late results between the cases treated surgically and those treated conservatively. However, more cases with concomitant disorders were found among the patients who remained dependent on care.

Haematoma recurred in 1 of 15 cases.

7.5.1 Discussion

F. Danke, Würzburg

Many patients present for psychiatric treatment because of a variety of unspecific symptoms and syndromes, which may be caused by vascular disease of the central nervous system. The diverse clinicial findings do not immediately enable an accurate diagnosis to be made, particularly when one considers the variety of pathological conditions that may develop with advancing years. Psychiatry is essentially a conservative field so that a wide range of ancillary diagnostic methods is essential.

We have in the last 6 years investigated 232 patients by angiography and have found a wide variety of conditions, resulting from cerebral vascular disorders.

However, a spontaneous intracerebral, space-occupying haemorrhage was found in only one of these 232 angiograms. This involved a 55-year-old woman who developed abnormal obsessional behaviour, with disorders of speech and right-sided signs. Consciousness was unimpaired and there was no vascular hypertension. The EEG indicated a left temporal lesion and the midline echo was displaced. Isotope scan indicated pathological activity in the left temporal region. An angiogram showed vascular displacement and an avascular area in the posterior temporal region (Fig. 1). An air encephalogram was also done and it was decided to treat the patient conservatively. She showed a remarkable improvement with return of speech and normal orientation and regression of the neurological signs on the right side. She was discharged after 10 weeks with minimal residual disability.

Five months after the acute onset an angiogram showed that conditions were nearly normal (Fig. 2). When examined more than 5 years later, she showed no signs of speech disturbance, although there was some mental slowing, lability and a tendency to perseverate.

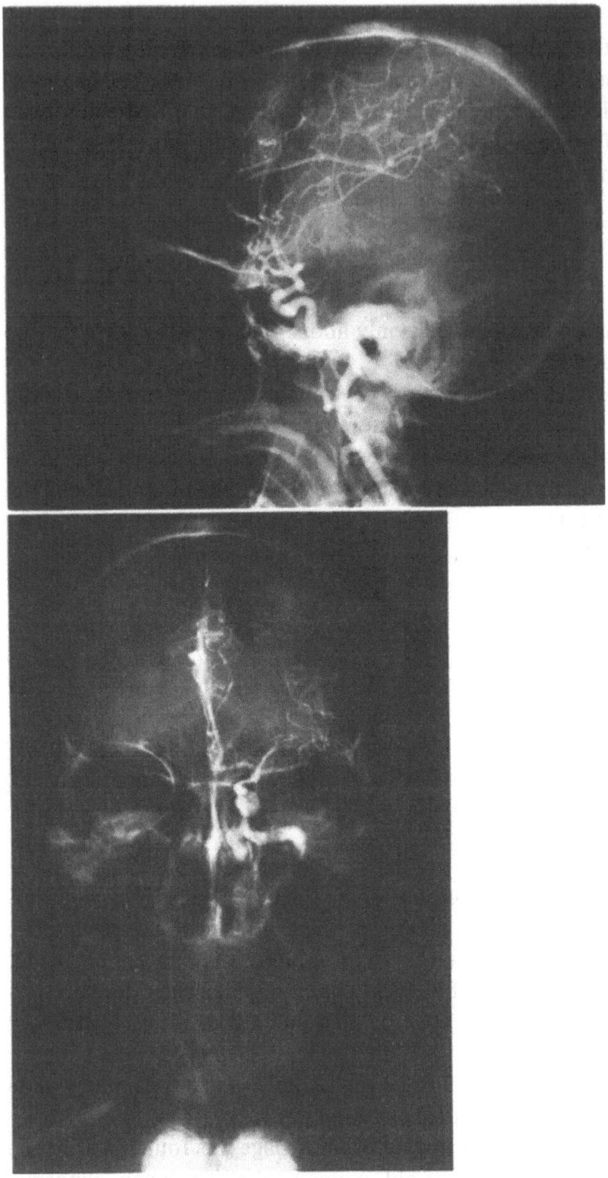

Fig. 1. Cerebral angiography of left carotid artery, 4 October 1972, frontal and lateral view. Elevation of the middle cerebral artery, avascular area in the temporal region left side, rarefication and calibre variety, no delay in cerebral flow. Female, 55-years-old, spontaneous intracerebral haemorrhage left side temporal region

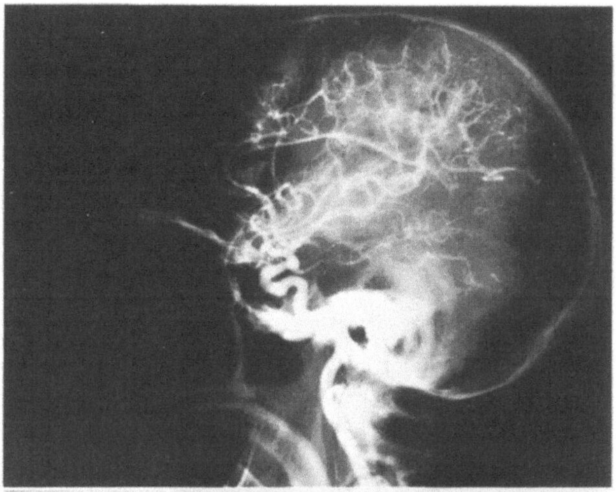

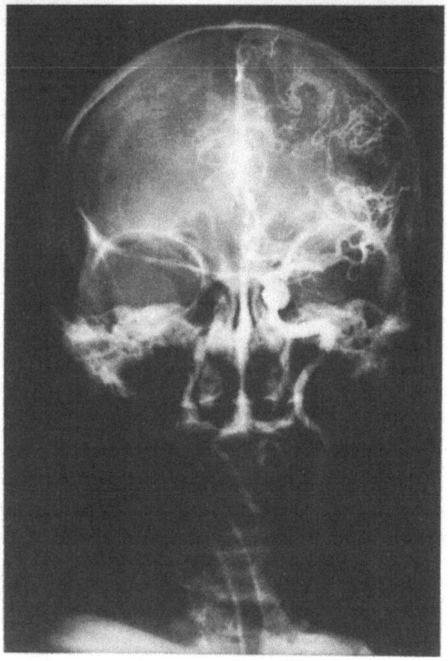

Fig. 2. Cerebral angiography of left carotid artery, 21 February 1973, frontal and lateral view. Remission of the temporal changes, clinical improvement (cf. Fig. 1)

It is of interest that vascular disease should produce such an essentially psychiatric disorder. It emphasizes the need for full investigation of such cases, as well as the value, on some occasions, of conservative treatment.

8 Operative Treatment

8.1 General Surveys

8.1.1 Experiences with Operation in 149 Cases of Spontaneous ICH (1966–1977)

B. Guidetti and F. Gagliardi, Rome

The increased mortality and morbidity of spontaneous intracerebral haemorrhages has encouraged neurosurgeons to intervene and the relevant literature is full of valuable contributions that have allowed us during these recent years to take a more critical attitude in deciding on the correct line of treatment (Arsenjo and Fierro 1958; Lazorthes 1959; McKissock et al. 1959; 1961; Mitsuno et al. 1966; Pagni et al. 1969; Becks and Marguth 1974; Arana Iniguez et al. 1976; Kaneko et al. 1977; Janny et al. 1978).

Today it is clear that treatment can be conservative or surgical according to the location of the haematoma, its dimensions and the condition of the patient (Cuatico et al. 1965; Luessenhop et al. 1967; Ransohoff et al. 1970; Pia 1972; Paillas and Alliez 1973; Tedeschi et al. 1975). Computerized tomography (CT) had shown itself to be the most successful means of investigation, allowing us to identify with precision the location and dimensions of the haematoma, and also to follow its evolution in time, hence permitting a more skillful therapeutic approach.

Clinical Material

The basis of this contribution are 149 consecutive patients affected by spontaneous intracerebral haematoma not caused by detectable aneurysms, angiomatous malformations, trauma or neoplasm, observed in the last 12 years. The series comprises 93 males and 56 females and the greatest frequency is in the fifth and sixth decades. Only 77 patients presented with an arterial pressure above 150 mm Hg (Table 1). We realize that these data appear unusual considering the frequency of arterial hypertension reported in other case studies, but in

Table 1. Incidence of intracerebral haematomas relative to age, blood pressure and site of lesion

Age (yrs.)		Total	10–29	30–39	40–49	50–59	60–69	70–79
No. cases		105 (44)	18	15	20	31 (6)	17 (14)	4 (24)
	< 150	72	18	12	15	16	10	1
BP	150–180	17 (15)	–	1	2	7 (6)	4 (4)	3 (5)
	< 180	16 (29)	–	2	3	8	3 (10)	(19)
Site of lesion	lobar	76 (8)	18	10	11	24 (4)	11 (2)	2 (2)
	capsular	29 (36)	–	5	9	7 (2)	6 (12)	2 (22)

Within brackets, patients not operated upon

evaluating the material it is necessary to note that our institute is a specialized hospital where we admit, preferably, selected patients in whom there is the possibility of surgical treatment.

In the entire series of 149 cases, angiography had been performed in all the cases, except in four, and this investigation was performed as soon as the neurovegetative condition of the patient appeared stabilized. The data furnished by the neuroradiological examinations, by the clinical state and by the surgeon's medical reports have allowed us to classify the haematomas, as had been done by other observers (Cuatico et al. 1965; Luessenhop et al. 1967; Benes et al. 1972) into lobar (84 cases) and "capsular" (65 cases) haematomas. This information about the location and size of the haematoma, the presence or non-presence of herniation of the midline structures under the falx and/or the tentorium and about the physical condition of the patient is used to decide on the treatment thought suitable for each individual case. As a general rule patients in whom the haematoma involved the basal nuclei were usually subjected to conservative treatment. The majority of these patients reach us in a state of profound stupor or coma and operation seemed of doubtful value. Those patients with a large lobar haematoma have been mainly subjected to surgical treatment, especially if not of an advanced age and in good neurovegetative condition. In young patients, with a fair-sized haematoma, even if the haematoma was capsular, intervention was thought to be advisable.

Results

To assess our results we took advantage of some tables already employed by Luessenhop et al. (1967) and Cuatico et al. (1965). Table 2 classifies patients operated on and treated conservatively into three groups according to their condition at the time of intervention. One can see that more than half (28 of 44) of the patients not operated on were classified in group C and it was these moribund or gravely ill patients in whom operation appeared to be totally unjustifiable. All 28 patients died at various intervals after their admission to the clinic, and autopsy obtained in 18 cases confirmed the futility of surgical treatment. Of the other 16 patients who underwent conservative treatment only, in half the haemorrhage was classified as lobar and in the remainder capsular. Operation was thought to be unjustified either because the haemorrhage was of modest dimensions, or because there was a clinical picture of continuous and progressive improvement associated with normal intracranial pressure.

Table 2. Classification of patients with primary intracerebral haemorrhage

	Group A	Group B	Group C
Surgical	17	56	32
Non-surgical	6	10	28
State of consciousness	Alert or drowsy	Drowsy to stuporous; purposeful response to pain	Unresponsive to voice; decorticate or decerebrate response to pain
Motor symptoms	Minor or subjective	Mild paresis to complete hemiplegia	Unilateral decorticate or decerebrate
Pupils	Normal	Normal to small and reactive	Unilateral dilatation; disconjugate with head turning or small with disconjugate movement; mid-position and fixed
Respirations	Normal	Eupnoeic or dyspnoeic	Eupnoeic to apnoeic

Of 105 patients who underwent surgical treatment and were observed for a period of from 1 to 12 years (Table 3), 15 (15.2%) died after the intervention and 15 of these belonged to group C and one to group B (Table 4). Of the other 89 patients 49 can be considered healed (excellent, i.e. the patients regained their pre-haemorrhage condition); 29 show minor deficits but have still achieved a full recovery in social life (good); and finally 44 have marked and crippling neurologic deficits (poor).

As regards the location of the haemorrhage (Table 5), it can be seen that of the cases operated on and healed, in 45 the haematoma was lobar and only in 4 was it capsular. Of those patients discharged with minimum neurological disturbances in 22 the haematoma was lobar and in seven capsular. Among those discharged with grave neurological deficits only in four was the haematoma lobar, while in seven was it capsular. Finally of the deceased, in 11 cases the haematoma was located in the basal nuclei and only in five in the white substance of the hemispheres.

Concerning the *timing* of the operation (Table 6) we found that of 22 patients operated on in the first three days, seven died, while of 85 patients operated on later than this, nine died. Also

Table 3. Mortality and morbidity in surgical and non-surgical cases

	Surgical cases	Non-surgical cases
Excellent (without deficit)	49 (46.7%)	4 (9.2%)
Good (some neurological deficit)	29 (27.6%)	6 (13.6%)
Fair (severe neurological deficit)	11 (10.5%)	6 (13.6%)
Died	16 (15.2%)	28 (63.6%)
Total	105	44

Table 4. Pre-operative condition and results of operation

	Exellent			Good			Fair			Died		
	A	B	C	A	B	C	A	B	C	A	B	C
Surgical (105 cases)	17	31	1	–	19	10	–	5	6	–	1	15
Non-surgical (44 cases)	4	–	–	4	2	–	–	5	1	–	–	28

Table 5. Results in relation to anatomical location

Class	Capsular (no. cases)		Lobar (no. cases)	
	Surgical	Non-surgical	Surgical	Non-surgical
Excellent	4	–	45	4
Good	7	4	22	2
Fair	7	4	4	2
Died	11	28	5	–
Total	29	36	76	8

Table 6. Time between last haemorrhage related to results of operation

Days after haemorrhage	No. of cases	Results			
		Excellent	Good	Fair	Died
1	8	1	1	2	4
2–3	14	4	5	2	3
4–7	26	10	8	3	5
7–10	18	11	2	1	4
Over 10	39	23	13	3	–
Total	105	49	29	11	16

as far as the functional results are concerned these were a great deal more favourable in patients operated on after the first days of the haemorrhage. Our results correspond to those reported in the literature and strengthen the belief that an immediate intervention brings about a higher mortality and morbidity than operating after a period of 4–5 days or later and when the neurovegetative condition of the patient was stabilized (Cuatico et al. 1965; Ransohoff et al. 1970; Paillas and Alliez 1973).

Discussion and Conclusion

A review of recent literature suggests that most workers in this field favour conservative rather than surgical treatment. It appears clear that the indications for any particular form of treatment vary according to the location of the haematoma and the condition of the patient. Thus, the efficacy of medical treatment should not be compared with that of surgical treatment, both are complementary and the one precedes or follows the other. Surgical treatment can offer nothing to the patient in a state of profound stupor or coma, with a considerable haematoma that mainly involves the basal nuclei, whereas it can offer much to the patient in good general condition and with a clinical picture of progressively deteriorating consciousness in which the haematoma is situated in the white substance acting mainly as an expanding lesion. Conservative therapy is the procedure of choice in the first circumstance. In the second it can be of great help in that it allows the patients to overcome the first dramatic post-haemorrhage days and to be operated on later with better results. We believe that conservative therapy should be much more aggressive than it usually is today. The reasons for this are that patients with a cerebral ictus are, if conscious, admitted to general medical wards, but if in coma or deep stupor they go into an intensive care ward. In the first circumstance it usually happens that too little is done for this type of patient. In the second case much is done, but with inexact notions concerning the treatment of patients affected by complex lesions of the central nervous system. The ideal would be admission to special centres equipped for the medical and surgical treatment of cerebral vascular disease and where, as in coronary units, more specialists are working as a team to deal with the same therapeutic problems.

On the basis of our experience and the data collected from the literature, our attitude to treatment can be summarized as follows:

1) In patients affected by a massive haemorrhage involving the basal nuclei occurring acutely, usually in old patients with arterial hypertension and generalized arteriosclerosis and in a state of coma or deep stupor from the onset, treatment is exclusively conservative and surgical treatment does nothing but aggravate the damage already done by the haemorrhage.

2) In patients with a progressively deteriorating consciousness and in whom the haematoma is mainly collected in the white substance and acts almost solely as an expanding process, once the autonomic condition has been stabilized, operation is the best treatment.
3) In haemorrhages of moderate dimensions, if herniation under the falx is absent or moderate, conservative treatment is indicated. The same applies to haematomas of major dimensions that reach the surgeon some days after the haemorrhage has occurred and are already showing a marked and progressive degree of improvement. However if the CT scan shows a marked herniation of the midline structures towards the opposite side, even if the patient is in a good condition we believe that operation is valuable not only for preserving the life of the patient, but also for securing a good functional recovery.

As regards the time of the intervention, immediate operation is rarely indicated and the optimum time is when the neurovegetative condition has been well stabilized. Today CT scan controls and ICP monitoring allow a better indication for the therapeutic procedure to be adopted.

8.1.2 Experiences with the Surgical Treatment of 156 ICH (1955 – 1977)

E. Pásztor, D. Áfra, and É. Orosz, Budapest

Introduction

From a surgical point of view it would certainly be desirable to achieve a consensus regarding the main indications for operation, the contra-indications and the optimum timing.

To get some fundamental evidence towards this end we examined the records of consecutive patients who presented with intracerebral haematomas and were operated on in our institute during the last 23 years. In this study, analysis of the pre-operative state and postoperative mortality is emphasized.

Material

Of patients above 14 years of age, 156 presented with supratentorial space-occupying intracerebral haematomas and were operated on. This material does not include haematomas of traumatic or tumourous origin or those due to aneurysm or angioma rupture. Differential diagnosis was established on the basis of clinical history, neurological, angiographic and isotope scan investigations.

Sex and Age

Haematoma was found in 110 males and in 46 females, i.e. a ratio of 2.5 males to 1 female. This ratio was greater under 30 and above 60 years of age (Table 1). The highest incidence was in the fifth decade in both sexes.

Table 1. Age and sex distribution

Age (years)	Sex	
	Male	Female
15 – 20	4	2
21 – 30	14	5
31 – 40	20	13
41 – 50	34	14
51 – 60	27	11
61 – 70	11	1
Total	110 (71%)	46 (29%)

Onset of Symptoms

The onset was abrupt in 69%, and in about half of these cases consciousness was lost immediately (Table 2).

Table 2. Onset of symptoms

	No.	%
Acute	107	69
Subacute	27	17
Chronic	22	14
Total	156	100

Risk Factors

These were found in 60%. Hypertension seems to be the most significant (Table 3).

Table 3. Risk factors

	No.	%
Hypertension and/or arteriosclerosis	70	45
Heart failure	12	8
Alcoholism	10	6
Chronic anticoagulant therapy	2	1
Total	94	60

Pre-operative State of Consciousness

Coma or stupor was present pre-operatively in 24% of the patients, while 23% were fully conscious (Table 4).

Table 4. Pre-operative state of consciousness

	No.	%
Coma	21	13
Stupor	17	11
Somnolence and/or disorientation	82	53
Full consciousness	36	23
Total	156	100

Focal Symptoms

Apart from six patients, focal neurological deficits, such as hemiplegia, hemiparesis, aphasia were always detectable (Table 5).

Table 5. Pre-operative focal symptoms

	No.	%
Hemiplegia	58	37
Hemiparesis	92	59
No focal symptoms	6	4
Total	156	100

Site and Size of Haematomas

Since angiography may not show precisely the size of the haematoma (Butzer et al. 1976; Müke et al. 1978) extending towards the midline and into the ventricles, many haematomas which had ruptured into the ventricles were also operated on. The site of the haematoma was defined according to the lobe harbouring the main space-occupying lesion. A predominantly frontal space-occupying haematoma spreading into the temporal lobe is allocated to the frontal group. The most frequent location was temporal, then frontal and rarely occipital (Table 6).

Table 6. Site of haematoma

	No.	%
Frontal	51	33
Temporal	83	53
Parietal	18	11
Occipital	4	3
Total	156	100

Time Elapsed from the Onset of Symptoms Until Operation

This period of time was determined by various factors, partly outside our control. (1) Among the patients operated on in the first three days 65% were in coma or stupor from the very onset and had failed to respond to all medical management. (2) Thirteen patients with seriously impaired consciousness were transferred late to our institute only after 1 or 2 weeks of unsuccessful treatment. (3) Twelve patients after 2–4 weeks of transitory improvement became rapidly semicomatose again and were then transferred to us (Table 7).

Table 7. Period of time between onset of symptoms and operation

			Coma or stupor at time of operation	
	No.	%	No.	%
3 days	20	13	13	65
4–14 days	49	31	13	27
2–4 weeks	50	32	8	16
More than one month	37	24	4	11
Total	156	100	38	24

Histopathological Evaluation of Micro-angiomas

At 68 operations the haematoma specimen was submitted for histological examination and micro-angioma was proved in 21 cases. This incidence of small vascular malformations is nearly identical with previously reported series (Luyendijk and Schven 1964; Krayenbühl and Siebenmann 1965; Van der Ark and Kahn 1968) (Tables 8, 9).

Among these patients males predominated more than in the whole material. The highest incidence was found in the second and third decades.

Table 8. Histopathology

	Number of examination	Micro-angioma verified	
		No.	%
Histology	68	21	31

Table 9. Analysis of micro-angioma cases

	No.	%		No.	%
All cases	21	100	Hypertension	2	10
Male	18	86	Chronic onset of symptoms	5	24
Female	3	14	Coma	0	0
Age over 50	2	10	Hemiplegia	20	95
Age under 50	19	90	Occipital loc. of haematoma	2	10
Age under 30	13	62	Operated later than 1 month	9	43

Hypertension was only one-quarter as frequent in this group, as in the whole material. A chronic onset preponderates. A higher percentage of these patients was operated on at a later stage.

Operation

Craniotomy was performed in all cases.

Operative Results

Results were excellent or good in 83%. The operative mortality was 17%. Mortality was three times lower under 50 years than over. No sex difference was detected with respect to mortality (Table 10).

Table 10. Postoperative mortality

	Number of patients	Died	
		No.	%
Whole material	156	27	17
Under the age of 40	58	5	9
Under the age of 50	106	11	10
Over the age of 50	50	16	32
Male (Total)	110	19	17
Female (Total)	46	8	17
Male over 50	38	12	32
Female over 50	12	4	33

Discussion

Comparing normal and hypertensive groups, mortality is three times higher in the latter. While the mortality of patients in coma is 62%, all conscious patients survived (Table 11). This fact also confirms earlier conclusions (Davidoff 1958; McKissock et al. 1959). Mortality is high in comatose patients regardless of their blood pressure, but hypertension, associated with the slightest disorder of consciousness, increases mortality. Table 12 summarizes all factors that significantly influence mortality: age over 50, hypertension and serious disorders of consciousness. When all of these conditions are present improvement may be expected only in 12% – 17% of operated cases. At the same time it is obvious that serious disorders of consciousness are overwhelmingly the most important among those factors influencing mortality.

The site of a space-occupying haematoma (Table 13) does not bear any significant relation to the postoperative mortality, contrary to some authors. But, if the haematoma penetrates into the ventricles it is an aggravating factor (Benes et al. 1972; Pia 1972).

Analysing the relation of the time preceding operation to the postoperative mortality revealed the following: Mortality is highest when surgical intervention is performed within the first

Table 11. Postoperative mortality

	Number of patients	Died	
		No.	%
Whole material	156	27	17
Normotension	86	8	9
Hypertension and/or arteriosclerosis	70	19	27
Coma	21	13	62
Stupor	17	5	29
Somnolence	82	9	11
Full consciousness	36	0	0

Table 12. Postoperative mortality

	Number of patients	Died	
		No.	%
Whole material	156	27	17
Normotension + coma	9	5	56
Hypertension + coma	12	8	67
Normotension + stupor	10	1	10
Hypertension + stupor	7	4	57
Normotension + somnolence	42	2	5
Hypertension + somnolence	40	7	18
Hypertension + coma or stupor, under 50 years	7	2	29
Hypertension + coma or stupor, over 50 years	12	10	83
Hypertonia + coma, over 50 years	8	7	88
Micro-angioma	21	1	5

Table 13. Postoperative mortality

	Number of patients	Died	
		No.	%
Whole material	156	27	17
Site of haematoma:			
frontal	51	9	18
temporal	83	14	17
parietal	18	3	17
occipital	4	1	25
Time elapsed until operation			
3 days	20	10	50
coma or stupor	13	7	54
4 – 14 days	49	11	22
coma or stupor	13	6	46
2 – 4 weeks	50	5	10
coma or stupor	8	3	38
over 1 month	37	1	3
coma or stupor	4	1	25

3 days, decrease after 1 – 2 weeks, reaches its minimum with 3% after 3 – 4 weeks or a month. However, if one looks at the mortality rate of those patients, within the four previously mentioned groups, who presented with stupor or coma, the figures are high and astonishingly similar (Table 13).

Our experience does not support the view of Lazorthes (1959) that the best result may be achieved by operating within the 1st week, i.e. within a fixed, determined interval. Our opinion is that independent of the time, the success of operation depends primarily on the patient's pre-operative state. Furthermore, when symptoms and a high intracranial pressure can be influenced by medical treatment, a postponed operation gives better result.

The group of histologically verified micro-angioma cases has to be considered separately. Mortality is least within this group, only 5%. These patients usually are young, mostly in their twenties or thirties, hypertension was present in only two cases and chronic onset of symptoms was more frequent. It seems to be another entity and represents a completely different group among the cerebral haemorrhages, which can be explained by another aetiological factor.

Sussmann et al. (1974) described that apart from pressure or other recognized mechanism, the haematoma exerts some unexplained adverse effect upon adjacent brain tissues. He showed that pO_2 in brain tissues adjacent to haematoma decreases, a fact which cannot be explained sufficiently on the basis of increased intracranial pressure or reduced cerebral perfusion. These data support the idea of more active operative intervention, even if there is no intracranial hypertension (ef. Suzuki and Ebina, p. 121 – 128).

Summary

After having analysed the history of 156 patients treated by operation we concluded that operation is indicated in any case of supratentorial space-occupying haematoma, when the patient fails to respond to active medical treatment or is deteriorating. Only in total ventricular tamponade is any operation contra-indicated. Hypertensive patients, over 50 and in a state of coma, have little chance of survival in spite of surgical intervention (12%). Patients not in coma or stupor may benefit from operation independent of hypertension or age. No death occurred in the fully conscious patients. The best operative results are found in the micro-angioma group. The patients status is of the greatest importance in deciding the time of operation.

8.1.3 Experience with the Treatment of 48 Hypertensive ICH (1968 – 1978)

A. Erbengi, K. Benli, V. Bertan, S. Saglam, and O. Gurcay, Ankara

A series of 48 hypertensive intracerebral haematomas diagnosed and treated between 1968 and 1978 is presented as a retrospective clinical study. The number of one to three cases per year showed a marked increase in the last two years to seven per 7 year. There were 18 females and 30 males. There was a marked increase in incidence in the fifth, sixth and seventh decades. Only four patients were below the age of 40.

Complaints, Signs and Symptoms

There was a change in the level of consciousness from drowsiness to coma in 30 cases. Complaints of motor weakness of varying severity were noted also in 30 cases. Headache was the third most frequent symptom in 27 cases, and nausea and vomiting were present in 14 cases. In the history of 13 cases there was some degree of speech disorder. Coronary ischaemic attacks were described in six patients. Three patients had one or more epileptic attacks prior to admission, and one had urinary infection.

Clinical neurological findings at the time of admission showed loss of motor function varying from slight hemiparesis to profound hemiplegia in 41 cases. Pathological reflexes were found in 30 cases. There were changes in the level of consciousness in 30 cases, seven of them were drowsy, eight were in stupor and the remaining 15 were in coma. Cranial nerve involvement was present in eleven cases; these were mostly central-type facial palsies and in seven a third nerve palsy was present. Stiffness of the neck was found in only eight cases, while seven patients came in with anisocoria and tentorial herniation. Five cases were aphasic and there was hemianopia in another five. Papilloedema was found in four cases, spasticity and decerebrate rigidity were found in three cases and respiratory difficulties with apnoeic periods in another three.

The interval between the ictus and hospital admission was within 24 h in 29 cases, 1 week in 16, 4 weeks in two and more than 3 months in one.

Diagnostic Studies

Routine X-ray studies were done in all cases (Table 1). Sixteen of them were abnormal with non-localizing positive findings. Radio-isotope scintigraphy was done in two cases, both being non-diagnostic. Lumbar puncture showed a pressure above 200 mm H_2O in all 11 cases in which it was done and the CSF was bloody in nine. Angiography was performed in 30 cases and in about three-quarters of the cases gave mostly indirect signs of an avascular space-occupying lesion. It was not possible to demonstrate a circumscribed space-occupying lesion in the rest of the cases and the diagnoses were in doubt. CAT scans done in 26 cases were all positive.

There were slightly more haematomas in the right hemisphere, but the difference was not significant. The haemorrhage from the internal capsule extended to the temporal lobe in 38 cases and to the parietal and frontal lobe in each of five cases. Only two cases had occipital haematomas.

Treatment

Of 48 cases, 31 were treated surgically. Burr-hole exploration and subtotal evacuation using a brain cannula was performed in 14 cases. Most of these patients had severe neurological deficits

Table 1. Diagnostic procedures performed in hypertensive intracerebral haematoma cases

Diagnostic examination	Frequency
Skull X-ray	48
EEG	21
Angiography	30
Computerized axial tomography	26
Brain scanning	2
Lumbar puncture	11

and changes in vital signs prior to operation. Craniotomies were performed in 17 cases. Seventeen patients with a small deep-seated haematoma without significant midline shift were selected for conservative treatment, including bed rest, control of vital signs, maintenance of fluid and electrolyte balance combined with administration of gluco-corticosteroids. Anti-fibrinolytic agents were not used.

Results

There was an overall mortality rate of 48% (23 cases). Although nine patients were lost to follow-up, 16 came for regular examinations. Three of 16 recovered completely and resumed their normal life. Twelve patients improved, with some degree of neurological deficit (such as slight hemiparesis, speech disturbance, mental slowness). One case showed no significant change in the neurological state and remained permanently hemiplegic.

There were no complications in 15 of the entire group of 48 patients. Fever and mostly respiratory and urinary system infections were seen in 24 cases. Severe respiratory distress was also observed in 24 cases and serious electrolyte imbalance in three. One case had a fatal gastro-intestinal haemorrhage.

Of the 32 cases in the last 3 years which had been diagnosed by the CT scan, 17 were treated conservatively; many of them were small deeply seated lesions. Four of them died, and of the remaining 15 cases who were treated by operation eight died.

The correlation of clinical findings in fatal cases treated by operation, and conservatively, showed that all patients with uncal herniation died, whether treated surgically or conservatively (Table 2). No patients with minor neurological deficits such as isolated speech disorders and papilloedema died. Surgical mortality was 42.85% in cases with only motor neurological deficit and 25% in the conservatively treated group. The surgical mortality rate was 72% in cases with marked changes in consciousness and 20% in cases treated conservatively. It was 66% in patients with stiff neck, marked neurological deficit and coma when treated surgically, whereas all the conservatively treated patients died. Of the surgically treated patients with hemiparesis and changes in consciousness we lost two-thirds and of those who had no operation, one-third.

Table 2. Findings in fatal surgical and non-surgical hypertensive intracerebral haematoma cases of the years 1976, 1977 and 1978 (correlation)

Findings	Mortality rate	
	Surgical (%)	Non-surgical (%)
Hemiparesis and hemiplegia	42.85	25
Changes in consciousness		
Stupor – Coma	72.72	20
Papilloedema	0	1 (1)
Speech disorders	0	0
Loss of consciousness (coma) and anisocoria	100	100
Hemiplegia, loss of consciousness (coma) and stiff neck	66.66	100
Loss of consciousness (coma) and spasticity	100	0
Hemiparesis and changes in consciousness	66.66	33.33

Discussion

It is recorded in the literature that about 10% of all spontaneous intracranial haemorrhages are located in the cerebellum (Richardson 1976; Little et al. 1978; Yoshida et al. 1978). Surprisingly enough, we did not see any hypertensive cerebellar haemorrhages in this series. It could be said that the diagnosis was missed for one reason or another, but despite CAT scan examination in all suspected cases since 1976, no cerebellar haemorrhages were demonstrated. It is hard to believe that cerebellar haemorrhages are rare in Turkey. In reality we believe that those cases which are often fatal did not have a chance to be transferred to our institution from the local hospitals. In spite of the improvements in diagnosis achieved by the CT scan (Richardson 1976; Backmund 1978; Becker 1978; Humphreys 1978; Little et al. 1978), it is our practice to perform angiography whenever possible to find whether the haemorrhage is spontaneous or caused by aneurysm, angioma, AV malformation.

What we have learned from our limited experience and from the vast experience of others as recorded in the literature is that the indications for operation must be very carefully considered and it should be avoided in those patients admitted in deep coma with severe neurological deficit without any sign of improvement. In these there is very little hope of avoiding a fatal outcome. However, better surgical results can be obtained if the surgeon is patient enough to wait until the clinical state becomes stabilized or if there is little or no change in the level of consciousness in a patient who has a space-occupying haematoma.

8.1.4 Surgery in Spontaneous ICH

H. A. D. Walder, Nijmegen

My personal experience with 51 patients treated by operation is as follows:

The series includes only patients with no history of trauma, tumour or vascular anomaly. Included are patients with a raised blood pressure and/or coagulopathy, congenital or artificial.

In Fig. 1 is shown the distribution according to sex and age; mortality is also shown. The highest incidence, as well as the highest mortality rate, is in the fifth and sixth decades.

Figure 2 indicates the site, the mortality and the presence of coma pre-operatively. There is no specially favoured site, but occipital and cerebellar ones are quite uncommon.

Table 1 shows details regarding those who survived the bleeding and the operation. Although most of them had a good level of consciousness, there were five patients in pre-operative coma who survived and made a good recovery.

The recovery rate of those patients with a severe neurological deficit was quite significant (7 of 13). Of the 34 patients, 27 had a complete recovery, i.e. 51% of the total.

The average volume of the haematoma was 30 cc (10 – 60 cc). In nine of 34 patients there were definite clinical signs of raised intracranial pressure.

Table 2 gives some information about mortality. In 12 cases an autopsy was performed with the following findings: recurrence of the haematoma, 3 times; haemorrhagic infarct, four times; basal ganglia involvement, 2 cases; and one case of postoperative infection.

Fifteen patients were in coma and the remaining three in subcoma; all patients with coagulopathy died. Nine of the 18 patients showed clinical signs of raised intracranial pressure. The average volume of the haematoma was 40 cc (15 – 80 cc).

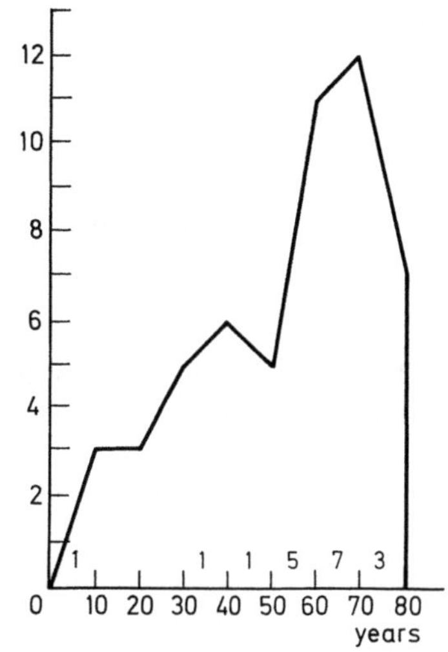

Fig. 1. Age distribution and mortality

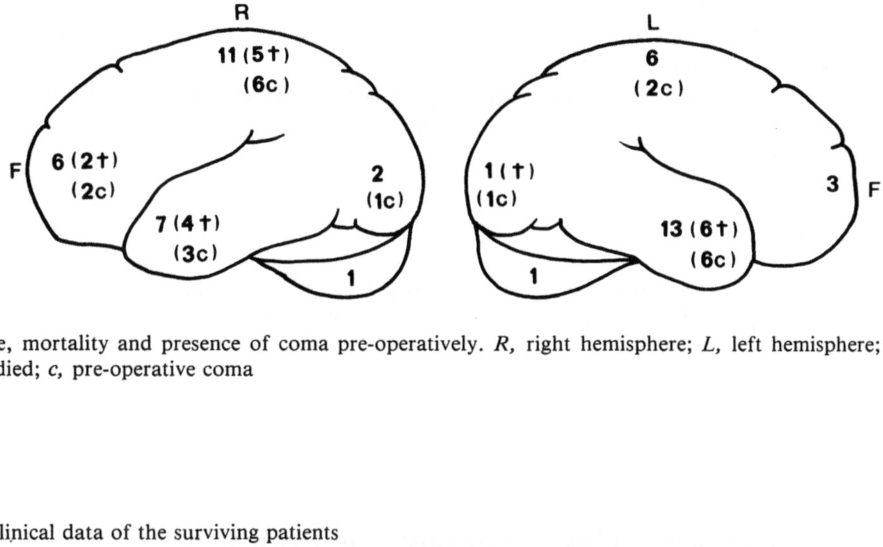

Fig. 2. Site, mortality and presence of coma pre-operatively. *R*, right hemisphere; *L*, left hemisphere; †, patient died; *c*, pre-operative coma

Table 1. Clinical data of the surviving patients

				Patient's condition		
Number	Site	Right	Left	Pre-operative	Post-operative	Cause
34 (65.3%)	Frontal	4	3	Coma 5		Hypertension 14
	Parietal	6	6	Subcomatose 11		
	Temporal	3	7	Conscious 18		
	Occipital	2	0	Hemiparesis 11	5	
	Cerebral	1	1	Aphasia 2	1	
				ICP 9		

Table 2. Mortality

Number	Site	Right	Left	Pre-Operative	Cause
18 † (34.7%)	Frontal	2		Coma 15	Hypertension 4
	Parietal	5		Subcomatose 3	Anticoagulability 2
	Temporal	4	6	ICP ↑ 9	Haemophilia 1
	Occipital	0	1		

The data in Table 3 indicate that:

1) The pre-operative state of consciousness is very important, yet 5 of 20 patients in coma survived.
2) Six of 13 patients recovered completely from a severe neurological deficit.
3) Clinical signs of raised intracranial pressure give some guide as to the prognosis.

On the basis of these findings, we can give some indications for operation and a guideline for our clinical procedure.

However, it seems better to establish some more objective criteria such as:

1) CT scan for better information about the extent of the haematoma (especially whether the basal ganglia are involved) and whether we are dealing with a haemorrhagic infarct or a haematoma in the strict sense.
2) A more appropriate objective measurement of the intracranial pressure (extradural or intraventricular).
3) The cerebral blood flow measurements around the haematoma in relation to the prognosis and the indications for operation.

A combined study by various neurosurgical centres, which aim to apply those objective criteria, will probably help us to establish more fundamental guidelines for the treatment of these patients.

Table 3. Mortality

Coma	20 → 15 †	Hemiparesis	11 → 5	Hypertension	18 → 4 †
Subcomatose	14 → 3 †	Aphasia	2 → 1	Anticoagulability	2 → 2 †
Conscious	18 → 0 †			Haemophilia	1 → 1 †
ICP ↑	18 → 9 †			No cause	31 → 11 †

8.1.5 Spontaneous ICH – Prognosis and Discussion

W. Piotrowski, Mannheim*

In the last 5 years we have operated on 36 spontaneous intracerebral haematomas. Among these were 12 with hypertension, three with brain tumour (two gliomas and one metastatic melanoma) and three patients who were undergoing anticoagulant therapy. In 18 cases the cause was unknown.

* In Collaboration with K. Tornow and M. Kröger

We did not consider haemorrhage caused by vascular malformations. Only three patients with hypertension survived, while no patient with a tumour and only one patient under anticoagulant therapy did, but where the cause was unknown 14 patients survived.

The average age of our patients was 46.2; there were more men than women. As might be expected the average age of the 18 surviving patients (43.7 years) was distinctly lower than the age of those who died postoperatively (51.9 years).

Table 1 shows the age distribution of our patients. The youngest was 8 years old, the oldest 75. Two patients who were older than 60 years survived.

Most of the haemorrhages were temporal (Table 2). These had the worst prognosis. Of 16 patients, 11 died. We did not see any spontaneous intracerebellar haemorrhages.

With regard to the operative technique, craniotomy was considered superior to a burr-hole because of better haemostasis. But, in any case we always do a burr-hole first.

The later we operated on a haematoma (Table 3), the lower was the mortality and the better was the quality of recovery of the surviving patients. If the operation was later than ten days after the onset of the bleeding seven of ten patients survived, of whom five were able to resume their normal work once more. Two of three surviving patients with hypertension recovered fully.

Table 1. Spontaneous intracerebral haemorrhage, 1973 – 1978

Age		Postoperative	
		Surviving	Deceased
0 – 20	3	2	1
21 – 40	7	4	3
41 – 60	19	10	9
>60	7	2	5
Total	36	18	18

Table 2. Spontaneous intracerebral haemorrhage, 1973 – 1978

Location mostly			Postoperative	
	Right	Left	Surviving	Deceased
Frontal	2	5	7	0
Parietal	9	4	5	7
Temporal	17	19	10	18

Table 3. Spontaneous intracerebral haemorrhage, 1973 – 1978

Time before operation (days)	Able to work	Incapable of working	Postoperative	
			Surviving	Deceased
1	0	2	2	7
2 – 10	3	6	9	8
11 – 60	5	2	7	3
Total	8	10	18	18

Of our patients, 31 had a disturbance of consciousness, and some had neurological deficits. Four of our patients who had extensor spasms pre-operatively did not survive.

The best prognosis was in those:

1) Whose cause of bleeding was unknown;
2) In whom the haematoma was in the frontal lobe;
3) In whom we did a craniotomy;
4) Who were not older than 60 years;
5) Who where operated on not earlier than 11 days after the onset of the haemorrhage.

8.2 Grading and Timing

8.2.1 Grading and Timing of Operative Treatment

F. J. Gillingham and K. Satyanarayana, Edinburgh

Spontaneous intracerebral haematomas are high-risk lesions, and operative treatment, to be successful, has to be considered in the light of the factors which have already largely determined that risk, e.g. site and size of the clot, age and cardiovascular status of the patient. Our series is relatively small because of the conservative attitude of referring physicians and is therefore selective. One hundred and two consecutive patients have been referred over the past 27 years (Fig. 1). All showed no evidence of a causative lesion apart from some with hypertension and each patient was investigated clinically with echo-encephalography, plain X-ray, angiography and more recently CT scan.

We have looked at some of the problems involved and in particular the timing of operation. In some respects, we have also counted the cost – to the patient, his relatives, and to a national health service, inevitably the cost to the state with a limited budget for health. If we spend resources on the irretrievably damaged through costly surgical intervention and prolonged convalescence, then help may have to be restricted for those with a better outlook. If, therefore, at this symposium, we can define with reasonable clarity in which groups of patients we can achieve a good quality of life, rather than poor survival, by immediate or delayed operative or other treatment, then we shall have made a significant contribution. Even after referral, some patients were managed by us conservatively, either because they were moribund or after some delay in referral they were obviously improving and did not require operation. In our analysis of the outcome of conservative and operative treatment, we have graded their clinical status on admission and at intervals thereafter according to the level of consciousness and also, but separately, limb, visual and speech deficits (Tables 1, 2). The results of treatment have been measured in practical terms of independence, i.e. quality of life, at the time of discharge of the patient (usually in 1 month) and subsequently over the years up to the longest follow-up of 16 years (Table 3).

Consideration of the results 24 h after the ictus (Table 4, 5) suggests that on the basis of mortality, operative treatment is better than conservative management (22.4% and 34%, respectively).

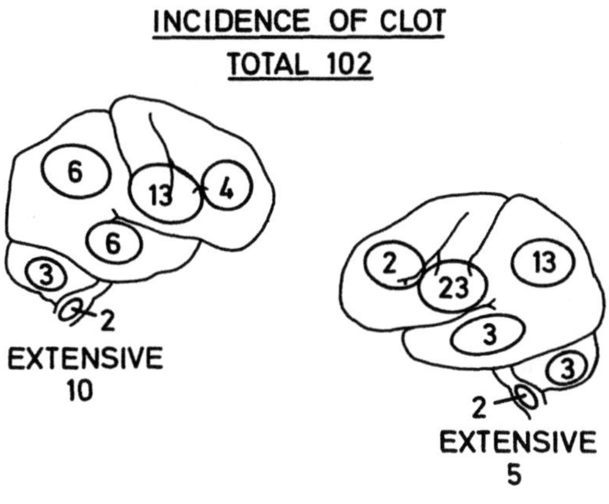

Fig. 1. Distribution of haematomas. In nine patients the haematoma could not be located with certainty and these have been left out

Table 1. Level of consciousness

Grade I:	alert, oriented, coherent in speech
Grade II:	confused, disoriented
Grade III:	drowsy, responds to verbal commands
Grade IV:	semicomatose, responds only to pain
Grade V:	comatose, decerebrate, response to pain, no response

Table 2. Neurological deficits[a]

	Motor	Sensory	Speech	Visual
Grade I:	None	None	No deficit	No deficit
Grade II:	Minimal and/or reflex changes	Minimal	Minimal	Minimal
Grade III:	Moderate	Moderate	Moderate	Moderate
Grade IV:	Severe	Severe	Severe	Severe
Grade V:	Hemiplegia	Hemianaesthesia	Aphasia	Hemianopia

[a] Grading of the maximum neurological deficit of any of the above clinical features

Table 3. Degree of recovery

0:	Full social and economic independence
A:	Slightly disabled
B:	Disabled but independent
C:	Disabled and dependent[a]
D:	Death

[a] In general grade C represents a poor quality of life and, if speech and language functions are involved, it is probably intolerable

Table 4. Spontaneous intracerebral haematomas (no demonstrable lesion)

Age group	No. of patients	Conservative treatment	Operative treatment
0–9	2	1	1
10–29	7	2	5
30–49	25	8	17
50–69	62	30	32
70 and above	6	3	3
Total	102	44	58
Mortality	28 27.6%	15 34%	13 22.4%

Table 5. Level of consciousness 24 h after ictus: treatment, mortality, morbidity

Grading of level of consciousness	No. of patients	Conservative treatment	Operative treatment	Degree of recovery with conservative treatment				Degree of recovery with operative treatment			
				0 + A	B	C	D	0 + A	B	C	D
I	16	8	8	5	2	1	–	4	4	–	–
II & III	48	21	27	7	2	9	3	7	8	11	1
IV & V	32	11	21	–	1	3	7	1	–	10	10
Total	96	40	56	12	5	13	10	12	12	21	11

[a] Patients died within 24 h after ictus and admission

If considered only in terms of conscious level it is apparent that operative treatment gives slightly better results than conservative management in the alert patient. However, six patients had already died between the time of admission and 24 h in hospital, two from early operation and four with conservative treatment. In the less conscious patients, the same pattern follows, but in the deeply unconscious patient there is no significant difference. If we look at the results in the lower grades of consciousness, what is gained by operation with respect to reduction of mortality is lost by increased and severe morbidity and is of doubtful benefit. This may reflect primary diencephalic injury or irreversible disruptive haemorrhage or dislocation and compression by the more deeply sited clot. Very early operation does not therefore at first seem helpful. Alert patients do well with conservative treatment as well as with operation and the unconscious ones do badly whatever treatment is employed. If however we look at a longer time interval between the ictus and operation (Table 6), it is evident that results of operation improve conspicuously after 72 h and particularly after 5 days. Only 5% of those deeply unconscious 24 h after admission made a useful survival by 1 month after operation, whereas 54% of those alert or with moderate depression of consciousness did well. Disturbance of consciousness is a direct reflection of diencephalic injury, and poor results may depend considerably upon whether the damage is irreversible or not. The problem is to assess when injury by clot is irreversible, depending on destruction or compression. In their paper, McKissock et al. (1961) observed that, "An alert patient with a severe hemiplegia has a better chance of survival than a drowsy patient with minimal signs", but their follow-up was relatively short – only 6 months. We have therefore analysed short-term and long-term results separately on the basis of neurological deficits as well as disturbance of consciousness (Tables 7, 8). Short-

Table 6. Time interval between ictus and operative treatment; level of consciousness at operation and degree of recovery on discharge

Time interval	No. of patients	I+II+III	0+A+B	C	D	IV+V	0+A+B	C	D
Less than 24 h	14	2	1	0	1	12	0	4	8
24–28 h	6	4	1	3	0	2	0	2	0
48–72 h	2	2	1	1	0	0	0	0	0
4 days	3	2	1	1	0	1	0	0	1
5–7 days	14	12	6	5	1	2	0	1	1
8–14 days	13	11	5	5	1	2	1	0	1
More than 2 weeks	6	6	6	0	0	0	0	0	0
Total	58	39	21 54%	15 38.5%	3 7.5%	19	1 5%	7 35%	11 58%

Table 7. Principal sites of intracerebral haematomas and outcome on discharge

Sites of ICH	No. of patients	Degree of recovery			
		0 + A	B	C	D
1. Hemispheric lobes	34	15	9	7	3
2. Anterior basal ganglia and basal ganglia/internal capsule and external capsule	36	4	5	21	6
3. Massive ICH	15	0	0	0	15

Table 8. Spontaneous intracerebral haematomas: prognosis and long-term follow-up[a]

Sites of ICH		Neurological deficits at admission			Recovery on discharge			Recovery at follow-up		
		I	II + III	IV + V	0 + A	B	C	0 + A	B	C + D
Hemispheric lobes	16	0	7	9	8	6	2	9	2	5
Basal ganglia/ int. capsule/ ext. capsule	15	0	2	13	3	3	9	8	3	4

[a] Average follow-up, 5 years 8 months

term follow-up on the basis of these factors supports McKissock's observations, but long-term follow-up shows less support. But of course after 5 or more years the numbers become smaller, some dying of old age.

The site and size of the haematoma also has a bearing with respect to neurological deficit; for example, 9 of 16 lobar haematomas showed gross deficits on admission and seven had moderate disabilities. On discharge from hospital, eight showed little disability, six were independent and only two showed a poor quality of life. Some years later, there was some further though slight overall improvement. One patient improved from being disabled and dependent to minimal disability, but five patients who had reached independence subsequently died – all from a second or third spontaneous intracerebral haemorrhage, one 10 years after operation, in the opposite hemisphere, a hypertensive patient. These patients were older (60–70+). Surprisingly, survivors from basal ganglia–capsule haematomas did well after prolonged follow-up when they had shown only modest recovery at the time of discharge (Table 8).

In summary, timing of operation is not the only consideration in the management of spontaneous intracerebral haematomas. There are many other factors, including hypertension (Tables 9, 10). On the basis of this analysis the ideal time for evacuation of clot would seem to be between the 3rd and 5th day. However, it has to be said that this study covers many years of work and there have been many recent advances. Experience with complete and definitive evacuation of clot using the microscope leads me to believe that earlier operation may be more successful under these conditions, even in some of the larger haematomas. Yet, some selection for operation would seem to be necessary and patients with massive, more medially placed, intracerebral haematomas admitted in deep coma with major deficit are best left to die. If they survive, they exist with a poor quality of life. All the others, including those with haemorrhage in the basal ganglia capsular region in whom consciousness is only moderately depressed should be pursued with vigour and for the moment as early as possible. The presence of vascular hypertension does not materially affect the result of operative treatment compared with conservative treatment in the long term, but the initial response to operation is better than conservative management at the time of discharge.

Table 9. Vascular hypertension and outcome on discharge

Normotensive/ Reactive hypertensive	Degree of recovery				Hypertensive	Degree of recovery			
	0 + A	B	C	D		0 + A	B	C	D
40	12 30%	6 15%	12 30%	10 25%	62	12 19%	11 18%	21 34%	18 29%

Table 10. Spontaneous intracerebral haematomas and vascular hypertension: long-term follow-up[a]

Normotensive	Degree of recovery at follow-up				Hypertensive	Recovery at follow-up			
	0 + A	B	C	D		0 + A	B	C	D
16	10	3	1	2	19	10	3	3	3

[a] Average follow-up: 5 years and 8 months

8.2.2 Grading and the Indications for Treatment in ICH of the Basal Ganglia (Cooperative Study in Japan)

H. Kanaya, H. Yukawa, Morioka; Z. Itoh, H. Kutsuzawa, Akita;
M. Kagawa, Tokyo; T. Kanno, Toyoake; T. Kuwabara, Yokohama;
M. Mizukami, G. Araki, Isezaki; and T. Irino, Osaka

In Japan, cerebrovascular diseases are the main cause of death, and among such diseases, the mortality due to hypertensive intracerebral haemorrhage is one of the highest. Putaminal haemorrhage is the most common type of hypertensive intracerebral haemorrhage, accounting for 60% – 70% of the total. There have been reports by McKissock et al. (1961), Cuatico et al. (1965), and Paillas and Alliez (1973) concerning the indications for operating on patients with putaminal haemorrhage. However, since the above reports showed a high operative mortality, surgical indications have been discussed in only a few of the reported cases. There are also few reports of comparisons with medical treatment as a control study.

As shown in Table 1, three co-operative studies have been performed in Japan: by Mitsuno in 1971 which included 514 surgical cases in 78 institutions, by Kanaya and Handa in 1974 consisting of 1558 cases in 75 institutions, and by Kanaya et al. in 1978 involving 410 cases in six neurosurgical departments. In this paper, indications for surgical treatment of putaminal haemorrhage are discussed on the basis of the above-mentioned study by Kanaya et al. (1978). This was performed by experts in this field in Japan, and comparisons were made with results obtained by medical treatment.

Table 1. Results after operation in patients with hypertensive intracerebral haemorrhage in basal ganglia on the co-operative study in Japan

Authors	No. of cases	No. of dead cases (%)
Mitsuno[a] (1971)	514	180 (35.0)
Kanaya and Handa[b] (1974)	1558	476 (30.6)
Kanaya et al.[c] (1978)	410	106 (25.9)

[a] 78 neurosurgical clinics. Mortality within 1 month after operation
[b] 75 Neurosurgical clinics. Follow-up period: 2 months to 13 years (Av. 2.1 years)
[c] Six neurosurgical clinics. Follow-up period: at 6 months

Clinical Materials and Methods

The neurological grading for surgical risk made by the authors was used in this research (Table 2). The grading consists of 6 grades: grade 1 is fully conscious; grade 2, somnolent; grade 3, stuporous, grade 4a, semicomatose without herniation signs; grade 4b, semicomatose with herniation signs; and grade 5, deep coma. The relation between our neurological grading and the surgical results showed statistically significant differences ($p \geqslant 0.01$) at each grade for mortality and activities of daily living (ADL) at 6 months after operation. In this research on the indications for operation in relation to the neurological grade, 410 surgical cases were used. In

Table 2. Neurological grading according to surgical risk of hypertensive intracerebral haemorrhage

Grade	Criteria
1	Alertness or confusion
2	Somnolence
3	Stupor
4a	Semicoma without herniation signs[a]
4b	Semicoma with herniation signs[a]
5	Deep coma

[a] Herniation signs: (1) unilateral or bilateral mydriasis (over 5 mm) and no reaction to light; (2) unilateral or bilateral decorticate or decerebrate rigidity

Table 3. CT classification of putaminal haemorrhage

Type	Criteria	Cases
Ext. C	Localized in the outside of internal capsule	68
Ca	Extending to anterior limb of internal capsule	59
Cp	Extending to the posterior limb of internal capsule	91
Ca + p	Extending to the ant. and post. limb of internal capsule	66
Th	Extending to the thalamus or hypothalamus	57

the control studies, 204 medical cases in three neurological departments in Japan were examined. For research on surgical indications on the basis of the location of haematoma on computed tomography (CT), 145 surgical cases and 196 medical cases in three neurological departments in Japan were compared. The CT classification of putaminal haemorrhage consists of the five types (Table 3). The follow-up periods for both surgical and medical treatment were 6 months after the completion of treatment. The follow-up results were estimated by ADL: I, full work; II, minimal disability; III, partial disability; IV, total disability; and V, vegetative state.

Results

Surgical Indications by Neurological Grading

As shown in Table 4, the patients who returned to full work and minimal disability after surgery included 33 of 37 cases of grade 1 (89.2%) and 63 of 107 cases of grade 2 (58.9%). Statistically there was no absolute significant difference when compared with cases treated medically. However, the surgical results in grades 3 and 4a were 35 of 107 cases (32.7%) and 40 of 85 cases, respectively, as compared with 2 of 38 cases and 1 of 12 cases, respectively, for medical treatment. These results showed an absolute significant difference, and it was clear that better results were obtained with surgical treatment. However, among the cases of grades 4b and 5, there were almost no patients returned to full work and with minimal disability after either surgical or medical treatment (Fig. 1).

Table 4. Correlation between neurological grading and results 6 months after surgical and medical treatment

Grade	Treatment	No. of cases	ADL					No. of deaths	Mortality (%)
			I	II	III	IV	V		
1	Surgical	37	14	19	3			1	2.7
	Medical	61	31	17	6	4		3	4.9
2	Surgical	107	14	49	28	5	1	10	9.3
	Medical	58	9	18	13	9		9	15.5
3	Surgical	107	6	29	43	8	2	19	17.8
	Medical	38	1	1	5	11		20	52.6
4a	Surgical	85	7	33	19	2		24	28.2
	Medical	12		1	1	3		7	58.3
4b	Surgical	42	1		9	5	3	24	57.1
	Medical	6						6	100.0
5	Surgical	32	1		1		2	28	87.5
	Medical	29						29	100.0

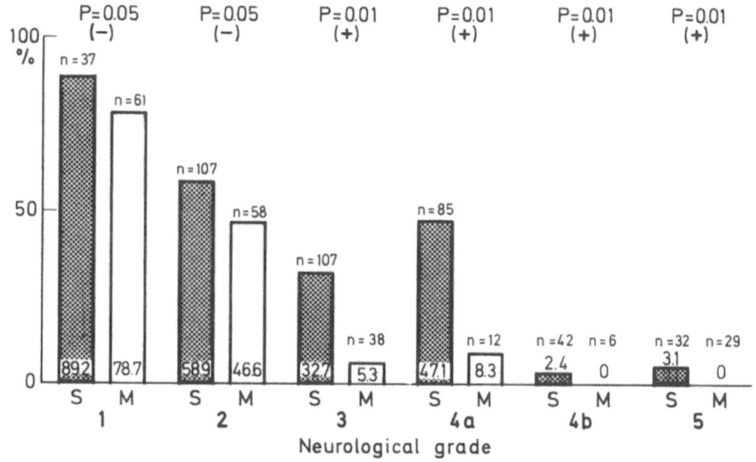

Fig. 1. Results of full work and minimal disability 6 months after surgical (*s*) and medical (*m*) treatment

In partial disability, the results did not show the difference between surgical and medical treatment in grades 1 and 2, but the surgical results in grades 3 and 4a were 48.9% and 31.1%, respectively, as compared with 27.8% and 20%, respectively, for medical treatment. Cases showing total disability and vegetative state after surgical treatment in grades 3 and 4a were fewer than those for medical treatment. The mortality after operation was 2.7% of the grade 1 cases and 9.3% of the grade 2 cases. However, there were no absolute significant differences between these mortalities and those for medical treatment. However, the grade 3 mortality in surgical treatment was 17.8%. For grade 4a, it was 28.2%, for grade 4b, 57.1%, and for grade 5, 87.5%, compared with 52.7%, 58.2%, 100% and 100%, respectively, in cases treated medically. In cases of grades 3 – 5, there were absolute significant differences between these and the medically treated cases.

Surgical Indications by CT

The time of the CT scan is within 1 week of the haemorrhage. As shown in Table 5, cases showing full work and minimal disability after surgical treatment included seven of eight cases (87.5%) of the Ext. C type, and 14 of 21 cases (66.7%) of the Ca type. There were no differences in the results for these two types between surgical and medical treatment. In the Cp and Ca + p type cases, full work and minimal disability was achieved in 16 of 44 cases (36.4%) and 12 of 36 cases (33.3%), respectively, after surgery, compared with only 8 of 47 (17.4%) and 3 of 30 (10%), respectively, after medical treatment. The results of surgical treatment were better in these types. In the Th type, the percentages were low for both surgical and medical treatment (Fig. 2).

Mortality 6 months after surgery was 0% and 9.5% for types Ext. C and Ca, respectively. These figures did not differ from those for medical treatment. The mortality among the Cp and Ca + p types was 15.9% and 11.1%, respectively, for surgical treatment, but 34.0% and 60.0%, respectively, for medical treatment. The mortality was much lower in the cases undergoing surgical treatment. In the Th type, the mortality was 41.7% for surgical treatment, while almost all of the patients treated medically died.

Table 5. Correlation between CT-types on cerebral haemorrhage and results 6 months after surgical and medical treatment

Grade	Treatment	No. of cases	ADL I	II	III	IV	V	No. of deaths	Mortality (%)
Ext. C	Surgical	8	4	3	1				
	Medical	60	45	7	5	3			
Ca	Surgical	21	6	8	4	1		2	9.5
	Medical	38	13	18	3	2		2	5.3
Cp	Surgical	44	1	15	15	5	1	7	15.9
	Medical	47	3	5	12	10	1	16	34.0
Ca + p	Surgical	36	1	11	12	7	1	4	11.1
	Medical	30		3	2	7	0	18	60.0
Th	Surgical	36		4	11	3	2	15	41.7
	Medical	21		1		1		19	90.5

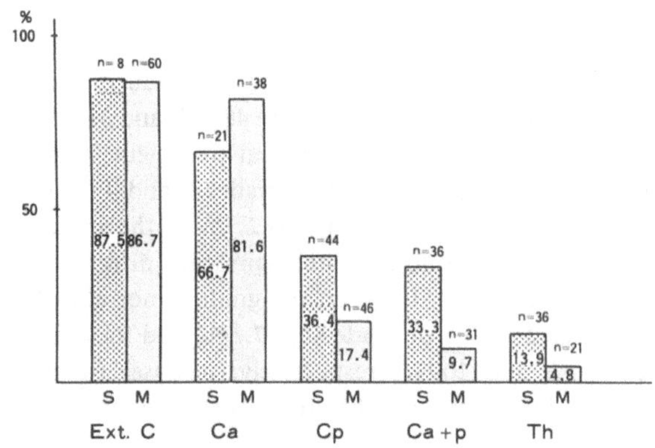

Fig. 2. Location of haematoma and results 6 months after surgical and medical treatment; full work and minimal disability. *S*, surgical treatment; *M*, medical treatment

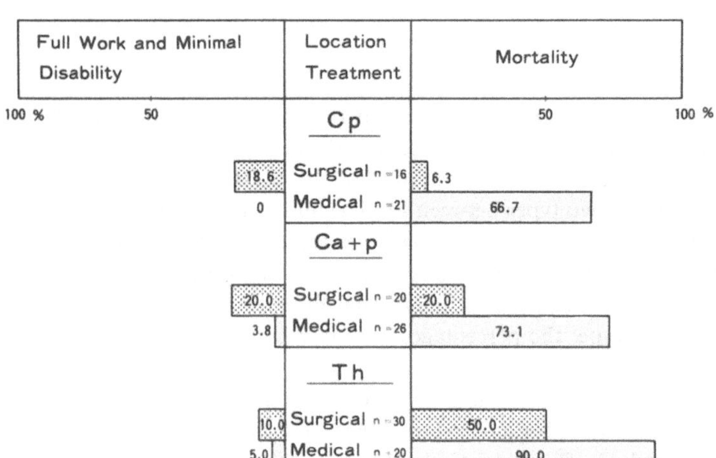

Fig. 3. Location of haematoma with ventricular haemorrhage and results 6 months after surgical and medical treatment

The results of surgical and medical treatment in patients with ventricular haemorrhage among the putaminal haemorrhage cases are as follows: Since there were no differences in mortality and ADL between surgical and medical treatment in the Ext. C and Ca types, the Cp, Ca + p and Th types were investigated (Fig. 3). Patients showing full work and minimal disability after surgical treatment accounted for 3 of 16 cases (18.6%), 4 of 20 cases (20%) and 3 of 30 cases (10%) of the Cp, Ca + p and Th types, respectively. There were slight differences from the figures for medical treatment. The mortality was 6.3%, 20% and 50%, respectively, for the Cp, Ca + p and Th types undergoing surgical treatment. Among the medically treated cases, the mortality was higher in all three types of patients. These results show that surgical treatment is clearly better.

Discussion

From the above surgical and medical results in mortality and ADL, it appears that the absolute indication for operation based on the neurological grade is grades 3 and 4a. For grade 4b, full work and minimal disability cannot be expected, but about 60% of those undergoing surgical treatment survived when compared with 100% mortality in medically treated cases. To clarify the indications for operation in patients, the correlation between neurological grades and CT classifications was investigated in a total of 341 patients undergoing surgical and medical treatment. The results obtained are shown in Table 6. Grades 1 and 2, which showed no differences between surgical and medical results as described previously, included many of the Ext. C and Ca types which also showed no differences between surgical and medical results. However, the Cp and Ca + p-type cases which showed better results for operative than for medical treatment accounted for 11 of 65 cases of grade 1 and 49 out of 109 cases of the grade 2. There were many Cp and Ca + p types but few Ext. C and Ca types among the grades 3 and 4a cases which showed better results for surgical treatment than for medical treatment. Most of the Th types were found among cases of grades 4b and 5 which showed extremely bad results for both surgical and medical treatment. As indicated above, there is a certain degree of correlation between the neurological grade and the location of the haematoma, but it is necessary to investigate both neurological grade and the site of haematoma when deciding on the surgical indications. The authors are now studying this point.

Table 6. Correlation between neurological grading and location of cerebral haemorrhage on CT

Grade	No. of cases	Location of cerebral haemorrhage				
		Ext. C	Ca	Cp	Ca + p	Th
1	65	39	15	10	1	0
2	109	24	32	30	19	4
3	66	2	10	27	21	6
4a	38	1	2	13	10	12
4b	29	1	0	3	4	21
5	34	1	0	8	11	14
Total	341	68	59	91	66	57

Summary

From a comparison of the results obtained by medical treatment and those obtained by surgical treatment under the same conditions, the following can be concluded concerning indications for operation employed in patients with hypertensive intracerebral haemorrhages in the putaminal region:

1) Medical treatment should be employed on patients of neurological grades 1 and 2, except for those with haematomas extending to the posterior limb (Cp) or the anterior and posterior limbs of the internal capsule (Ca + p).
2) Surgical treatment should be adopted on patients of neurological grades 3 and 4a, except for those with haematomas localized outside of the internal capsule (Ext. C) or extended to the anterior limb of the internal capsule (Ca).
3) Surgical treatment in patients with neurological grades 4b and 5 can promise almost nothing with respect to ADL, but it is probably best to attempt surgical treatment just with the idea of preserving life.

8.2.3 Grading and Timing of Operation in Putaminal ICH

J. Suzuki and T. Sato, Sendai

Introduction

The results of operation for hypertensive intracerebral haemorrhage, following the first attempt by H. Cushing (1903) were poor, and the opinion was often expressed that it was useless (Craig and Adson 1936; Penfield 1953). Even for those actively pursuing a policy of such treatment, the hospital death-rate was between 30% and 50% (Lazorthes 1959; Luessenhop et al. 1967; McKissock et al. 1959). For some reason about 70% of hypertensive intracerebral haematomas arise in the area around the internal capsule (Russell 1954).

In order to cause little or no damage to the brain when removing haematomas in the putaminal region, we have developed the trans-Sylvian approach (Suzuki and Sato 1972, see p. 345 and 384) and have used it in 52 cases between 1970 and December 1975.

Material

There were 37 males and 15 females, between 25 and 67 years of age. The age distribution is shown in Fig. 1. The interval from onset until operation varied from 1 day to 51 days (Fig. 2). Our results (Fig. 3) show that an extremely good outcome is possible. We have lost only one patient subsequently. Here our indication was incorrect and we operated on a patient in deep coma.

Three patients died later between 6 months and 4.5 years after discharge, one case from rebleeding after gastrectomy, one case gradually weakened and died and a 36-year-old woman died of an unrelated lesion.

In the light of these findings, it is thought that excellent results can be obtained, provided that the indications for operation are accurately determined.

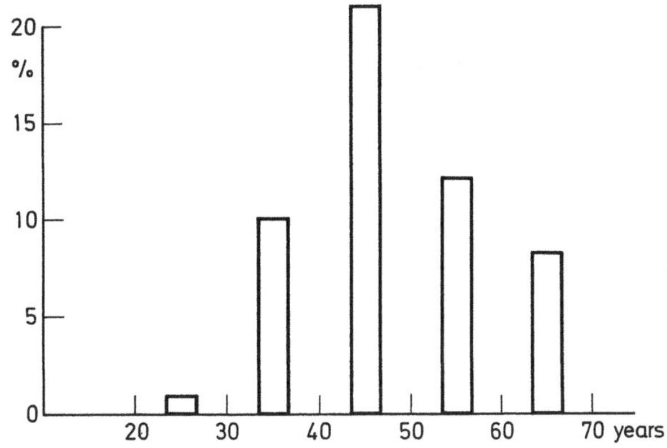

Fig. 1. Age distribution

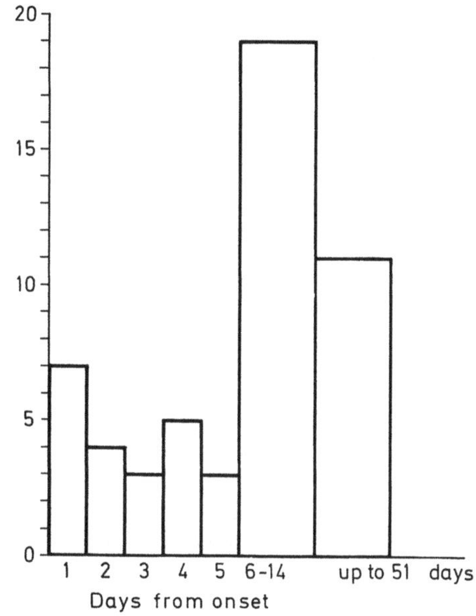

Fig. 2. Interval from onset until operation

The state of consciousness was considered the next most important factor (Table 1). In spite of semicoma in seven, drowsiness in 19 and confusion in 14 cases, 46 patients returned to normal, while four of five improved to the state of confusion at the time of discharge. At the time of the follow-up studies (6 months to 4 years and 1 month), all surviving 48 patients were conscious.

Motor function (Table 2) was variable at the time of follow-up depending on the site and the degree of brain damage resulting from the haematoma. Twenty-nine patients returned to work or could follow their normal daily activities. Fifteen needed some help with dressing and other functions; however, they could walk without help. Four patients were bedridden, but three of these were over 60.

Concerning timing the most surprising observation was that the recovery of normal consciousness and motor function was rapid in cases operated on within 24 h of onset (Fig. 4). The later the timing of operation (Figs. 5, 6), the slower was the recovery, particularly for the cases operated upon on the 34th and 51st days (Fig. 7), both of whom were found at follow-up to need help in their day-to-day life, despite their relatively young ages.

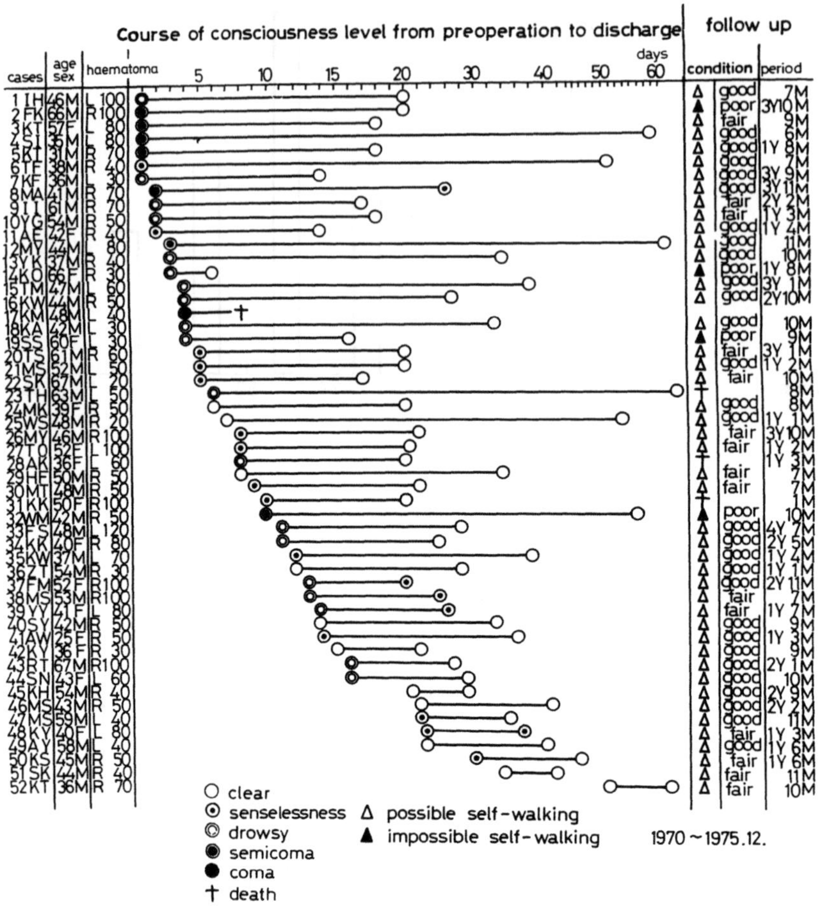

Fig. 3. Hypertensive intracerebral haematoma; cases operated on by the trans-Sylvian approach. The first circles indicate the consciousness level just before operation and the timing of the operation after the onset. The second circles indicate the conscious level at time of discharge and the duration of stay in hospital

Table 1. Conscious level of 52 operated cases pre-operatively, on discharge and at follow-up

Consciousness	Pre-operative	Discharge	Follow-up
Clear	11	46	48
Confused	14	5	0
Drowsy	19	0	0
Semicoma	7	0	0
Coma	1	0	0
Death		1	3
Total	52	52	51

Table 2. General condition of 51 follow-up cases

Condition	
Good	29
Fair (unaided walking possible)	15
Poor (unaided walking impossible)	0
Vegetative	0
Death	3
Total	51

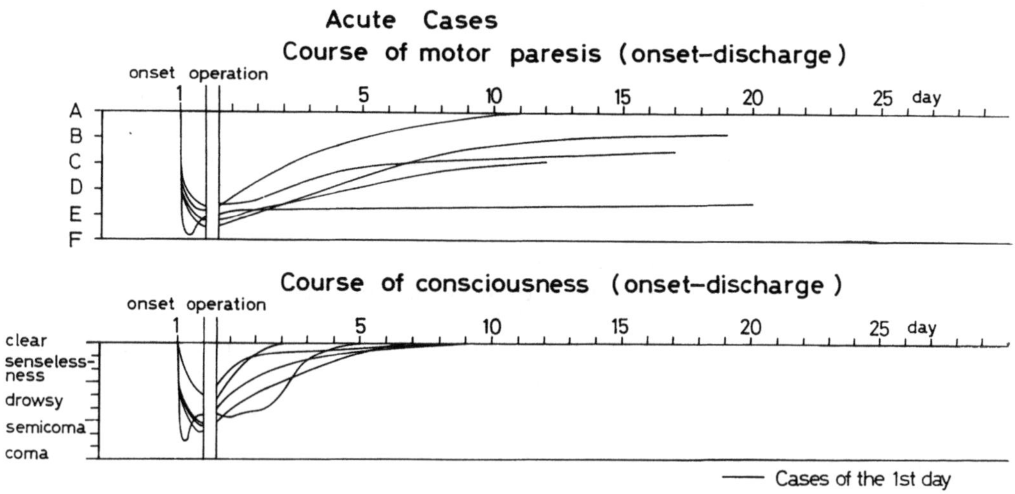

Fig. 4. Pre-operative and postoperative courses of five cases which were operated on in the acute stage within 1st day of onset. Motor paresis was classified as follows (in Figs. 4, 5, 6, 7): *Group A:* The patients had hemiparesis, but were capable of walking without assistance; *Group B:* The patients had hemiparesis, but were capable of walking or standing with assistance; *Group C:* The patients had hemiparesis, but were capable of flexing and extending their knees; *Group D:* The patients had hemiparesis, but were capable of maintaining flexed knees; *Group E:* The patients had hemiparesis, but were capable of reacting to pain; *Group F:* The patients had complete hemiplegia

There were no striking differences in the follow-up results according to sex; it could be shown, however, that the men were in better condition than the women.

A precise determination of the size of the haematoma was impossible. A rough classification into those haematomas greater than 100 cc, those between 50 and 100 cc and those less than 50 cc showed no significant differences. Probably as a result of the location of the haematoma there were severe cases who had small haematomas and cases without sequelae who had large haematomas. Nevertheless, it was found that of the nine cases with large haematomas, three were in fair, one in poor condition and one was dead. Six of the 15 cases with middle-sized haematomas were in fair condition and one was dead; six of the 27 with small haematomas were in fair, three were in poor condition and one was dead, indicating that the smaller the haematoma the better the condition at follow-up.

From these results it is thought that in elderly patients over the age of 60 in a semicomatose state who are admitted on the 2nd or 3rd day after onset, it is best to observe the general

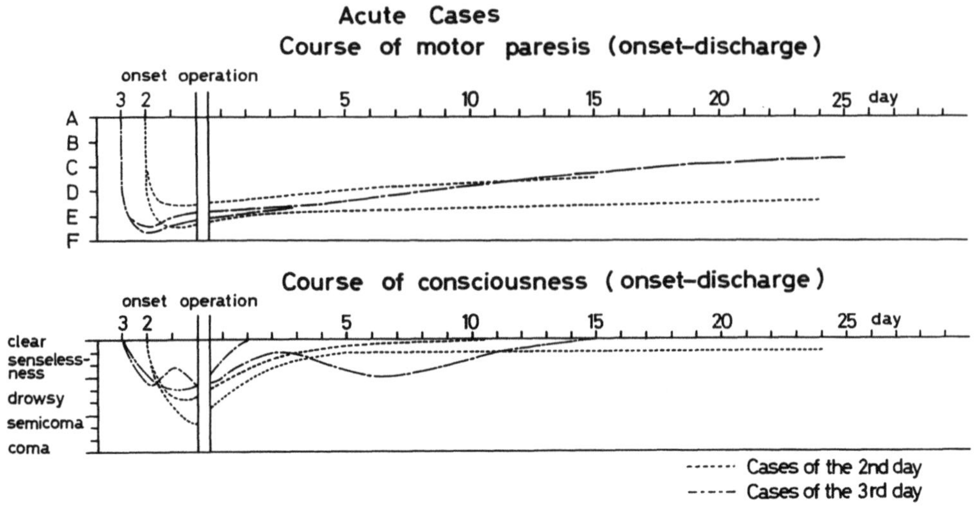

Fig. 5. Pre-operative and postoperative course of four cases operated on 2nd or 3rd day after the onset

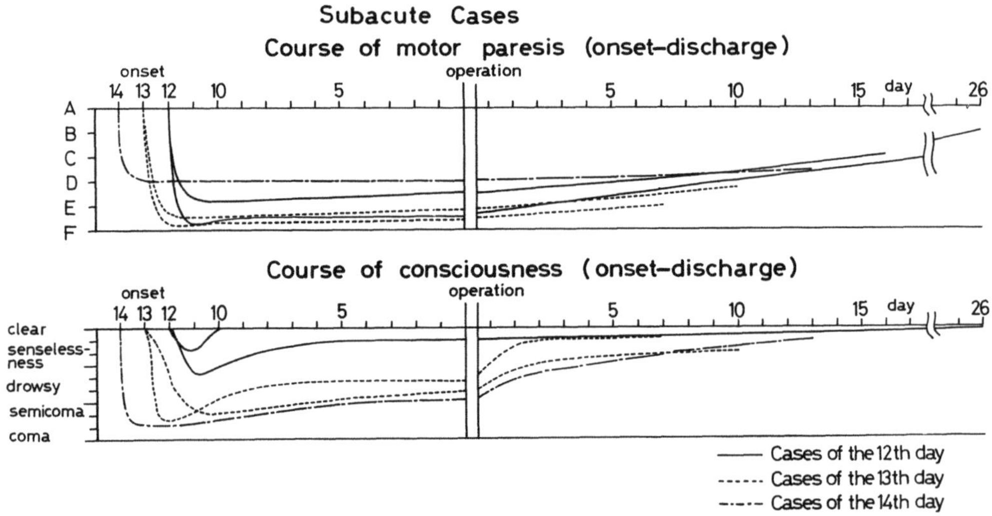

Fig. 6. Pre-operative and postoperative course of five cases operated on in the subacute stage

condition before performing the operation. It thus becomes necessary to ask why such favourable results are obtained by operation within 24 h. We believe that with the formation of a haematoma in the putaminal region, surrounding brain tissue is compressed, causing impairment of the circulation in the tissue surrounding the haematoma and gradually resulting in necrosis. Provided that extirpation of the haematoma alone is accomplished without causing further brain damage and while the area of necrotic change is still small, the results of operation are clearly good. However, the longer the period that has elapsed from onset until operation, the larger the layer of necrotic matter and the slower the postoperative recovery will be, even if the haematoma is completely removed.

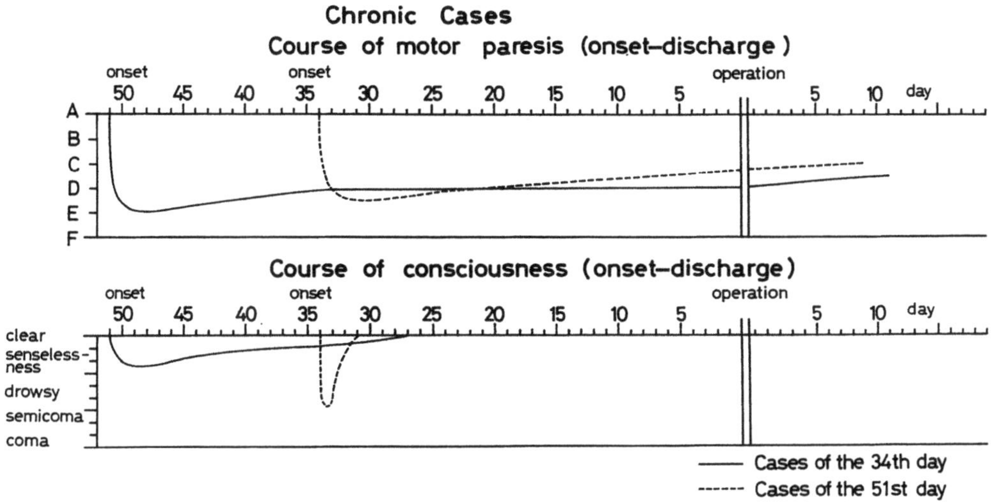

Fig. 7. Pre-operative and postoperative course of two cases operated on in the chronic stage

Since it is a fact that at the present time operation cannot be performed within 24 h of onset except in a few lucky patients, establishment of emergency facilities for apoplexy is urgently needed.

However, if the surgical method outlined is used at an early stage, effective results can be achieved in cases of hypertensive intracerebral haematoma.

8.2.4 Discussion

H. W. Pia, Giessen

In my experience with 364 intracerebral haematomas of differing aetiology in the years 1954 – 1976 (Table 1), the main criteria for operative treatment independent of the aetiology are the presence of a well-defined space-occupying haematoma, progressive neurological signs and local or general increase of the intracranial pressure with or without symptoms of midbrain or tonsillar herniation, provided the central regulation remains intact.

Concerning the timing of the operation our results from 1972 (Table 2) showed that all the haematomas with hyperacute course and signs of central dysregulation occurring immediately after rupture of the vessel have an extremely bad prognosis. Of 67 patients with hyperacute bleeding, 31 died without, and 27 died with operative treatment and only nine patients (14%; 7/27 operated cases) survived. The causes of death were tamponade of the ventricular system, haemorrhagic destruction of the thalamus and hypothalamus, haemorrhages in the brain stem and secondary cerebral lesions, less frequently extracerebral lesions.

The prognosis of patients with an acute, subacute or chronic course is better. Spontaneous death occurred less frequently, i.e. 6 of 59 between the 1st and 3rd day, 7 of 33 between the 4th

Table 1. Spontaneous intracerebral haematomas

Aetiology	Haematomas			Died	
	Number	% of total	Survived	Number	% of total
Aneurysms (N = 450)	78	21	27	51	65
Angiomas (N = 206)	93	26	84	9	10
Intracran. A. (N = 166)					
Micro-angiomas	36	10	26	10	28
Hypertension	86	24	34	52	60
Other aetiology	71	19	32	39	55
Total	364	100	203	161	44

Table 2. Onset and course of symptoms

	Number	Survived	Number	Died (%) of total number	% of operated cases
Hyperacute – 24 h	67	9	58[a]	86	40
Acute 1–3 days	59	38	21[b]	35	25
4–7 days	15	10	5	27	[c] 20
1–2 weeks	18	14	4		
2–4 weeks	36	25	11	27	
Chronic >1 month	46	35	11		

[a] Thirty-one without operation
[b] Six without operation
[c] Seven cases without operation

day and the end of the 2nd week. Treatment between the 1st and 3rd days saved 38 of 59 (75%). Operations performed later than this produced surprisingly similar and not, as previously expected, better results. When considering spontaneous haematomas in general there are no definite criteria to indicate an optimum timing for the operation.

In hypertensive haematomas, of 86 patients with long-lasting arterial hypertension 52 died; of 31 with the hyperacute form, 29 died, while 8 without and 21 with operation of different type died. Only two patients survived. Of 25 patients with an acute course and treatment between the 2nd and 7th day, 14 died and, of 30 patients in whom the interval between the haemorrhage and the operative treatment was longer than 1 week, 11 died. Among these there were nine, all in grade III, in whom removal of the angiographically diagnosed space-occupying haematoma 2–6 weeks after the haemorrhage resulted in an unfavourable outcome. Six patients died, two deteriorated and one showed no significant improvement. In spite of the mass of the haematoma all patients had a non-progressive neurological deficit and no signs of increased intracranial pressure. Our results proved that in general it is raised intracranial pressure which is the decisive indication for operation. Operating on hypertensive haematomas with a hyperacute course, at least their evacuation, during the 1st day has no effect and has been completely abandoned. Later, during the second half of the 1st week and the 2nd week, seems to be the optimal time for evacuating the clots associated with raised intracranial pressure.

I think that grading of patients with hypertensive haematomas is essential to assess the methods of treatment and their results. I propose to follow the same guidelines which have been worked out for deciding the operative treatment of aneurysms.

Patients in grades I and II with absent or mild neurological signs and intact central regulation are exceptional. Isolated lobar haematomas with a mild subacute or chronic pseudo-tumoural course belong to this category. Patients in grade III are characterized by a localized neurological deficit due to capsular involvement with slight or no disturbances of consciousness. Those in grade IV represent severe neurological, psychic and central vegetative and metabolic disturbances and finally patients classified as grade V are moribund. The level of the intracranial pressure is another important factor. Age, the premorbid status, disturbances of the heart, lung, kidney and liver function and metabolic disorders all additionally influence the degree of risk. Because of these numerous factors it is extremely difficult in my opinion to establish a true grading. The most important factors are the state of consciousness and intracranial pressure, the state of the central regulation and the general arterial and circulatory system, the site and extension of the haematomas and the age of the patient.

Cases in grades I and II with localized lobar haematomas and mild intracranial pressure are optimal and show the best results from an evacuation. Patients in grade III with haematomas in the internal capsule and the basal ganglia may be operated upon.

An unsolved problem concerns the so-called late operation, by which I mean operation performed 4 – 6 weeks after the onset of the bleeding. I am not speaking here about tumour-like cases with oedema and progressive deterioration. I have in mind those patients who after an acute onset improved very slowly and may remain without further improvement for days and weeks. They are admitted to hospital and a space-occupying lesion is found. I have operated on ten such patients; two died, four deteriorated and four improved. In these cases I have learned that intracranial pressure is no longer the problem and all I have achieved was to interfere with the normal process of healing. I was faced with this problem particularly in older hypertensive patients.

Another problem is the acute operation, using the trans-Sylvian approach in cases without disturbances of consciousness, but with hemiparesis. In such patients it is not the saving of life which is more important, but the preservation of function. Such a concept puts the principles of treating intracerebral haematomas in a new light. I wonder if the early operation, inaugurated and recommended by J. Suzuki (p. 384) has better results in the lights of CT findings than the conservative treatment. However, I think that we should follow his recommendations to acquire proven evidence of the effectiveness of early operation.

8.3 Aetiology – Indications and Prognosis

8.3.1 Hypertensive ICH

8.3.1.1 Possibilities of Operative Treatment and its Limitations

F. Loew and H. Jaksche, Homburg

The selection of patients for operative treatment has become more difficult since the old rule (Lazorthes 1956, 1959; Ransohoff et al. 1970) has been increasingly abandoned. The tendency nowadays is to operate only on those patients with hypertensive intracerebral haematoma, who are not in coma, without signs of decerebration, and even showing a tendency to improve spontaneously (Mitsuno et al. 1956; Luessenhop et al. 1967; Pia 1972; Kaneko et al. 1977). In this paper we shall not deal with the question of whether such patients need operative treatment at all (McKissock et al. 1961) or under what conditions it might be done. Our aim has been to determine some criteria which might make it easier to decide against operation because such patients are likely to die in spite of all efforts.

We have also had the idea that perhaps in some situations it might be possible to predict an outcome which for the surviving patient would be worse than death. For instance we considered that the combination of aphasia, hemiplegia and general decrease of mental faculties resulting from larger haematomas in the dominant hemisphere could produce intolerable suffering. Surprisingly enough, we have been unable to confirm this idea in our patients. During the last 4 years, eight patients with such a syndrome survived, but in all these cases the general cerebral impairment prevented real suffering. In some instances it has been the relatives but not the patients themselves who regarded the situation as intolerable. On the other hand, Paillas and Alliez (1973) reported a 5% incidence of suicide in their patients, which is doubtless much higher than in the general population. But even this number, in our opinion, does not justify a general rule not to operate upon larger haematomas on the dominant side. A possible exception may arise when somebody who knows about such situations clearly expresses his will before such an event and specifically forbids any active treatment under the above-mentioned circumstances.

To find an answer to the first question of whether there are signs which allow the prediction that even operative treatment will not save the patient's life, we analyzed the findings in our patients of the last 4 years. All cases with real space-occupying haematomas have been operated upon as emergencies without regard to how bad their condition had been at the time of admission and diagnosis.

Of those patients with hypertensive intracerebral haematoma, who on admission were in deep coma with decerebrate signs and were older than 55, none survived. But coma and decerebrate state alone did not prove to be a reliable sign of an unfavourable outcome.

Another indicator seems to be the circulation time in the serial carotid angiogram. Of 19 angiograms suitable for such an evaluation, 12 showed a circulation time of 8 or more sec measured from the beginning of the arterial to the beginning of the venous phase. Of these 12 cases, 10 died in spite of operative treatment, and the two survivors developed an apallic syndrome.

A third situation which seems to justify a decision against operating is when there are large haematomas in both hemispheres. In our material none of these patients survived.

Intracranial pressure measurements alone, as recently confirmed by Janny et al. (1978), do not seem suitable for predicting an unfavourable outcome. The same is true as regards the location of a single haematoma. As shown by Luessenhop et al. (1967), even patients with haematomas of the basal ganglia, which on admission are in a decerebrate state, can in some rare cases be saved by operation.

If we are to give any guidelines at all for action in this difficult field, we can mention the three unfavourable factors which we have found in our material. These are:

1) Decerebrate state in patients older than 55 years;
2) Circulation time from the arterial to the venous phase in the angiogram longer than 8 sec; and
3) Large bilateral haematomas.

8.3.1.2 Indications and Contra-Indications

R. Lorenz, Giessen

High blood pressure, whether it is associated with vascular anomalies or diseases, plays a significant role in the genesis of so-called spontaneous intracerebral haematoma. From the pathogenic point of view high blood pressure is easily the most frequent cause of intracerebral haemorrhage (Luyendijk 1972). The suggestion of Russell (1954) is that only those lesions should be designated as intracerebral haemorrhages which have a diameter of at least 3 cm and when in the brain stem, a diameter of 1.5 cm.

According to the statistics in West Germany, about 7500 died from a brain haemorrhage in 1976. In 45% of these there was evidence of high blood pressure. There is no doubt that these statistics regarding the cause of death are not always reliable, a fact which is supported by the details given on the death certificates. According to figures collected by Luyendijk (1972), there were haematomas caused by hypertension in 50% – 71% of the cases in post-mortem material and in 29% – 80% of clinical cases.

We recently treated a 40-year-old doctor (I. No. 080938371) who had been admitted to a local medical clinic with a diagnosis of high blood pressure and cerebral ischaemia due to a thalamic haematoma. His blood pressure initially was 230/140 mmHg and only returned to normal in the course of 3 weeks. It was later learned that even lower blood pressures had been previously recorded and that 20 years and 4 years before the present illness there had been fleeting pareses involving the right side of the body. Only 3 weeks after the haemorrhage in a control angiogram was there an area suspicious of a micro-angioma in the distribution of the middle cerebral artery.

On the basis of the course of the illness, the control angiography and the additional details of the previous history, the original assumption that this was a hypertensive intracerebral haematoma could no longer be supported. It seemed rather that he had a central failure of blood pressure regulation in the sense of a Cushing response, as Auer (1978) had also described in hypertensive encephalopathy.

Material

Over a period of 25 years we have seen 71 intracerebral haematomas associated with hypertension. Of these, 45 (63.4%) were in men and 26 (36.6%) occurred in women. The greatest incidence was in the sixth decade (Fig. 1).

The surgical findings indicated that the haematomas were sited mainly in the temporal lobes, in the parieto-occipital junction and also in the frontal lobes (Fig. 2). The rest were distributed through all parts of the brain. Four patients were not operated on, as they died a short time after admission.

Thirty-nine patients died after, or in spite of, the operation, corresponding to a total mortality of 60.6% (Fig. 3). In 59 (83%) the course was acute; in ten (14%) it was slowly progressive. At the time of admission 24 patients were comatose, 19 somnolent and 15 showed mental slowing (Table 1). (In the tables only those patients are shown in whom the level of consciousness had been reliably recorded.) In 53 (74.6%) there was a hemiparesis; in 22 (30.9%) a more or less complete aphasia; in 13 (18.3%) there were visual field defects; and in 11 (15.5%) a definite anisocoria. Associated complications included respiratory or cardiac failure in 11 (15.5%), renal failure in seven (9.8%), diabetes mellitus in 11 (15.5%), and in 15

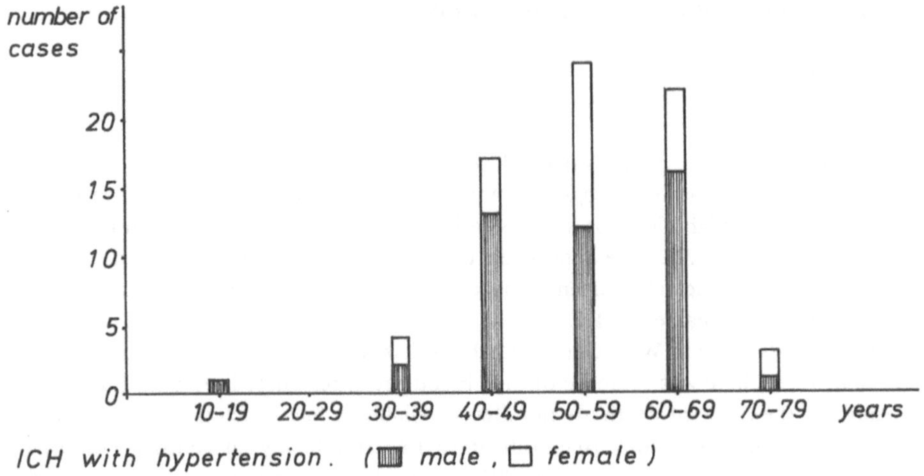

Fig. 1. Age and sex distribution in 71 patients with hypertensive haemorrhage

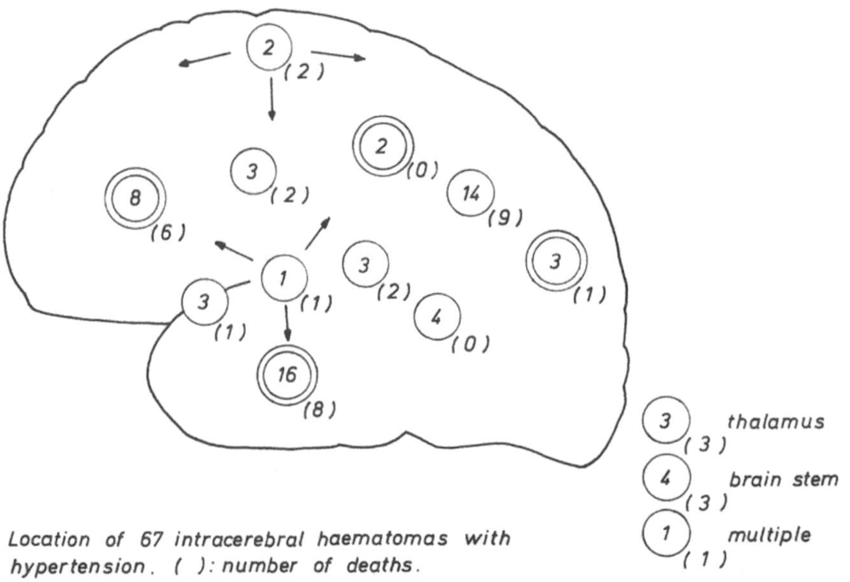

Fig. 2. Site of intracranial haemorrhages, corresponding to operation findings in 67 patients

(21.1%), there were other significant associated diseases, e.g. marked obesity. We have examined only ten patients since the advent of computer tomography. In the remainder the diagnosis was established by angiography. Further details about the diagnosis will not be discussed here.

Among the cases treated by operation, 40 had a craniectomy (56.3%), 26 cases (36.6%) a burr-hole and three patients (4.2%) had ventricular drainage. Of the patients, 28 (39.4%) survived and 43 (60.5%) died. If one relates the site of the haematoma to the involvement of

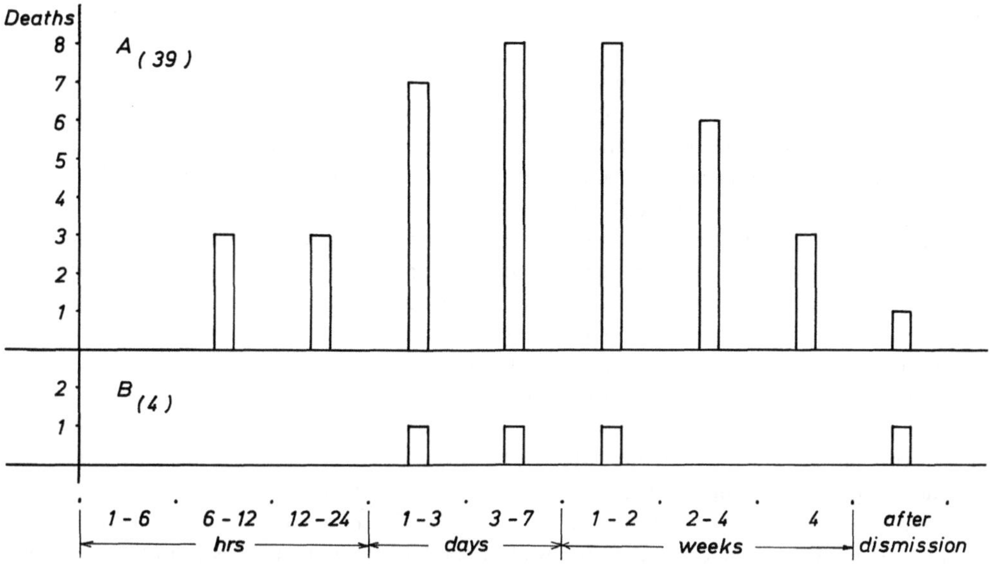

Death after operation (A), without operation (B)

Fig. 3. Interval between onset and death in fatal cases, with and without operation

Table 1. State of consciousness at the time of admission and before the operation

Level of consciousness	On admission	At operation
Attentive	12	12
Drowsy	15	11
Somnolent	19	9
Coma	24	24
with reaction to pain stimuli	5	5
with decerebrate rigidity	14	14

central areas of the brain, or the penetration of the haemorrhage into these central parts, it is seen that the prognosis is much worse when these parts are involved (Table 2). Thus, of 23 patients in whom the hypertensive bleeding had involved the basal ganglia 19 died. The main explanation for this is the destructive effect of the haemorrhage in the region of the central structures. On the other hand, in those cases where the main effect is that of a shift, the situation is reversible.

Table 2. Relation of the haematoma to the central brain structures[a]

Site	Died	Survived	Total
Perforation into the ventricles	19	8	27
Capsula interna	15	7	22
Basal ganglia	17	2	19
Thalamus	3	–	3
Brain stem	3	1	4

[a] Prognosis of ICH with hypertension (43 of 71 patients died whilst in hospital)

Discussion

Neurosurgical material represents only a small fraction of spontaneous cerebral haemorrhages, if one compares the existing statistics of the cause of death with the average figures for treatment in neurosurgical units. The experiences reported here regarding the collection of material, the site of the haematoma and symptoms and prognosis, correspond essentially with those in the literature (see Luyendijk 1972).

Although the introduction of computer tomography has significantly broadened our knowledge concerning the location, development and prognosis of intracerebral haemorrhage, from our personal experience, we have not so far been able to propose any definite guidelines for operative treatment. The careful weighing of the indications and contra-indications for operation is closely related to the difficulty in differentiating between the destructive and/or the displacing effects of the haematoma (Stochdorph and Meessen 1957). The destructive component leads to destruction or loss of cerebral tissue (Neubürger 1930) and, in the central white matter, this can dominate the picture. Mostly, however, it is overlaid by the displacing effect of the haematoma. According to Stochdorph and Meessen, the wall of the haematoma cavity is frequently shaggy and lacerated and this suggests that in these cases, there is a pre-existing *status lacunaris* or similar change. If the wall of the haematoma cavity is smooth, one often finds a ragged circumscribed area which corresponds to the point of origin of the bleeding, or the remnant of a localized lacunar area.

At all events, these pathological observations indicate that the condition of the wall of the haematoma cavity may give a hint regarding the prognosis. It still remains an open question to what extent the CT scan makes possible any pre-operative differentiation. An irregular appearance in the marginal zones and also in the centre of a haemorrhage may well suggest its destructive character. Á rapid deterioration or a quick transition to a decerebrate state is a contra-indication, as a rule, to any operation, while a gradual deterioration or a static clinical state should encourage operative intervention. The absence of any gross shifts indicates, rather, the destructive character of the haemorrhage (although one should take note of such details as an atrophic brain and widened – internal and external – fluid spaces), while evidence of substantial shifts indicates a displacing process which should, of course, be distinguished from cerebral oedema, e.g. as the result of uncontrolled high blood pressure. If the haemorrhage is situated in the cerebral hemisphere or individual lobes, this facilitates the decision regarding operation. On the other hand, haemorrhages in the basal ganglia, the thalamus or brain stem should only be operated on if there are particular factors such as a gradual progress of previously slight neurological signs (Table 3). One could consider that operation is indicated if the diagnosis is uncertain, if a tumour or an AV malformation is suspected, as well as when the pre-morbid blood pressure is unknown. Severe cardiac circulatory or respiratory diseases, as well as severe cerebrovascular arteriosclerosis and uncontrolled high blood pressure should also be regarded as contra-indications to operative treatment. In my opinion it is still an open question whether old age constitutes a contra-indication to operative treatment. The increase of more encouraging and favourable results after operative intervention in older subjects allows one to expect wider indications for operation in the future than have been customary so far.

The prognosis in spontaneous intracerebral haematomas from hypertension is determined by the following points:

If the haemorrhage has led to destruction of brain tissue, the symptoms are as a rule more marked and the clinical picture is unlikely to improve. Haemorrhages which produce a shift have a more favourable prognosis.

The more central the haemorrhage, the worse is the prognosis. On the one hand, this is because in the central regions the destructive element predominates and on the other hand, because important regulation mechanisms are located in the central parts of the brain.

Table 3. Review of indications and contra-indications for operation in cases of spontaneous intracerebral haematomas with hypertension

Indications	Contra-indications
Slow deterioration	Hyperacute deterioration
Mass shift	No signs of mass shifts
Localization in the hemisphere or lobes	Location in basal ganglia, thalamus and brain stem (relative contra-indication)
Suspicion of tumour or AV malformation (uncertain diagnosis)	Severe cardiac, circulatory and respiratory diseases
Unknown premorbid blood pressure	Severe cardiovascular arteriosclerosis
	High levels of blood pressure
	Senility?

The speed with which the symptoms develop is decisive for the prognosis. The more rapidly the symptoms increase or the more marked they are at the onset, the more unfavourable is the prognosis. Hence, it is irrelevant in the first place whether there appear to be local symptoms or remote symptoms related to cerebral shifts.

The older the patient, the more unfavourable in general is the prognosis, for not only does the ability of the brain to compensate diminish, but also the possibility of further complications in peripheral organs substantially increases. Of course, these boundaries have been gradually pushed back in recent years so that even old age cannot be regarded as an absolute contra-indication.

The extent and degree of the associated complications often determine the fate of the patient, regardless of any improvement in the cerebral functions. This applies particularly to respiratory diseases, cardiovascular disturbances and disorders of metabolism.

Apart from any indications and contra-indications for operation and the prognosis of hypertensive haemorrhages, the most important thing will be in what way cooperation can be brought about between physicians, neurologists, neurosurgeons and geriatricians, if we are to improve the hitherto unsatisfactory results of the treatment of intracerebral haemorrhages in hypertension.

8.3.1.3 Discussion

C. Arseni and A. Gontea, Bucharest

Arterial hypertension may be considered the determinant cause of primary intracranial haematoma only when it is higher than 180 mm Hg before the haematoma develops. Arterial hypertension developing in the course of a haematoma is considered secondary to the autonomic disorders produced by the haematoma and especially by hypoxia of the vasomotor centres (Kreindler and Voiculescu 1963). Of the 364 haematomas studied, 43.59% were assumed to be caused by arterial hypertension (Istrati 1975). If to this one adds the cases in which arterial hypertension was associated with other factors, the proportion is 47.76%. In nine cases arterial hypertension was associated with one factor and in three cases with two factors. In one case of intraparenchymatous haematoma with arterial hypertension, the patient had suffered 2 years previously from cerebral haemorrhage on the opposite side.

Our statistics show that primary haematoma and cerebral haemorrhage in the cerebral hemispheres are more frequently produced by arterial hypertension than by other causes. In the cerebellum both vascular accidents are frequently caused by benign arterial hypertension.

Brain stem haematomas are not associated with arterial hypertension, but haemorrhage in the pons is frequently produced by high blood pressure, a fact of importance for differential diagnosis.

The prognosis of primary intraparenchymatous haematoma does not depend upon arterial hypertension, but that of cerebral haemorrhage does.

Paroxysmal arterial hypertension was encountered in 18% of cases, and varied between 180 and 300 mm Hg. In such cases the prognosis of haematoma is severe because recurrences, always accompanied by marked cerebral oedema, may occur. In three cases of haematoma situated in the insula, operation was uneventful, but afterwards blood pressure oscillations up to 300 mm Hg abruptly developed; two of the patients developed haematomas a few hours later, were reoperated on and the haematomas evacuated, but they died after 2 – 3 days from marked cerebral oedema. The third patient was reoperated on twice (at 2 days and 1 week) and survived but with serious sequelae.

Arterial hypotension may also be the cause of subacute or chronic haematomas due to venous stasis, but the prognosis is always favourable.

K. Schürmann, Mainz: I will start with contra-indications with regard to the localization of spontaneous intracerebral haematomas. In my opinion, no operation is indicated in the typical haemorrhage in which the central areas of the brain and the basal ganglia are destroyed, especially when combined with evidence of compression and shifting of the brain. There are no indications for operating on patients with intrapontine and intramedullary bleeding. Surgery should not be performed on patients in deep coma, patients in the very acute phase of haemorrhage or patients over 70 years of age. Operation should also be avoided in patients under cumarin therapy and whose Quick index is below 15%. They must be treated immediately by PPSB and vitamin infusions and eventually operated on when the coagulation disturbances have been satisfactorily dealt with. Other contra-indications are serious insufficiency of heart, kidneys, lungs or liver, particularly when combined with venous congestion. The risks of operation under such conditions, in hypertensive patients, are in my opinion much higher than the chance which the patients is given by the operation.

There is a relative indication for operation in patients in whom neither the space-occupying haematoma nor the perifocal or general oedema of the affected hemisphere regresses under intensive therapy and the brain thus continues to remain under compression. This is an important point for me. The above situation usually occurs a few days after the onset of the haemorrhage. In these conditions it seems to be advisable to reduce the compression in the brain by timely evacuation of the haematoma to avoid the danger of further secondary lesions which would result from this untreated compression. If stabilization of the vegetative state is achieved, operation performed at that stage yields better results.

An absolute indication is when there is a progressive increase in an originally slight disturbance of consciousness, with an increase in the neurological signs, and when substantial brain compression and shifts occur in spite of intensive treatment and high doses of dexamethasone. After rapid and so-called atraumatic emptying of the haematoma the decompressed brain may have a chance of recovering. However, it must be noted that the prognosis is better the longer the interval between the acute bleeding and the time of operation. In other words, the more acutely one must intervene immediately after the onset of the bleeding because of acute progression of clinical symptoms, the poorer is the prognosis. In this acute phase of instability of vegetative state and still extreme vulnerability of the brain tissue swelling can occur during the operation or shortly afterwards with very unfavourable effects. As far as possible one should wait for at least a few hours before operating and, if possible, for a few days. In all cases we carry out a plastic widening of the dura with a galea-periosteal flap to provide sufficient space for the anticipated brain swelling.

In Mainz we have operated on 74 patients with spontaneous intracerebral haematomas. Among them were 29 patients with hypertension and 12 who were under long-term anticoagulant therapy. Twenty-one patients underwent acute operation within 24 h of bleeding, and 35 patients were treated by delayed operation after 24 h – 5 days after bleeding. Thirty-five patients had slight disturbances of consciousness, whereas 28 underwent operation in a comatose state. Twenty-five patients died, nine remained in a bad condition with severe neurological and mental deficits and 22 patients recovered with only slight neurological deficits. The latter group had delayed operations. The largest group of patients was aged between 55 and 65 years, and nine patients were older than 65 years. The highest mortality was found in the oldest patients and in those with arterial hypertension.

J. Haftek, Lódź: In the Department of Neurosurgery, Military Ácademy in Lódź, we have operated on 29 cases of spontaneous intracerebral haematoma. Our mortaliy was 25%. We evacuate the haematoma through a craniotomy, cortical incision and removal of blood and clots under direct visual control.

Late results. Nineteen cases have been followed up for a period of 2 – 11 years. Three patients were completely free of symptoms and signs. Eleven patients had slight neurological deficits and/or epileptic seizures. Five patients had severe deficits. As far as indications and contra-indications for operation are concerned, I think that the clinical course is more important than the condition of the patient at the time of examination. In other words, a patient with signs of involvement of the brain stem, who has been in this condition for several hours or days, will not be operated on, but a patient even if comatose and with signs of brain stem involvement will be investigated and possibly operated on, if the condition is of recent onset. It seems to me that this is the only way to help the patient who is deteriorating. However, I agree with many speakers who have already stressed that better results are to be expected if there is some delay before operation is performed.

B. Pertuiset, Paris: In considering the surgical treatment of haemorrhage one must take account of failures, because only they allow us to give a prognosis of the spontaneous evolution.

It is better to postpone the operation when the outcome can be regarded as poor in any case. This is the case when the haemorrhage is dissecting, involves the midline structures and is not due to a vascular malformation. Patients in grades I – III with haematoma or haemorrhage in the hemisphere should be operated on immediately. There will be a large number of patients who will not fall into these two categories, and it may be difficult to decide on the best form of treatment for them.

The clinical grade of the patient is of the utmost importance and must be given first consideration. The surgical treatment of intracerebral haemorrhage requires more clinical experience than surgical expertise. We must distinguish between compression which can be relieved by operation and destruction, which cannot. A patient with a dissecting haemorrhage in grade III or IV will not be operated upon, but a patient with a haemorrhage in the cerebellum should be operated on because we find that in every case there is direct compression of the brain stem.

H. Penholz, I. P. McCarthy, and H. Braunke, Heidelberg: From 1970 to 1978, 36 patients suffering from spontaneous ICH and with the diagnosis of elevated blood pressure were treated. Their ages ranged from 34 to 66 years. Most of the females (15) were aged 40 – 44 years, while most of the males (21) were between 45 and 49 years.

As regards the hemispheric location of the haematomas our figures were comparable with those of other authors, i.e. 58% (21) right-sided, 34% (12) left-sided. In 8% (3) of the cases the haematoma was located in the pons region with rupture into the ventricular system. Haematomas were commoner in the temporal and parietal lobes; 56% (20) of the cases had temporal lesions; approximately 22% (8) had parietal or parieto-occipital lesions; and approximately 14% (5) frontal and 8% (3) in the pons.

Operation was performed in 75% (27) of the cases and the rest was treated conservatively. Mortality after conservative treatment was 67% (6) and 25% (7) after surgical intervention.

For prognostic purposes we divided the conscious level of the patients into four grades:

1) Awake
2) Somnolent
3) Unsconscious without brain stem symptoms
4) Unconscious with brain stem symptoms.

A significant rise in mortality occurs with impairment of consciousness both in the surgically and the conservatively treated groups (Fig. 1).

If one analyses the chance of survival in relation to the time of operation there is a mortality rate of about 56% (n = 4) when the operation is performed within 24 h of the ictus (n = 7). With the exception of one patient, all operations performed within the first 24 h after haemorrhage were, in fact, carried out within 8 h. If operation is postponed the chances of survival increase (Fig. 2), reaching a survival rate of 100% after the 10th day. If both the time of operation and grading of consciousness are considered, the grading is more important for prognostic purposes than the time of operation (Fig. 3). There is a high mortality in grade 3 and 4 patients if an early operation is performed. A high mortality was not only seen in grade 3 and 4 patients who underwent early operation but also in those who were operated on later thȧn 24 h, so that the state of consciousness is apparently the most important factor in determining the outcome.

In the follow-up of those treated surgically (n = 20), there is at the time of discharge an improvement of the motor deficit in about 50% in the hemiparesis group as well as in the hemiplegia group (Table 1). In reviewing the results 6 months to 6 years after operation we

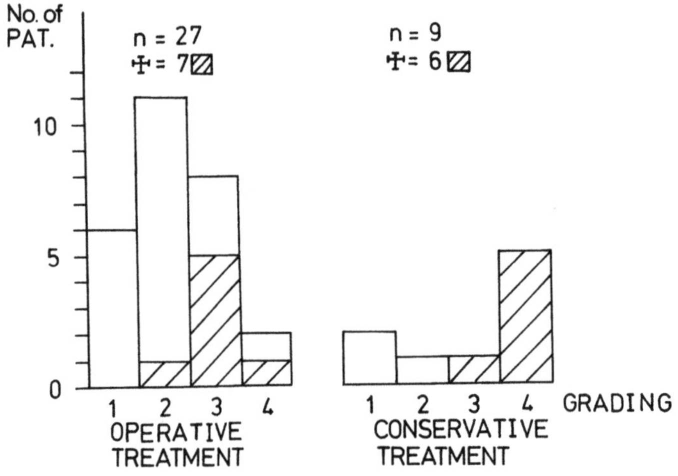

Fig. 1. Mortality in relation to grade of consciousness

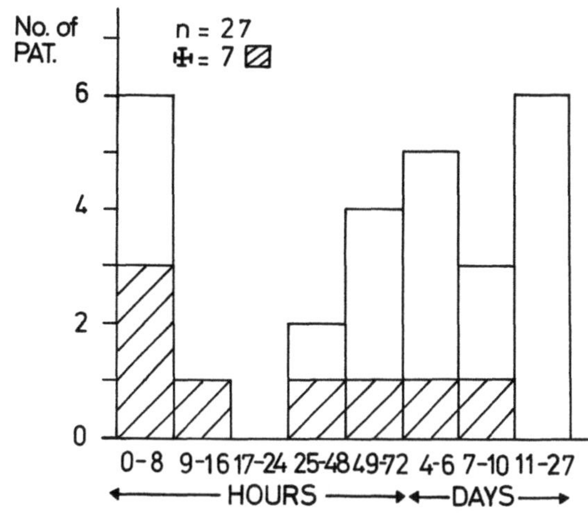

Fig. 2. Mortality in relation to time between ictus and operation

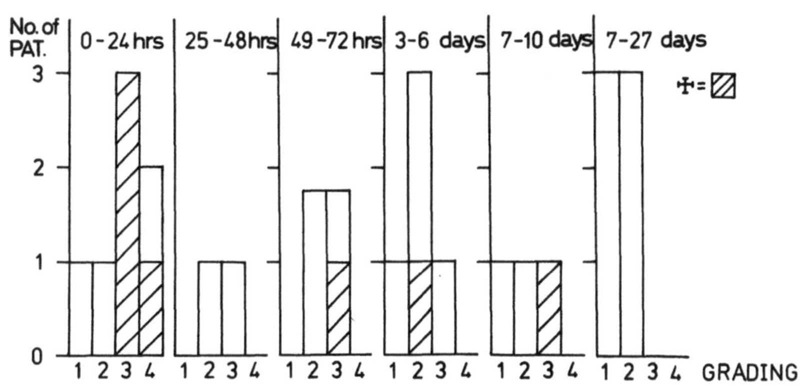

Fig. 3. Mortality in relation to operation time and grade of consciousness

Table 1. Postoperative results

On admission	On discharge		
	Symptom-free	Improved	Unchanged
Hemiparesis (n = 9, 100%)	2 (22%)	3 (34%)	4 (44%)
Hemiplegia (n = 11, 100%)	–	6 (55%)	5 (45%)

Table 2. Follow-up results 6 months – 6 years after discharge

On admission	On discharge			Follow-up results		
	Symptom-free	Improved	Unchanged	Symptom-free	Improved	Unchanged
Hemiparesis (n = 6)	2 (33%)	1 (17%)	3 (50%)	3 (50%)	2 (33%)	1 (17%)
Hemiplegia (n = 5)	–	2 (40%)	3 (60%)	–	2 (40%)	3 (60%)

found in a questionnaire study that patients with dense hemiplegia had not improved whereas in the hemiparesis group there was a further increase (from 50% to 83%) in the number of improved and symptom-free patients (Table 2).

Summary

The prognosis of spontaneous ICH in patients with raised blood pressure depends to a considerable degree on the level of consciousness. We feel that the mortality rate in patients with severe disturbance of consciousness can rarely be influenced by early surgical treatment. Operation during the subacute or chronic phase seems to give better results.

R. Nagpal, Bombay: Of 109 patients of spontaneous intracerebral haemorrhage, 66 had haemorrhage due to hypertension. The blood pressure varied from 280/180 to 150/100 mm Hg. The largest group of patients belonged to the fifth and sixth decades. Of these 66 patients, 45 expired, and in four the fate is unknown. The mortality in relation to sex was 2 males to 1 female. Of the 66 hypertensive haemorrhages 43 were males.

Prognosis in Relation to Duration of Symptoms

Six patients with symptoms of less than 24 h died; 23 of the 36 patients in whom the duration was greater than 48 h died. Amongst the 24 in whom this information was not available, 16 died. The fate of four is unknown.

Prognosis in Relation to Level of Consciousness at the Time of Admission

Nine of the 15 conscious, 8 of the 12 drowsy, 8 of the 12 semiconscious and 20 of the 23 unconscious patients died.

Relation to Location of Clot

Of the 37 with clots in and around the basal ganglia, 33 died. The five patients with thalamic haemorrhages who expired have been included in these 37 cases. Of the 23 subcortical haemorrhages 10 expired. One patient with a clot in the cerebellum and brain stem died. Of the 45 patients who expired, 20 were shown at autopsy to have intraventricular haemorrhage.

Prognosis in Relation to Form of Therapy

Surgical evacuation of the clot gave the best results. Ten of the 22 patients so treated survived, whereas only 4 of the 17 patients treated by aspiration survived. Conservative treatment yielded very poor results and, of the 23 patients treated conservatively, 20 died.

In summary, we found that younger patients, with a longer duration of symptoms (i.e. a less acute onset), conscious, with a clot in the subcortical areas which is surgically evacuated have a better chance of surviving a hypertensive intracerebral clot.

R. Müke, Hamburg: In discussing the prognosis of patients with intracerebral haematomas and hypertension it is also necessary to consider the time of operation, age of the patient, the extension of the haematoma and the level of consciousness. The statistics from all our surgically treated patients since 1976 shows the relationship of the various factors.

Timing of Operation

If we have to operate within 12 h after the onset of bleeding, the prognosis is poor; only 8 of 21 survived. If we can wait 24 h, the prognosis improves considerably; seven of nine survived (Table 3).

Table 3. Spontaneous intracerebral haematomas – prognosis

Time of operation	
12 h	21 cases (8 survived)
12 – 24 h	12 cases (7 survived)
after 24 h	9 cases (7 survived)

Age

Of 16 patients older than 50, only five survived; of 26 younger than 50, 17 survived (Table 4).

Table 4. Spontaneous intracerebral haematomas – prognosis

Age	Survived	Died
Younger than 50 yrs	17	9
Older than 50 yrs	5	11

Level of Consciousness

All four patients without signs of intracranial pressure survived; of 24 with signs of intracranial pressure, 9 died and, of 14 deeply comatose, 11 died (Table 5).

Of seven patients operated on with a known history of hypertension, all died despite operation. But all these patients were deeply comatose on admission and had to be operated on within 12 h of the bleeding. Probably the results of operation would look more favourable if we

Table 5. Spontaneous intracerebral haematomas – prognosis

Level of consciousness	Survived	Died
No signs of intracranial pressure	4	0
With signs of intracranial pressure	15	9
Deeply comatose	3	11

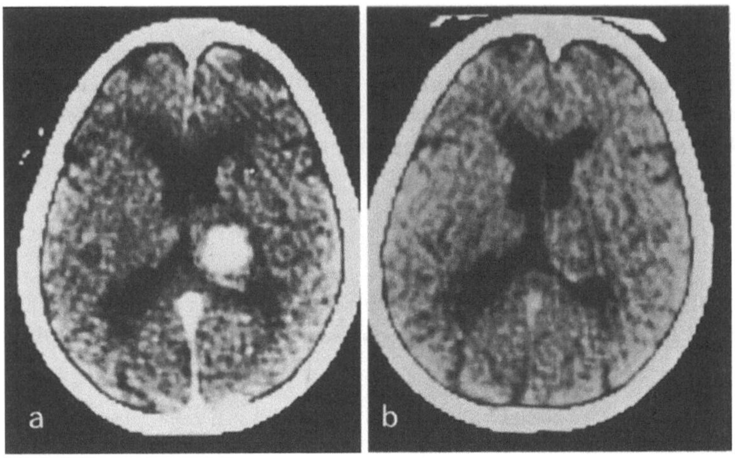

Fig. 4. a Haematoma in the area of the basal ganglia, the thalamus and the internal capsule, **b** 18 days later, the haematoma has spontaneously resolved

had operated on patients in better condition. On the other hand, five patients not operated on because there was no vital risk involved, survived. Figure 4 shows the CT of one of these patients with a haematoma, in the area of the basal ganglia, the thalamus and the internal capsule, that resolved spontaneously within 2 weeks. This agrees with the results of McKissock (1959) who reported that the outcome in patients with a haematoma due to hypertension is worse after operation than after conservative treatment. Hence, we do not think that a hypertensive haematoma of the basal ganglia should be operated on.

8.3.1.4 Prognostic Factors in the First 48 Hours in Spontaneous ICH and Spreading Haemorrhages*

B. Pertuiset, A. Yacoubi, J. P. Sichez, and D. Gardeur, Paris

During the last 30 years reaching an agreement about a clear definition of the various types of spontaneous intracerebral haemorrhages has been a challenge to pathologists, neurologists, neurosurgeons and neuroradiologists. The words haematoma and haemorrhage have been used indiscriminately, leading to considerable confusion when one tries to compare different papers.

* In the CT pictures of this report the left side as seen by the reader corresponds to the right side of the craniom

According to Greek etymology, a haematoma is a full-blooded tumour, while a haemorrhage is an outflow of blood coming from an artery. In other words, a haematoma is a clearly outlined clot and remains in a static condition, while a haemorrhage is an active phenomenon.

Misunderstandings arise in cases in which, even though the haemorrhage is arrested, blood continues to spread into the brain tissue with a blurred outline. We propose in such cases to use the term "spreading haemorrhage" to define this unstable condition.

In the past the confusion in terminology as well as the difficulty of clinically analysing an intracerebral haemorrhage, regarding its location and spread, has increased the differences of opinion concerning prognosis and therapy.

Information from CT scans has helped us to understand the situation in every patient since a correlation can be made between the pathology (CT scan), the clinical condition and the aetiology. Therefore, it is now possible to try to analyse the prognostic factors during the first 48 h after the onset of the stroke.

During the last 6 months of 1978 we have been able to collect in the University Clinic of la Pitié full records on 41 patients. They were selected because an angiogram was performed in every case as well as a CT scan with a scanner of the new generation (Neurodensitome N.D. 8000). Data on haemorrhages occurring in tumours were discarded.

All patients were investigated between 10 and 48 h after the onset of the haemorrhage, thanks to the medical manning of ambulances and our special intensive care unit for comas.

Material (Table 1)

There were 25 males and 16 females, the ages ranging from 20 to 80.

Table 1. Spontaneous intracerebral haematoma and spreading haemorrhage

	Haematomas (N = 25)	Spreading Haemorrhages (N = 16)
Aetiology		
Hypertension	1	10
Coagulation defect	3	1
AVM	8	2
Aneurysms	10	–
Unknown	5	3
Clinical grade		
1	9	3
2	8	3
3	4	2
4	4	8
Location		
Frontal lobe	9	–
Temporal lobe	10	–
Parietal lobe	4	–
Occipital lobe	1	–
Cerebellar hemisphere	1	–
Basal ganglia [a]	–	9
Central sulcus [a]	–	4
Brain stem [a]	–	2
Cerebellar vermis [a]	–	1
Mortality	9 (36%)	8 (50%)

[a] Site of original haemorrhage

We have analysed four essential factors:

A) The Aetiology of the Haemorrhage

Vascular malformations (ten saccular aneurysms and eight AVM) were separated from those of medical origin: arterial hypertension (11), coagulation defect (4), unknown (8).

Ruptured vascular malformations appeared between the ages of 20 – 70, with a maximum between 20 and 30.

Patients with "medical" haemorrhages ranged from 40 to 80, with a maximum between 60 and 70.

B) The Clinical Grade

This was considered according to the aetiology of the haemorrhage:

Vascular malformations: grade 1 (alert, oriented, coherent in speech), five cases; grade 2 (drowsy, with or without neurological deficit), five cases; grade 3 (comatose, with no response to verbal command), three cases; grade 4 (comatose, with decerebration), five cases.

Medical aetiologies: grade 1, seven cases; grade 2, six cases; grade 3, three cases; grade 4, seven cases.

It can be stated that in this series there is no relation between the clinical condition and the aetiology. Consequently, the grade is related to the rapidity of the onset, to the location of the haemorrhage and its extension as well as to the age of the patient.

The angiogram has been performed in all cases after the CT scan and for this reason was selective. It has shown the vascular malformation and the vascular displacements provoked by a space-occupying lesion.

We consider the angiogram as a necessary investigation which can reveal the aetiology, but it cannot give in a particular case any useful information about the characteristics of the haemorrhage.

It must be stated that in some cases an AVM does not show itself on the angiogram, but the CT location of the haemorrhage may suggest such a diagnosis.

C) The CT Scan (Figs. 1, 2, 3, 4)

This investigation gives information on four major points:

1) Location of the Haemorrhage

Because the CT scan is performed during the first 48 h after the onset of the haemorrhage, the blood gives a high density picture in all cases. It was easy to identify the haemorrhage in the white matter of the hemispheres (28), in the grey nuclei (9), in the cerebellum (2), and in the brain stem (2).

2) Outline of the Haemorrhage

It was possible to separate two types:

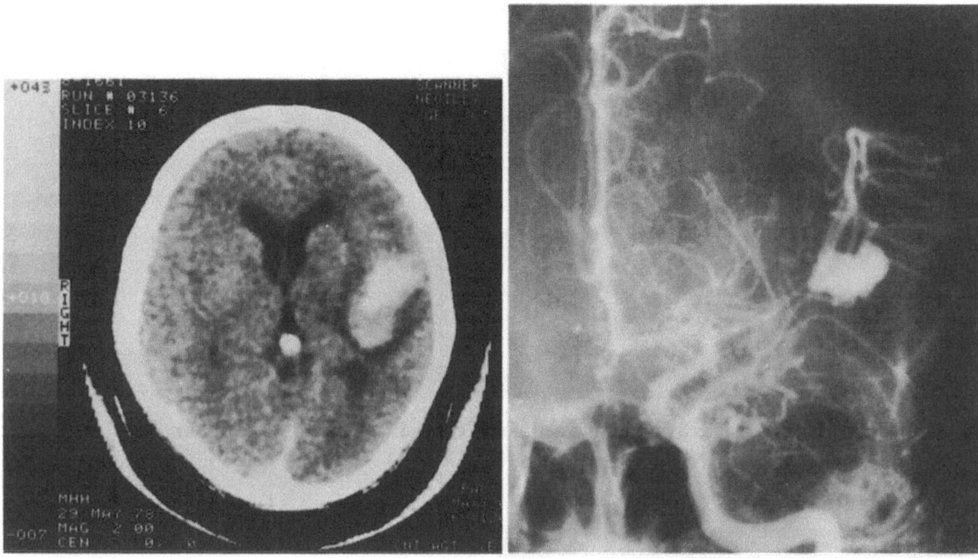

Fig. 1. Ruptured saccular aneurysm of the left middle cerebral artery with temporal haematoma (3rd day after rupture)

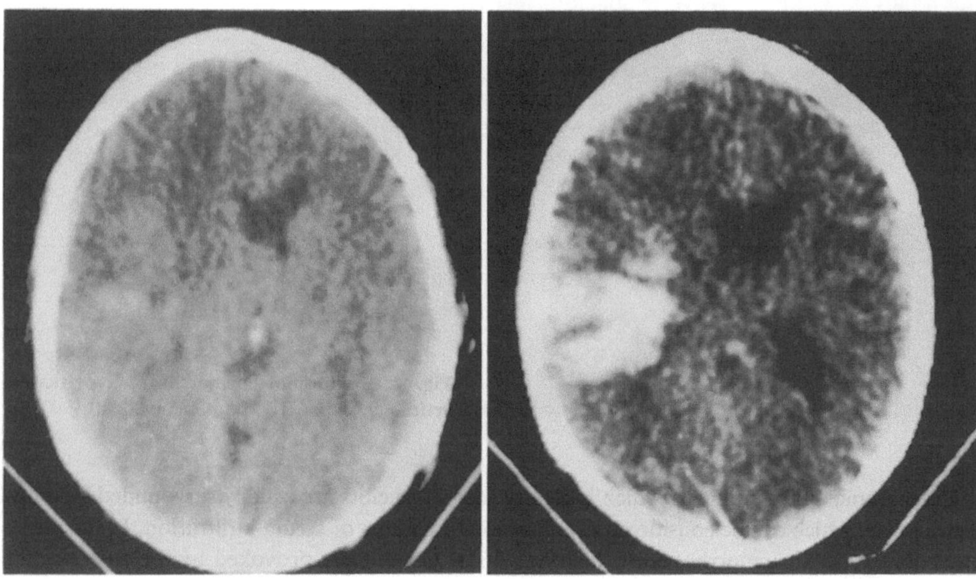

Fig. 2. Frontal and parietal haematoma; hypertensive aetiology. Left deficit, recovery after surgery

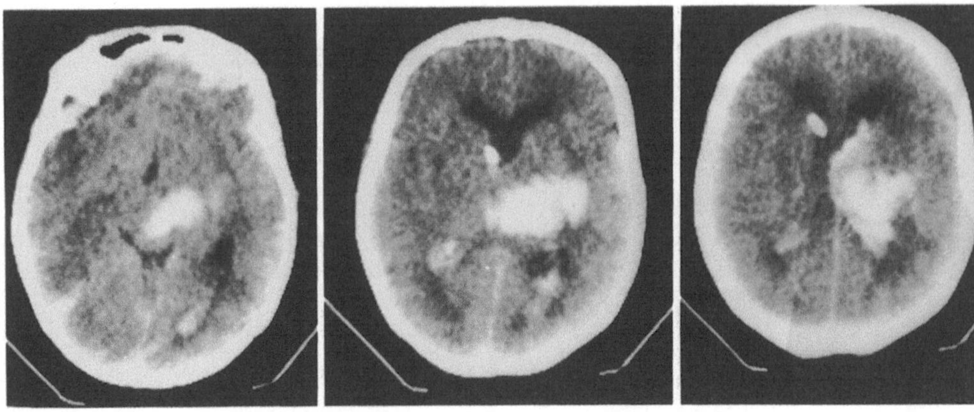

Fig. 3. Spreading haemorrhage; hypertensive aetiology, coma II; death after operation

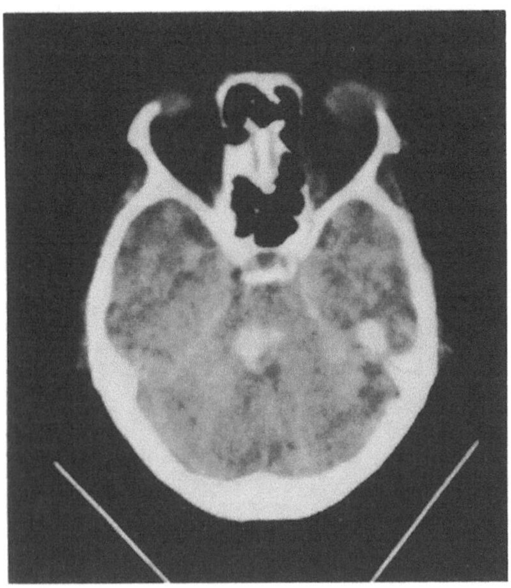

Fig. 4. Brain stem haemorrhage; hypertensive aetiology, coma III; spontaneous death

Haematomas, the outline of which is clearly seen. The clots are usually surrounded by a low density zone which can be considered as ischaemia or an area of serum infiltration. In this series were observed 25 haemorrhages of this type, 16 of which were provoked by the rupture of a vascular malformation.

Spreading haemorrhages, the outline of which can be well delineated on one scan, while on the others they appear as extensions in the white matter or in the grey nuclei. In most cases the outline is irregular. The clots can be surrounded by oedema in the white matter which usually is more diffuse than in haematomas. During the first 48 h this oedema is usually of less importance than later. In this series there were 16 cases of this type, only two of which came from a vascular malformation which was an AVM.

Therefore, it can be stated that haematomas occur mostly from rupture of vascular malformations and spreading haemorrhages of medical origin.

3) Intraventricular Haemorrhage

When the haemorrhage has ruptured into the ventricular system it is worthwhile noting that blood in the lateral ventricles can provoke an oedema around the cavities. The haemorrhage can be localized or fill the entire ventricular system, worsening the prognosis.

4) Hydrocephalus

This complication of the haemorrhage can be clearly seen on the scan. When the pressure in the ventricle is higher than it is normally, there is usually an image of diffusion of CSF around the frontal horns (low density image). In this series only one such case was observed.

Thus, it is obvious that CT scan is able to give information which we never obtained before. It is comparable with pathology and is of great value in deciding prognosis and treatment when compared with the help given by the clinical condition and the aetiology.

D) Prognosis

Mortality (Table 2)

In our series mortality has been spontaneous or after operation which in all cases was performed through a small flap.

Spontaneous Mortality

It has been very variable, according to the type of haemorrhage: in cases of haematoma, 1 of 25 (4%) and, in spreading haemorrhage, six of sixteen (37%).

Postoperative Mortality

Figures have been the reverse: haematomas, 8 of 25 (32%) and, in spreading haemorrhage, 2 of 16 (12%).

Table 2. Intracerebral spontaneous haemorrhages: spontaneous and postoperative mortality

Type and aetiology	Mortality	
	Spontaneous	Postoperative
Haematomas (25)		
Vascular malformations	1	7
Other aetiologies	0	1
Spreading haemorrhages (16)		
Hypertension	4	1
Unknown	1	1
Coagulation deficit	1	0
AVM	0	0

Table 3. Spontaneous intracerebral haemorrhages: epidemiology of mortality in 17 cases

	Mortality	%
Localization		
Sub-tentorial	3 of 4	75
Basal ganglia	4 of 9	44
Hemispheric	10 of 28	36
Nature of the haemorrhage		
Spreading haemorrhage	8 of 16	50
Haematoma	9 of 25	36
Clinical grade		
1	1 of 11	10
2	3 of 9	33
3	3 of 8	37
4	10 of 13	76
Spontaneous death	7 of 17	41
Postoperative death	10 of 17	59

These findings have confused our opinion; to clarify, we have analysed the 17 fatal cases.

Epidemiology of Mortality (Table 3)

This has been analysed according to:

Location; the highest mortality occurred in the posterior fossa lesions (75%), but the number of cases has no statistical significance. The lowest mortality occurred in hemispheric lesions (36%).

Types of haemorrhage; the highest mortality occurred in the spreading haemorrhages (50%, compared with 36% in haematomas).

Clinical grade; grade 4 patients had the highest mortality.

Spontaneous or postoperative evolution; the postoperative mortality has been higher (59%), due to the other factors (location, type of haemorrhage and clinical grade).

Therefore, from this series it can be stated that posterior fossa and grey nuclei haemorrhage as well as spreading haemorrhages are the more serious lesions, especially when the patient is in grade 4 condition, is suffering from hypertension and is over 50.

Discussion

We knew from pathology that spreading and medial spontaneous haemorrhages had a serious prognosis but we have not previously been able to analyse the characteristics of the haemorrhage in a patient during the first 48 h.

The information given by CT scan has changed our position. It is now possible to approach the prognosis and consequently to advise treatment.

We think actually that the surgical treatment of an intracerebral haemorrhage must take into account the figures which indicate the prognosis of its spontaneous evolution.

On one hand it is better to postpone the operation when the evolution can be considered as very poor anyway.

We must now consider haematomas and spreading haemorrhages:

Haematomas. When there is a vascular malformation the patient will be operated on anyway, but the timing of operation will be related to the clinical grade.

When no vascular malformation is seen on the angiogram we suggest waiting if the patient is in grade 1.

The operation will become necessary if an aggravation of the clinical condition occurs (ingravescent apoplexy).

Spreading Haemorrhages. In patients with involvement of the grey nuclei, over the age of 50, in grade 3 or 4 and hypertensive, the prognosis is poor; an operation will precipitate the fatal issue. In patients with haemorrhage in the posterior fossa, the prognosis is poor but we continue to operate on these patients unless there is a hydrocephalus which requires external ventricular drainage.

In patients with haemorrhage in the hemispheres, therapy will be decided according to the clinical grade, the aggravation and the previous history.

Special Problems. When there is a haematoma of the thalamus it is necessary to wait as in haematomas of the brain stem. In these particular patients it is necessary to repeat the CT scan to decide if external ventricular drainage is necessary.

Summary

Thanks to the CT scan it now seems possible to predict the outcome of patients who are seen during the 48 h following a stroke caused by a spontaneous intracerebral haemorrhage.

The age of the patient, the clinical grade, the aetiology and the type of haemorrhage allows one to classify the patients into three main groups:

Patients who will die anyway (those over 50, hypertensive, in grades 3 – 4, with spreading haemorrhage).

Patients who will survive without operation (those under 40, non-hypertensive, in grade 1, with haematoma).

Patients who will survive after operation (those under 50, vascular malformation, in grades 1 – 2, with haematoma or spreading haemorrhage).

A fourth group is under discussion: those patients with posterior fossa and brain stem haemorrhages.

This approach to the prognosis will probably have to be revised in the coming years after the analysis of a larger series.

8.3.1.5 Haemorrhage and Haematoma

C. Arseni and A. Gontea, Bucharest

We would like to discuss some data concerning the pathological anatomy, aetiology and clinical aspects related to primary intraparenchymatous haematomas of the brain.

Morbid Anatomical Data

Cerebral haemorrhagic accidents (or blood extravasates) result in cerebral haemorrhage or in intraparenchymatous haematoma (Fig. 1). A cerebral haemorrhage is a diffuse blood extravasate that infiltrates and lacerates the cerebral tissue. It is most frequently located in the areas involved in important vegetative functions, such as the region of the basal ganglia and the brain stem (Figs. 2, 3). Other characteristics are a serious clinical state (coma), severe vegetative disorders, poor chance of spontaneous recovery (namely, if not too many important autonomic centres are damaged). A haematoma is a well-circumscribed collection of blood localized in the white matter (Figs. 4, 5). It develops suddenly, evolves clinically like an intracranial expanding process over a variable period of time, without apparent cause, increasing in volume by an osmotic process. This is why haematomas cannot be treated conservatively. Operation is the only possible treatment. The occurrence of one or other anatomical type depends on various factors, such as:

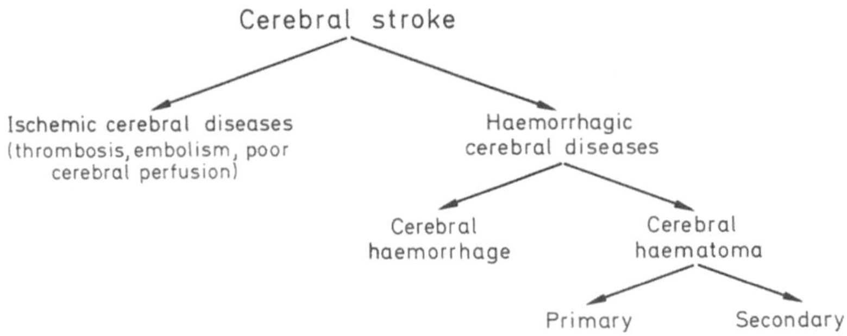

Fig. 1. Classification of cerebral strokes

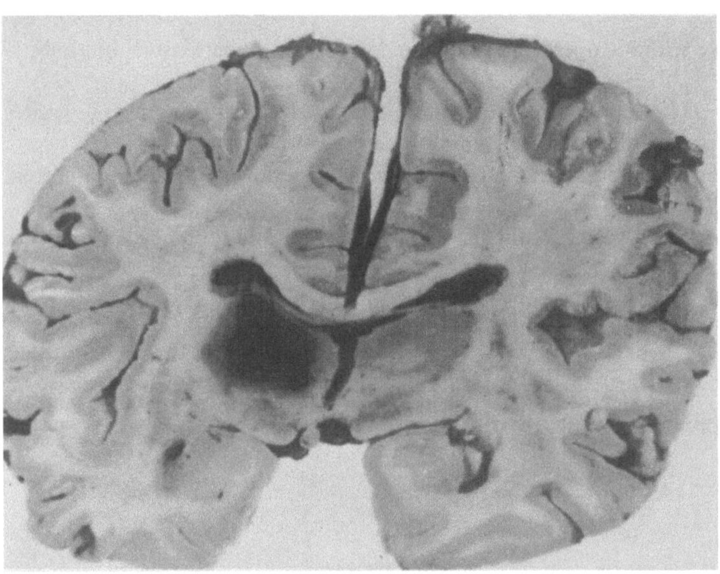

Fig. 2. Haematoma of the thalamus

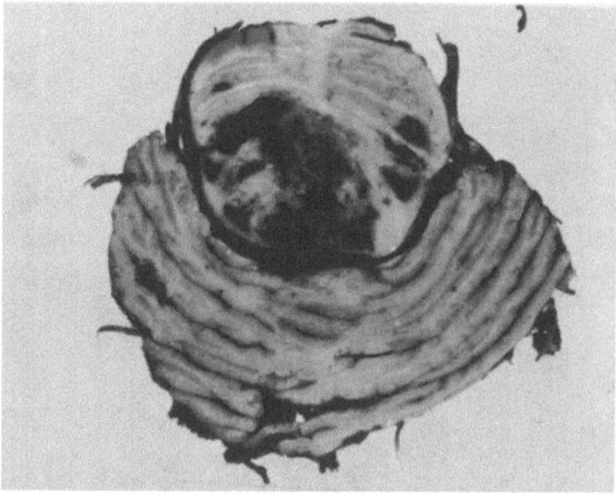

Fig. 3. Pontine haemorrhage

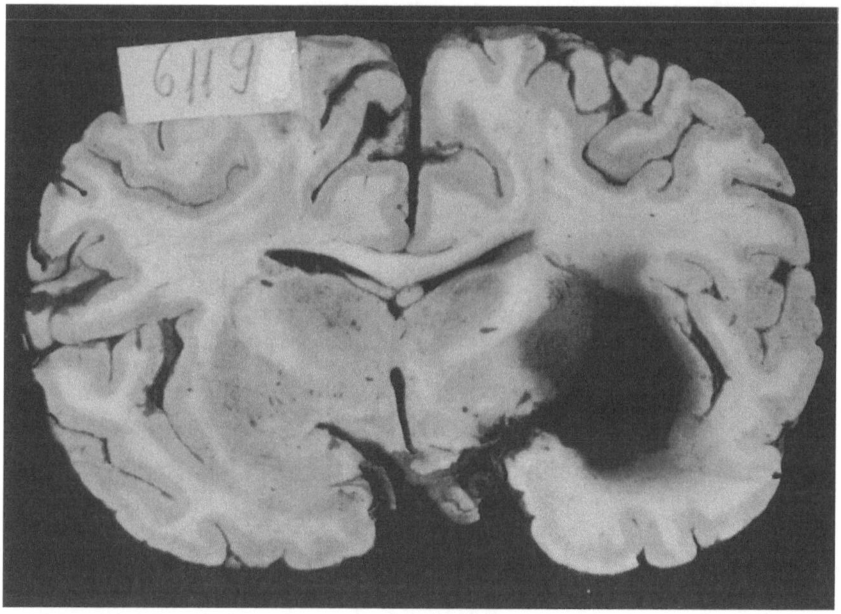

Fig. 4. Haematoma of white matter, temporomedial

The structure of the site where they occur; the blood extravasate becomes diffuse in the basal nuclei and pons because of their dense structures, whereas it coalesces when localized in the white matter;

The source of the haemorrhage; it is arterial in the basal nuclei, but venous in the white matter;

The pattern of vascularization in the basal nuclei; the arterioles run at a right angle and the arterial blood pressure is equal to that in the carotid (Fig. 6), while in the white matter the arterial tension is low, vascularization is poor with inadequate anastomoses (Fig. 7).

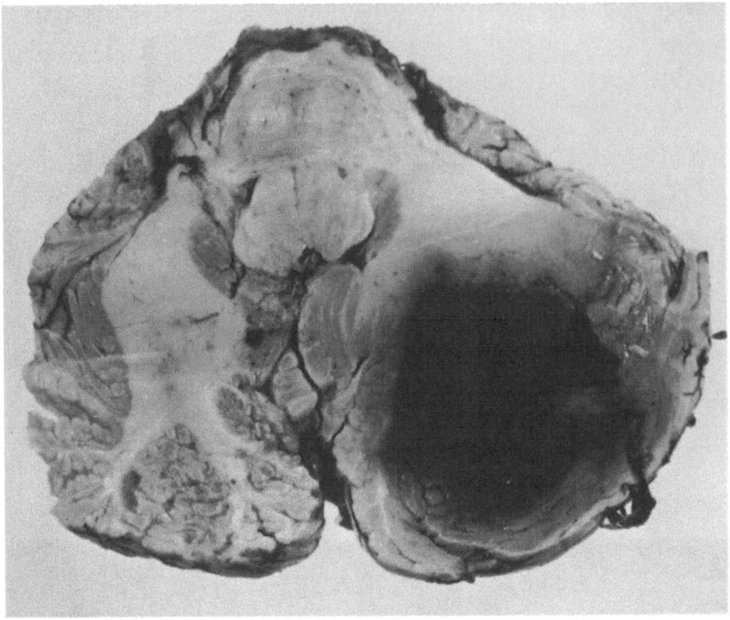

Fig. 5. Haematoma of white matter in the cerebellum

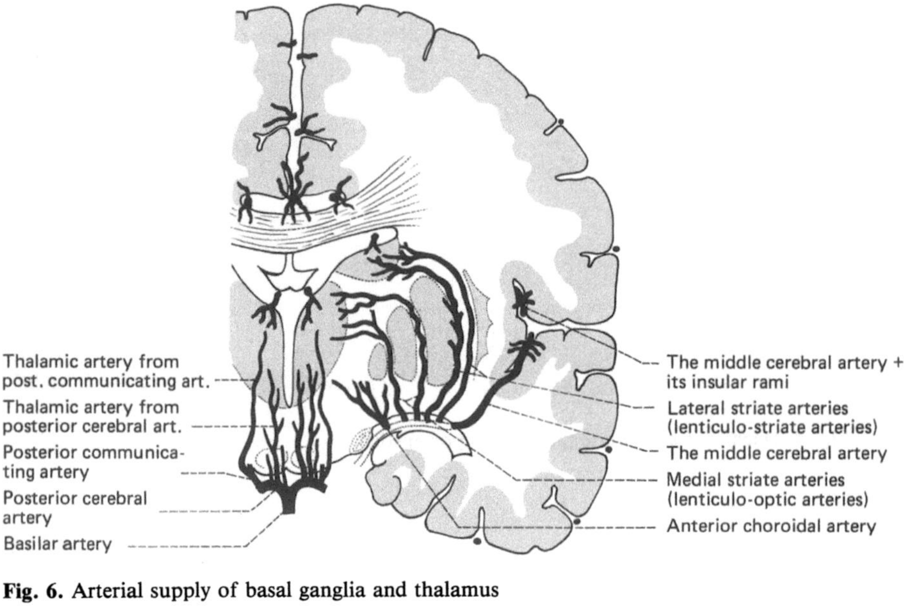

Fig. 6. Arterial supply of basal ganglia and thalamus

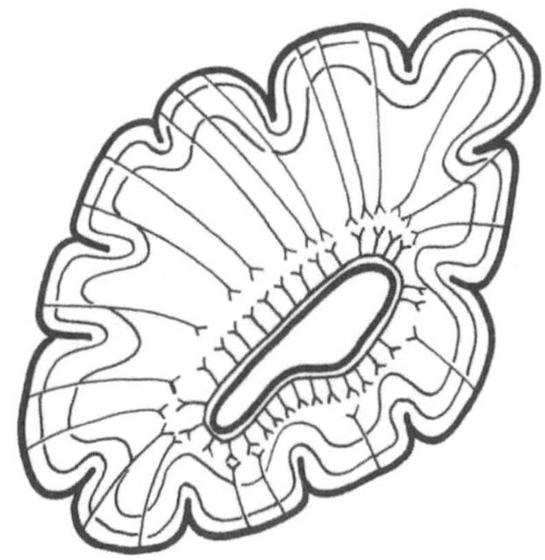

Fig. 7. Schematic representation of the periventricular (centrifugal) circulation and its relation to the deep penetrating (centripetal) supply

When there is no apparent cause for the blood extravasate it is called primary. Bleedings resulting from craniocerebral trauma, rupture of some cerebrovascular malformation or from a metastasis, are secondary intracerebral haematomas accompanying the primary lesion. They cannot be distinguished as clinical entities and must, therefore, be considered together with the basic disease. From the therapeutic point of view, the secondary haemorrhage and its cause should be dealt with together.

The designation of primary intracerebral haematoma is meant on the one hand to distinguish the haematoma proper from the secondary one, and on the other hand to replace the term spontaneous haematoma which would imply that the haematoma occurs by itself, without any cause. The truth is that no disease can occur without aetiology and although no definite aetiology is known in primary intracerebral haematoma the term spontaneous, used so far for this disease with multiple predisposing causes, is undoubtedly wrong.

Some authors have put forward the idea that some transitional forms might exist between primary haematoma and cerebral haemorrhage, which would imply that these two processes are two stages of one and the same disease (Pilcher 1941; Fasano and Broggie 1956; Pecker 1957). We do not agree with this view because of the morbid anatomical appearance of the lesion. Pathological and clinical findings in our cases have shown that cerebral haemorrhages exist with mild alterations of vegetative functions, associated with neurological signs and that both the vegetative and the neurological signs may worsen within a variable time interval – from hours to days. On necropsy, apart from a haemorrhage in the basal nuclei with or without ventricular haemorrhage, a large haematoma was found in the white matter (Figs. 8, 9). In these cases, cerebral haemorrhage became associated with an intracerebral haematoma rather than developing into it as the above-quoted authors maintain. Certainly, if the patient's general state is not much impaired, though with neurological signs, operation for removal of haematoma may be performed. In these cases angiography, and particularly the CT, show at the onset a cerebral haemorrhage, but later after deterioration, repetition of these examinations will also reveal a haematoma.

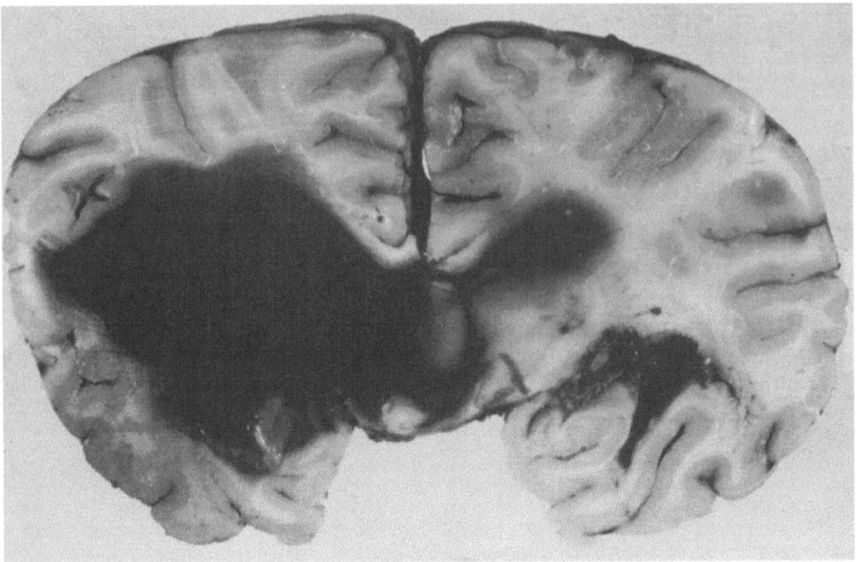

Fig. 8. Haematoma of basal ganglia, white matter and the ventricles

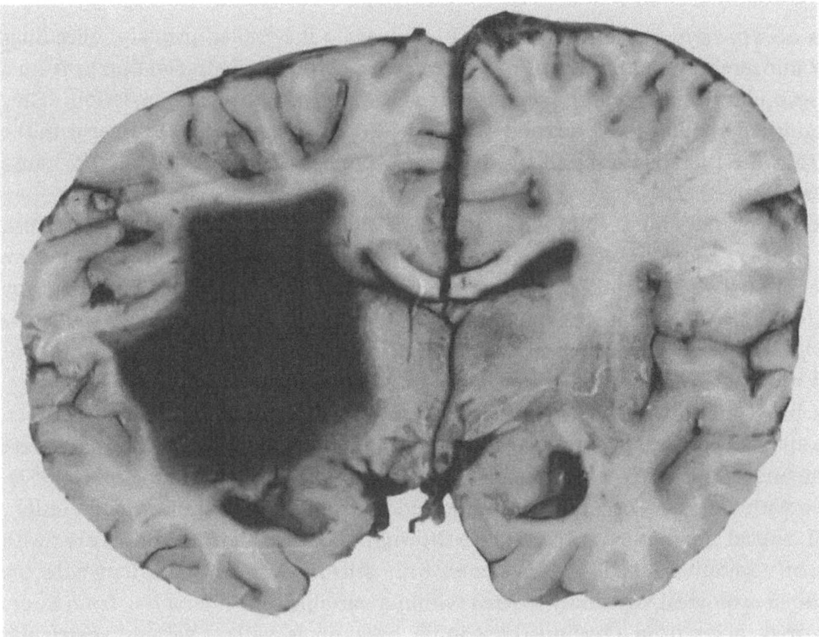

Fig. 9. Small haemorrhage of the basal ganglia with large haematoma in the white matter. Surgical intervention indicated

Aetiology of Primary Intraparenchymatous Haematoma

The clinical and laboratory examinations could establish the cause in 60% – 70% of cases with hemisphere haematoma and in 10% – 20% of those with cerebellar or brain stem haematoma. The percentage of cases of haematoma of obscure origin is still very high.

What is certain is that several aetiological factors – determinant, predisposing or occasional and precipitating – are incriminated in the origin of haematoma. The cause determining primary haematoma is vascular fragility. This can be congenital (vascular aplasia) or acquired. However high the arterial blood pressure, it cannot break a structurally normal vessel. The acquired vascular fragility may come from any cause (traumatic, toxic, infectious, degenerative or endocrinal).

Predisposing causes are the high or low arterial blood pressure, increased tension in the pulmonary circulation (mitral stenosis), meteorological factors, blood dyscrasia and iatrogenic haemorrhagic syndrome. High arterial blood pressure determines lesions in the vessels. According to Zülch (1971), arterial hypertension produces arteriosclerosis in the proximal segment and hyalinosis in the distal segment of the lenticulostriate artery. With the patient's aging the proximal segment becomes dilated and sinuous (tortuous). Persistence of arterial hypertension results in progressive narrowing and occlusion of distal small branches with consequent increase of blood pressure in the proximal segment; the thin walls break and a haemorrhage occurs in the proximal segment. High arterial blood pressure in the benign form may produce rupture of muscle fibres in the vessels and consequently, rupture of vessels. In malignant hypertension a process of necrosis occurs. Arterial hypertension may produce alterations of the elastica, lesions of the intima and of the adventitia. Among the eliciting causes, we would mention paroxysmal arterial hypertension and also physical or intellectual strain.

Frequently, several factors are associated. Among the cases in which predisposing factors were identified, we found two and three factors in 85% and 11% of patients, respectively.

Clinical Picture

In the literature (David and Hecaen 1945; Guillaume and Joinville 1945; Paillas et al. 1952; Lazorthes 1956; Petrovici 1960), intraparenchymatous haematoma is described clinically under four headings: classical (in two stages), "ingravescent apoplexy", pseudo-tumoural and stagnant.

In our opinion the above classification is inappropriate. In fact, any of the above forms may be acute, subacute or chronic, which is of great importance in making the prognosis; prognosis in the acute form differs from that in the subacute or chronic form.

As the prognosis and even the timing of operation depends on the clinical form of intraparenchymatous haematoma, we have drawn up a classification in the light of our experiences, based on (1) The duration of the disease (acute, subacute or chronic clinical form) and (2) the clinical picture during the course of the disease (hence, variants with symptom-free intervals, with a progressive or a static course).

The results depend on the clinical type. Thus, operation in the acute forms showed poorer results; there were more severely marked neurological sequelae and the postoperative mortality was high (30%). In the subacute forms the mortality was lower (8%), and 70% recovered with slight or no sequelae; in chronic haematoma, they recovered with some deficits, and there was no operative mortality (Table 1).

Table 1. Cerebral haematoma – comparative results

Clinical aspects	Mortality	Cured without sequelae	Minor sequelae	Major sequelae
Acute haematoma	30%	10%	25%	65%
Subacute haematoma	8%	40%	30%	30%
Chronic haematoma	0%	80%	20%	–

8.3.2 Clotting Disorders

8.3.2.1 Indications and Prognosis

E. Grote, Giessen

Any indication for operation is mainly dependent upon the judgement of the surgeon, and is not primarily influenced by the state of clotting. We think that a single intracerebral lobar haematoma due to a clotting disorder should be evacuated, if it is a space-occupying lesion leading to a local or generalized shift. This is particularly true for those patients whose consciousness and neurological state are gradually deteriorating. Eventually some of these will recover with conservative management alone, but in our opinion their rehabilitation will take longer. In most instances there will be a better functional neurological improvement after surgical evacuation. A minor symptomatic haematoma does not require operation and all multiple haematomas, particularly those encountered in thrombocytopaenic conditions, should not be treated surgically.

Almost all coagulation disorders may be controlled immediately. All heparin- and dicumarol-dependent coagulopathies are treated with fresh plasma, concentrated coagulation factors and antidote, respectively. With careful control of haemostasis, operation may be started without delay. It is essential that therapy and substitution of factors are continued until the wound is soundly healed.

There may be troubles in thrombocytopaenic haematomas, which have to be operated on quickly. For technical reasons, substitution of fresh concentrate of thrombocytes takes time. The operation may be postponed. Additional therapy with corticoids may succeed in mobilizing the patient's own thrombocytes within some days.

There are contra-indications in relation to the neurological state and also regarding haemostasis. In our opinion any patient who is already comatose and showing evidence of midbrain compression for more than a few minutes will probably not recover at all in spite of clot evacuation and relief of pressure. The clotting disorders will cause additional small bleeding in the brain stem, particularly in the midbrain, if the latter is compressed or the venous drainage is impaired. We know that these haemorrhages occur in any long-standing midbrain syndrome, but in a coagulation disorder they are numerous and early. Not one patient in this condition could be saved. The haemorrhages are very small, and will not necessarily be demonstrated by computer tomography.

With regard to haemostasis any consumption coagulopathy and any untreated fibrinolysis are contra-indications to operation. First, underlying causes of consumption such as shock, sepsis ect have to be treated. After this, interruption of intravascular clotting by heparin and substitution of coagulation factors are mandatory. Operation has to be postponed until this moment. In this situation, antifibrinolytic drugs have to be used cautiously because fibrinolysis of intravascular clots is of great importance for survival of tissues.

Uncontrolled fibrinolysis of other origin has to be treated in advance. The operative situation with increased fibrinolysis is often disastrous, because after the initial clotting, dissolution will soon lead to a rebleed and formation of a haematoma from many injured vessels. High doses of antifibrinolytic drugs with appropriate control and administration of fibrinogen will clear the situation before operation is undertaken.

Prognosis

All patients with clotting disorders and intracerebral haematomas showing midbrain herniation died, mainly because of secondary bleeding into the brain stem. However, because of the slow progress and tumour-imitating course, many haematomas are recognized and operated upon before such a catastrophe occurs. Their long-term survival and neurological function are dependent upon the extent and location of the evacuated haematoma. In particular, some patients with severe pre-operative hemiplegia demonstrated very adequate restoration of function a few weeks later, mainly because these haematomas tend to produce compression and displacement of brain tissue rather than destruction.

Underlying diseases such as leukaemia, liver cirrhosis and metastatic disease can lead to coagulation deficits and thus determine the patient's fate and terminate life. In these cases, successful operative treatment and intra-operative management of clotting disorders are merely treating a complication of a potentially fatal situation.

8.3.2.2 Haematomas Due to Anticoagulant Treatment

J. Iizuka, Bonn

I am not quite convinced that there are any cases of intracerebral haematoma which are exclusively caused by anticoagulant treatment. According to the haematological tests, all nine patients with intracerebral haematoma had been receiving cumarin at the optimal rate of prothrombin time i.e. 20% – 30% (H. G. Lasch) at the time the haemorrhage occurred. This is why I think anticoagulants must not necessarily be regarded as solely responsible for any intracerebral haematoma. In other words, there is no specific prognosis for an intracerebral haematoma which developed during anticoagulant therapy, because a vascular lesion or vascular hypertension might also possibly contribute to such a condition to some extent.

Apart from the intracerebral haematoma which happened to develop during cumarin therapy, there were nine cases in which the intracerebral haematoma occurred during treatment with heparin. From a prognostic viewpoint, there is a considerable difference between these two groups.

In my own experience and as reported by others the outcome in patients previously treated with cumarin was rather poor, and only two of our nine patients survived after the surgical intervention. On the contrary, the patients who had been receiving heparin showed a much better prognosis. In our series, seven of nine patients recovered fairly well after surgical evacuation of the intracerebral haematoma.

This fact, however, does not necessarily indicate the advantage of heparin over cumarin as an anticoagulant. It may, perhaps, mean different conditions of treatment in the two groups of patients, since heparin was given to inpatients usually by means of injections, while cumarin was given by mouth to outpatients. The prognosis of an the intracerebral haematoma may well depend on the duration of cerebral compression.

It is felt that in outpatients, it usually takes much more time to reach a diagnosis of intracerebral haematoma and to organize surgical treatment than it does in patients who are under close observation in a ward or even in an intensive care unit of a hospital.

As was stressed by Prof. John Gillingham, the timing of operation is one of the most important factors for a favourable outcome in all cases of intracerebral haematoma, but in particular in those patients with intracerebral haematoma following or during anticoagulant therapy. In conclusion, I am sorry not to have more cases to allow me to give a clear-cut idea of the prognosis. I am, however, not all that unhappy to report so few cases in view of the clear evidence that the use of anticoagulants has significantly reduced the mortality from vascular thrombosis and its complications.

8.3.3 Traumatic ICH

8.3.3.1 Comparative Study of the Results in Spontaneous and Traumatic ICH

A. Karimi-Nejad and E. Hamel, Cologne

The early and late results of 104 surgically treated spontaneous intracerebral haematomas have been analysed and compared with the results of 121 operated traumatic haematomas. This study contributes to the question of the early prognosis of spontaneous haematomas and the indications for surgical treatment.

Clinical Material

This study presents the clinical course of 104 patients in whom, before the era of computer tomography, the indication for surgical treatment was determined exclusively by angiography. Forty-seven patients (45%) were known to suffer from hypertension, but only 17 of them had received previous treatment for this.

In 13 patients (12%), coagulopathy is believed to have caused the haemorrhage. In the case of nine of these patients, haemorrhage was caused by previous treatment with anticoagulants. In four patients the primary cause was haemophilia.

In 44 patients (42%) the aetiology of the haematoma remained unknown as angiography showed no trace of either an aneurysm or any micro-angiomas.

Figure 1 shows the age distribution in relation to aetiology of the haematomas. Table 1 relates the location and aetiology of the haematomas.

Ten of the frontal haematomas (three hypertensive, one coagulopathic, six unknown) and 37 of the temporal ones (21 hypertensive, five coagulopathic, 11 unknown) were either primarily deep haematomas or, in the case of a massive haemorrhage, had penetrated into this region.

In 27 mainly temporal cases, the haemorrhage had penetrated into the ventricular system. This happened only in cases of deep frontal haematoma.

To make things clearer the postoperative outcome and late results have been graded as follows:

1) Patients who, later on, showed no neurological and/or psychological deficit and were fit for work;
2) Patients with slight neurological and/or psychological deficit who remained moderately disabled;
3) Patients who remained in need of care; and
4) Patients who died after operation.

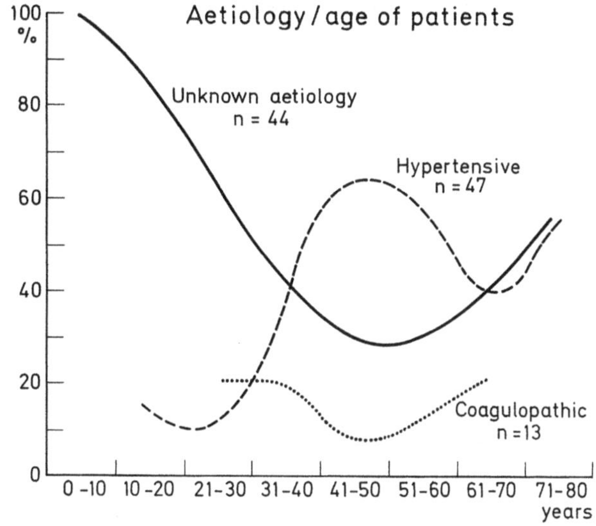

Fig. 1. Age distribution in spontaneous intracerebral haematomas

Table 1. Spontaneous intracerebral haematomas – aetiology and location

	Hypertensive		Coagulopathy		Unknown aetiology		Total	
	No.	%	No.	%	No.	%	No.	%
Frontal	6	24	2	8	17	68	25	24
Temporal	31	56	8	15	16	29	55	53
Parietal	9	47	1	6	9	47	19	18
Occipital	1	1	1	1	2	2	4	4
Posterior fossa	0	0	1	1	0	0	1	1

Results

The postoperative results of 104 patients with spontaneous intracerebral haematomas, grouped according to aetiology of the haematoma, and of 121 traumatic haematomas have been compared (Fig. 2).

In only 16% of the spontaneous and only 7% of the traumatic intracerebral haematomas could complete restoration of deficits and fitness for work be achieved after operation. The mortality in both groups which is as high as 61% is, apart from other factors, mainly due to the fact that in former years indication for an operation was much less restricted, and even patients in deep coma (stages III or IV; cf. Frowein 1978) were operated on. Moreover, before the era of computer tomography, diagnosis was based exclusively on angiography, so that before an operation, neither the depth nor the extent of a haematoma could be verified exactly, as can now be done.

Factors Which Influence the Course of the Condition

With both spontaneous and traumatic intracerebral haematomas the main factor determining their subsequent course proved to be the speed at which clinical symptoms developed and demanded quick diagnosis and subsequent operation. If a haematoma developed within the

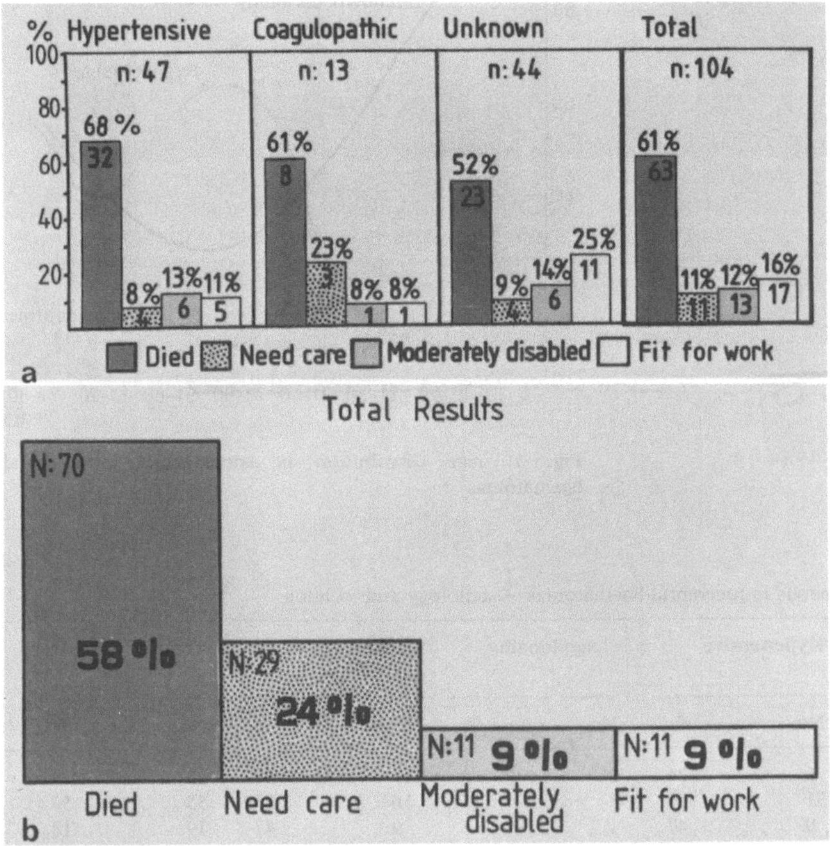

Fig. 2. Outcome and late results in relation to the aetiology of haematoma. **a** spontaneous ICH; **b** Traumatic ICH

first 4 h after trauma or onset, the patients died, irrespective of immediate operation, their age or the aetiology of their haematomas. Results were much better in those cases where clinical symptoms did not develop so very dramatically but more slowly and where the haematoma was verified later on and operated on accordingly.

In Fig. 3 the results obtained with spontaneous and traumatic intracerebral haematomas have been compared according to their speed of development and the timing of operation.

Satisfactory results were only achieved in those cases where spontaneous haematomas were operated on within the 1st and 2nd week after onset. Complete recovery and fitness for work was achieved in 30% or 31%, respectively. With traumatic haematomas, similarly favourable results were obtained only in those cases where a period of 3 weeks had elapsed between trauma and diagnosis of the haematoma with subsequent operation.

Results in Relation to Pre-Operative Impairment of Brain Function

Prognosis was influenced considerably by the pre-operative presence of a general disorder of brain function, i.e. impairment of consciousness. In cases of either spontaneous or traumatic haematomas the mortality reached 84% and 74%, respectively, if the patients were unconscious before the operation. With spontaneous haematomas, however, late results were also rather

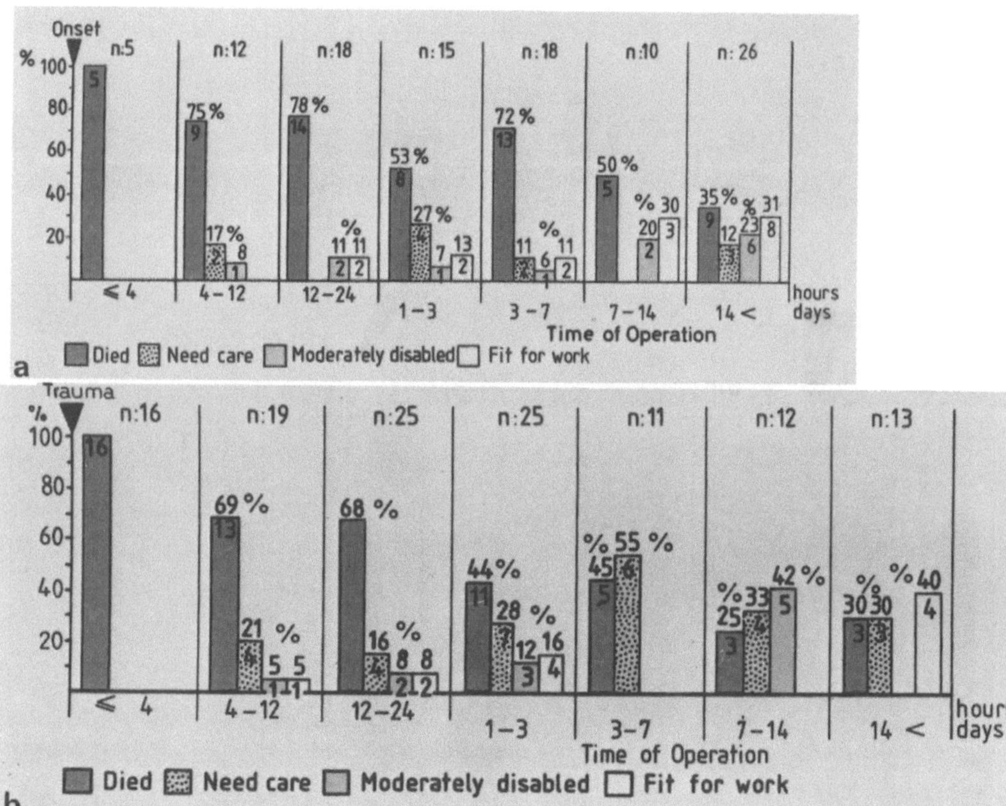

Fig. 3. Outcome and late results of ICH in relation to timing of operation. **a** Spontaneous ICH, **b** Traumatic ICH

bad with patients who had a relatively slight pre-operative impairment of consciousness, either confusion or a clouding of consciousness. Thus, for example, the mortality was 58% in patients with clouding of consciousness and 35% with patients with confusion.

Figure 4 shows the early and late results compared with the pre-operative level of consciousness.

Location

The most favourable postoperative results were obtained with parietal or occipital haematomas of atypical location where the results were satisfactory in 54% (13 of 24 patients), although no type of haemorrhage showed any special frequency (10 hypertensive, 3 coagulopathic and 10 unknown ones). When comparing the frontal and temporal lesions, results were slightly better

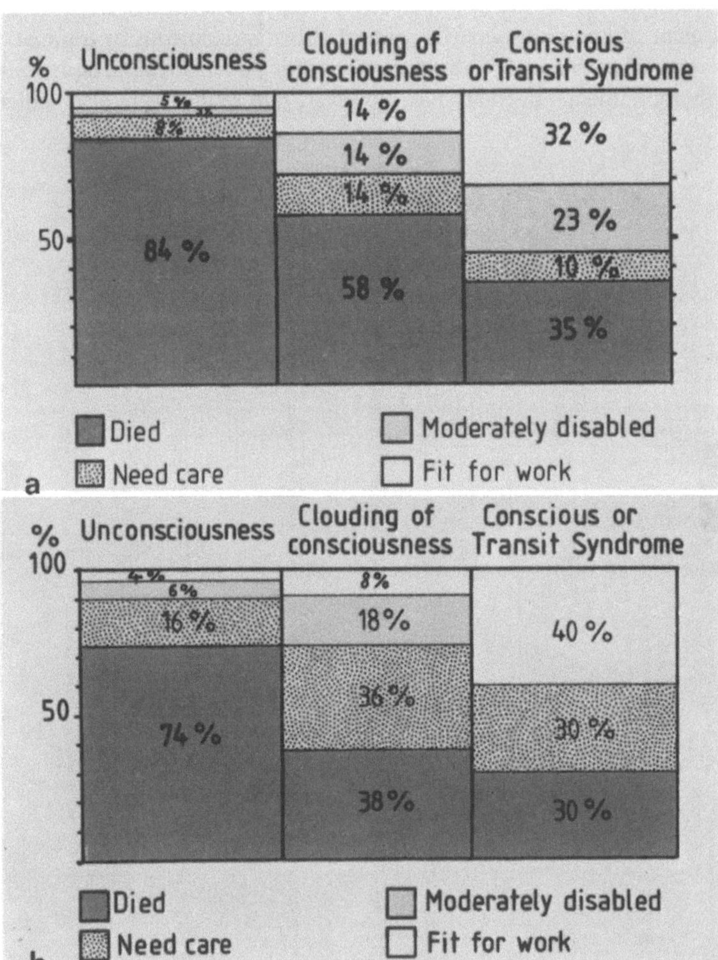

Fig. 4. Results in relation to pre-operative disorders of brain function. **a** Spontaneous ICH, **b** Traumatic ICH

with frontal haematomas, being satisfactory in 28% frontal but only 18% temporal and showing a mortality of 68% frontal but 71% temporal.

The disappointing early and late results with spontaneous intracerebral haematomas cannot be explained only by the pre-operative general disorder of brain function, for even in patients with little or no clouding of consciousness, results with spontaneous haematomas were unsatisfactory (cf. Fig. 4). Investigations to find the reason for these disappointing results revealed that it is the depth of the lesion rather than its actual size which influences the late results. Table 2 compares the results obtained with lobar and deep haematomas in different sites. With deep haematomas, especially temporal ones, the mortality was enormous at 86%, and the late results were also disappointing, so that in practice a recovery up to moderate disability could be achieved in rather less than 10%. Of 27 patients suffering from haematomas with penetration into the ventricular system, 22 (81%) died. The five survivors had frontal haematomas. The disappointing results with spontaneous intracerebral haematomas of medial location are even more striking if one considers the pre-operative general disorder of brain function or state of consciousness of these patients.

Figure 5 relates the results of operation in cases of deep temporal spontaneous intracerebral haematomas (gangliobasal) to the pre-operative general disorder of brain function. Of five patients with reduced brain function, in the sense of confusion without clouding of consciousness, three died. One patient remained disabled. Only in the case of one patient, aged 45, with confusion, severe headache and a brief period of unconsciousness, who was operated on 2 days after onset, recovery up to fitness for work was achieved after an operation on his mediotemporal haematoma. During the 1st year after operation, however, he suffered from

Table 2. Spontaneous intracerebral haematoma – results in relation to location

	Frontal		Temporal		Parietal		
	Lobar	Deep	Lobar	Deep	Lobar	Deep	Other locations
Fit for work	3 (20%)	1 (10%)	7 (39%)	1 (3%)	4 (27%)	0 0	1 (20%)
Moderately disabled	2 (13%)	1 (10%)	2 (11%)	0	5 (33%)	1 (25%)	2 (40%)
Needed care	0 0	1 (10%)	2 (11%)	4 (11%)	3 (20%)	1 (25%)	0 0
Died	10 (67%)	7 (70%)	7 (39%)	32 (86%)	3 (20%)	2 (50%)	2 (40%)

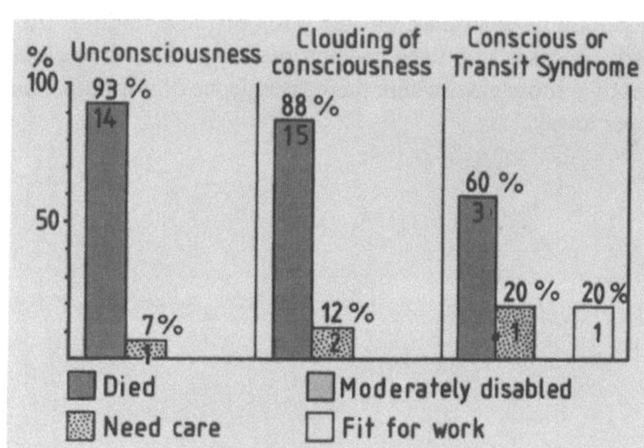

Fig. 5. Results of gangliobasal spontaneous ICH related to general pre-operative state of consciousness

four generalized cerebral seizures, which led to the need for regular anticonvulsant treatment. Of ten patients with clouding of consciousness, eight died and two remained in need of care. Of 15 patients who were unconscious pre-operatively, only one survived, and remained disabled. In comparing the results with the clinical course (decreasing, increasing and constant symptomatology), one finds that of eight patients with pre-operative impaired brain function but with no clouding of consciousness, three died from recurrent haemorrhage after operation.

Conclusion

The results show that operating on deep haematomas, especially temporal and dorsomedial ones with a frontal location, is no longer advisable. This operation seems the more pointless, if pre-operatively there is only a local syndrome as indicated by neurological deficits but no clouding of consciousness which might indicate serious general brain disorders. The indication for an operation could be restricted even more if one excludes those patients who show clinical improvement spontaneously before the operation. If there is persistent unremitting unconsciousness or if acute deterioration occurs in the condition of unconscious patients, surgical treatment might be advisable, as with these patients there is nothing to lose, there is only something to gain.

Summary

The early and late results of 104 patients with spontaneous intracerebral haematomas treated by operation and of 121 patients with traumatic haematomas are reported on and compared. The spontaneous haematomas were due to hypertension, coagulopathies and haemorrhage of unknown aetiology. Haematomas due to angiomas or aneurysms are not included in this report. The inquiry shows that none of these patients survived if a haematoma had developed quickly within the first 4 h after onset or trauma. Quite obviously, the prognosis was influenced considerably by pre-operative disturbances of consciousness. In spontaneous haematomas in patients with or without any significant clouding of consciousness both mortality and late results are very unsatisfactory. These unfavourable results were mainly caused by deep or gangliobasal haematomas. Results that were satisfactory both from the neurological and the social point of view were achieved mainly with parietal or occipital and frontal or temporal lobar patients who were neither hypertensive nor coagulopathic. Prognosis is worse with medial temporal haematomas. On the basis of these findings the operative indication should be very strict in cases with deep haematomas, especially coagulopathic or hypertensive ones, and even more in those cases where there is evidence of a spontaneous improvement in the condition pre-operatively.

8.3.3.2 Indications and Operative Treatment of Traumatic ICH

D. Parkinson, E. G. Newry, and D. Tubman, Winnipeg

The comparison of the non-operative mortality rate of 33% with the operative mortality of 77% gives a misleading impression. The non-operative series includes those so badly injured and those with associated fatal injuries such as ruptured spleen or ruptured aorta that operation was never considered. These mortality figures represent the mortality of patients selected for operation opposed to those not selected and it can just as well indicate that fewer should have been operated upon or that more should have been operated upon.

Indications

The absolute indication for operation is seen in a young individual who is deteriorating after an interval of normality in the presence of a large, superficial, solitary intracerebral haematoma which is behaving as a space-occupying lesion. Conversely a senile patient with continuing coma and multiple small deep haematomas would be an absolute contra-indication to operation. One other absolute contra-indication that will appear more frequently is the intracerebral haematoma as an incidental finding by CT scan (Table 1). Between these three extremes are multiple permutations of the various factors. This emphasizes the need for decisions regarding operation to be made by surgeons rather than by some individual with a set of books and charts. From all the information available at present it appears that the best chance for an optimal survival with a given intracerebral haematoma is obtained by avoiding operation. This presumption is made without knowing two factors. We do not know what proportion of the total volume of a clot is represented by destroyed brain tissue. Does a 30 cc clot represent 30 cc of destroyed brain tissue? We would think not and would estimate that approximately one-third to one-half the volume of the clot represents destroyed tissue and the remaining volume corresponds to compressed, stretched and displaced cerebral tissue. This factor becomes important if decisions to operate are qualified by the concept that additional surgical destruction is insignificant in view of the total destruction already present. The other unknown factor concerns the viability of inactive neurons. We know that large numbers recover function over a period of weeks and even months, but we do not know whether some live neurons fail to recover function or whether viability is jeopardized by the continued presence of the clot or its breakdown products. Should operation be performed to preserve function, short of the point where it is mandatory to preserve life? Without these two factors, i.e. the amount of destroyed tissue associated with any given clot and the viability of nerve tissue after prolonged pressure, one cannot possibly formulate an equation that will be any more helpful and reliable in deciding the advisability and timing of operation. If it appears that the best result is obtained by avoiding operation and its necessary additional brain damage (which is considerable with a deep clot), then the surgeon is for ever between the Scylla of operating unnecessarily and the Charybdis of waiting until the sudden onset of deep coma with its near 100% operative mortality (Tandon and Kristensen 1965). If it can be proved that operation is indicated with a clot greater than a given diameter to preserve function, then the surgeon is relieved of his dilemma. He is in the same relatively comfortable position as when dealing with an extracerebral collection, realizing that he should operate once such a lesion is demonstrated. However, no figures currently available answer these questions. They may be answered in the future with careful CT monitoring of the size, course, resolution or expansion of clots, together with meticulous

Table 1. Absolute indications and contra-indications for operation. The elderly deteriorating patient in continuing coma with small multiple deep lesions represents an absolute contra-indication whereas the young individual slowly deteriorating after a lucid interval, with a large, single, superficially located, intracerebral haematoma behaving as a space-occupying lesion represents an absolute indication for operation. Another absolute contra-indication at the present time is the incidental finding on a CT scan

No	Operation	Yes
Elderly	Age	Young
Deteriorating	Course	Deteriorating slowly
Continuing coma	Interval	Lucid
Small, multiple, deep	Haematoma	Large, single, superficial
Incidental finding		

clinical observations and a follow-up (Ransohoff and Randt 1965) of large numbers with particular attention to the function referrable to the clots location. There are no silent areas in the brain, but only areas whose function we are unable to demonstrate.

Some further factors require consideration. On occasions the surgeon removes an extracerebral clot and finds beneath it an unsuspected but contiguous intracerebral clot which may deliver itself almost like an afterbirth. On such occasions the surgeon never feels that his original indication for operation was any less because he also encountered an intracerebral clot. If we recognize the inherent differences between traumatic and spontaneous cases we also have the additional evidence of Pia's pioneering breakthrough, where he pointed out that the spontaneous intracerebral haemorrhages even when massive and filling ventricles could and should be operated upon with a rather striking recovery rate (Pia 1959, 1968). McLaurin and McBride (1956) demonstrated a significant recovery rate operating on patients with traumatic intracerebral clots and persistent coma.

We recognize that operation itself carries a mortality rate over and above that of the surgical problem. If it is performed we agree with the principles that a sufficient opening must be made to enucleate the clot either with finger or spoon, irrigate the bed and control the oozing (McLaurin and McBride 1956; Botterell 1958; Pia 1959, 1968; Stender and Schulze 1965). It is not infrequent for such cavities to refill with clot by the time the wound is closed. The decision to use a drain is up to the individual surgeon, but we must recall Cushing's statement that a drain never prevents the formation of a clot but will merely give another clue that it is forming. It is only rarely, and never in our series, that a clot will run out through a brain cannula. Intracerebral endoscopy is not developed to the level where it can deal with these satisfactorily. Conservative management in our centre includes the honouring of standard neurosurgical precepts, judicious use of dehydrating agents and spinal fluid drainage, careful pressure monitoring, while following the mass effect with the CT scan and recognizing that the clot may become isodense. We have no evidence that steroids are helpful and we do not use hypothermia.

Summary

Apart from the absolute indications for operation, which in our centre include evidence of a progressive lesion in any individual with no contra-indications for operation, it seems possible that we should be more aggressive in attacking more of those cases in the doubtful group. We must not be afraid of an increased operative mortality if it means decreasing the overall mortality. Should figures ever become available to indicate that operation is indicated to preserve function, short of the point where it becomes mandatory to preserve life, then the surgeon will be relieved of the dilemma presented so far by these traumatic intracerebral haematomas. However, we must avoid drawing conclusions without supporting figures. The scan will artificially reduce mortality by picking up smaller lesions, but it will be of tremendous help to the surgeon in showing the size, progress and exact location, including the area closest to the surface.

8.3.3.3 Prognosis in Traumatic ICH

D. Parkinson, E. G. Newry, and M. West, Winnipeg

Prognosis is determined largely by factors beyond the surgeons control, by the nature of the injury, and to a lesser degree by the patient's age, coexisting disease and delay in arriving at a neurosurgical centre (Donaghy et al. 1965; Gurdjian and Thomas 1965; Sano 1965; Tandon and Kristensen 1965). The prognosis for survival is fairly constant in the various series. In our own, the overall mortality is 64%; our operative mortality was 33%. The non-operative mortality was 78%, but nearly one-fifth of these patients died in less than 12 h, many with severe associated damage including ruptured liver, ruptured aorta, crushed chest, etc., and these might be deleted from the figures. The non-operative mortality will become progressively lower as more incidental haematomas are added to the figures by the increasingly routine use of the CT scan. The difference between operative and non-operative mortality does not mean that more should be operated on any more than it might mean that fewer should be operated on. It merely reflects the selection of cases for operation excluding the most severely damaged. While mortality is reported as increasing by each decade (Voris 1945; Devet 1965; Gurdjian and Thomas 1965), age in our series had no statistical significance on the prognosis. The site of the lesions had an enormous influence on the outcome (Table 1), with 15% of patients with temporal lobe lesions dying, 56% of those with frontal lobe lesions, 66% with ventricular haemorrhages, and 100% of those with cerebellar haemorrhages. Another factor of great prognostic value is the association of basal fractures in whom 17 of 18 patients died (Fig. 1) (Chi square = 15.03; $p >$ .001). The association of fractures in all locations by decades is shown in Fig. 2 for the intracerebral haematomas. The overall mortality at our centre for basal fractures including those with intracerebral haematomas is 8%. The tremendous mortality with the association of basal fracture and intracerebral haematoma is not really a summation of the mortality rate of the two conditions but more probably a factor of the responsible forces producing this combination of lesions.

Table 1. Mortality and location of haemorrhage in 70 intracerebral traumatic haematomas. The total is greater than 70 as combined sites are included under the bottom column of "other"

Site	Total	Deaths	%
Temporal	34	5	15
Frontal	16	9	56
Cerebellar	10	10	100
Ventricular	12	8	66
Other	10	5	50

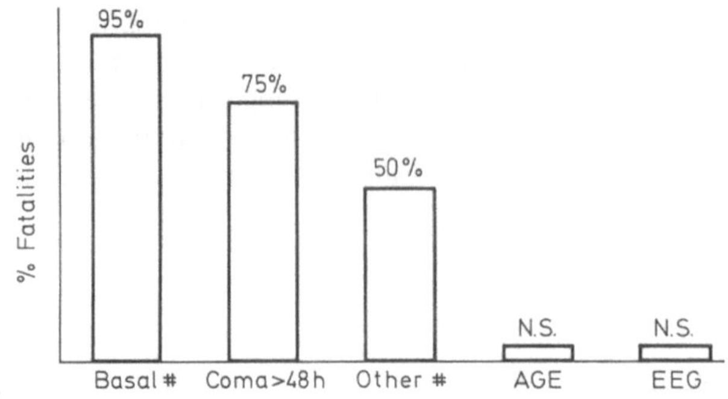

Fig. 1. High mortality rate associated with basal fractures as opposed to the mortality with associated fractures, in general, which is no more than 50%. Age does not appear statistically significant, nor does an EEG abnormality

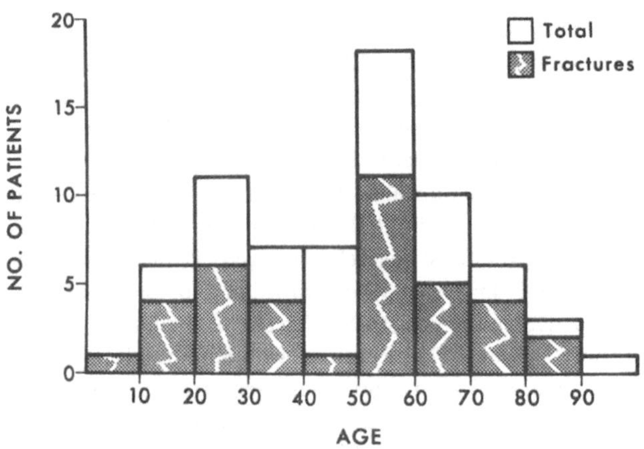

Fig. 2. Distribution by decade of associated fractures of all types including basal fractures

There were associated extracerebral collections in 27 patients; 16 of these were moribund and were never considered for operation. The other ten all survived after removal of both the extra- and intracerebral collections. It is thus evident that a combination of basal fracture with profound and continuing coma all carry a very poor prognosis. The poor prognosis with the frontal and, in particular, the cerebellar haemorrhages may represent less than adequate recognition and treatment on our part. Although the use of alcohol featured prominently in the aetiology, we have no statistical evidence that it influenced prognosis.

The quality of survival is not available from any of the published series apart from McLaurin's (1956) report in which 9 of the 14 followed were symptom-free. A high proportion of our patients were in a socio-economic category that required few or none of the higher intellectual and cognitive functions to return to their usual activities and quite possibly neither the patient nor the examiner would recognize some deficits. There are no truly silent areas in the brain, only areas whose function we cannot demonstrate (Fig. 3). Although seizures would seem a likely complication (Jennet 1975), none of McLaurin's (1956) had seizures as did none of ours. We would agree with Walker's (1957, 1960) observation that neither abnormal EEGs nor

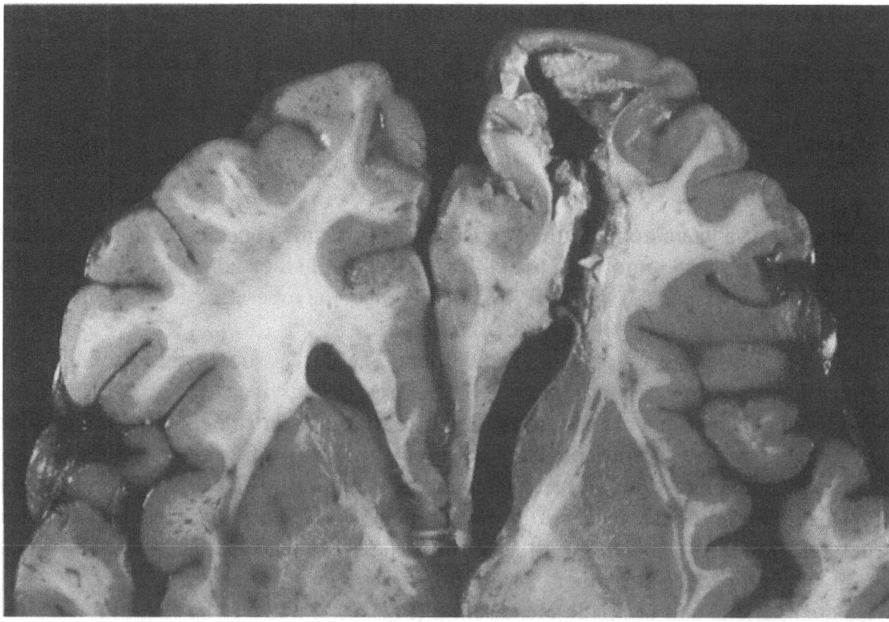

Fig. 3. Autopsy specimen of individual who died of a second head injury many months after recovering from a frontal lobe intracerebral haematoma. This individual was considered to have made a complete recovery by himself, his friends and employers and the attending medical staff. This indicates the extent of damage that may exist in a so-called silent area

the occurrence of a few seizures after the accident mean the patient is going to be a life-long sufferer from seizures. We have no information that a better survival is obtained by removing a haematoma that is not life-threatening. Reliable information may eventually be available with CT scan, by monitoring changes in clot size along with careful detailed follow-up studies of a large series, searching in particular for neurological deficits referrable to the lesion site (Ransohoff and Randt 1965). If we report that an individual is symptom-free after recovering from a 150 cc intracerebral clot, it merely reflects our inability to recognize the deficit. In the absence of such data we must be very cautious not to allow a few scattered opinions to assume the mantle of dogma as they are published repeatedly.

Beyond honouring the standard neurosurgical techniques it is evident from our overall head injury study that the most significant factor under our control which influences prognosis is the behavior of the physician and the attending staff from the moment the patient arrives; this includes contact with the relatives. If the attitude of all concerned is that with recovery the patient is best up and about and doing his usual work the patient is left with a vastly different life-long attitude than if the physician prolongs bed rest and warms that the patient must "take it easy" after going home, awaiting for we know not what. Such an attitude leaves the patient with the impression that something might happen inside his head if he uses it too much, an attitude that can be anything but helpful in his recovery and usefulness. The most effective therapy is a return to his usual activities.

8.4 Location – Indications and Prognosis

8.4.1 Haematomas in Hemispheric Lobes

J. Zierski, Giessen

The location of a haematoma in the hemisphere is generally considered as the most favourable for permitting surgical removal of the clot with acceptable mortality and morbidity. There are, however, many associated factors which influence the operative indications. The Giessen material of 103 cases form the basis of this report.

The site and extension of the haematoma (Table 1) shows that isolated monolobar haematomas have the best prognosis. Of 23 cases, 16 survived. However, the fact that the haematoma occupies one or more lobes seems to play a lesser role than the involvement of the basal ganglia and the rupture into the ventricles. Of 53 patients with monolobar haematomas, 26 died while among 49 multilobar haematomas, there were 28 deaths. The mortality rate was much higher in those cases in which the haematoma involved also the capsular and paracapsular structures. Among 45 patients with subcortical haematomas, 17 died and of 57 haematomas also involving the deep structures, 38 did not survive.

Isolated parietal and occipital haematomas (Figs. 1, 2) had a more favourable outcome than temporal and frontal ones (Figs. 3, 4), although one has to take into account that they produced much less displacement of major vessels and that none of the patients belonging to this group was in coma or in a decerebrate condition at the time of operation, which is in sharp contrast to the group of frontal and temporal haematomas. In the first group the operative indication is debatable. The functional defect will not be influenced by evacuation of the clot. On the other hand these are the most easily accessible haematomas. In case 3 the marked compression and shifting of the hemisphere due to the surrounding oedema demands the evacuation in spite of the smallness of the haematoma. Huge haematomas (case 4) have always been evacuated.

There was no direct relationship between the volume of haematoma and mortality. For reasons which we still are not able to determine, the degree of oedema surrounding the haematoma is very variable and can contribute decisively to the amount of shift produced.

Table 1. Haematomas in hemispheric lobes and basal ganglia [a]

Site	Survived	Died	Total
Subcortical			
Monolobar	16	7	23
Multilobar	12	10	22
Total	28	17	45
Capsular, paracapsular and with ventricular rupture			
Monolobar	10	20	30
Multilobar	9	18	27
Total	19	38	57

[a] Neurosurgical University Clinic, Giessen; 1956 – 1977

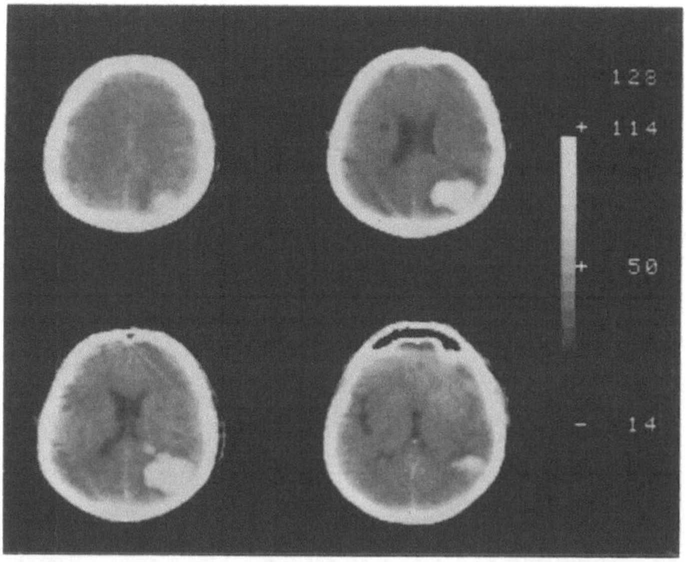

Fig. 1. Occipital haematoma with slight oedema without major displacement. The bleeding occupies the occipital horn, but has not spread into the whole ventricle

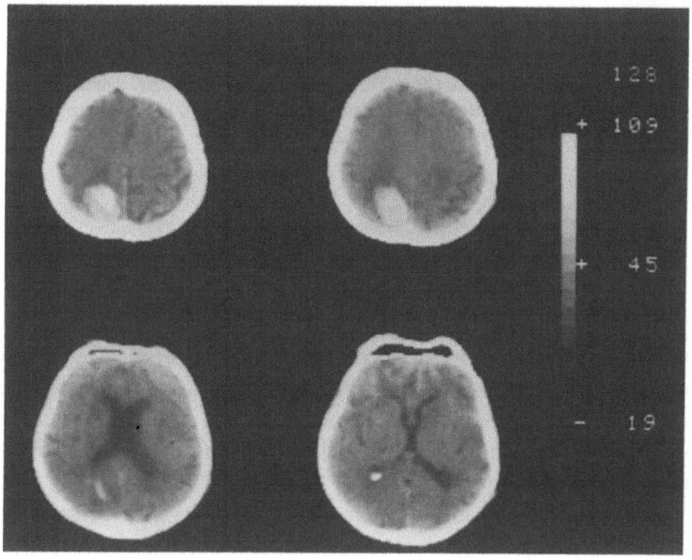

Fig. 2. A similar case of an occipital haematoma with no displacement and only slight oedema

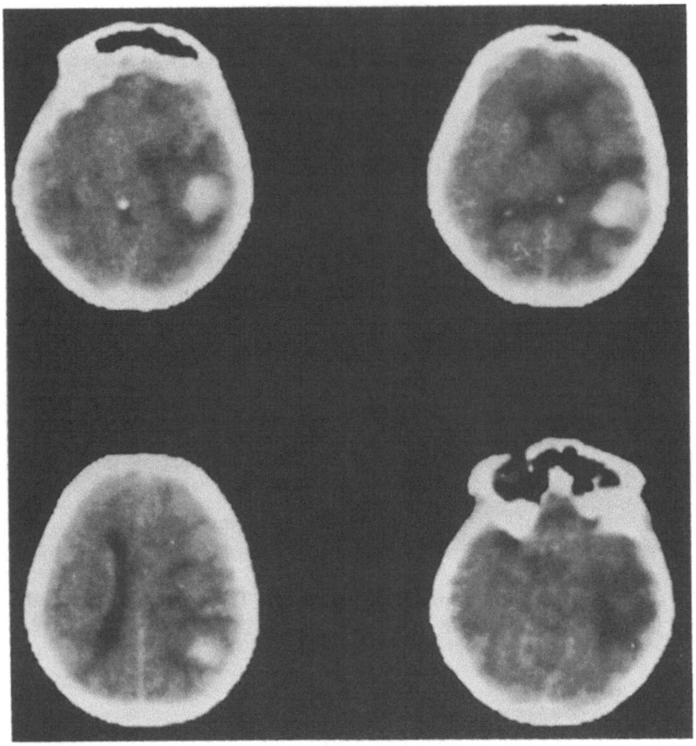

Fig. 3. A case of a haematoma of lesser volume than the previous ones, but with considerably more surrounding oedema which is spreading from the parietal to the temporal region and causing considerable compression and shift of the ventricular system

No great differences between monolobar and multilobar haematomas were found as far as the timing of operation is considered (Table 2). Monolobar haematomas seem to do slightly better than multilobar when operated after the 1st week. The inverse mortality for haematomas operated between 1 and 3 days after ictus remains unexplained. Generally better survival rates for patients not operated on immediately do not allow a true correlation, because in the majority of them the level of consciousness was much better than in those patients who were operated on within the first 24 h.

As have all other authors, we have found the level of consciousness at the time of operation as the most important single factor influencing mortality (Table 3). There will always be exceptional cases surviving the decerebrate state at the time of operation. Patients who are drowsy or fully alert at the time of operation have the best chances of survival; the fact that the haematoma is monolobar or multilobar is less important.

On comparing the change of the level of consciousness between the onset of the haematoma and the time of operation, we found that the operation proved to be life-saving in less than one-quarter of 30 patients deteriorating into the stage of coma, with unpurposeful reaction to pain or decerebration (Table 4).

As expected there was a definite correlation between increasing age and mortality rate both for monolobar and multilobar haematomas.

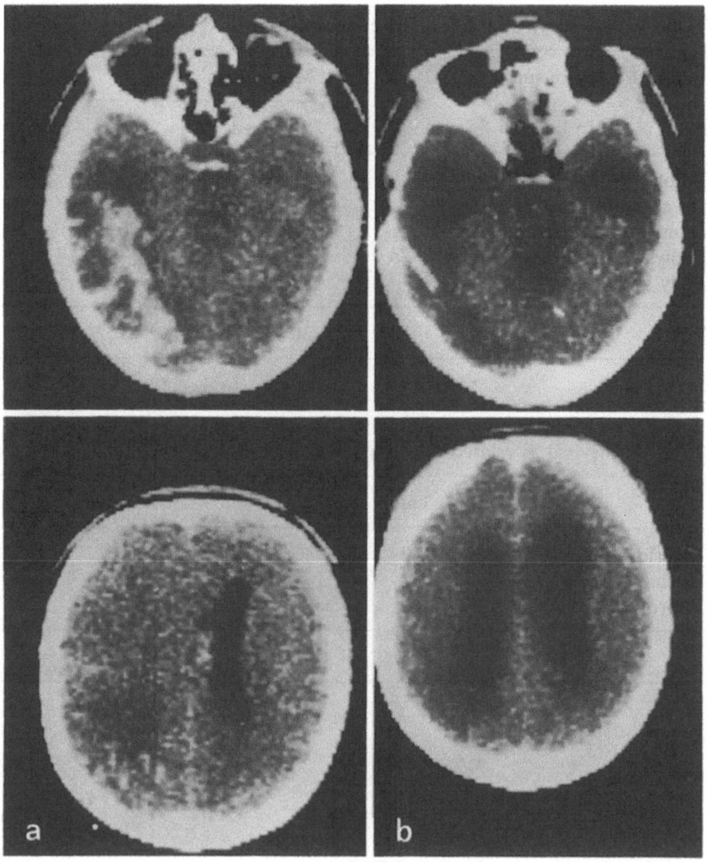

Fig. 4a, b. Huge paraventricular haematoma extending temporally, before **a** and after **b** evacuation of the clot. Note the enlargement of the ventricular system

Table 2. Site, survival and timing of operation

Interval between ictus and operation	Monolobar		Multilobar	
	Survived	Died	Survived	Died
1 – 6 h	1	2	1	6
6 – 24 h	2	10	3	11
1 – 3 days	1	6	5	1
3 – 7 days	3	1	3	2
1 – 2 weeks	7	4	3	4
2 weeks – 1 month	12	4	6	4
Total	26	27	21	28

Table 3. Site, survival and level of consciousness

Level of consciousness	Monolobar		Multilobar	
	Survived	Died	Survived	Died
Bulbar	1	1	0	2
Decerebrate	1	11	3	15
Coma without decerebration	1	6	2	3
Drowsy	15	7	12	5
Fully alert	8	2	4	3
Total	26	27	21	28

Table 4. Survival as related to change in consciousness level between ictus and operation

	Total	Survived	Died
Deterioration	30	7	23
Unchanged	67	34	33
Improved	6	5	1
	103	46	57

8.4.2 Intraventricular ICH

8.4.2.1 Surgical Treatment

F. Loew and H. Jaksche, Homburg

For diagnostic, therapeutic and also prognostic reasons, it is important to follow the classification of intraventricular haemorrhages, which was proposed by Pia in 1968. He distinguishes three forms: haematocephalus totalis, i.e. haematomas of the whole ventricular system, haematocephalus partialis which occurs when blood clot fills only circumscribed portions of the ventricular system, and intraventricular haemorrhage without real haematoma. The last-mentioned form is not a space-occupying lesion. Its therapy is not concentrated upon the blood in the ventricular CSF, but upon the source of the bleeding. Fig. 1 gives an example. The angiogram has demonstrated the rupture of an aneurysm, originating from the carotid bifurcation, into the lateral ventricle with subsequent "transarterial" ventriculography. In spite of the acute intraventricular bleeding the patient was relatively well, grade II – III, and it was possible to clip the aneurysm during the acute stage with a good result. Similar situations may occur after rupture of angiomas of the choroid plexus or the ventricular wall. If such a haemorrhage stops spontaneously without producing a space-occupying haematoma, it can be treated conservatively until the situation becomes stable and only then should operation upon the underlying pathology be done.

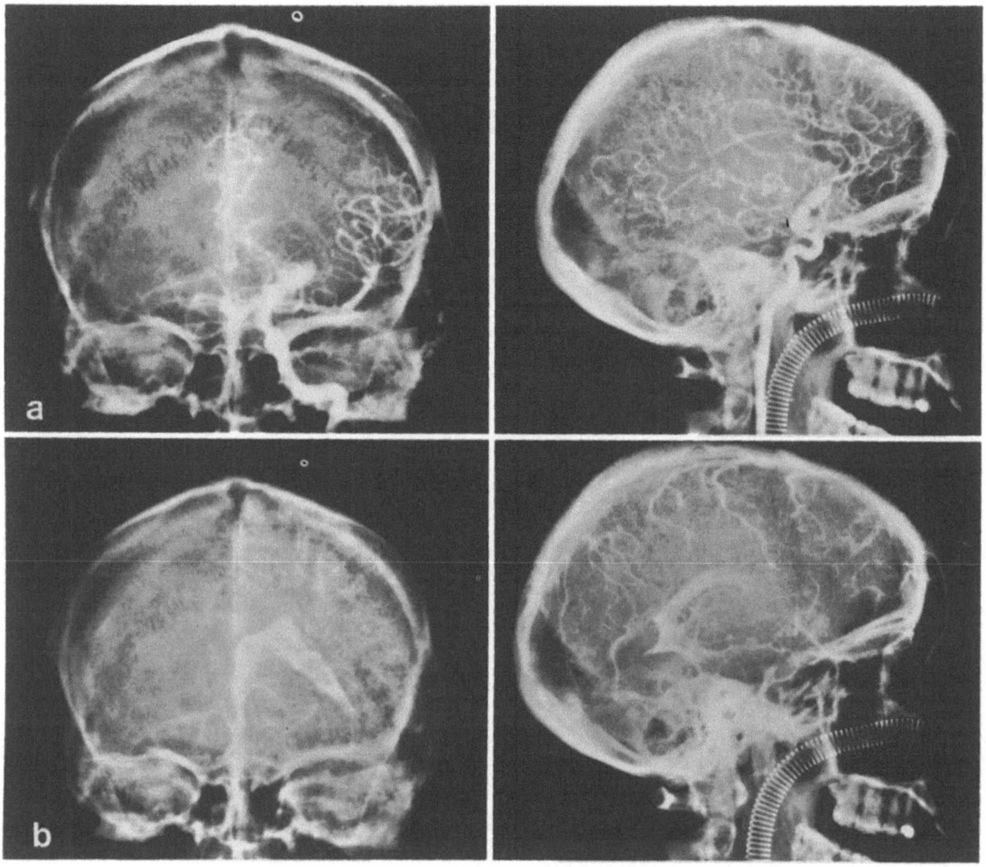

Fig. 1a, b. Angiogram of ruptured aneurysm of the carotid bifurcation. **a** Arterial phase. **b** Venous phase. Note the filling of the ventricle with the contrast medium injected into two carotid arteries

Real haematomas of the ventricular system may occur not only from such angioma bleedings but also from primary intraparenchymal haemorrhages, which only secondarily perforate into the ventricular system. These act locally as space-occupying lesions and furthermore produce a tamponade of the CSF pathways with enlargement of the ventricles and generally raised intracranial pressure. In such cases, besides the evacuation of a local space-occupying clot, it has proved useful in our experience to perform external CSF drainages of both lateral ventricles. It is well known (Little et al. 1977) that such drains tend to be clogged. We therefore irrigate the ventricles for several days and in this way have been able to avoid a clogging of the external drainage system. The drainage should be continued until CSF resorption has returned to normal, which means mostly for 1 to several weeks.

Another example is shown in Fig. 2. The patient was in deep coma with decerebrate rigidity and inadequate respiration. We immediately performed ventricular drainage and irrigation, artificial respiration for more than 1 week, temperature control and all other intensive therapy and during this stage the patient was delivered of a healthy child in the neurosurgical intensive care unit. After several weeks of CSF drainage the patient regained consciousness. Morphologically, a slight ventricular dilatation remained (Fig. 3). The patient is now able to do her housework with only minor to medium impairment of initiative and activity.

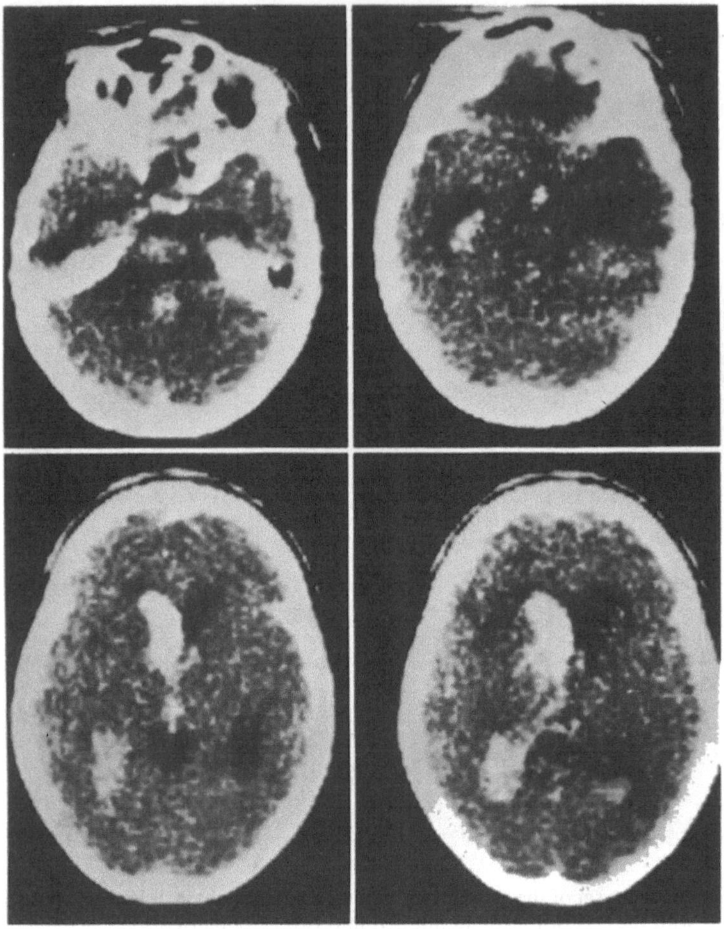

Fig. 2. Intraventricular haemorrhage. Blood clot in the lateral, third and fourth ventricles

Before the introduction of long-term ventricular drainage and irrigation therapy, all patients with haematocephalus totalis died. The same is true in the series of other authors (Janny et al. 1966; Pia 1972; Little et al. 1977). After introducing this treatment, three of five such patients survived.

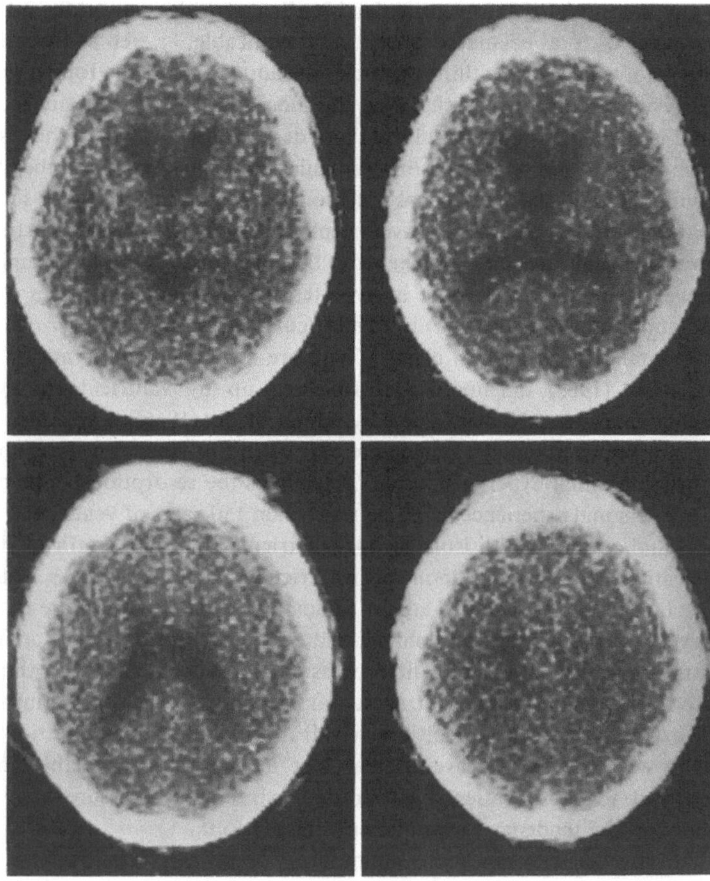

Fig. 3. The same patient as in Fig. 2. Slightly dilated ventricular system several weeks after haemorrhage and drainage

8.4.2.2 Location, Indication and Prognosis

H. W. Pia, Giessen

Indication and contra-indication for operative treatment of intraventricular bleeding have been discussed from different points of view and with conflicting results. The main reason has been the inadequacy of diagnosis and the lack of true criteria to establish the course of the natural history as well as the effect of operative procedures. This has been changed fundamentally by the CT scan.

My present statement has to be regarded therefore as an historical one. I believe, however, that the clinical findings, symptoms and signs will remain the fundamental basis for deciding the best method for treating ICH associated with intraventricular bleeding and especially isolated ones.

The prognosis of intraventricular bleeding provides important information (Table 1). The prognosis of total haematocephaly is unfavourable, as well as that of partial haematocephaly with involvement of the third ventricle, the aqueduct and the fourth ventricle. All patients died, nearly all spontaneously within 24 h and those few treated by drainage, during the 1st week. The onset is acute with coma, local signs and decerebration – often the result of associated pontine haemorrhages and severe central dysregulation, as has been described by Sanders (1881). In the group of partial haematocephaly of the lateral ventricle, 14 of 25 survived. The outcome was favourable in the group of intraventricular haemorrhage; it is nearly the same as in ICH without intraventricular bleeding. In general the prognosis is best in angiomatous haemorrhages. However, we should say that in hypertensive bleeding some cases of partial haematocephaly and about half of those with intraventricular haemorrhage survived.

Spontaneous remissions occur. There are instructive observations as in a case of Ojemann and New (1963) diagnosed and followed up by ventriculography, or in cases of open haematomas already mentioned by Janny et al. (1966). They wrote, "Here the ventricular rupture brings about the immediate and definitive cessation of all the phenomena associated with intracranial hypertension and accelerates the resorption of the haemorrhage."

My personal experience based on more than 150 cases of ventricular bleeding, associated with ICH and about 20 with isolated intraventricular bleeding confirms that in general there is no indication for operating upon intraventricular haemorrhage. As I have previously described, the choroid plexus seems to adhere almost immediately to the site of rupture into the ventricle preventing dangerous tamponade and, at the same time, it permits washing-out of the extraventricular blood clot. The process of spontaneous healing is thus accelerated and is more effective. In many cases of intracerebral haematomas the rupture into the ventricle seems to be the explanation of the patient's survival. It remains an open question whether it is necessary at all to evacuate the extraventricular clot in such cases, whether the evacuation should be confined to those patients with raised intracranial pressure and whether it facilitates or improves the tendency to spontaneous resolution.

Another question is whether a temporary open ventricular drainage should be set up to lower the raised intracranial pressure and at the same time to diminish the meningeal reaction and prevent the development of hydrocephalus. My personal experience is limited and does not allow one to give any clear guidance about this.

In the group of partial haematocephaly with tamponade of the lateral ventricle, spontaneous resolution of the clot has been observed by many authors as well as in our own cases. However, we have proved the life-saving effect of the acute removal and rinsing-out of the intracerebral and intraventricular clot. In 1968 I reported on 16 patients who had been operated upon, nine on the day of the haemorrhage and seven on the day after. Eight patients survived and six

Table 1. Intraventricular bleeding

	Hypertension		Aneurysms		Angiomas		Total[a]	
	N	†	N	†	N	†	N	†
Haematocephalus totalis	8	8	9	9	8	8	32	32
Haematocephalus partialis	9	5	4	2	9	2	25	11
Haemorrhagia intraventricularis	23	11	2	2	35	4	68	19
Total	24	12	32	16	33	6	119	47

[a] Including other groups

became symptom-free. Of these, only two were the result of hypertension, the rest being caused by angiomas or other unknown vascular pathology.

My present strategy is determined by the clinical signs and progress. Space-occupying haematomas with signs of local damage which are progressive, manifest, or not decreasing and with a general increase of intracranial pressure should be operated upon. There is an absolute emergency indication in haematomas caused by angiomas, whereas with the typical hypertensive haematomas I became less and less active and almost completely abandoned any procedure in the acute stage. Patients in coma and with decompensation of central regulation, associated with complete haematocephaly, do not have any chance of surviving. This is an absolute contra-indication to operation.

Solitary intraventricular localized haematomas should be treated, starting with open drainage and followed in angiomatous cases by evacuation with extirpation of the angioma at the same stage. I do not know if there is any indication in hypertensive cases, if those cases arise at all; I would try at least to rinse out the intraventricular blood by a temporary catheter.

In summary, intraventricular haemorrhage does not require any active procedures; its existence means facilitation of the spontaneous resorption of a haematoma in the basal ganglia. In cases of partial tamponade of a lateral ventricle with raised intracranial pressure the evacuation of both the extra- and intraventricular clot is indicated. Isolated intraventricular clots should be washed out. In total haematocephaly, there is no indication for operative treatment. Ventricular drainage should be performed and has proved effective in several cases.

8.4.2.3 CT Scan and Treatment

W. J. Stendel, E. Schneider and H. Becker, Frankfurt

Since the introduction of computer tomography (CT), intraventricular haemorrhages can be more easily demonstrated in patients and the clinical course related to the extent and location of the bleeding (Steiner et al. 1975; Steudel et al. 1979). The present study describes the prognosis in relation to the extent and location of intraventricular haemorrhages in 90 cases.

Patients and Methods

In 11 000 CT-examinations 90 patients with intraventricular bleeding of varying aetiology were found. The aetiology, the age and the outcome is shown in Table 1.

The level of consciousness was classified into five categories (modified from Hunt 1968): grade 1 (no disturbance); grade 2 (the patient can be aroused to a normal level of awareness from somnolence); grade 3 (stupor – the patient may be aroused to some extent but cannot reach or sustain a normal level of consciousness); grade 4 (coma – the patient cannot be aroused even by painful stimuli); grade 5 (deep coma – no longer any reaction to painful stimuli, dilated pupils, areflexia).

The CT was first performed with the Siretom prototype (matrix 80 × 80, 4000 examinations) and later with the Siretom I (matrix 128 × 128, 7000) in the period from 1974 to 1978.

Table 1. Intraventricular haemorrhage

Aetiology	N	Age Median	Interval from first symptom to death (days) Median (Range)	Surviving patients
Trauma	26	40	7 (1 – 52)	6
Aneurysm	17	42	27 (1 – 155)	2
Angioma	3	28	(1.5)	1
Tumour	4	53	6 (3 – 7)	–
Hypertension	21	51	2 (1 – 4)	7
Haemorrhagic disorders	7	45	(1.9)	5
Unknown	12	50	7 (1 – 25)	2

The CT-findings were classified into three categories (according to Pia 1972): a mixture of cerebro-spinal fluid (CSF) and blood clot which can either partially or totally fill the ventricles.

Results

CT Findings. Clotted blood and CSF-blood mixture can be distinguished by the CT. Freshly clotted blood is shown with density values from +40 to 80 units in the Siretom. Density values of +20 to +40 units are recorded for the CSF-blood mixture. The CSF-blood mixture discernible in the CT scan is frequently found in the occipital horns because of the supine position of the patient during the examination and it displays a surface reflection. We have not so far been able to detect CSF-blood mixture below the specified density values.

Hypertensive Haemorrhages. Of 21 patients with known hypertension four had no disturbances of consciousness or somnolence or stupor (Table 2). Seventeen patients were comatose; eight of these were in deep coma. Three of the four patients who were not comatose showed a tiny haemorrhage in one part of the ventricular system and survived.

Table 2. Hypertension (N = 21)

Level of consciousness	CT findings		
	CSF blood mixture	Clotted blood	
		Partial	Total
I (Normal)		● ●	
II (Somnolence)	● [a]		
III (Stupor)		●	
IV (Coma)	○	● ● ● ○ ○	○ ○
V (Deep coma)	○	○ ○ ○ ○ ○ ○ ○ ○	○

[a] ●, surviving patient

In the other eight patients, a complete intraventricular blood clot was shown three times, a partial one 13 times and in addition on two occasions CSF-blood mixture in the occipital horns. These patients survived the bleeding by only a few days (see Table 1). Only three patients with ventricles partially filled with clotted blood survived.

Bleedings in Haemorrhagic Disorders. Intraventricular haemorrhages occurred six times in connection with anticoagulant treatment and in one case there was haemophilia. Five patients were somnolent on admission and survived (Table 3). CT showed an intracerebral haematoma in five cases and in one an extensive intracerebellar haematoma combined with a clot in the fourth ventricle; this patient died.

Haemorrhages of Unknown Aetiology. In 18 cases, the aetiology remained unclear. Two of these patients with an intraventricular haemorrhage in which only parts of the ventricular system were involved, survived (Table 4). Neither of these patients was comatose at the time of CT examination.

Table 3. Haemorrhagic disorders (N = 7)

Level of consciousness	CT findings		
	CSF blood mixture	Clotted blood	
		Partial	Total
I (Normal)			
II (Somnolence)	● ● [a]	● ●	
III (Stupor)		●	
IV (Coma)		○ ○	
V (Deep coma)			

[a] ●, surviving patient

Table 4. Unknown cause (N = 12)

Level of consciousness	CT findings		
	CSF blood mixture	Clotted blood	
		Partial	Total
I (Normal)			
II (Somnolence)			
III (Stupor)	● [a]	●	
IV (Coma)		○ ○ ○ ○ ○ ○	
V (Deep coma)		○ ○ ○ ○	

[a] ●, surviving patient

Discussion

Follow-up studies of intraventricular haemorrhages are possible using computer tomography. Our study shows (as has been known for a long time) that patients do not survive extensive intraventricular haemorrhages. Haemorrhages with unilateral or partial intraventricular involvement and with CSF-blood mixture may survive. Our findings support the classification of intraventricular haemorrhages into haematocephalus totalis et partialis and haemorrhagia intraventricularis (Pia 1972, 1975).

Summary

Ninety patients with intraventricular haemorrhages were examined and the extent of bleeding compared with the clinical course. With the help of computer tomography it is possible to distinguish between intraventricular clotted blood and CSF-blood mixture.

The clinical course of intraventricular haemorrhages is largely related to the extent and to the location of bleeding. In our study, with only two exceptions patients with clotted blood in the third ventricle died. Only patients who were not comatose and who showed intraventricular CSF-blood mixture or partially filled ventricles had a good prognosis.

8.4.3 Basal Ganglia and Thalamus

8.4.3.1 Indication for Operative Treatment of Hypertensive ICH in the Basal Ganglia and Thalamus

K. Kitamura and M. Kagawa, Tokyo

Introduction

Many opinions regarding the indications for operative treatments of hypertensive intracerebral haematoma have been reported; however, this particular subject is still being debated (Lazorthes 1959; McKissock et al. 1961; Luessenhop et al. 1967; Richardson 1969; Paillas and Alliez 1973; Ojemann and Mohr 1975; Tedeschi et al. 1975).

In this paper, we will discuss the indications for operative treatment and the prognosis of hypertensive intracerebral haematoma in the basal ganglia and the thalamus. (The technical aspects have been discussed on p. 383.)

Indications for Operative Treatment

The clinical details recorded in 133 consecutive cases with haematoma in the basal ganglia or in the thalamus were studied. We have tried to establish what are the main prognostic factors indicating the outcome of surgical or medical treatment (Table 1).

In this study, a statistical method of Spearman's coefficients of rank correlation was utilized.

Table 1. Distribution of hypertensive intracerebral haemorrhage[a]

Type	Surgical	Conservative	
Putaminal	61	29	90 (52.3%)
Thalamic	9	34	43 (25.0%)
Subcortical	17	7	24 (14.0%)
Cerebellar	5	0	5 (2.9%)
Pontine	0	10	10 (5.8%)
Total	92	80	172

[a] Haemorrhage in the basal ganglia, 133 of 172 (77.3%)

According to this investigation, the important factors influencing prognosis and operative results were found to be the CT findings including the location and size of a haematoma, as well as the rapidity and the direction of its evolution (Table 2, 3; Figs. 1, 2).

The level of consciousness and neurological deficits such as hemiparesis, signs of herniation also showed a closer correlation with the prognosis than many other factors (Table 4).

According to the data obtained by statistical study, the cases of hypertensive intracerebral haematoma in the basal ganglia and the thalamus were graded as follows. This grading proved of value in predicting the prognosis.

Table 2. Classification of thalamic haemorrhage

Type	Description
Localized (T1)	Haematoma is located in the lateral or medial nuclei, expands in a small ovoid haematoma with its centre remaining at the site of origin
Thalamo-capsular (T2a)	Haematoma enlarges laterally, spreads against and into the internal capsule
Subthalamo-midbrain (T2b)	Haematoma spreads infero-medially into the subthalamus and midbrain
Ventricular cast (T3)	The massive haematoma involves the adjacent structures, and most ventricular systems, particularly the third ventricle are filled by haematoma

Table 3. Classification of putaminal haemorrhage

Type	Description
1. Localized (P1)	Haematoma is located in the putamen or expands in a ball-like fashion with its centre remaining at the site of origin. The actual diameter of the haematoma is less than 3 cm
2. Putamino-capsular (P2a)	The actual diameter of the haematoma is more than 3 cm. The haematoma extends forwards and backwards; the posterior limb of the internal capsule is partially involved
3. Advancing (P2b)	The internal capsule is totally destroyed, the haematoma spreads upwards through the corona radiata into the centrum semiovale, and then through the isthmus of the temporal lobe to produce a large mass in the posterior temporal white matter, or ruptures into the ventricular system
4. Ventricular cast (P3)	The haematoma occupies most of the ventricular system, and particularly the third ventricle is obstructed

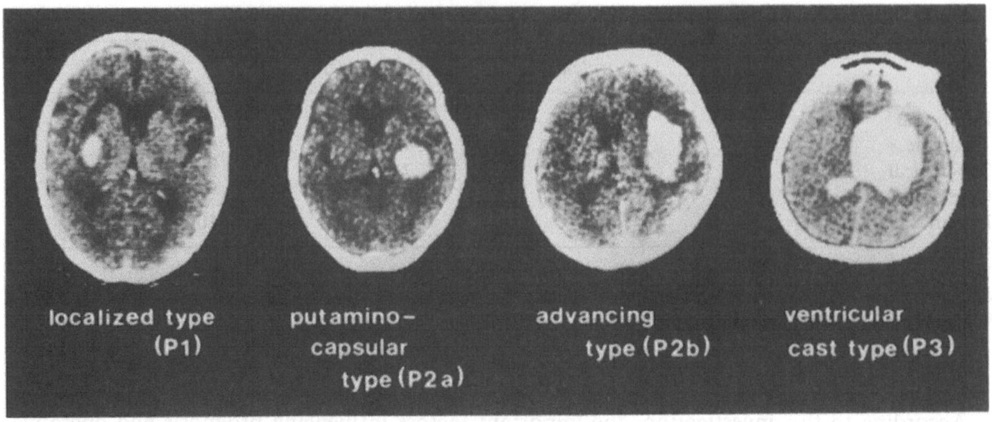

Fig. 1. Classification of putaminal haemorrhage

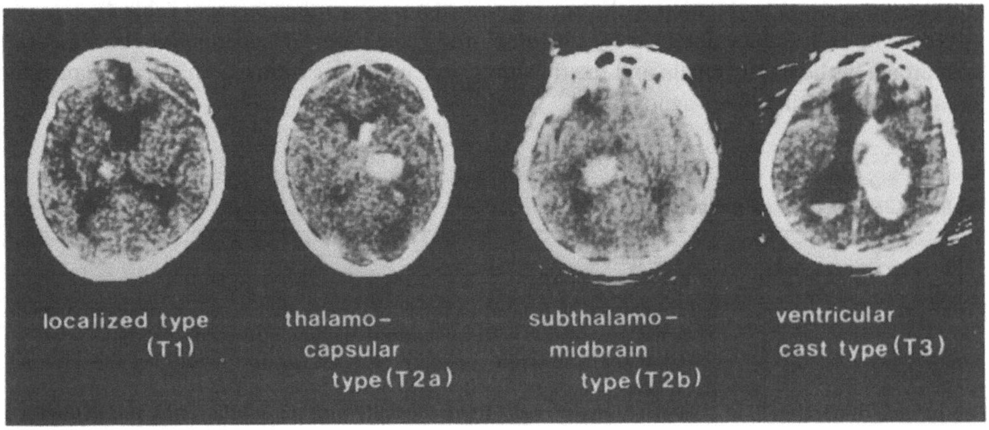

Fig. 2. Classification of thalamic haemorrhage

Table 4. Statistical analysis of prognostic factors

Factor	Spearman's coefficient τ_0
Level of consciousness	0.7114[a]
Neurological deficit	0.7507[a]
Classification of CT scan	
Putaminal	0.4893[a]
Thalamic	0.6291[a]
Early signs of herniation	0.4389[a]
Amount of haematoma	
Putaminal	0.5142[a]
Thalamic	0.5643[a]
Ventricular rupture	0.3209[b]
Complication	0.2010[b]

[a] $p \leq 0.01$; [b] $p \leq 0.05$

Grade I,	alert or drowsy, with or without a slight neurological deficit. Localized type of the putaminal and thalamic haematoma.
Grade II,	drowsy or stuporous, with a slight to moderate stable neurological deficit. The putamino-capsular or the thalamo-capsular type. The patients of Grade I who, over the course of several hours, progressively worsen, increasingly developing further neurological deficit.
Grade III,	drowsy or stuporous, with a moderate to severe neurological deficit. The advancing type of the putaminal haemorrhage or the thalamo-capsular type.
Grade IV,	semicomatose, with a stable moderate to severe deficit or early signs of herniation; the subthalamo-midbrain type of thalamic haemorrhage.
Grade V,	comatose, with decerebrate posture; the ventricular cast type of the putaminal and thalamic haemorrhage.

Our general guidelines for operative treatment are as follows:

For patients with a thalamic haematoma, direct evacuation of the haematoma is not advisable. Only ventricular drainage or a subsequent shunt operation is indicated.

For patients in grade I, who are alert or drowsy with little or no neurological deficit, conservative medical treatment is indicated. There is no difference in the outcome between those treated surgically and medically.

For patients in grade II, operative treatment is strongly indicated. In the patient who does not show any improvement, operation may be beneficial even in the subacute stage. For patients in grade III, operative treatment is superior to medical treatment. For patients in grade IV, an emergency operation is indicated in the cases with putaminal haematoma. For patients in grade V, operation is not advisable. All except one of the patients in grade V died even after operative treatment, so that in this grade, operation is contra-indicated (Fig. 3).

In general, age is not an important factor as long as there are no coexisting complications, but in the case of those over 70 years of age, they must be carefully assessed before considering operative treatment.

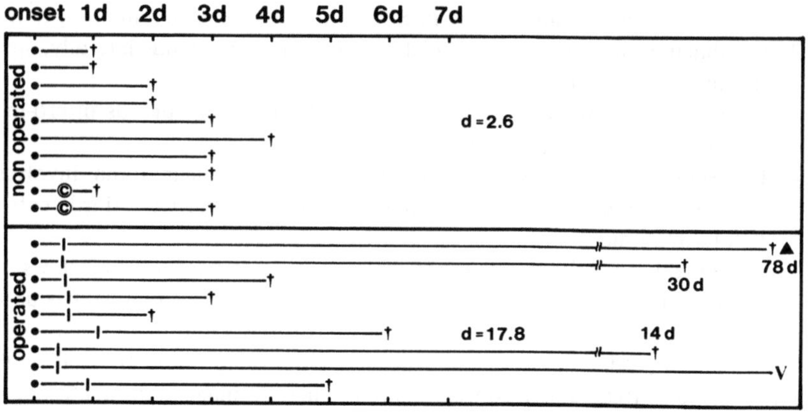

Fig. 3. Outcome of treatment in patients in grade V. †, died; ©, continuous ventricular drainage; I, operation; ▲, died from complications

Table 5. Statistical analysis of prognostic factors

Factor	Spearman's coefficient
Age	−0.0368[a]
Dominancy of cerebral hemisphere	−0.0358[a]

[a] $p > 0.10$ (not significant)

In our statistical analysis, dominance of the involved cerebral hemisphere is not a major factor in deciding on operative treatment. There is no significant difference between dominant and non-dominant cerebral hemispheres as far as mortality is concerned. A haematoma in the dominant hemisphere does not provide an absolute contra-indication to operation, although cerebral dominance affects the quality of recovery. In our series, operative cases with a haematoma in the dominant hemisphere have not recovered to their previous normal social life (Table 5).

Another important factor relating to the outcome is the timing of operation. Our experience showed that the best results were obtained by immediate operation, and favourable results were obtained when the interval between ictus and operation did not exceed 24 h.

Thalamic Haemorrhage

In our series, about 25% of hypertensive intracerebral haematomas occur in the thalamus. The location, the direction and the size of thalamic haemorrhage were investigated in 43 consecutive cases in which CT scan was performed.

This study shows that thalamic haemorrhage arises in the inferior medial and the lateral nuclei of the thalamus. The thalamic haemorrhage may extend laterally to the internal capsule, and spread infero-medially towards the upper brain stem, or into the hypothalamus (Figs. 4, 5).

Thalamic haemorrhage is grossly classified into four types based on CT findings of haematoma advancement (Fig. 2).

1) The localized type, in which the haematoma is situated in the medial or in the lateral nuclei, expands in a small ovoid haematoma with its centre remaining at the site of origin.
2) The thalamocapsular type, in which the haematoma extends laterally, spreads against or into the internal capsule.
3) The subthalamic-midbrain type, where the haematoma spreads infero-medially into the hypothalamus or the midbrain.
4) The ventricular cast type, in which the massive haematoma involves the adjacent structures, and most of the ventricular system, particularly the third ventricle, is occupied with haematoma.

Our guidelines for the treatment of thalamic haemorrhage are as follows:

For patients in grade I (the localized type), conservative treatment is absolutely indicated. Good results were obtained with conservative treatment and there was no mortality.

Patients in grade II (the thalamocapsular type) or in grade III (the subthalamic-midbrain type) should be treated with continuous ventricular drainage in the acute stage and a subsequent shunt operation if necessary.

For patients in grade IV (the ventricular cast type), only conservative treatment is indicated as a fatal outcome may be expected in this group regardless of any kind of treatment.

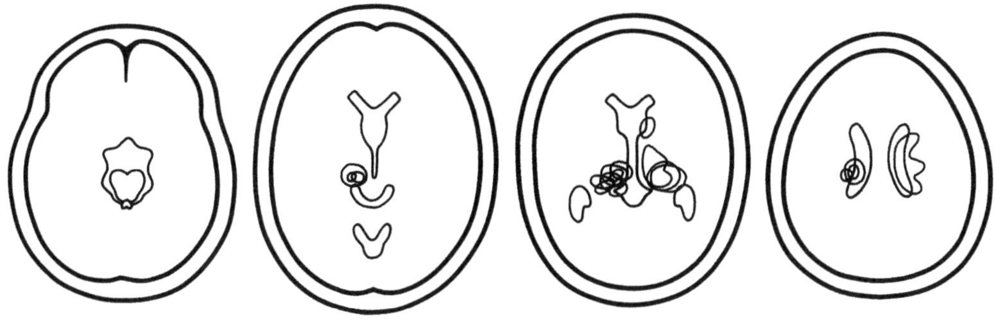

Fig. 4. Thalamic haemorrhages, localized and thalamocapsular type

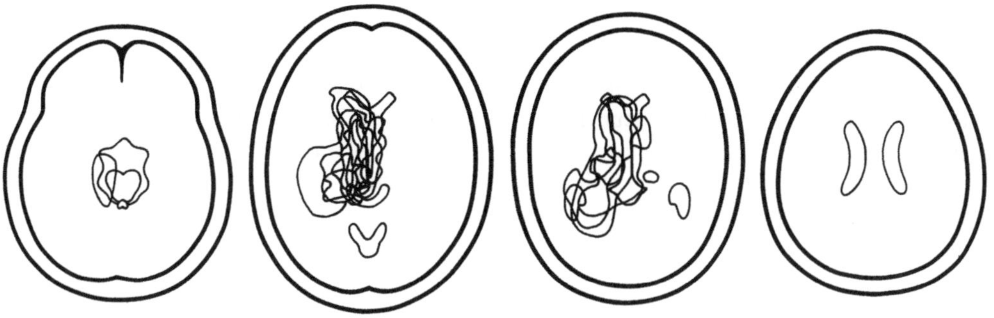

Fig. 5. Thalamic haemorrhages, subthalamo-midbrain and ventricular cast type

Prognosis

The results were reviewed in 133 cases with hypertensive intracerebral haematoma in the basal ganglia and the thalamus. Of these 63 were treated conservatively and 70 were treated surgically. The overall mortality of the patients treated conservatively was 30% and that of the patients treated surgically was 29% (Table 6).

To investigate the difference between the results of surgical and medical treatment, we selected 46 surgical and 27 conservative cases in whom operation appeared to be absolutely necessary according to our grading. This study showed that the mortality of the patients in

Table 6. Prognosis of hypertensive intracerebral haematomas in the basal ganglia and thalamus (overall management of patients)

	Total	Recovery to					
		Social life	Independent daily life	Daily life partly assisted	Daily life totally assisted	Vegetative state	Dead
Surgical	70	–	24%	21%	19%	7%	29%
Medical	63	11%	22%	29%	5%	3%	30%

Table 7. Comparison of prognosis with surgical and medical treatment

	Independent daily life	Daily life partly assisted	Daily life totally assisted	Vegetative state	Dead
Patients in grade II					
Surgical	63%	25%	12%	0%	0%
Medical	26%	47%	5%	5%	17%
Patients in grade III & IV					
Surgical	16%	29%	29%	13%	13%
Medical	0%	37%	12%	13%	38%

grade II was 17% and that in grades III and IV was 38%, whereas in the surgical cases the mortality was 0% in grade II and 13% in grades III and IV, respectively.

The morbidity of patients treated surgically was superior to that of conservative cases in grades II, III and IV.

The follow-up periods ranged from 6 months to 3 years. Of the surgically treated cases in grade II, 63% recovered to an independent existence while only 26% of conservative cases in the same grade recovered to similar quality. No vegetative patient was noted in the surgical cases.

In grades III and IV, 16% of patients treated surgically recovered to an independent existence, while no patient treated conservatively showed a similar recovery (Table 7).

Discussion and Conclusions

Hypertensive putaminal haematomas should be operated on in accordance with the indications as described. The proposed grading, or similar systems, seem to be the most important point.

Whether thalamic haematomas should be treated surgically or conservatively is still being discussed. Only a few surgical cases with thalamic haematoma have been reported. We had several cases in the earliest trials in which direct removal of the thalamic haematoma was performed. These efforts at removal of a haematoma from the thalamus failed to produce good results.

With regard to surgical intervention in thalamic haematoma, many problems arise because of its deep location and the existence of important and inaccessible structures. For this reason direct attack on a thalamic haematoma should be avoided and only ventricular drainage or a subsequent shunt operation are indicated.

Concerning the timing of operation, in our series, good results were obtained when the interval between ictus and operation did not exceed 24 h. Therefore, we prefer the immediate to the delayed operation.

The operative approach and technique are based on haematoma size and location. In the most recent cases we have used a large craniotomy. Our experience showed that the whole of a solid haematoma could not be removed through a burr-hole or trephine opening, whereas craniotomy offered the advantages of a wide operative field and the possibility of subsequent external decompression in cases with a massive haematoma or extensive brain oedema. For this reason a trephine opening or burr-hole should not be used.

Our comparative study of the results of surgical and medical treatment revealed that there were no differences as far as overall mortality and morbidity were concerned, as described by McKissock and Richardson (1961). However, operative treatment offered significant advantages when operations were performed in accordance with our clearly defined indications.

8.4.3.2 Putaminal ICH with Regard to its Size in CT Scanning

Y. Matsukado and N. Sakurama, Kumamoto

Several neurosurgeons, especially in Japan, have tried to classify hypertensive cerebral haemorrhage in relation to angiographic findings, level of consciousness and other neurological signs, or various laboratory examination. In hypertensive cerebral haemorrhage, estimation of the haematoma volume during operation was found to be quite useful in evaluating the subsequent prognosis. We have found that CT scan estimation of the haematoma volume is more accurate than intra-operative aspiration techniques and has disclosed several interesting findings.

Materials and Method

Twenty-six cases of hypertensive putaminal haemorrhage, excluding the cases with thalamic extension, were examined by CT scan to estimate the volume of the haemorrhage. The cases are summarized, but one was omitted because of inadequate scanning. To determine the precise relationship between the estimated size of haematoma and the postoperative morbidity, thalamic haemorrhage, intraventricular haemorrhage and the putaminal haemorrhage of any combination of these were excluded from the present study. For the same reason patients comatose after an apoplectic attack were not included. The age of the patients ranged from 27 to 75 years, with an average of 47.7. Two patients were markedly younger (27 and 35), and this accounted for the low average age.

All the patients were right-handed, and ten (40%) had haemorrhage in the left cerebral hemisphere. Thirteen (52%) of 25 operated patients underwent craniotomy within 7 h of the onset. Duration of the follow-up study ranged from 2 months to 1 year, with an average of 6.4 months. Five patients (20%) died within the period of follow-up study. Postoperative morbidity and recovery were examined periodically and the activities of daily living (ADL) score was obtained. Of those patients in ADL 1, 28% died, while of those in ADL 2, ADL 3 and ADL 4, 12%, 20% and 20%, respectively, died.

Level of consciousness before operation is listed in Table 1 and the ADL score was classified in the surviving patients. One patient, who was operated on on the 5th day because of hemiplegia, showed only minimal impairment of consciousness, and 13 patients (52%) in a lethargic state survived. Two patients in a state of impaired consciousness died 14 and 64 days

Table 1. Level of pre-operative consciousness and ADL

	State of disturbance			
	Slightly impaired	Lethargic	Semicomatose	Comatose
ADL 1	1	6		
ADL 2		1	2	
ADL 3		4	1	
ADL 4		2	3	
Total	1	13	6	0

after craniotomy, from pulmonary and renal complications. Six patients survived from a semicomatose condition and three patients died 2, 3 and 41 days, respectively, after operation. As mentioned above comatose patients were not included in the present study because they might have some other neuronal involvement such as cerebral herniation. To simplify the analysis in reviewing the estimated size of the haematoma, examination was limited to the above-mentioned group of patients.

Recovery of the ADL in relation to the time of surgical intervention is summarized in Table 2. Sixteen cases (64%) were operated on within 24 h of onset, and three patients (12%) expired 2, 3 and 14, respectively, days after operation. Actually these three cases belonged to the group in which operation was performed within 7 h of onset and there was no death in the cases who were operated on between 7 and 24 h. Six patients (46%) of 13 who were operated on within 7 h showed satisfactory recovery of ADL and, in all, 10 cases (40%) of 25 showed recovery to ADL level 1 or 2.

The location of haemorrhage was in the putaminal region of either the left or right cerebral hemisphere; however, the shapes of the haematomas in the brain were never alike and showed irregular expansion. Estimation of the haematoma diameter at a certain slice does not make any sense in this aspect, and extension of the haematoma to any particular structure should be carefully analysed. Structural characteristics of the haematoma in regard to morbidity and mortality of hypertensive cerebral haemorrhage can be drawn and reconstructed very easily by CT scan. At present we have estimated the volume of haemorrhage with pre-operative CT scan, and quite useful information was obtained for the surgical prognosis. All of the slices in which the haematoma was demonstrated were collected and the size of the haematoma was estimated by measuring the extent of the high density area in each 1 cm slice. Then the value was summed up and magnified according to the actual scale. Concomitantly computer programming for the estimation of the haematoma volume is now in progress and the comparative study with the data obtained from a print-out digital display was made. There was still some inaccuracy of counting the marginal high density zone, but the error was less than 5%.

In all patients, the haematoma was surgically removed through the Sylvian fissure, and the volume of the haematoma content was measured by aspiration. A remarkable inconsistency of the haematoma volume was encountered in several cases and measurement of the haematoma volume during operation was found to be quite inaccurate. As shown in Table 3, six cases had a haematoma of less than 30 ml, although the level of consciousness was lethargic or semicomatose and hemiplegia was pronounced in all cases. In particular, three cases in the same group were considered to have about 15 ml haematomas by CT scan estimation. It is not surprising that the volume of haematoma in those patients was overestimated during operation, and it is worth noting that haematomas of only 15 ml in the putaminal region could produce

Table 2. ADL recovery and time from onset to operation

	Within 7 h	Within 24 h	Within 3 days	Within 5 days	Within 1 week
ADL 1	5	–	1	1	–
ADL 2	1	1	1	–	–
ADL 3	3	2	–	–	–
ADL 4	1	–	4	–	–
Died	3	–	1	–	1
Total	13	3	7	1	1
ADL 1 or 2	46%	30%			

Table 3. See text

Name	Age	Sex	Onset to operation	Volume of haematoma (ml)	Conscious level	Side	Postoperative follow-up	ADL	Complication
U.T.	52	Male	5 h	14.4	Lethargic	Right	6 months	1	
T.K.	66	Female	7 h	14.8	Semicomatose	Left	1 year	2	
H.A.	53	Female	5 h	16.6	Lethargic	Right	7 months	1	
H.K.	35	Male	5 h	19.2	Lethargic	Left	6 months	1	
T.S.	59	Male	5 h	23.6	Lethargic	Left	7 months	1	
M.I.	42	Male	7 h	29.2	Lethargic	Left	9 months	1	
S.T.	48	Female	5 days	32.3	Almost clear	Right	11 months	1	
Y.M.	47	Female	5 h	39.6	Semicomatose	Left	4 months	3	
Y.T.	47	Female	6 days	39.8	Semicomatose	Left	41 days	Dead	
O.T.	75	Female	3 days	41.4	Lethargic	Right	8 months	4	
K.Y.	48	Male	5 h	42.7	Lethargic	Right	4 months	3	
T.N.	56	Female	3 days	45.2	Lethargic	Left	7 months	1	
H.K.	60	Male	17 h	54.3	Lethargic	Right	10 months	3	
T.M.	42	Male	2 days	55.0	Lethargic	Right	64 days	Dead	Kidney
S.Y.	45	Male	18 h	60.0	Lethargic	Left	1 months	2	
H.J.	27	Male	3 days	62.2	Semicomatose	Right	7 months	2	Kidney
T.H.	40	Male	5 h	63.4	Lethargic	Right	14 days	Dead	Lung
K.Y.	48	Male	5 h	69.4	Lethargic	Left	11 months	3	Stomach
N.S.	73	Female	2 days	79.1	Lethargic	Right	2 months	4	
M.T.	56	Male	2 days	82.3	Semicomatose	Right	2 months	4	Heart
H.R.	45	Female	17 h	91.1	Lethargic	Right	5 months	3	
K.I.	66	Female	6 h	91.4	Semicomatose	Right	2 days	Dead	
M.A.	73	Male	3 days	101.7	Lethargic	Right	4 months	4	
M.T.	48	Male	5 h	135.3	Lethargic	Left	4 months	4	
N.A.	59	Female	5 h	142.2	Semicomatose	Right	3 days	Dead	

complete hemiplegia and severe impairment of consciousness. It is still a subject of controversy whether these patients require surgical removal of the haematoma. All the patients in this group were operated on within 7 h of onset and recovery was found to be excellent in the follow-up study. As described before 13 cases were operated on within 7 h and 3 patients died (Fig. 1). Those patients had haematomas of 63.4, 91.4 and 142.2 ml, respectively, by CT scan estimation. No patients with ADL 3 or 4 were found in the follow-up study if the volume of haematoma was less than 35 ml, and we could expect recovery of ADL up to grade 2 if the volume of haematoma was less than 60 ml. The estimated haematoma volume in the CT scan and the recovery of ADL was fairly well correlated, irrespective of the side of the haemorrhage or the cerebral dominance. Although in three patients the volume of haematoma was about 60 ml or less, they died of postoperative complication in the kidney or chest. One of these was operated on 6 days after the onset, which was the longest interval from onset to operation in the present study. Among ten cases of ADL 1 or 2 group, seven were found to have a haemorrhage of less than 35 ml and two cases of ADL 3 or 4 showed a haemorrhage of less than 40 ml (Fig. 2) (Table 4).

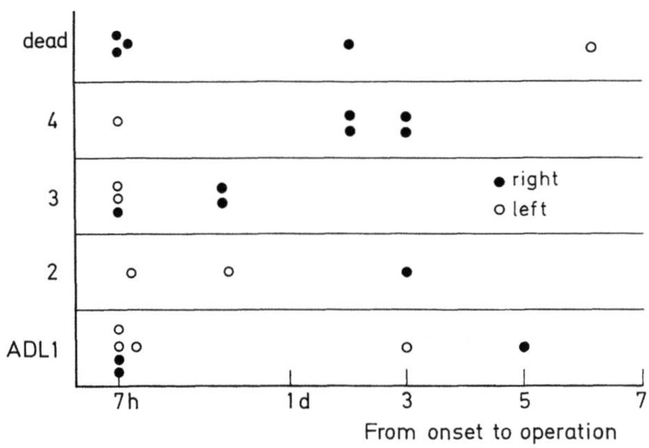

Fig. 1. Postoperative ADL in relation to interval between onset and surgery

Table 4. Size of haematoma and ADL

Grade	Number	Average age[a]	Size of haematoma[b]
ADL 1			25.8 ml
ADL 2	10	47.7	45.7 ml
ADL 3	5	51.8	59.4 ml
ADL 4	5	65	88 ml
Expired	5	51	78.4 ml

Size	ADL 1	ADL 2	ADL 3	ADL 4	Died
⩽30 ml	5	1			
30 – 50	2		2	1	1
50 – 70		2	2		2
⩾70			1	4	2

[a] Two cases of six (50 – 70 ml) patients belong to younger age group
[b] Seven cases of ten (ADL 1 or 2) patients less than 35 ml

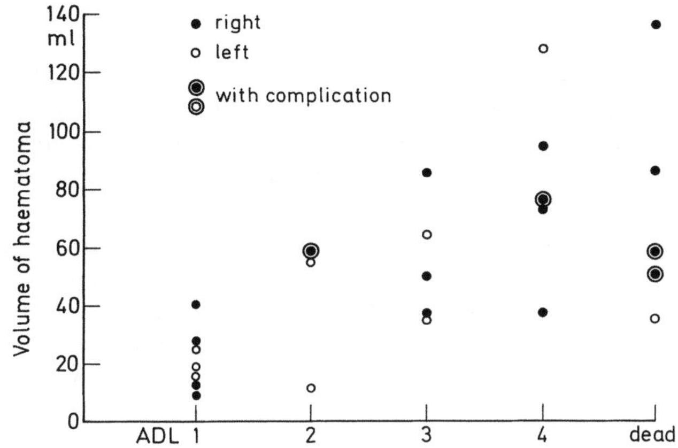

Fig. 2. Relation of postoperative ADL to volume of haematoma

Discussion

Much criticism could be made of the results of our present study and it should be reviewed after a randomized comparison of a larger number of cases. The principal aim of operative treatment for hypertensive haemorrhage is to improve the functional disability, and it is particularly important to restore the speech and the motor function on the side of handedness. The surgical treatment of hypertensive cerebral haemorrhage has achieved satisfactory recovery from those disabilities in a fair number of cases. However, it does not necessarily prove the overwhelming superiority of surgical treatment compared with medical treatment. Some of the patients showed really rapid recovery of function after surgical evacuation of the haematoma, but some did not. There are many other factors which complicate the postoperative course of hypertensive cerebral haemorrhage, such as advanced arteriosclerosis with cardiorenal failure or increased intracranial pressure and subsequent cerebral oedema. The most important question in the surgical treatment of hypertensive cerebral haemorrhage is to know how to select the patients for the operation.

Computerized analysis of the structure and size of the haematoma has been in progress and we expect in the near future to know which patients should be operated on immediately. Our present study is simply concerned with the volume of the putaminal haemorrhage in relation to the ADL recovery, and it showed that there was a satisfactory recovery of function when the volume of the haemorrhage was under 35 – 40 ml.

8.4.3.3 Trans-Sylvian Approach in Putaminal ICH with Mild Symptoms

J. Suzuki and T. Sato, Sendai

In addition to our previous report on 52 cases of hypertensive intracerebral haematoma in the putaminal region we would like to discuss here those 25 cases with mild symptoms, particularly as regards their state of consciousness. Fourteen were in a confused state and 11 were fully conscious. The results of these investigations, including the findings in 25 additional cases treated in 1976, and especially in three non-operated cases, are briefly summarized to highlight our policy for mild cases.

Among the non-operated cases there was a 31-year-old female with slight evidence in the CT scan of haemorrhage in the vicinity of the caudate nucleus. A right-sided hemiparesis and language deficit gradually improved, and she was able to walk again after 40 days. When we first saw her on the 66th day she had only slight motor paresis. She was discharged after 10 days in good condition.

The second case was a 45-year-old man with impairment of consciousness and marked motor paresis of the right limbs which was already showing marked improvement on admission. The angiograms showed slight lateral deformation of the lenticulostriate artery, and a CT scan revealed a haemorrhagic focus in the thalamic region. He recovered consciousness in 4 days, and he could walk by the 12th day after admission. He was discharged on the 23rd day with only sensory deficits.

The third case, a 56-year-old male, lapsed into unconsciousness 1 h after onset and was immediately admitted to hospital, where we saw him on the 5th day with the diagnosis of subarachnoid haemorrhage. He had marked headaches and neck rigidity and was confused. There was no motor deficit. CT scan revealed a haematoma in the vicinity of the caudate nucleus and there were also signs of bleeding into the ventricles. As the patient's level of consciousness worsened on the 2nd and 3rd days, bilateral ventricular drainage was performed. This resulted in a rapid improvement in consciousness and disappearance of the headache. The drainage was removed on the 8th day and the patient was discharged on the 32nd day, able to walk without assistance.

Indications for Operation in "Mild" Cases

The category of so-called mild cases of hypertensive intracerebral haemorrhage is itself somewhat vague. In general, they are classified according to the degree of impairment of consciousness, but a time factor also comes into play (Fig. 1). Patients who are semicomatose immediately after the onset and who subsequently improve should be operated on without hesitation, but in cases in which there is no paresis and the state of consciousness is good, it is questionable whether operation should be performed.

We have made an investigation of the mild cases operated on in our clinic (Tables 1, 2) and have found that even in those cases of putaminal haematomas, where walking is impossible due to motor paresis and in cases with mild motor paresis even with impaired psychic function or aphasia, postoperative recovery is marked, so that radical operation is thought to be worthwhile. Moreover, the postoperative recovery of cases operated on at an early stage was better the earlier the operation, as judged from the pattern of recovery and the follow-up studies; the postoperative recovery of patients operated on more than 1 month after the onset was not good. In the light of these facts concerning postoperative functional recovery, it is thought that operation should be performed at an early stage when possible (Suzuki and Sato 1976).

With regard to cases not considered suitable for radical operation, it is thought that operation should be postponed when there is almost no motor paresis and the state of consciousness is good, or in cases in which a considerable time has elapsed between onset and admission, during which time the clinical state has improved. It also applies in cases in which the state of consciousness was good, and the haematoma was near the thalamus, so that there was a risk of the radical operation causing additional deficits. When intracranial pressure was increased because of rupture of the haematoma into the ventricular system, we immediately performed

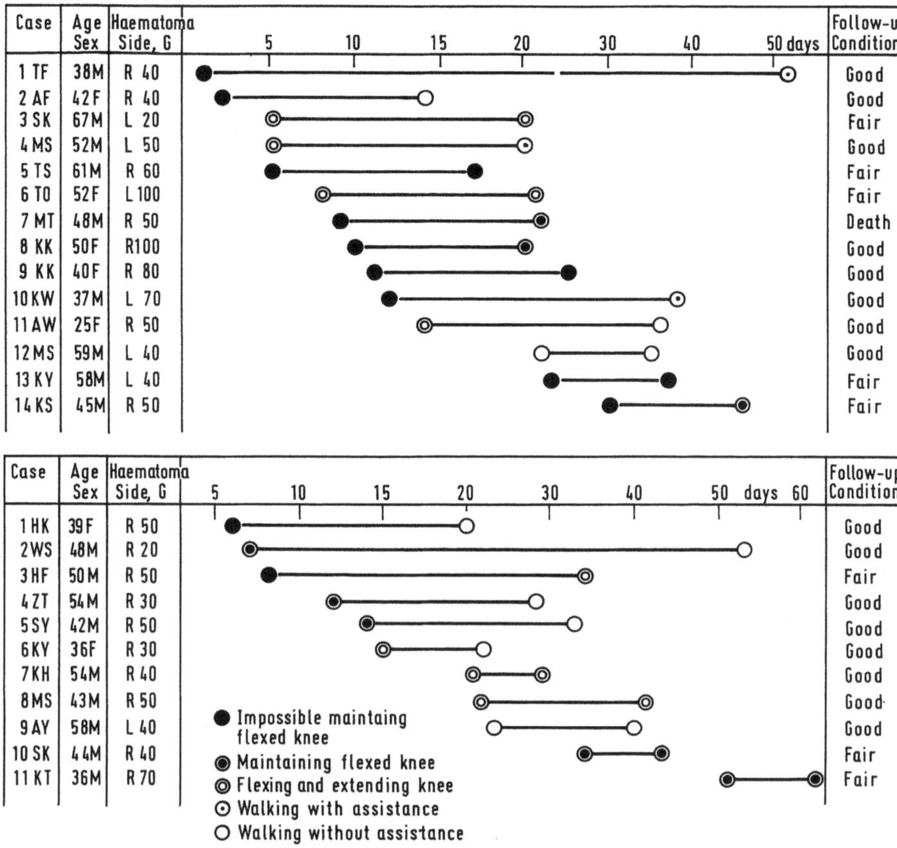

Fig. 1. Extent of motor paresis of the legs in mild cases (*Upper*, patients in a confused; *Lower*, patients with clear level of consciousness). *Initial circles*, paresis before surgery and timing of operation after onset. *Second circles*, paresis at time of discharge and duration of stay in hospital

Table 1. States of motor paresis of legs in confused patients

	Before operation	Discharge	Follow-up
Walking without assistance	1	3	13
Walking with assistance	0	3	0
Flexing and extending knee	4	2	0
Maintaining flexed knee	0	3	0
Impossible to maintain flexed knee	9	3	0
			1 (Death)

bilateral ventricular drainage, inserting a large tube into the anterior horns from the frontal region. In whatever type of case, i.e. in mild as well as severe cases, operation should be performed at an early stage when adequate removal of the haematoma can be achieved without producing further damage to the brain. When significant damage to the brain might be produced, the operation should be postponed.

Our aim in performing any operation should be to avoid any increase of the existing brain damage.

Table 2. States of motor paresis of legs in fully conscious patients

	Before operation	Discharge	Follow-up
Walking without assistance	1	6	11
Walking with assistance	0	0	0
Flexing and extending knee	3	3	0
Maintaining flexed knee	5	2	0
Impossible to maintain flexed knee	2	0	0

8.4.3.4 Discussion

J. W. F. Beks, Groningen

Spontaneous Haematomas in the Basal Ganglia

Despite numerous publications, there is no unanimity of opinion regarding the management of spontaneous intracerebral haematomas, especially when the lesion is located in the central grey matter of the brain. Some neurosurgeons think that conservative measures are better than surgical removal (McKissock et al. 1961), whereas others hold that operation should only be done under certain circumstances (Cook et al. 1965).

Paillas et al. (1973) argue for operation in those patients who are not immediately in a deep coma and in whom there is some chance of later rehabilitation. His goal was total removal of the clots by the least traumatic operative technique. This is, of course, a general principle, that any surgical procedure should always be as atraumatic as possible.

Backlund and Von Holst (1978) suggest that these patients may best be treated by aspiration through a burr-hole by stereotactic technique. This method though, would mean that a total evacuation was not possible in a number of cases. According to Backlund et al. (1978), that is not the aim of the operation, but rather to evacuate that volume, which is considered threatening to the vitality of the brain. Furthermore, subtotal evacuation should prevent rebleeding, particularly as Luessenhop et al. (1967) report that the most important surgical complication is reaccumulation of the clot. Others (Zwetnow 1976) say that the evacuation of a haematoma should be radical, as the presence of clots within the brain may produce some chemical influence upon the brain that is responsible for the surrounding oedema. Nevertheless, it is my opinion that under certain conditions, when it is decided that a clot should be evacuated, the stereotactic technique should be given a fair chance in the treatment of intracerebral haematomas, especially when they are located in the basal ganglia.

8.4.4 Cerebellar Haematomas

8.4.4.1 Indications and Prognosis

K. Sano and S. Yoshida, Tokyo

Cerebellar haemorrhage is reported in about 10% of all spontaneous intracranial haemorrhages at autopsy (Dinsdale 1964) and in about 7% of those in computed tomography (CT) according to Aizu Central Hospital (one of our affiliated community hospitals).

This paper is based upon our experience of 39 cases of cerebellar haematoma treated in our clinic and our associated hospitals. Among 39 cases, 30 were considered hypertensive cerebellar haemorrhage, because they had hypertension higher than 150/190 mm Hg prior to the haemorrhage and had no other suspected cause. Nine cases were regarded as cerebellar haemorrhage due to rupture of cryptic angiomas (vascular malformations), because in seven cases those angiomas were verified in surgical specimens and in the other two cases angiography and CT revealed small venous angiomas. Cases with trauma, tumours, blood dyscrasia, clearly demonstrated arteriovenous malformations and aneurysms were all excluded. The emphasis here is on a comparison of the hypertensive group and the angioma group.

Age and Sex

As seen in Table 1, the male to female ratio was 2:1 in both groups. The age of onset, however, was different in both groups. It was higher than 40 years in the hypertensive group and was mostly lower than 40 years in the angioma group. The mean age of onset was 64 years in the former and 37 years in the latter. This age distribution is clearly demonstrated in Fig. 1.

Initial Signs and Symptoms

In both groups, the most frequent initial symptoms were sudden outbursts of nausea and vomiting accompanied by severe headache and vertigo (Fig. 2). An immediate loss of consciousness was unusual. Cerebellar signs were more marked in the angioma group than in the hypertensive group.

Signs and Symptoms on Admission and Whilst in Hospital

In the hypertensive group, 40% of the cases manifest severe disturbance of consciousness (stuporous, 20%; comatose, 20%), whereas in the angioma group there was no comatose case and only two patients (22%) were stuporous. A fully conscious state was found in 27% of the

Table 1. Age and sex in 39 patients with cerebellar haemorrhage

	Hypertension (30 cases)	Angioma (9 cases)
Male/female	20/10	6/3
Range of ages (mean)	42 ~ 77 years (64)	16 ~ 56 years (37)

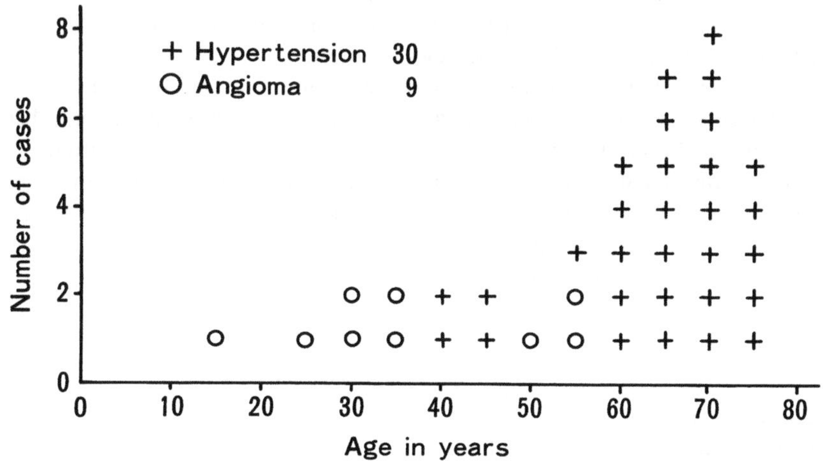

Fig. 1. Age distribution of 39 patients with cerebellar haemorrhage

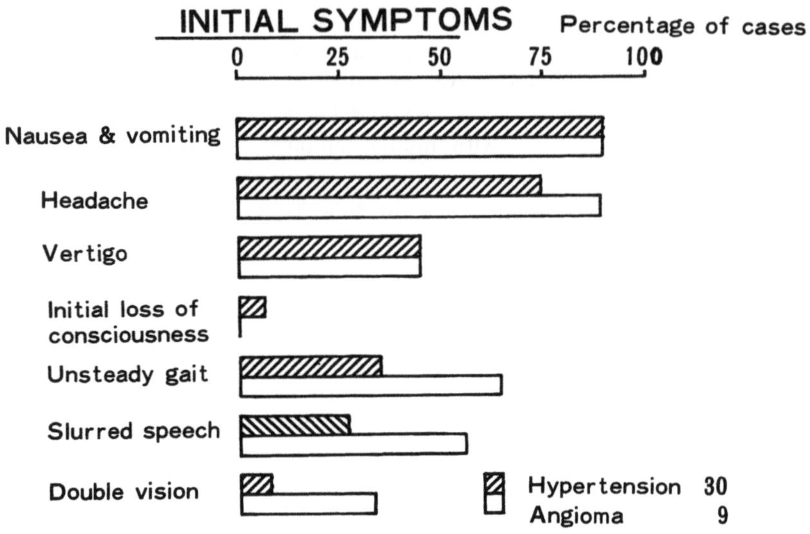

Fig. 2. Frequency of symptoms in 39 patients with cerebellar haemorrhage

hypertensive group and in 44% of the angioma group. In both groups 33% were drowsy.

Nuchal rigidity was found in 30% of the hypertensive group and in 22% of the angioma group. Myotic pupils (smaller than 2 mm) were noted in 57% of the hypertensive group and in 22% of the angioma group. In most of these, pupillary reaction to light was preserved. Respiratory disturbance was noted in 7% of the hypertensive group, but not in the angioma group. Motor weakness was found in 13% of the hypertensive group and in 11% of the angioma group. Conjugate deviation of the eyes, abducens palsy and facial palsy were found in a small number of the cases of both groups.

Syndromes of cerebellar haematomas during their stay in hospital can be classified into three types.

Type 1, vertigo syndrome, was seen only in small cerebellar haematomas. This syndrome consists of vertigo and vomiting on head movement. There may be mild dysarthria; there is no disturbance of consciousness.

Type 2, cerebellar dysfunction syndrome, consists of truncal and limb ataxia and cerebellar speech. There may or may not be some disturbance of consciousness. There may be a vertigo syndrome before this syndrome becomes manifest.

Type 3, brain stem compression syndrome, consists of severe disturbance of consciousness (stupor or coma), myosis and pyramidal tract signs such as a Babinski sign. There may be vertigo syndrome and cerebellar syndrome before this syndrome becomes manifest.

Type 1 was found in 20% of the hypertensive group, but in no case of the angioma group. Type 2 was noted in 23% of the hypertensive group and in 78% of the angioma group. Type 3 was seen in 57% of the hypertensive group and in 22% of the angioma group. The size of haematoma was the largest in Type 3 and smallest in Type 1.

Table 2. Surgical procedures in 27 patients with cerebellar haemorrhage

	Hypertension (18 cases)	Angioma (9 cases)
Removal of clot	10	6
Ventricular drainage and removal of clot	5	3
Ventricular drainage	3	0

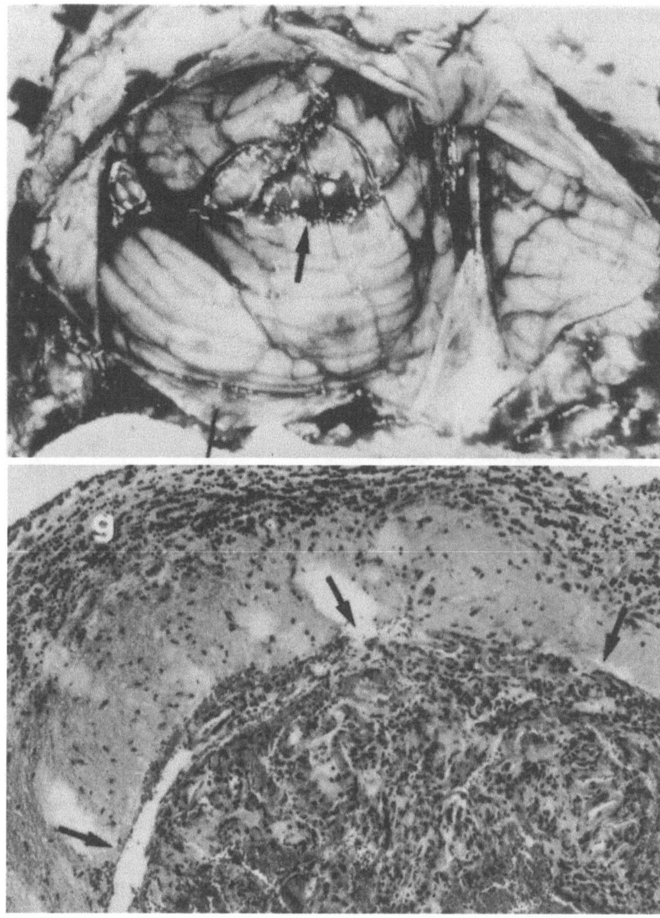

Fig. 3. Cerebellar haemorrhage caused by small angioma

Treatment

All the cases of the angioma group were submitted to operation. Of the hypertensive group 18 cases were operated on and 12 cases were not. Operation was done within 2 days of the onset in nine cases of the hypertensive group and in none of the angioma group. In five cases of the hypertensive group and in three cases of the angioma group, operation was done from 2 to 7 days after the onset. In four cases of the hypertensive group and in six cases of the angioma group operation was performed later than 1 week after the onset. The surgical procedures are listed in Table 2. Removal of clot means suboccipital craniectomy and removal of haematoma from the cerebellum. Figure 3 illustrates a case of cerebellar haematoma caused by cryptic angioma (indicated by an arrow). The histology (the lower half of the figure) reveals a small arteriovenous malformation (arrows).

The operative mortality according to the pre-operative level of consciousness is shown in Table 3. There was no mortality in the angioma group. In the hypertensive group, the operative mortality was 39% and this mortality was well correlated with the pre-operative level of consciousness.

Table 3. Surgical mortality in 27 patients with cerebellar haemorrhage

Pre-operative level of consciousness	Hypertension mortality	%	Angioma mortality	%
Awake	0	–	0	0
Drowsy	0	0	0	
Stuporous	3	50	0	
Comatose	4	57	0	–
Total	7	39	0	0

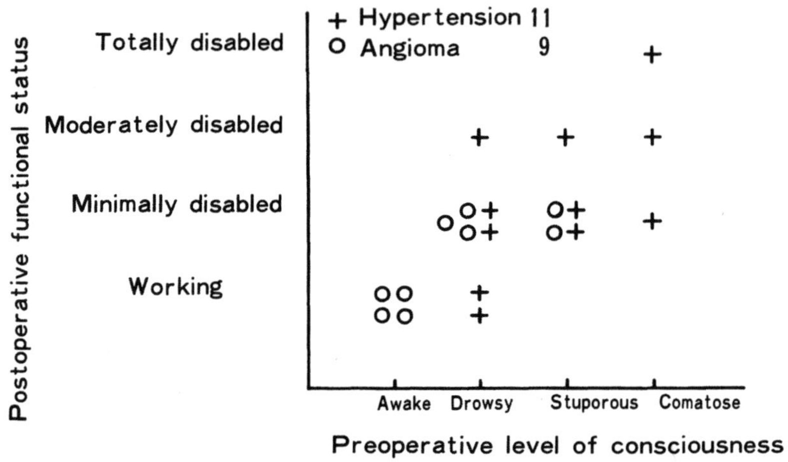

Fig. 4. Postoperative functional status according to pre-operative level of consciousness in 20 patients with cerebellar haemorrhage

Outcome of Cases

The quality of survival in cases submitted to operation according to the pre-operative level of consciousness is shown in Fig. 4. Cases of the angioma group are well and working (four cases) or only minimally disabled (five cases), but all are leading useful lives. Among the hypertensive group, two cases are well and working, five are minimally disabled, three are moderately disabled and only one is totally disabled. Therefore, 64% are leading useful lives. The quality of survival was roughly proportional to the pre-operative level of consciousness, namely, when the consciousness was clear, then the quality of survival was good; when the former was disturbed, the quality of survival was poor, as is clearly shown in Fig. 4. In general, the surgical results were far better in the angioma group than in the hypertensive group.

The outcome of 12 cases of the hypertensive group which were not submitted to operation is shown in Table 4. Here also, the pre-operative level of consciousness influenced the mortality and the quality of survival, i.e. six patients without disturbance of consciousness are well and working; of five patients in a drowsy state two died and of the survivors, one is working, one is minimally disabled and one is moderately disabled.

CT Findings and Outcome

CT is the most useful tool for the diagnosis of cerebellar haemorrhage. Twenty-three cases of the hypertensive group and two of the angioma group in our series were examined by CT within

Table 4. Outcome of 12 cases not submitted to surgery

Level of consciousness on admission	Mortality	%	Functional status of survivors
Awake	0	0	Working (6)
Drowsy	2	40	Working, 1; minimally disabled, 1; moderately disabled, 1.
Stuporous	0	–	
Comatose	1	100	
Total	3	25	

1 week of the onset. It was found that the size of a haematoma as estimated from CT findings correlated closely with the results of therapy and the eventual outcome in patients with hypertensive cerebellar haematoma.

The largest diameter of the cerebellar haematoma in the CT (transverse section) was measured. If the diameter was 2 cm or less, the haematoma was called small (Fig. 5). If the diameter was more than 2 cm and less than 3 cm, the haematoma was called medium sized (Fig. 6). If the diameter was 3 cm or more, the haematoma was called large (Fig. 7).

Most of the cases with large haematomas showed a severe disturbance of consciousness (coma or stupor) within 2 days of the onset. Therefore an emergency operation, namely, removal of haematoma, is necessary even if the patient is fully consciousness when first seen.

Cases with small haematomas showed a favourable outcome, because small haematomas were apt to be absorbed within 2 – 3 weeks without leaving any neurological deficit.

Table 5 shows CT findings (size of haematoma), ventricular dilatation, intraventricular haematoma, levels of consciousness, whether operation was performed or not, and the final outcome in 23 cases with hypertensive cerebellar haematoma.

As seen in this table, all cases with a small haematoma (2 cm or less in diameter) survived, whether operation was performed or not. This implies that operation is not necessary for cases with small haematomas.

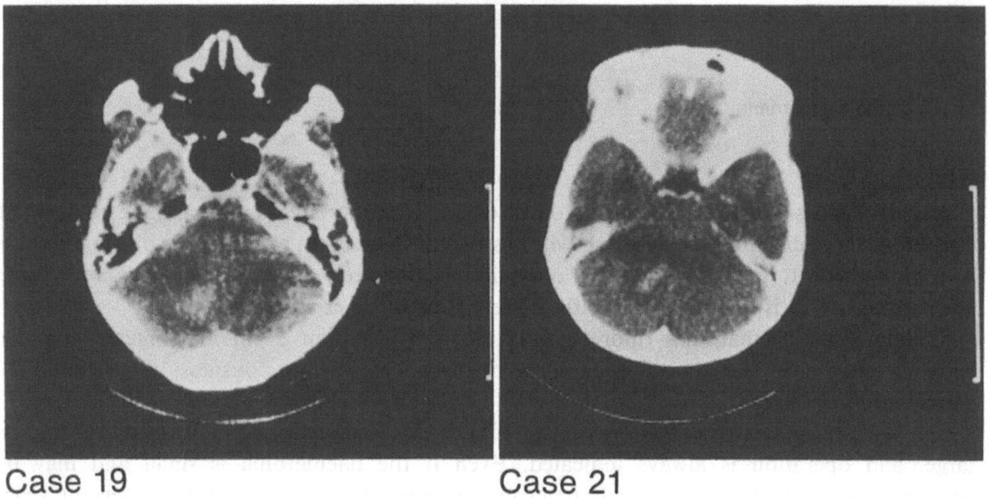

Fig. 5. Small haematoma, ⩽2 cm

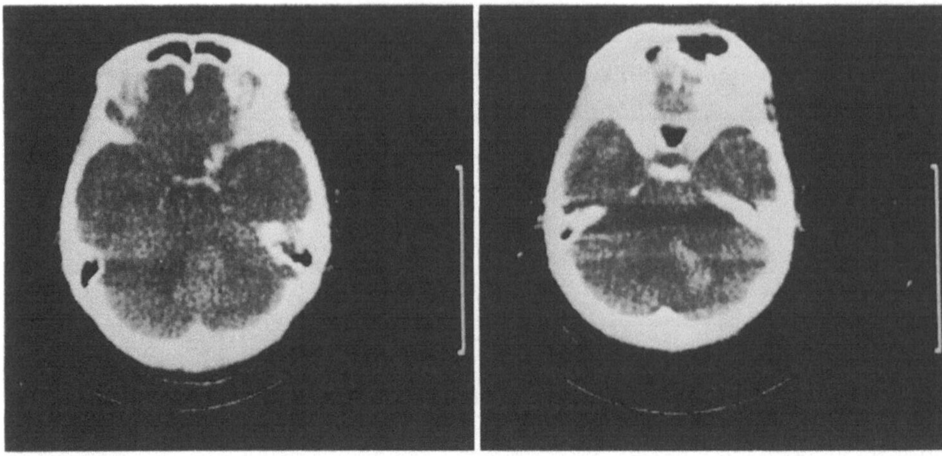

Case 11 Case 16

Fig. 6. Medium-sized haematoma, 2 – 3 cm

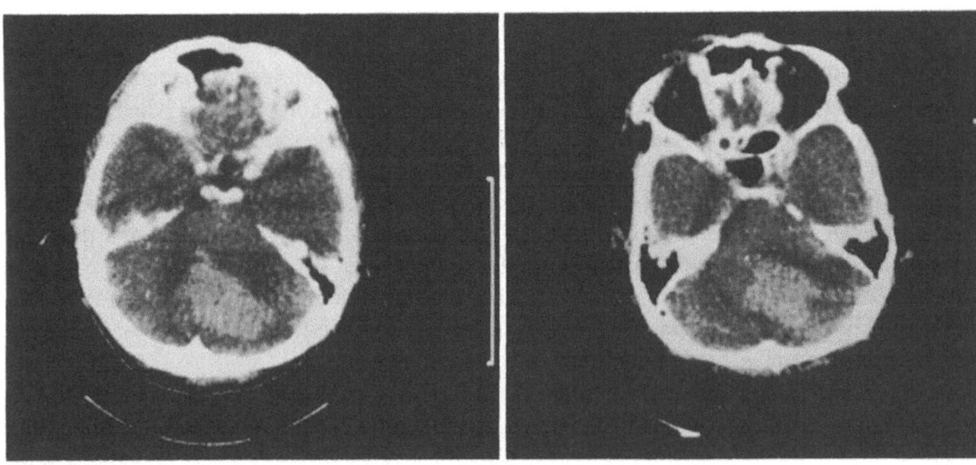

Case 4 Case 6

Fig. 7. Large haematoma, ⩾3 cm

Among 12 cases with large haematomas (3 cm or more in diameter), nine underwent operation, three died and six survived, whereas two of three cases which were not submitted to operation died. It may be said that operation is definitely indicated in cases with large haematomas. This is in accordance with the report of Little et al. (1978).

Medium-sized haematomas (more than 2 cm and less than 3 cm in diameter) may be spontaneously absorbed, but if they show disturbances of consciousness, they should be submitted to operation.

Cerebellar haematomas caused by rupture of a cryptic angioma are usually medium-sized or large, and operation is always indicated. Even if the haematoma is small and may be spontaneously absorbed, rebleeding from cryptic angiomas may occur after several years (Odom et al. 1961). Therefore, it is better to operate for removal of the haematoma and of the

Table 5. CT findings and outcome in 23 patients with cerebellar haemorrhage

Case No.	Size of clot (cm)	Ventricular dilatation	Intraventricular haematoma	Change in level of consciousness	Surgery	Outcome
1	5.0	+	+	Coma	+	Died
2	5.0	–	+	Coma	+	Died
3	4.5	+	+	Coma	–	Died
4	4.5	–	+	Awake→Stupor	+	Survived
5	4.0	+	–	Coma	+	Survived
6	4.0	+	+	Stupor→Coma	+	Survived
7	4.0	+	+	Drowsy→Stupor	+	Died
8	3.5	–	+	Stupor	+	Survived
9	3.0	+	–	Drowsy→Coma	–	Died
10	3.0	–	–	Drowsy	–	Survived
11	3.0	+	–	Drowsy	+	Survived
12	3.0	–	–	Awake	+	Survived
13	2.5	–	–	Stupor	+	Died
14	2.5	+	+	Drowsy	+	Survived
15	2.5	–	+	Awake	–	Survived
16	2.5	–	–	Awake	–	Survived
17	2.5	–	–	Awake	–	Survived
18	2.0	+	–	Stupor	+	Survived
19	2.0	–	–	Awake	–	Survived
20	2.0	–	–	Awake	–	Survived
21	2.0	–	–	Drowsy	–	Survived
22	2.0	+	+	Awake	–	Survived
23	1.5	–	–	Drowsy	–	Survived

angioma on the haematoma wall, even in cases of small haematomas, to prevent rebleeding. Cerebellar haematomas in younger subjects without hypertension should be submitted to operation for this reason.

Site of Hypertensive Cerebellar Haemorrhage

It has been reported that most hypertensive cerebellar haemorrhages arise in the region of the dentate nucleus (Dinsdale 1964; Fisher et al. 1965), and the vessels responsible are thought to be branches of the superior cerebellar artery. The ruptured vessel, however, was identified only in the report of Ito et al. (1973). In our series there were two cases in which haematomas were localized in the inferior portion of the vermis. In these cases, haemorrhage may have occurred from the vermian branches of the posterior inferior cerebellar artery.

Summary and Conclusion

Thirty cases of hypertensive cerebellar haematoma (hypertensive group) were compared with nine cases of cerebellar haematoma caused by rupture of cryptic angiomas (angioma group). The former were found above the age of 40 years (the average, 64 years) and the latter mostly below 40 years (the average, 37 years). In both groups the male to female ratio was 2:1.

In both groups initial signs and symptoms were most frequently sudden onset of nausea and vomiting accompanied by severe headache and vertigo. An immediate loss of consciousness was unusual.

Syndromes of cerebellar haematomas can be classified into 3 types: type 1, vertigo syndrome; type 2, cerebellar dysfunction syndrome; and type 3, brain stem compression syndrome, according to the size of the haematoma. The incidence of these syndromes in the different lesions is shown in Table 2.

In all nine cases of the angioma group, suboccipital craniectomy and removal of the haematoma with or without ventricular drainage was performed with no operative mortality. The same procedure was done in 15 cases of the hypertensive group and ventricular drainage only was performed in three cases of this group. The operative mortality in the hypertensive group was 39%. This mortality correlated well with the pre-operative levels of consciousness.

Quality of survival in the angioma group was good, all leading a useful life. That in the hypertensive group was roughly dependent on the pre-operative levels of consciousness, 64% of the cases leading a useful life. Among 12 cases of the hypertensive group which were not submitted to operation, pre-operatively awake patients (6 cases) showed good results, no mortality and all now lead useful lives; drowsy patients (5 cases) showed 40% mortality and quality of survival was not good; one comatose patient died.

The size of cerebellar haematomas, as revealed by CT within 1 week of the onset, was the most useful factor in determining the indications for treatment in the hypertensive group. When the largest diameter of the haematoma on CT (transverse section) was 2 cm or less (small haematoma), operation was not necessary and the haematoma was spontaneously absorbed. When it is 3 cm or more (large haematoma), operation should be done to save life and minimize neurological deficits. When it was between 2 and 3 cm, the existing level of consciousness determined the need for operation.

Operation was indicated in all cases of the angioma group. In our series we found no small haematoma. If, however, a small haematoma is found in cases without hypertension and below the age of 40, it is most probably caused by a cryptic angioma, and there is likely to be rebleeding from the angioma in the future. Therefore, a case of cerebellar haematoma thought to be caused by an angioma should be submitted to operation to prevent rebleeding, even if it is small.

8.4.4.2 Indications and Contra-Indications for Operation in Primary Haematomas of the Cerebellum and Brain Stem

C. Arseni and A. Gontea, Bucharest

The controversy that still persists today concerning the treatment of primary haematoma, at whatever site, results from confusion between the notion of haematoma and haemorrhage. As we have discussed in detail (Sect. 8.3.1.5) the difference between these two anatomoclinical entities with their different treatment is clearly understood. No form of haematoma recovers spontaneously. Operation is always indicated and has a good prognosis, whilst in haemorrhages the outcome is unfavourable with and without operation. Cerebellar haematomas show no differences from those in other parts of the brain. In Richardson's statistics (1972) there were 35 cases of cerebellar vascular accidents of which 17 were haemorrhages. Nine patients were operated on and one survived (operative mortality, 89%) and of the eight non-operated patients, two survived (mortality, 75%). Yoshida et al. (1978), in their statistics on acute cerebellar blood extravasation in severely ill patients, reported 14 cases of cerebellar haemorrhage proper of which five survived and nine died postoperatively (mortality rate, 64%). With conservative treatment, mortality was 36%. These data demonstrate that in cerebral haemorrhage, whatever the location, worse results are obtained by surgical than by medical treatment.

Once the diagnosis of haematoma of the cerebellum or brain stem has been established, the haematoma must be operated on and evacuated immediately. In severe cases the interval between admission and operation must be as short as possible, with a minimum of ancillary investigations. Numerous investigations require time and are not innocuous (e.g. puncture of the ventricles or drainage). Even arteriography may be a cause of aggravation (tetraplegia in the Yoshida data). The shortest interval between ictus and operation was approximately 1 h. In nine of our severe cases we operated only on the basis of clinical data (seven cerebellar and two brain stem haemorrhages). There are no contra-indications to operation except irreversible coma. Even in coma with respiratory arrest operation can be performed (Yoshida 1978).

Timing of the operation is the key to the prognosis. We believe that in primary haematoma of the cerebellum or brain stem the operation must be performed as early as possible because deterioration is progressive and a new haemorrhage is possible at any moment. Furthermore, the chances of recovery are greater at the beginning, as the cerebral parenchyma which is only compressed but not yet necrosed, maintains its functional potential and the pressure cone that often causes death of the patient is avoided. Operation gives good results, the mortality rate is low and the neurological sequelae are few and of lesser importance.

The operations performed according to our concepts yielded excellent results: In 25 cases of primary cerebellar haematomas operated on (8 acute, 5 subacute and 12 chronic) there was only one death from pulmonary complications in an aged patient with a subacute progressive haematoma; 17 patients recovered without sequelae, five with slight sequelae, two with marked sequelae but who may nevertheless be able to look after themselves (Table 1).

In three cases of primary brain stem haematoma (two subacute and one chronic form), one of the pons and two of the medulla oblongata recovered, two without sequelae and one with moderate sequelae (vertigo) who has also had a ventriculo-cardiac shunt performed. They are all alive after 5 years.

We do not agree with aspiration since the haematoma is not completely evacuated, herniation of the cerebellar tonsils persists with all the risk involved, a new haemorrhage may be precipitated and histological examination is not possible. Neither do we advocate ventricular

Table 1. Operative results

Clinical form	No. of cases	Operative results			Total	Dead immediately
		Complete recovery	Slight sequelae	Severe sequelae		
Cerebellar haematoma						
Acute haematoma	8	–			7	
Symptom-free int.	2	2			2	
Stationary form	2	1	1		2	
Progressive form	4	–	1	2	3	1
Subacute haematoma	5	–			5	
Symptom-free int.	1	1			1	
Stationary form	1	1			1	
Progressive form	3	–	3		3	
Chronic haematoma	12	12			12	
Total	25	17	5	2	24	1
Primary haematoma of the brain stem						
Subacute haematoma	2	1	–	1	2	
Chronic haematoma	1	1	–	–	1	

puncture with drainage, although moderate hydrocephalus develops within 3 h of the ictus; ventricular puncture is also liable to cause certain accidents (e.g. haemorrhage), especially as these patients may present vascular defects. The haematoma is evacuated by midline or unilateral craniectomy. As a rule we do not turn a flap.

8.4.4.3 Operative Treatment

M. Klinger and S. Kunze, Erlangen

As a rule, the treatment of choice for correctly diagnosed cases of cerebellar haematoma is a suboccipital craniectomy and evacuation of the clot (Table 1). This survey of cases in the literature, to which we have added our own cases, indicates the results of treatment in 109 cases of cerebellar haematoma, 99 of which were treated by operation with a survival rate of 70.7%. In other words, 70 of these 99 cases recovered. Fischer et al. (1965) strongly advocate immediate operation, particularly in cases of cerebellar haematoma due to hypertension, since the clinical course of these patients has a tendency to deteriorate rapidly and unexpectedly.

Computer tomography, however, has altered the attitude towards surgical treatment because this diagnostic procedure allows us to keep the patient under much closer surveillance than in the pre-CT era. The exact dimensions of the haematoma can be monitored and correlated with the clinical finding at any time. This may be illustrated by the following case:

Table 1. Results of treatment in cerebellar haematoma

	Number of cases	Form of treatment	Survival
Single case reports (1906 – 1948)	9	Surgical	9
Guillaume et al. 1949	5	Surgical	4
Single case reports from 1949 – 1959	16	Surgical	16
Arseni and Oprescu 1959	6	Surgical	5
McKissock et al. 1960	14	Surgical	9
Single case reports from 1960 – 1968	13	Surgical	9
Norris et al. 1969	19	9 conservative	3
		10 surgical	3
Nornes and Hauge 1972	5	Surgical	5
Rosenberg et al. 1976	18	Surgical	7
Klinger and Kunze (present series) 1979	4	3 surgical	3
		conservative	1
Total	109		77 (70.7%)

The patient (A H), a 13-year-old male, suffered a sudden attack of intense headache radiating into the neck on 27 December 1978. He did not lose consciousness and was not amnesic. On admission to hospital, the boy was found to have a stiff neck, and lumbar puncture revealed bloody CSF. Computer tomography showed a wedge-shaped area of increased density and early hydrocephalus (Fig. 1a). Angiography indicated that the source of the haematoma was an angioma. Since the boy remained conscious and the vital signs were stable, no operation was performed. The CT study was repeated 4 days later (Fig. 1b) and showed that the haematoma was somewhat smaller and that it was now surrounded by a border of oedema. After a further week of conservative treatment (Fig. 1c), another CT demonstrated that the density of the haematoma had decreased while the degree of hydrocephalus remained unchanged. As the clinical condition continued to improve steadily and there was no longer any nuchal rigidity, it was considered advisable to wait 2 weeks before making a new CT. On 22 January 1979, the CT showed that the density pattern in the vermis was becoming more normal, indicating that the haematoma was in the process of being absorbed (Fig. 1d). The degree of hydrocephalus was moderate and did not increase.

Since the absorption of intracerebral haematomas has been well documented (Weigel et al. 1978), we have adopted a similar attitude to cases of cerebellar haemorrhage if at all possible (Table 2). Our policy regarding the treatment of such lesions is summarized in this table. In patients with an intracerebellar haematoma who have lost consciousness, immediate operation is performed as a possible life-saving measure. Since we know that the prognosis of unconscious patients is poor, an operative procedure is their only chance. Fischer et al. (1965) report that even patients in a critical state with fixed pupils may be saved by the prompt surgical removal of such a clot. However, it is a feature of these haematomas that patients who are seemingly well may deteriorate to unconsciousness, coma and death within a few hours. Because of this lethal deceptiveness, patients in the second group, i.e. those who are well but deteriorating, should be operated on immediately. In other words, if the clinical status or the level of consciousness deteriorates, operation is essential. Those patients, however, who arrive at the hospital fully conscious and continue to remain stable may be watched closely and monitored by repeated computer tomograms. It is quite possible that they may recover completely without operation.

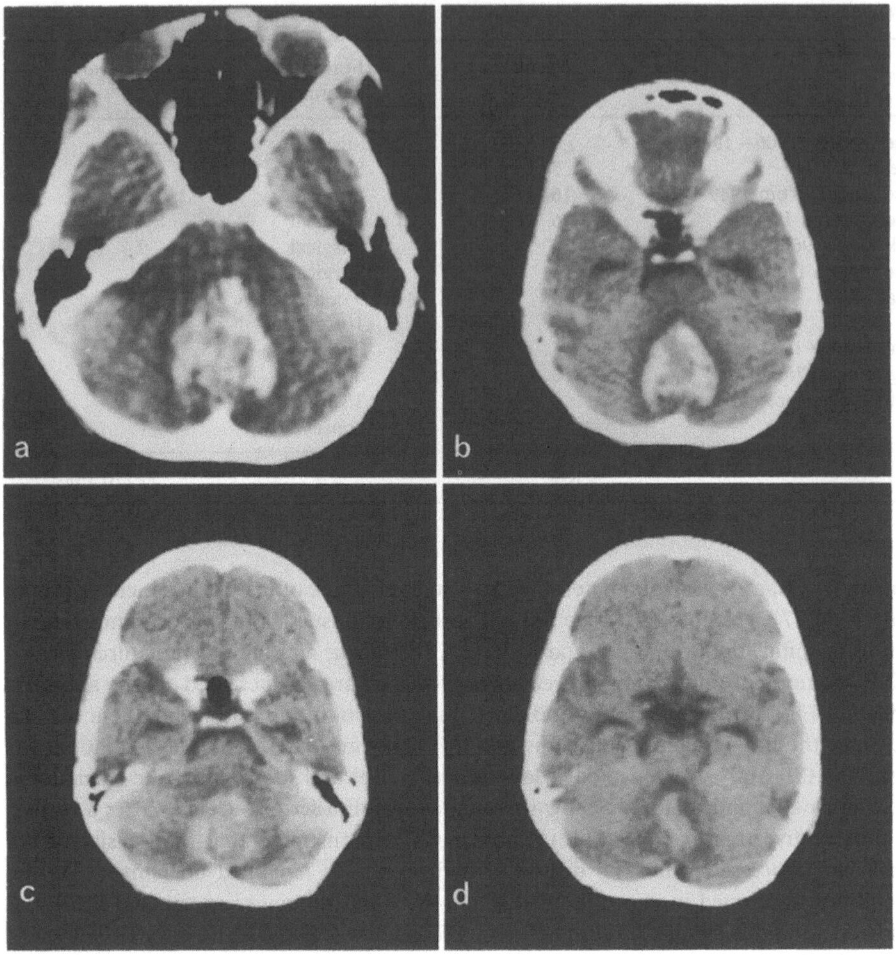

Fig. 1a – d. Follow-up of a 13-year-old male (A. H.) with a cerebellar haematoma, using computer tomography. No operation was necessary, **a** One day after acute onset of headache, CT shows circumscribed haematoma in the vermis. No loss of consciousness, **b** Four days later, a border of oedema is seen surrounding the haematoma, **c** One week later, the CT follow-up indicates that the density of the haematoma is decreasing. Nuchal rigidity has disappeared, **d** Four weeks after the acute onset of the haematoma, the resorption of the hyperdense area is in an advanced stage. The child continued to improve steadily

Table 2. Forms of treatment in cases of cerebellar haematoma

Level of consciousness	Treatment of choice
Patient unconscious	Operation
Patient awake, but deteriorating	Operation
Patient awake	Conservative (CT follow-up)

8.4.4.4 Intracerebellar Haematoma

T. Banno, M. Shibuya, M. Oda, and N. Kanie, Yokkaichi

It is generally agreed that the incidence of spontaneous intracerebellar haemorrhage is about 10% of all intracranial hypertensive bleeding. Of the 286 hypertensive haemorrhages reported from Boston City Hospital (Fang and Foly 1954), 231 (80%) were cerebral, 29 (10.1%) were cerebellar and 26 (9.6%) were pontine. Brown-Sequard (1861) described the first case of intracerebellar haemorrhage, but it was an autopsy case. Fisher in 1965 was probably the first surgeon to have operated on a patient with intracerebellar haematoma and the patient survived. Subsequently, many authors reported cases, but these reports consisted mostly of one or a few cases.

As regards the aetiology, the predominant cause of haemorrhage is hypertension. In the report by Dinsdale (1964), about 90% had hypertension, while the remaining 10% had a haemorrhagic diathesis, micro-angioma or aneurysm and so on.

As regards the location of the haematoma (Freemann et al. 1973), the most favoured site of haemorrhage is the paravermian portion of cerebellar hemisphere, where the dentate nucleus is, as is the basal ganglia in cases of haemorrhage in the cerebral hemispheres. The origin of bleeding is either the branches of SCA or PiCA.

The clinical symptoms of cerebellar haemorrhage are not so specific at the onset. According to the literature (Michael 1932; Friedman and Nielson 1941; Hyland and Levy 1954; Rey-Bellet 1960; Yoshida et al. 1978), the most frequent symptoms are impaired consciousness, headache, nausea and dizziness. Cerebellar dysfunction as a localizing neurological sign is rather rare. One characteristic sign is ocular disorder, that is paralysis of conjugate gaze to the side of the haematoma. The sixth and seventh cranial nerves on the side of the haematoma are often impaired.

Frequently, intracerebellar haemorrhages can be misdiagnosed as a normal subarachnoid haemorrhage resulting from a ruptured intracranial aneurysm, because the haemorrhages occur very near the fourth ventricle and easily rupture into the ventricle. In such a case the first symptom is sudden onset of headache, and a bloody CSF might be revealed on lumbar puncture.

The clinical course of the intracerebellar haematomas can be subdivided into the following three groups according to their site, size and the speed of growth of the haematoma:

1) Acutely progressive type, which presents signs of brain stem damage soon after the onset;
2) Subacutely progressive type, which presents signs of brain stem damage less rapidly; and
3) Chronic type, which presents minimal or no signs of brain stem damage.

Of these three types, acute and subacute progressive types could hardly have been treated surgically, but prompt diagnosis and immediate surgical exploration can cure these cases.

We have operated on 49 spontaneous intracranial haemorrhages in the last 4 years; three of these cases were cerebellar (Table 1).

Case 1: This 61-year-old female, who had been hypertensive for 3 years, was admitted to our hospital on 22 January 1976. Five days before admission she had sudden onset of severe headache followed by nausea and dizziness. She was examined by a practitioner, and bloody CSF was revealed on lumbar puncture. Her blood pressure was 200/130 mm Hg. She was sent to us with a diagnosis of subarachnoid haemorrhage. On admission she was stuporous and had a stiff neck. On neurological examination horizontal nystagmus to the left and conjugate gaze palsy to the right were noted. Papilloedema of 2.0 D was found bilaterally. Deep tendon

Table 1. Summary of three cases

Case	1	2	3
Age/sex	61♀	15♂	59♂
Hypertension	Yes	No	Yes
Onset	Headache	Headache	Dizziness
Course	Chronic	Subacute	Chronic
CSF	Bloody	Bloody	Clear
Conscious level	↓	↓	→
Signs	Nystagmus Dysmetria	VI, VII CN Hemiparesis	Nystagmus
Conjugate Gaze palsy	Yes	Yes	Yes
Hydrocephalus	Yes	Yes	No
Diagnosis	VAG VG	VAG VG	CT
Location of haematoma	Rt. paravermian	Rt. paravermian	Rt. hemisphere
Residual	Vertigo Ataxia	Vertigo Nystagmus	Vertigo

VAG = vertebral angiography; VG = ventriculography; CN = cranial nerves

reflexes were slightly reduced on the right. Cerebral angiography showed signs of marked hydrocephalus and suggested the presence of posterior fossa lesions (Fig. 1). Ventricular drainage through a right frontal burr-hole was instituted. After these procedures her conscious level improved remarkably. Ventriculography with Myodil (1 ml) showed signs of an intracerebellar space-occupying lesion (Fig. 2). On the morning of 25 January, dysmetria developed in her right upper limb. Suboccipital craniectomy in the prone position was carried

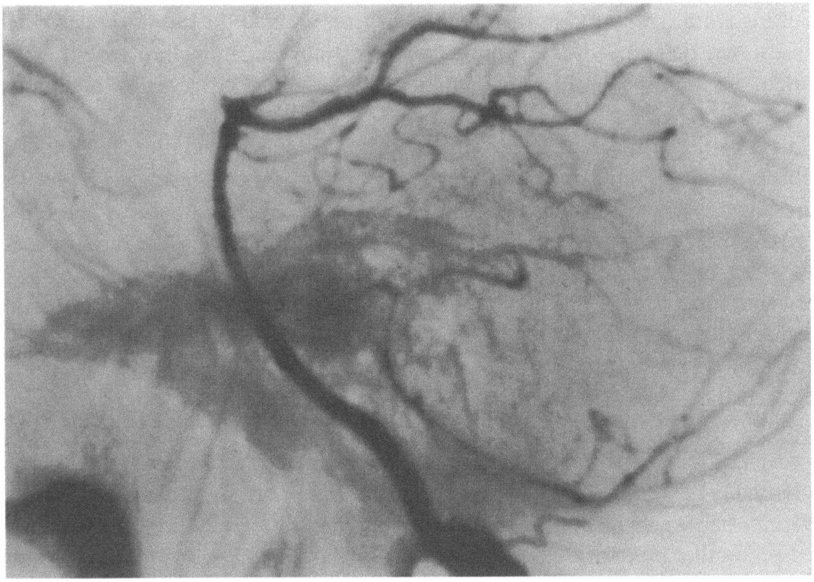

Fig. 1. Left vertebral angiogram in case 1. The basilar artery is stretched and pushed against the clivus, and the PiCA is markedly displaced anteriorly

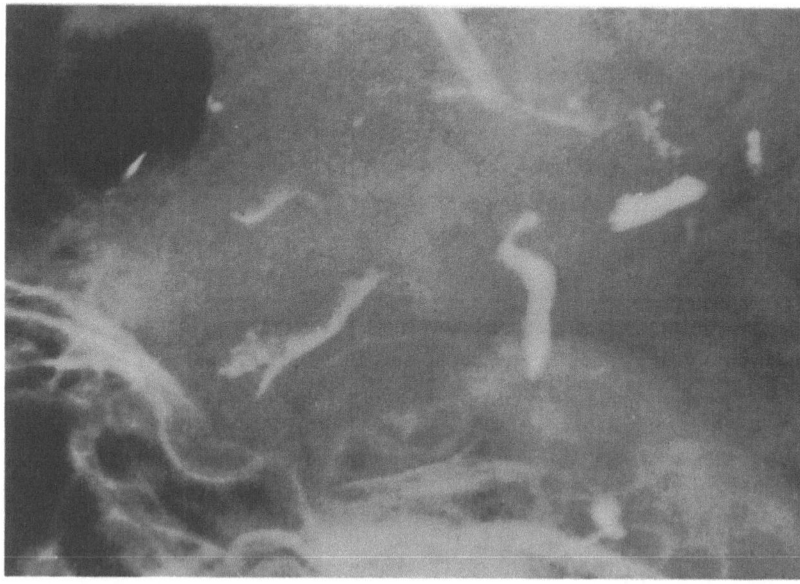

Fig. 2. Ventriculogram with Myodil in case 1. The aqueduct is kinked anteriorly at its upper portion and is obstructed at its end portion ("hockey stick" sign)

out in the afternoon of the same day. The right cerebellar hemisphere was markedly swollen. About 15 ml of haematoma was evacuated from the right paravermian region, part of which was shown to have ruptured into the fourth ventricle. Postoperatively, the signs of hydrocephalus disappeared. She was walking 1 month later and was discharged from the hospital with vertigo and an ataxic gait.

Case 2: A 15-year-old male had an acute onset of severe headache followed by nausea, vomiting and ataxia of gait on the way home from school on 9 May 1976. He had been suffering from intermittent headache for a few days. He was immediately admitted to another hospital and cerebral angiography was performed, which showed marked hydrocephalus. He was sent to us because of a progressively impaired level of consciousness on the following day. On admission to our hospital he varied from deeply stuporous to semicomatose. Pupils were anisocoric and hardly reacted to light; fundoscopic examination revealed petechial retinal haemorrhages, and respiration was irregular and ataxic. Ventricular drainage was inserted through a right frontal burr-hole soon after admission, and the ventricular pressure was reduced by the slow withdrawal of fluid, which was obviously bloody. After this he became more alert and could obey verbal commands. At this moment his pupils were isocoric, but reacted sluggishly to light, and horizontal nystagmus to the left and conjugate gaze paralysis to the right were observed. The sixth and seventh cranial nerves on the right were impaired. Moreover, left hemiparesis of moderate grade with a positive Babinski's sign were found. His blood pressure was 120/70 mm Hg. Ventriculography showed signs of an intracerebellar mass with a "hockey stick" sign of aqueduct and forward displacement of the fourth ventricle. At surgical exploration on 11 May, the right cerebellar hemisphere was remarkably swollen and about 20 ml of blood clot was evacuated from the right paravermian area. The haematoma was noted to have perforated into the fourth ventricle (Fig. 3). In this case, because of the unusual age of the patient, we inspected the haematoma cavity very carefully under the surgical microscope, but no vascular

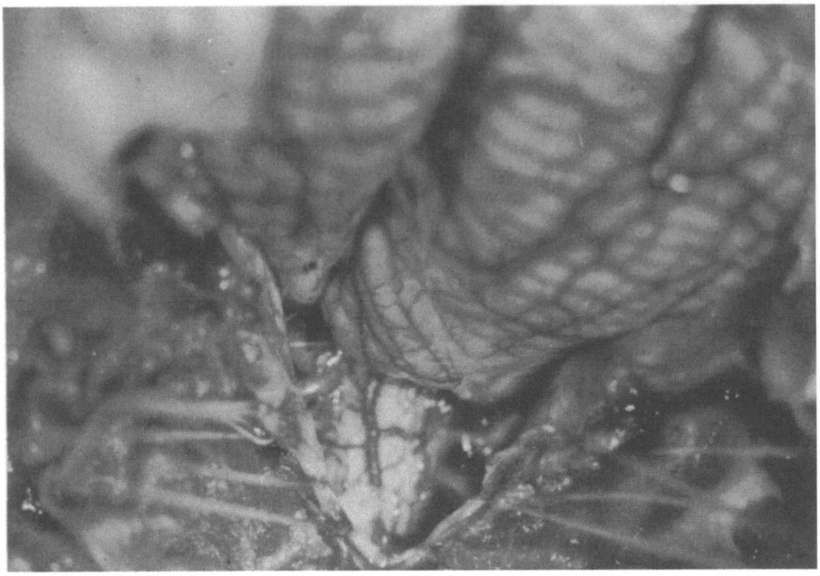

Fig. 3. Intra-operative photo of case 2. Marked swelling of right cerebellar hemisphere, and tonsillar herniation

abnormality was found, even by histological examination of the wall and the contents of the haematoma. However, the presence of micro-angioma or aneurysm could not be completely ruled out. The left hemiparesis of the patient resolved a few weeks later, and he was discharged on 10 July 1976, with subjective dizziness and horizontal nystagmus to the left.

Case 3: This 59-year-old male was admitted to our hospital because of severe left hemiparesis, which had suddenly occurred on 10 July 1978. Blood pressure was 190/120 mm Hg. Right serial carotid angiography showed minimal lateral displacement of the lenticulostriate arteries; a small haemorrhage in the right basal ganglia was diagnosed. As surgical intervention was not indicated, he was sent for physical therapy. His blood pressure was controlled to between 130 and 150 mm Hg systolic thereafter. Three months later he was able to walk with a stick, although a left hemiparesis with marked spasticity remained. On 14 October 1978, while he was still in the hospital, sudden dizziness attacked him in the early morning. Blood pressure was 190 – 210 mm Hg systolic, and nausea and vomiting followed. Blood pressure could not easily be controlled by antihypertensive drugs. Neurologically, horizontal nystagmus to the left and conjugate gaze palsy to the right were noted; otherwise no new focal deficits were observed. His left hemiparesis remained unchanged, and his consciousness remained clear throughout. Because his symptoms persisted, a cranial CT scan was made, which showed a large, round, high density area in the right cerebellar hemisphere (Fig. 4). On 17 October a suboccipital craniectomy was carried out with the patient prone. The right cerebellar hemisphere was markedly swollen, and the right cerebellar tonsil was displaced downwards, as it was in cases 1 and 2. About 20 ml of blood clot was evacuated, using the surgical microscope. The postoperative course was uneventful. Follow-up CT study on 10 November 1978, showed that the pre-operative high density area was replaced by a small low density area with ring-like contrast enhancement. Two months later his left hemiparesis was slightly improved and spasticity in left limb was markedly reduced. He could walk more smoothly with a stick.

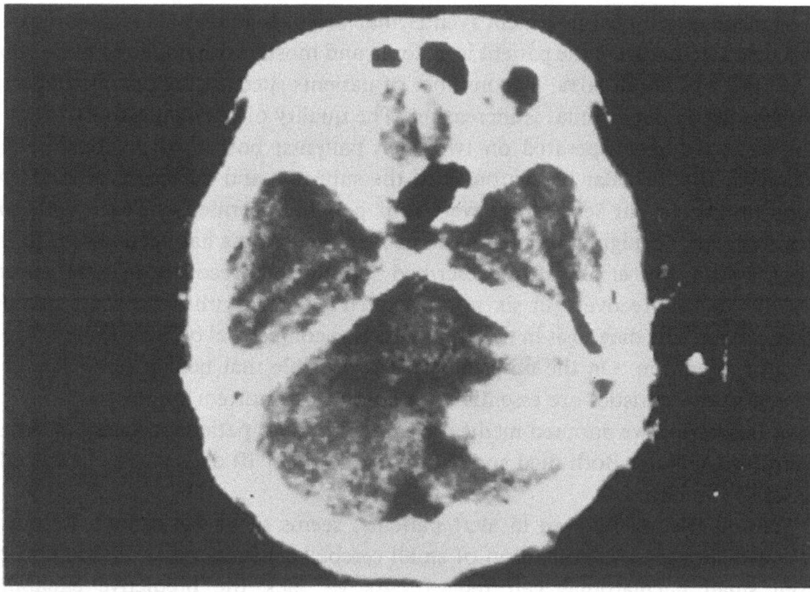

Fig. 4. CT image of case 3. Oval high density area with a little irregular margin in right cerebellar hemisphere. The fourth ventricle is displaced to the left and anteriorly

Discussion

Spontaneous cerebellar haematoma has been known for a long time, but its surgical treatment was developed only 25 years ago. Because its early symptoms are not so specific, immediate and correct diagnosis has been difficult. Furthermore, during the diagnostic procedures, such as angiogram or ventriculogram, irreversible brain stem damage might occur. But since CAT scanning was introduced, prompt and correct diagnosis can easily be obtained, without any hazard to the patient. There is not much to say about the surgical technique. This involves evacuation of the haematoma with a careful search for the source of haemorrhage such as micro-aneurysm or hidden angioma. Well-treated cerebellar haemorrhage leaves no major neurological deficits, such as the hemiparesia or aphasis which are commonly seen in cases of basal ganglia haemorrhages. Therefore, it is imperative to make the diagnosis as early as possible, and follow with prompt surgical exploration.

8.4.4.5 Operative Treatment

L. Calliauw and I. Dehaene, Bruges

Spontaneous intracerebellar haematomas are, according to their clinical signs and their natural history, divided into three types: the acute, the subacute and the chronic. Patients with haematomas of the acute type commonly die within 48 h if they receive only medical treatment or inadequate surgical treatment (ventricular drainage alone). The cases diagnosed during life and operated on when the patient is in coma and mostly with impaired brain stem reflexes, have a mortality of about 80%. The number of patients successfully operated upon, even when the patients are in deep coma, is increasing. The quality of survival is mostly very satisfactory. In our series we have operated on two such patients; both died postoperatively. The surgical treatment of cerebellar haematomas of the subacute and chronic type leads generally to very good results. In our series there were four patients operated on, each with good results. The possibility of a benign outcome of a cerebellar haematoma has been raised. In the period before the CT scan, Ott et al. (1974) described spontaneous recovery in nine patients. Richardson (1976) saw one recovery in six non-operated patients with a subacute or chronic cerebellar haematoma. The diagnosis in these patients was conjectural because there was no control by CT scan or operation. On the other hand, it is possible that benign cerebellar haematomas were missed as the statistics are essentialy based on post-mortem studies.

In this period we adopted medical treatment in two patients because of the stability of their neurological state. Both died suddenly, one of them 10 days and the other 30 days after the onset of the illness.

Medical treatment, even in alert patients, seems to be hazardous. Recently, CT scan has revealed spontaneous resolution of small cerebellar haematomas. It has also been shown that even small haematomas can rebleed. As we lack the predictive capabilities whereby a precipitous decline can be anticipated, we still adopt the policy that patients with any type of cerebellar haematoma should be promptly operated on. The only exception is in cases of haematoma of the fulminating type.

8.4.5 Brain Stem Haematomas

8.4.5.1 Clinical Aspects with Reference to Indications for Treatment

K. Sano and C. Ochiai, Tokyo

This paper is based on 25 cases of pontine haematomas encountered in our clinic and our affiliated hospitals from 1975 to 1978.

Age and Sex

The male to female ratio was about 7:1. Twenty-three patients were above the age of 40 and two were in their thirties; the average age was 52.9. One had malignant hypertension and the other one had rupture of a cryptic angioma (arteriovenous malformation) in the pons. There were 11 patients who were shown to have had hypertension prior to the haemorrhage. In the other 13 this information was lacking. One case which was confirmed as having no hypertension was that with the cryptic angioma mentioned above.

Initial Signs and Symptoms

Haemorrhage occurred when patients were working in ten cases, sleeping in four, eating or chatting in six and in an unknown situation in five. As an initial symptom, rapidly progressing loss of consciousness was predominant (60% of cases). There were, however, four cases which showed no disturbance of consciousness in the whole course of the disease. Nausea, vomiting and headache were symptoms next in frequency. In the four cases already mentioned, without loss of consciousness no headache was noticed (Table 1).

Table 1. Initial symptoms

Loss of consciousness	11
Nausea	8
Vomiting	8
Headache	7
Weakness of extremities	4
Dysarthria	4
Diplopia	3
Dizziness	2
Hyperhydrosis	1
Found to be comatose	4

Symptoms and Signs on Admission

Disturbance of consciousness was noticed in 84% of the cases. Motor disturbance, respiratory disturbance, abnormal pupils and abnormal ocular movement were also frequently seen (Tables 2, 3). Tetraparesis of alternating hemiparesis, Cheyne-Stokes respiration, pin-point pupils and skew deviation were characteristic signs. However, changes such as from tetraparesis to decerebrate rigidity, from pin-point pupils to anisocoria or mydriasis and so on, occurred quite rapidly in the course of the disease.

Table 2. Symptoms and signs on admission (25 cases)

Disturbance of consciousness	21
Motor disturbance	14
Tetraparesis	6
Hemiparesis	5
Hemiparesis alternans	2
Facial paresis	1
Sensory disturbance	4
Hemihypoaesthesia	2
Facial hypoaesthesia	1
Hemihypoaesthesia excluding the face	1
Respiratory disturbance (central neurogenic hyperventilation Cheyne-Stokes respiration, etc.)	9
Hyperthermia	2
Decerebrate posture	5
Gastro-intestinal bleeding	2

Table 3. Symptoms and signs on admission (25 cases)

Abnormal pupils	19
Pinpoint	10
Anisocoria	6
Mydriasis	3
Abnormal ocular movement	16
Skew deviation	6
Rowing eye movement	3
MFL syndrome, one and half syndrome	3
Nystagmus (vertical, rotatory)	3
Ocular bobbing	1
Absence of corneal reflex	4

CT Findings and the Outcome of Treatment

Of the 25 cases, 17 were examined with CT within 5 days of onset. All were regarded as the result of hypertensive haemorrhage. The cases were classified on the basis of the size of the haematoma as shown in a transverse section through the midpons. This classification and the fate of the cases is shown in Figs. 1 and 2. The number of slices demonstrating the haematoma is also recorded, but this has not been shown to be helpful.

Group A. The size of the haematoma was less than one quarter of the transverse section of the pons, or the largest diameter was less than 1 cm (Fig. 2a).

Group B. The haematoma covered more than one-third of the cross-section or the whole cross-section of the pons. In this group the largest diameter of the haematoma was more than 1 cm, but it did not extend beyond the pons (Fig. 2b).

sagittal☆ / horizontal	1	2	3	4	5
A	O (disabled)	O (disabled) O* O**	O	O (disabled)	
B		●	●●●●●●		
C			●	●	O (vegetative) ●

• O alive ● dead
* disabled (1.5M later rebleeding) ** disabled (4M later aspiration)
• ☆ Number of slices
• A B C

less than 1cm in diameter
more than 1cm without marked extension beyond the pons
extending beyond the pons with marked hydrocephalus and ventricular haemorrhage

Fig. 1. Extension of haematoma and outcome

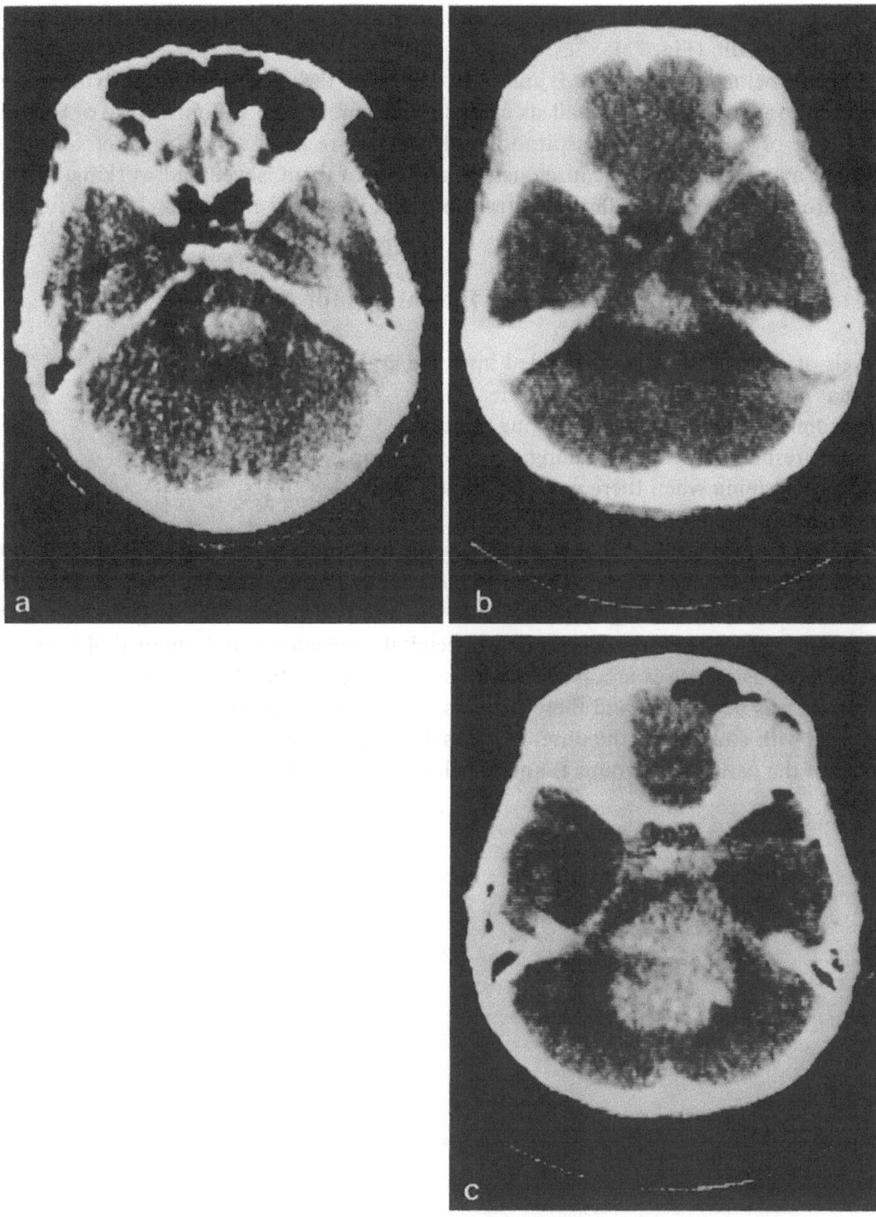

Fig. 2a – c. Classification of pontine haematomas. **a** Group A; **b** Group B; **c** Group C

Group C. The haematoma covered the whole tegmentum and the basis pontis and also extended to the cerebellum (Fig. 2c).

Patients belonging to groups B and C all died, with the exception of one living in a vegetative state. In contrast, in group A, all six cases survived more than 1 month. Two of them, however, died later of rebleeding and aspiration suffocation, respectively. The other four are all alive without any disturbance of consciousness and one of them is well and working. In these cases, haematomas were located in the rostral pons and the lower midbrain.

Disturbance of Consciousness and Indications for Operation

Levels of consciousness were divided into five grades:
Coma: not responding to any stimuli;
Semicoma: responding only to strong stimuli;
Stupor: responding to loud calling;
Drowsy: sleeping when there were no stimuli; and
Alert: normal consciousness.

In Fig. 3 the clinical course of all 25 cases is illustrated according to levels of consciousness (*ordinate*) and time (*abscissa*). The uppermost zone represents death. Cases examined by CT are marked with A, B, or C (group) and with the number of slices showing the haematoma.

In five cases, direct operation, i.e. suboccipital craniectomy and removal of haematoma, was performed. These cases are marked with solid circles in the chart. In seven cases, ventricular drainage was performed and these patients are marked with open circles. As seen in the chart, patients with coma from the onset or cases developing coma within 6 h all died within 1 week. Most of the patients in groups B and C belong to this category, except for one case in group C

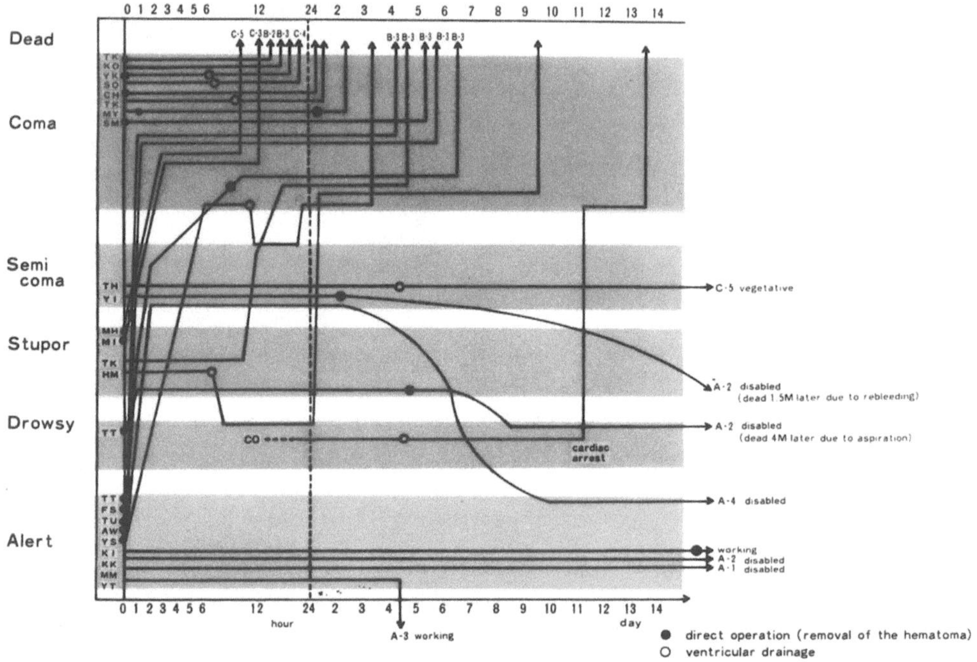

Fig. 3. Clinical course and level of consciousness

(TH) who is still living in a vegetative state. No patient in group A went into coma. Those in coma submitted to operation (two direct operation; four ventricular drainage) eventually died; all belonged to groups B and C.

Indications

From these results, it may be said that operation is not indicated for cases belonging to groups B and C, as shown in CT.

Among six cases in group A, two in semicoma or stupor underwent operation and survived 1.5 months and 4 months, but died of rebleeding and aspiration suffocation, respectively. One case with a cryptic vascular malformation (KI), who was not examined with CT but underwent direct operation 3 weeks after the onset, is well and working. Four cases in group A were treated conservatively and three are living with disability and one (YT) who was discharged on the 5th day is well and working.

Therefore, even in patients in group A, if they are hypertensive, operation is of doubtful benefit, except in instances of hydrocephalus for which ventricular drainage may be indicated. For those in group A without hypertension and below the age of 40, direct operation (removal of haematoma) may be indicated, because in such cases haemorrhage may be due to rupture of cryptic vascular malformations and rebleeding may occur unless an operation is done.

Summary and Conclusions

1) Clinical aspects of 25 cases of pontine haematoma seen from 1975 to 1978 were surveyed.
2) Among these, one had a haematoma caused by a cryptic angioma. The patient underwent direct operation (removal of haematoma) and is well and working.
3) In the other 24 cases, haematomas were probably of hypertensive origin. Among them, six with haematomas less than 1 cm in the largest diameter as shown on the CT (group A), survived more than 1 month and four of them are still living, one of them working.
4) In cases with a haematoma more than 1 cm in the largest diameter on CT (groups B and C), all died except for one living in a vegetative state.
5) The indications for operation are doubtful even for those in group A, except for patients with hydrocephalus or with suspected cryptic angiomas.

8.5 Special Technical Problems

8.5.1 General Remarks

F. J. Gillingham and K. Satyanarayana, Edinburgh

The objective of operation for spontaneous intracerebral haematomas is to remove as much of the clot as possible with minimal disturbance, to reduce local and generalized pressure. If haemostasis is required, the cause of bleeding is usually deep and focal, and a limited surface approach is sufficient. The securing of haemostasis is usually not a problem for active bleeding has often stopped by the time the patient has been admitted to hospital. Of course, if a causative lesion such as a very small arteriovenous malformation or a telangectasis is found, then it has to be removed or coagulated to reduce the risk of a recurrence of bleeding. Experience has led me away from burr-hole aspiration, for in most instances, only one-third of the volume of clot can be removed and in hypertensive patients, recurrent haemorrhage may be precipitated. In the past few years, I have preferred a small craniotomy or trephine hole of about 3 cm diameter placed over a "silent" cortical area as near to the haematoma as reasonably possible. The CT scan has helped greatly in siting the clot and its size and hence in determining the approach required. Similarly, the microscope gives good lighting and allows the definition and ablation of small vascular lesions. A narrow 5 mm speculum applied through a 2 cm cortical incision will give sufficient access to explore the clot cavity. It is entered by separating the overlying white matter with an insulated sucker following the track of a brain cannula inserted into the clot before making the cortical incision. The microscope is best used at this early stage. Low pressure suction with moderately large aperture will quickly clear the clot. High pressure suction is likely to damage the wall of the cavity, may destroy a lesion if present, and precipitate bleeding over a wide area of the wall – particularly when operation is early and associated with vascular hypertension. In fact, it pays to be fairly cautious when removing the last few millimetres of clot lining the wall. Intraventricular clots have to be followed and all the clot progressively cleared by suction and irrigation, taking care to avoid damage to ependyma, choroid plexus and veins. Small vascular malformations are sometimes discovered by removing a localized firm area of clot which covers them. They have to be excised and finally all oozing from the wall of the cavity should be stopped by gently packing with perforated nylon-covered patties. Ventricular or clot cavity drainage into a closed system at normal pressure is advisable for 72 h postoperatively to remove blood-stained CSF. It also provides the opportunity for intracranial pressure monitoring.

Careful observation over the next week is essential, especially in hypertensive patients when recurrent bleeding may sometimes be a problem. Drug control of vascular hypertension is essential.

Finally, in these severely ill and potentially disabled patients is there anything to be gained from disimpaction of tentorial and foraminal herniation after evacuation of the clot? There are two groups of patients for consideration. First, those who present as urgent problems with rapid deterioration a few hours after the ictus with evidence of midbrain ischaemia and a dilating pupil from a third nerve compression. Second, those who have major deficits including that of consciousness who have begun to deteriorate, or fail significantly to improve, after a few days. There is pathological evidence to show that although cerebral compression is generally relieved by effective removal of most of the clot, the herniations in both groups may become stuck, particularly at the level of the tentorial hiatus. Continuing midbrain ischaemia from direct compression may prevent the expected degree and speed of recovery which may be interpreted as a local disruptive effect of the initial haemorrhage. Autopsy evidence in some instances suggests otherwise. These dynamic factors are well known, but inadequately acted upon. Direct disimpaction by incision of the medial edge of the tentorium and lifting out the herniated brain has in my experience been a moderately damaging procedure. Norman Dott persuaded me some 26 years ago to deal with these problems indirectly. He gave a fairly rapid injection of 100 ml sterile Ringer's solution into the lumbar theca through a large-gauge needle after removal of clot and while the dura was still open. I speak with the tongue of the converted and use it routinely if there is evidence of midbrain compression. A degree of maintained impaction together with blood debris in the basal subarachnoid space is, of course, a cause of subsequent hydrocephalus. Fortunately, the CT scan may give us some indication of this tendency in the postoperative period (Isherwood 1976). It can confirm a clinical suspicion of hydrocephalus from failure of continuing improvement or deterioration in intellectual function.

We have already considered the results in the Edinburgh series in the light of timing of operation, and they are now being considered in relation to the operative approach used. As will be seen, this is dependent on the site and size of the clot and the means applied for its evacuation.

Burr-hole aspiration and evacuation give poor results, probably as a result of inadequate removal and haemostasis. The more definitive removal of the haematoma by craniotomy or craniectomy shows a greatly reduced mortality and morbidity. Of the 38 patients in whom this method was applied, 23 recovered well or fairly well, i.e. 60.5%. For burr-hole aspiration or evacuation, reasonably good or good survival occurred only in 1 of 20, i.e. 5%. However, there is no doubt burr-hole aspiration or evacuation was used as a desperate measure in more than half the patients (Table 1).

It is clear that lobar haematomas have the best prognosis, carrying an operative mortality of

Table 1. Degree of recovery at discharge – approximately 1 month from ictus

Type of operation	Total	0 + A	B	C	D
Burr-hole aspiration	14	0	0	5	9
Burr-hole evacuation	6	0	1	3	2
Trephine craniotomy	4	1	0	3	0
Craniotomy or craniectomy	34	11	11	10	2
Total	58	12 21%	12 21%	21 36%	13 22%

Table 2. Principal sites of intracerebral haematoma and outcome at discharge

Sites of ICH	No. of patients	Degree of recovery			
		0 + A	B	C	D
Hemispheric lobes	34	15	9	7	3
Anterior basal ganglia and basal ganglia/internal capsule and external capsule	36	4	5	21	6
Massive ICH	15	0	0	0	15

Table 3. Long-term recovery compared with recovery at discharge

Sites of ICH		Neurological deficits on admission			Recovery on discharge			Recovery at follow-up		
		I	II + III	IV + V	0 + A	B	C	0 + A	B	C + D
Hemispheric lobes	16	0	7	9	8	6	2	9	2	5
Basal ganglia/ int. capsule/ ext. capsule	15	0	2	13	3	3	9	8	3	4

8.8% and a reasonably good or good recovery in 71%. Operation for the massive haematomas was hopeless. It was poor for haematomas of the basal ganglia with a mortality of 16.7% and a reasonably good or good recovery on discharge (1 month from the ictus) of only 25%. However, in the long term, the poor survivors (grade C, 58.4%) did much better than expected, with only 27% severe morbidity or death (Tables 2, 3).

It confirms our impression of the need of definitive surgery through a trephine hole or craniectomy of adequate size or small craniotomy. The speed and extent of recovery after the more skilful and complete removal of the haematoma with the microscope in the last ten patients have been impressive. It is also clear that even in the long term, those with large or deep haematomas do badly and operation is of doubtful value, particularly when the quality of life and the human and financial cost to the patient, his relatives, and a Health Service are considered. However, abdication of the surgeon will not solve all the problems because conservative treatment will allow some of these patients to survive, although significantly fewer and often less well.

8.5.2 Craniotomy

R. Lorenz, Giessen

Independent of whether operative treatment of space-occupying intracerebral hypertensive haematomas is necessary and possible or whether conservative treatment is sufficient (see Sect. 8.3.1.2), there exists the problem of choosing the operative approach.

Computerized tomography forced us to re-evaluate the question of the operative approach for evacuation of haematoma. The extent and consistency of intracerebral haematoma and its relation to the subarachnoidal and subdural space, as well as to the ventricular system, can be much more easily evaluated than was ever possible with the help of neuroradiological and angiographic investigation. The analysis of our material is retrospective so the conclusions will have obvious limitations. Our material comprises 65 patients, 53 of whom were operated upon.

A vertical linear skin incision was used in 28 cases, and a skin flap was turned down in 25. For frontal and temporoparietal approaches the surgeon usually used the linear incision, whereas for temporal and occipital approaches, a skin flap was used (Table 1). There was no preference for either the burr-hole or enlarged burr-hole (osteoclastic craniotomy) nor for the normal craniotomy using the bone flap (Table 2). Table 3 summarizes the operative findings. The

Table 1. Type and site of skin incision

Location \ Approach	Longitudinal skin incision	Skin flap	Total
Frontal	13	3	16
Temporal	6	11	17
Temporo-parietal	4	1	5
Occipital	5	10	15
Total	28	25	53

Table 2. Type and site of craniotomy

Location \ Approach	Burr-hole	Enlarged burr-hole (craniectomy)	Bone flap	Total
Frontal	8	5	3	16
Temporal	1	4	12	17
Temporo-parietal	–	3	2	5
Occipital	2	3	10	15
Total	11	15	27	53

statement that the haematoma was liquid could be confirmed only in patients in whom the brain cortex was entered with spatulas, because simple puncture provides no information about the solid part of the haematoma. In patients in whom only burr-hole was performed it was often necessary to enter the brain to evacuate the haematoma (Table 4). In 15 cases craniectomy was performed (see Table 2); in ten the haematoma was composed mostly of solid clots. Among 27 patients in whom normal craniotomy was performed, mostly solid haematoma was found in 23. In 26 patients the lateral ventricle was entered independently from the approach used. In six patients the clots filled the ventricular system (partial ventricular tamponade) (Fig. 1). In seven patients the choroid plexus closed the site of perforation of the haematoma into the ventricle (Pia 1979). In one patient the haematoma perforated into the subdural space. The brain was entered with spatula in 37 patients (Table 5). Puncture only was performed in 14 patients. Very often before the incision of cortex, a puncture was made to release the dural tension. In two cases evacuation of the haematoma was completed with lobectomy, one temporal and one

Table 3. The form of haemorrhage and its relation to the ventricular system compared with the approach used

Type of haematoma \ Approach	Burr-hole and enlarged craniectomy (26)	Bone flap (27)	Total (53)
Liquid haematoma	16	2	18
Mostly solidified haematoma	10	23	33
Rupture into the ventricle	12	14	26
Ventricle filled with blood clots	2	4	6
Site of perforation covered by choroid plexus	2	5	7

Table 4. Approach and type of craniotomy

Approach \ Haematoma removal	Puncture	Incision of the cortex	Resection	Total
Burr-hole and craniectomy	14	11	1	26
Bone flap	–	26	1	27
Total	14	37	2	53

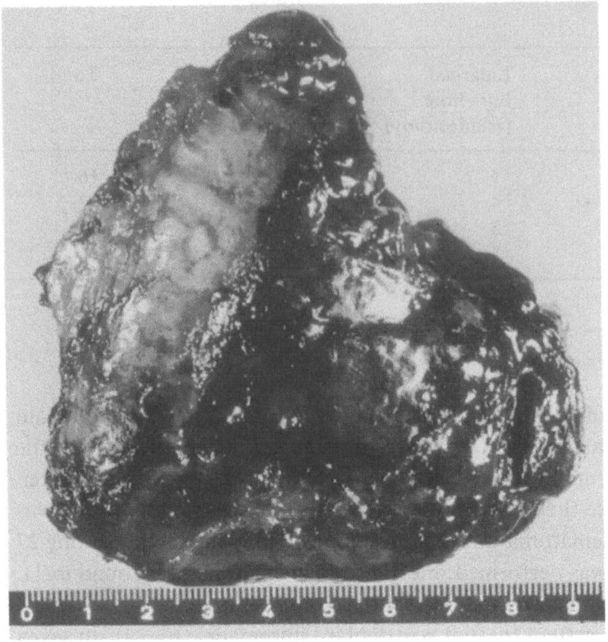

Fig. 1. Partial ventricular tamponade (ventricular clot)

Table 5. Choice of approach in relation to the timing of the operation

Approach \ History (duration)	Up to 24 h	2–7 days	>7 days	Total
Burr-hole and craniectomy	16	4	6	26
Bone flap	1	4	22	27
Total	17	8	28	53

occipitital. The choice of approach (burr-hole or craniotomy) depended strongly on the rapidity of the development of clinical signs. For operations performed in the acute phase, a rapid approach through the burr-hole was employed, whereas for patients operated on after the 1st week after the onset of bleeding, the approach through a bone flap was preferred.

The correlation between the way of approach and prognosis is a false one (Table 6). The

Table 6. Approach and early prognosis

Approach \ Result	Improvement		Died
	Rapid	Delayed	
Burr-hole and craniectomy	3	3	24
Bone flap	12	6	5
Total	15	9	29

Table 7. History and early prognosis

Prognosis \ History (duration)	Up to 24 h	2–7 days	>7 days	Total
Survived	3	2	19	24
Died	14	6	9	29
Total	17	8	28	53

clinical course is not very much influenced by an early operation performed in the acute phase. Of 17 patients operated on within 24 h after the onset of the bleeding, 14 died. Of 28 patients who survived the 1st week after the bleeding and were operated upon, only nine died (Table 7). In two cases death was caused by respiratory in sufficiency, in 2 cases by pulmonary embolism and 25 patients with hypertensive ICH died from raised intracranial pressure and/or central vegetative dysregulation, accompanied by cardiopulmonary complications.

Discussion

Stochdorph and Meessen (1957) stressed that the majority of intracerebral haematomas found at autopsy are mainly solid. In the neurosurgical material 64% of the patients had solid haematomas and of this number 17% of haematomas perforated into the ventricular system. The puncture of the haematoma without CT control must be regarded as insufficient for the evaluation of the true consistency of the haematoma. From the surgical point of view one therefore has to assume, that the cavity of the haematoma is filled with clots which cannot be aspirated in the large majority of cases. The aim of the operative treatment is:
The reduction of increased intracranial pressure;
Removal of clot and blood to diminish the cerebral reaction to the products of extravasated blood; and
Creation of conditions permitting the treatment of central dysregulation.

This aim can be accomplished only if blood has been cleared from the cavity of the haematoma and the possible source of bleeding has been stopped. It is mandatory to have an adequate approach to the haematoma cavity. It is of no great importance whether a bone flap (slightly more time-consuming) or enlarged burr-hole (craniectomy) is used.

Case Report

A 58-year-old female presented with headaches of 2 weeks duration, confusion and right-sided weakness with speech disturbances 24 h prior to admission. On admission there was a complete right-sided hemiplegia and complete aphasia and the patient was in coma. Computerized tomography showed a large parieto-occipital haemorrhage with perforation into the ventricular system (Fig. 2). The patient was considered to have an intracerebral haemorrhage, particularly as she was on warfarin therapy because of thrombosis, and she had a Quick test index of 19%. She had a cervical carcinoma 3 years before. A burr-hole of 3 cm diameter was made in the left occipital region, and the cavity of the haematoma was cleared of clots. The walls of the cavity were smooth. A small branch of the Sylvian artery which bled was clipped. The patient made an

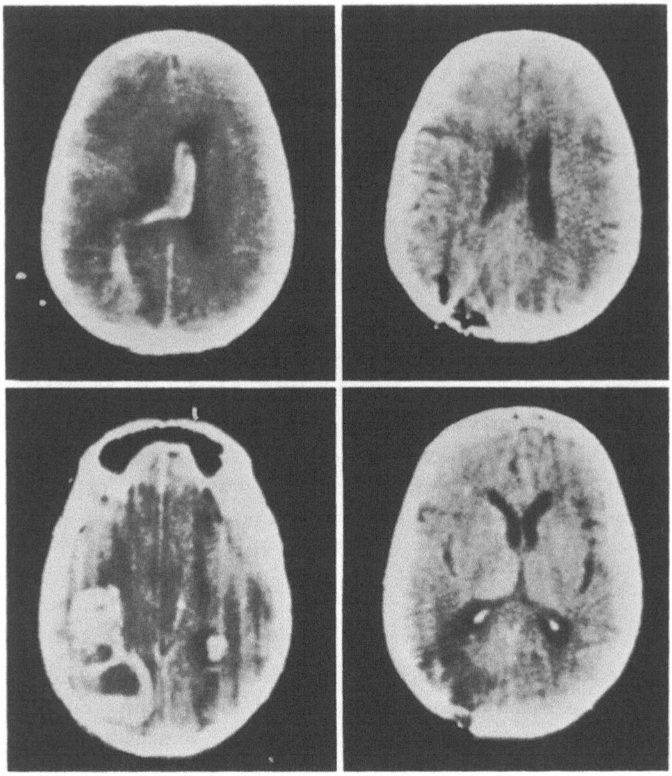

Fig. 2. CT in a case of large parieto-occipital haematoma with rupture into the ventricle, (pre-operatively (left) and postoperatively (right))

uneventful recovery, and the right-sided weakness and speech disturbances improved considerably. A check CT scan confirmed that the blood clots were almost completely removed.

It is preferable to perform an osteoplastic craniotomy particularly if one wishes to avoid later possible pressure variations and also for cosmetic reasons. Puncture of the haematoma permits the reduction of raised intracranial pressure for a short period, but it will not influence the course of the central dysregulation.

Computerized tomography permits:
Exact delineation, location and estimation of the extent of the intracerebral haematoma;
Visualization of the relation of the haematoma to the CSF spaces;
Visualization of the accompanying oedema and brain softening; and
Evaluation of the degree of displacement.

CT provides very important indices which help to decide the necessity and timing of operation with possible sequelae, and it helps to find the most direct approach to the haematoma cavity.

Summary

Of patients with hypertensive ICH, 76% had a haematoma composed mostly of blood clots. In 17% the ventricular system was filled at least partially with blood clots and in 50% a communication was present between the cavity of the haematoma and the ventricles. Osteoplastic craniotomy is the preferred way of approaching the haematoma cavity. Computerized tomography permits the choice of the most direct approach to the haematoma. Postoperative CT provides good control of the immediate result of haematoma removal.

8.5.3 Burr-Hole Evacuation

R. Müke, Hamburg

Before the introduction of CT scanning, only 70% of all intracerebral haematomas could be recognized as space-occupying lesions, and it was sometimes difficult to differentiate these lesions. The extent and limits of the haematoma was often uncertain. Therefore, it was only logical to make a big bone flap to get an adequate exposure for the removal of the haematoma. With the introduction of computerized tomography it became easy to recognize intracranial haematomas as zones of higher density in their location, extent and relation to the neighbouring structures. With the information provided by CT it seems to us that a burr-hole is big enough to reach the haematoma.

A second reason for making a bone flap was the idea that total removal of the haematoma should be performed; this reason also needs to be discussed. From the clinical course and CT follow-up of patients with large intracerebral bleedings – not operated on because they had no critical intracranial pressure – we know that spontaneous resorption of the haematoma and a total clinical recovery are possible. We have seen spontaneous recoveries even in cases with massive ventricular haematomas in a poor clinical state (Fig. 1). In addition, intracranial pressure measurements showed that in critical cases of raised intracranial pressure this could be relieved if only a few cubic centimetres of the haematoma were removed.

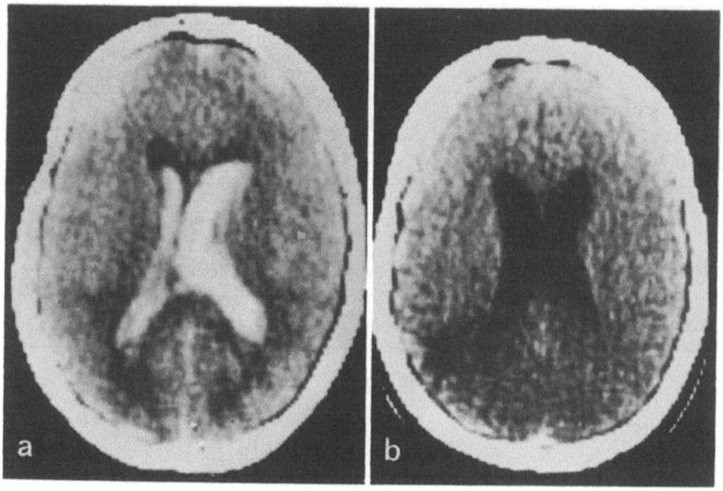

Fig. 1. a Massive intraventricular haematoma; **b** Spontaneous resorption

Therefore, we think that a subtotal removal of the haematoma through a burr-hole should be sufficient in most cases. Only if we intend to remove a tumour which is bleeding or to operate on an angioma or aneurysm in one procedure do we use a big bone flap.

A burr-hole can be done immediately under local anaesthetic without major preparation and with no stress for the patient. The burr-hole may sometimes be enlarged up to 2 or 3 cm in diameter. After coagulation and incision of the brain the haematoma is opened, using two small spatulas, and is evacuated by suction. We remove as much of the haematoma as is easily possible, often more than necessary to release the critical pressure. We prefer this method also in acute cases instead of aspiration with needle and syringe.

Since the introduction of the CT scan in July 1976 we have treated 42 patients with intracerebral haematomas in this way. In no case was a second operation necessary because of rebleeding. The prognosis of intracerebral bleedings after burr-hole evacuation seems by no means worse than after a bone flap, a fact, interestingly enough, already mentioned by McKissock in 1959. The prognosis depends on different factors: the aetiology, the age of the patient, the level of consciousness and the location of the bleeding. The principal points in the timing of the operation were the critical intracranial pressure and the loss of consciousness. Most of our operations (33 of 42) were done in the 1st day after the onset of the bleeding. We do not agree with postponing the operation in these cases until the end of the 1st or 2nd week, as Lazorthes (1959) has recommended. In cases without risk to life our decision to operate depends on the severity of the neurological deficit and its remission. We know from Sussmann et al. (1974) about the metabolic changes in the tissue adjacent to the haematoma. In these cases, however, the time factor is not so important.

One of the most important factors for the prognosis is the aetiology (Table 1). Of 15 patients with spontaneous intracerebral bleeding of unknown aetiology, possibly cases with so-called micro-angiomas, only one died. This was despite the fact that some of these patients were operated on when in a very bad condition and also that in six of these cases the intracerebral haematoma was combined with an intraventricular haematoma. Most of these cases were adults

Table 1. Spontaneous intracerebral haematomas – prognosis

Aetiology	Survived	Died
Hypertension	–	7
Aneurysm	3	4
Angioma		
Bleeding disorders	3	7
Tumour	3	1
Unknown	14	1

Table 2. Spontaneous intracerebral haematomas – prognosis

Quality of life	
Able to work	10
Take care of themselves	2
Need permanent care	8
Unknown	2
Total	22

younger than 50 (13 of 15). Of ten patients with bleeding disorders, seven died; of seven patients with hypertension all died.

Concerning the quality of life postoperatively, of 22 patients, ten are able to work and earn their living without limitation; two are out of work but can take care of themselves; eight need permanent care; and two have been lost to follow-up (Table 2).

To stress these points the CT scans are shown and the clinical course of three patients operated on with a burr-hole evacuation is indicated.

Case 1. A 47-year-old male with a large parietal haematoma (Fig. 2a), deeply comatose on admission, was operated on in July 1977 and re-examined 3 months later (Fig. 2b). At this time he was able to come by public transport and showed only a slight dysphasia.

Case 2. A 50-year-old male presented with a huge left-sided occipital haematoma which ruptured into the ventricular system (Fig. 3a). Stuporous before operation, he is now fully

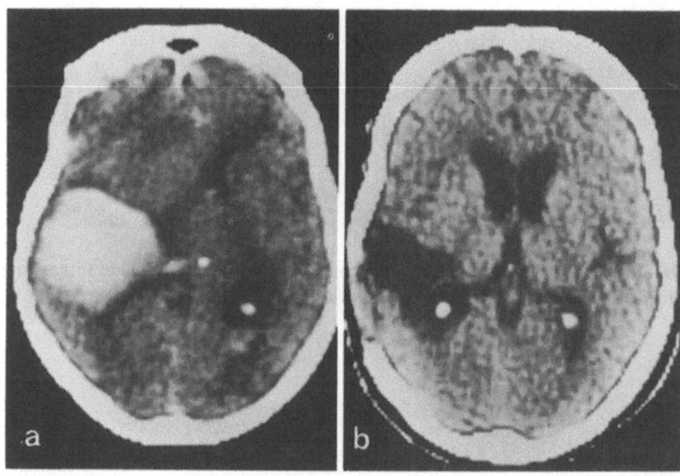

Fig. 2. a Large parietal haematoma; **b** Three months later, after subtotal burr-hole evacuation

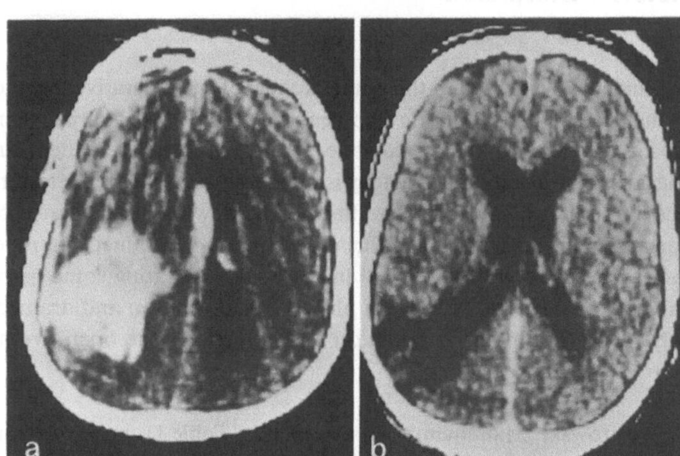

Fig. 3. a Huge left-sided occipital haematoma with rupture into the ventricular system; **b** Two months later, after subtotal burr-hole evacuation

conscious and ambulatory with only a slight right-sided hemiparesis which is still improving (Fig. 3b).

Case 3. A 36-year-old female presented with a right frontal haematoma combined with an extensive intraventricular haematoma (Fig. 4a). Comatose before operation, she is now without neurological deficits (Fig. 4b) and only a slight psychotic syndrome persists.

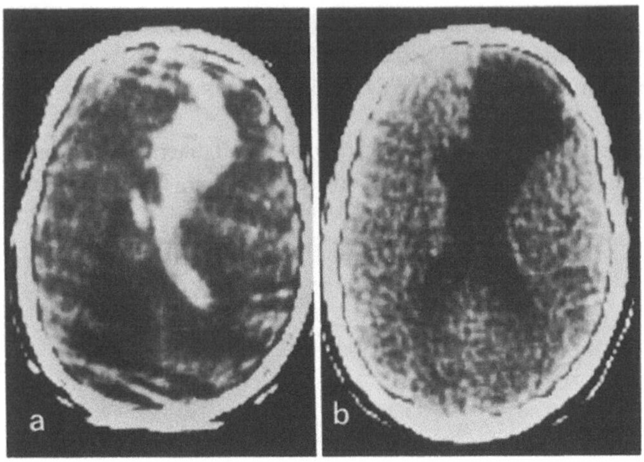

Fig. 4. a Right frontal haematoma combined with an extensive intraventricular haematoma; **b** Six weeks later, after subtotal burr-hole evacuation

8.5.3.1 Discussion

B. Guidetti, Rome: From the point of view of our operative technique we preferred in all cases to make a small osteoplastic flap centred on the cortical area where the haematoma appeared most superficial, avoiding damage to any important eloquent areas. Personally we do not consider that a trephine opening is adequate for the complete removal of a haematoma. On opening the dura we reach the haemorrhage with the guidance of a ventricular needle. The haematoma is then evacuated through a small cortical incision under direct vision. The walls of the cavity are carefully explored in the hope of locating some pathological tissue, the cavity is irrigated abundantly with warm physiological solution and drained through a silicone catheter for 24 – 48 h. Bipolar coagulation and sometimes the operative microscope are of particular help.

W. Piotrowski, Mannheim: Our experience (Table 1), however limited, proves that craniotomy gives the best results in the treatment of intracerebral haematomas. Of 25 cases, 14 survived. With evacuation through a burr-hole, only 4 of 11 patients survived. In spite of these findings we always started with burr-hole evacuation.

Table 1. Spontaneous intracerebral haemorrhage, 1973 – 1978

Surgical method	Postoperative	
	Surviving	Deceased
Burr-hole	4	7
Craniotomy	14	11
Total	18	18

8.5.4 Operative Technique in Putaminal and Thalamic ICH

K. Kitamura and M. Kagawa, Tokyo

A craniotomy should be used and not a trephine opening. A 2 – 3 cm cortical incision is made immediately over the clot, usually in the superior temporal gyrus. The haematoma is exposed through the cortical incision and removed by suction and saline irrigation.

Total removal of the mass of blood should be performed if possible, but the clot which adheres tightly to the wall of the haematoma cavity should be allowed to remain so that further injury to the surrounding brain tissue may be avoided.

Arterial bleeding may be noted during haematoma removal. This is probably the cause of the original haematoma. Arterial bleeding is controlled with bipolar coagulation or with a clip. Any area of venous oozing should be controlled with oxidized cellulose or gelatin sponge.

In many cases direct visualization with magnifying lens and headlight or an operating microscope might be helpful during this stage of the procedure.

Another technique used is the exposure of the insula by dividing the arachnoid membrane and opening up the Sylvian fissure. The haematoma is then removed through an incision of the insular cortex (cf. Suzuki 1977).

If excessive swelling or perifocal oedema of the brain are noted, the bone flap may be removed for external decompression.

The most important surgical complication is the re-accumulation of blood. Some authors suggested that a drain should be left in the haematoma cavity for 24 h. However, we do not use a drain except when ventricular drainage is necessary because of rupture of the haematoma into the ventricle.

Haematomas in the thalamus were rarely operated on. The technique adopted in the most early trials was a craniotomy. The haematoma was removed through either the transcallosal or the infratentorial-supracerebellar approach. A few cases were approached transcortically. However, recently we consider that a direct operation on the haematoma is not indicated in thalamic haemorrhage. In the case of massive intraventricular haematoma or acute hydrocephalus, ventricular drainage appears to offer some advantages not only in terms of reduction of intracranial pressure but also in the evacuation of the haematoma (Fig. 1).

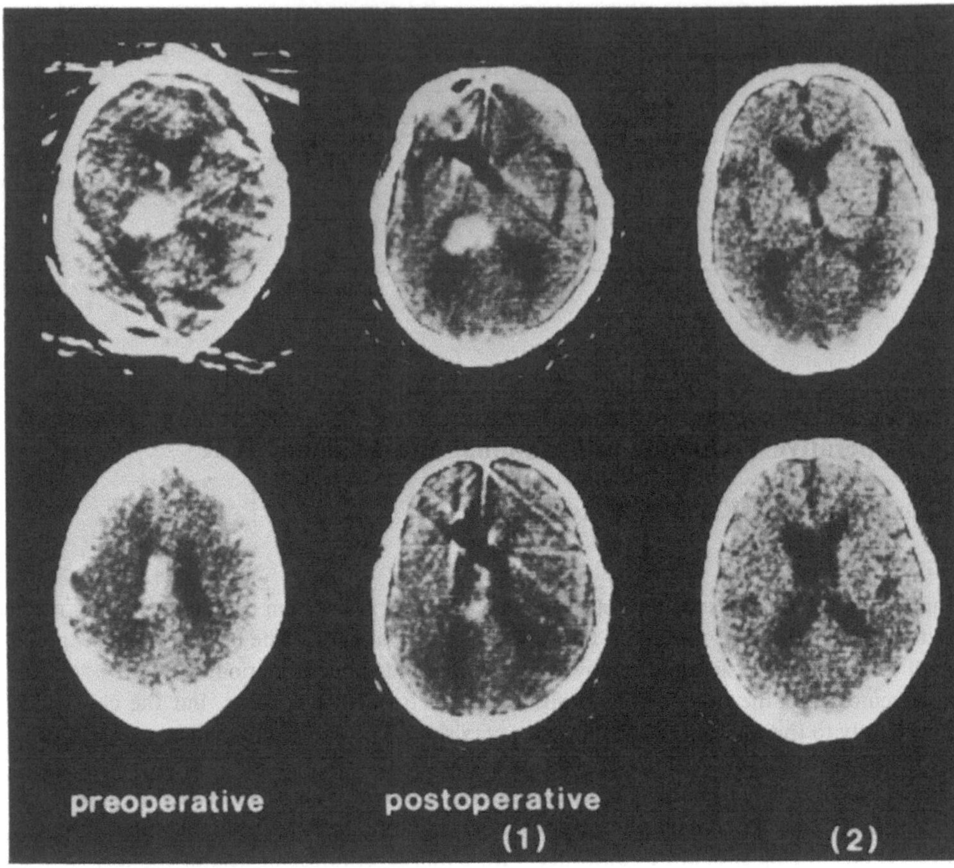

Fig. 1. Thalamic haemorrhage treated with continuous ventricular drainage

8.5.4.1 Trans-Sylvian Approach to Putaminal Haematomas

J. Suzuki and A. Takaku, Sendai

In 1972 we reported in the Japanese Journal of Surgery a new operative technique (Suzuki and Sato) for putaminal haematoma. This uses the trans-Sylvian approach, by which the haematoma can be evacuated with minimal or no brain damage. This short paper explains the key points in the technique of the trans-Sylvian approach.

Operative Procedure (Fig. 1)

Pre-operatively, 1000 ml 20% mannitol is usually administered intravenously. The patient is placed in the supine position with his head turned about 60° to the side. A linear skin incision

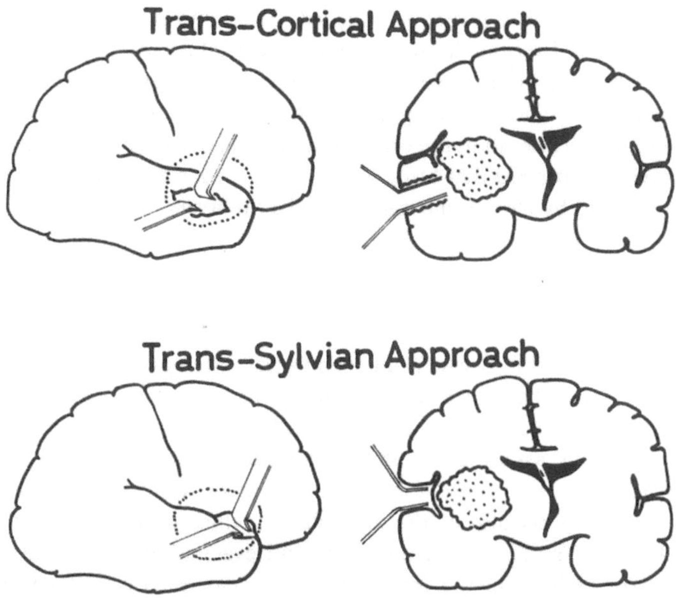

Fig. 1. Comparison of surgical approach to intracerebral haematoma. Upper, the conventional trans-cortical approach; lower, the new trans-Sylvian approach

about 6 cm in length from the hair-line is made on the line between the upper and outer border of the orbit and the anterior three-quarters point between nasion and inion. This line will be on the Sylvian fissure. After the dissection of the muscle and the periosteum from the skull surface, the bone of the frontotemporal region, particularly the sphenoidal ridge, is rongeured away to make an opening about 5 cm in diameter. The dura mater is then opened and the Sylvian fissure is exposed. Both sides of the Sylvian fissure are then lined with cotton swabs, producing pressure on the overlying arachnoid. Having raised the veins of this region, careful dissection is made of the arachnoid over the Sylvian fissure and an initial opening is made into the arachnoid. After dividing the arachnoid a further 2 cm, the deep portion of the Sylvian fissure is approached by gently separating its lips with a couple of spatulas 3-mm wide. Damage to the brain tissue and blood vessels is avoided by protective cotton swabs. The approach is easily accomplished if a 2 cm opening in the Sylvian fissure can be gently made. Continuing this approach, the insular cortex, over which run the middle cerebral artery and its branches, can be detected. The haematoma usually lies directly beneath the insular cortex, which is often slightly swollen and has a yellow tinge. By inserting a Dandy cannula posteriomedially so as not to damage blood vessels, if they have not already disintegrated because of the haematoma, the haematoma will be discovered at a depth of 1 cm at the most. Sufficient lighting is provided by using about 3 mm spatulas in the opening, and aspiration of as much as possible of the haematoma is undertaken.

At the time of evacuation of haematoma, the healthy and even softened brain tissue surrounding the haematoma should not be removed particularly at the bottom of the haematoma cavity where important regions such as the internal capsule, thalamus and hypothalamus usually lie. Immediately after the aspiration the white colour of "normal" brain tissue appears directly at the bottom of the haematoma, sufficient cotton swabs should be used to prevent any injuries of the important brain tissue. Absolutely none of the softened brain in that area should be aspirated. The internal surface of the brain should be protected by cotton swabs to which a thread is attached. The removal of the haematoma is completed, and the cavity rinsed repeatedly with physiological saline. As the cortical origin of the haematoma is directly behind the visible area, it is not easily aspirated. Its removal is facilitated by bending the suction tube and relying upon the sounds of suction to complete the evacuation. By the end of the surgical operation the brain volume will have decreased, facilitating the surgical procedure. Having confirmed that bleeding has stopped, the dura mater is tightly closed and the operation completed by closing the muscles and skin layers.

Discussion

During the last decade, many surgical attempts have been made to treat hypertensive intracerebral haemorrhages but the results have not always been satisfactory. Therefore, new surgical techniques and surgical indications must be considered.

Burr-hole aspiration of the haematomas, traditionally employed, is a convenient method which does not cause too much operative trauma. However, the method is not always satisfactory because of the difficulty in removing the clot completely and in controlling the bleeding points. Large craniotomy and evacuation necessitate a comparatively large incision and/or excision of the cortex over the haematoma cavity, causing further destruction of the normal brain tissue because of the great distance between the haematoma cavity and the brain surface. On the other hand, the transinsular approach through the Sylvian fissure which we propose makes it possible to reach the insular surface without causing any brain damage, and it greatly shortens the distance to be covered. Occasionally it is possible to observe on the surface of the insula the swelling caused by the haematoma, and in some cases the haematoma may spurt out spontaneously. The significant advantages offered by the new approach are that the brain damage inflicted during surgical intervention is reduced to the minimum of only a small incision over the cortex of the insula. A complete removal of the haematoma can also be easily achieved.

However, as we stress in this report it is necessary not to damage any healthy brain tissue. Satisfactory results can only be expected if the operation is performed with careful attention to the details of technique which we have outlined here (Suzuki and Sato 1976; see also Sect. 8.5.5.1).

8.5.5 Continuous Ventricular Drainage

E. Grote, Giessen

There are two indications for this procedure in treating spontaneous ventricular haematomas.

1) In all cases of ventricular haematoma obstructing the third and fourth ventricle, hydrocephalus may develop quickly and should be treated as we did in a case of an AV malformation of cerebellar origin completely blocking the fourth ventricle and causing obstruction. After drainage for a few days the ventricular size diminished considerably. However, particularly in patients with haematomas from AV angiomas and aneurysms, there are hazards in this procedure of lowering the pressure; rebleeding may occur after pressure

tamponade is relieved, as we found in a case of thalamic AV angioma. After bilateral frontal drainage, CSF was at first only blood stained; then arterial bleeding recurred and the pressure rose to 100 cm of water.

2) We are convinced that blood in the CSF contributes to vessel spasm, which may lead to functional deterioration and death. We are also sure that blood in the ventricular system causes diencephalic dysregulation which is often followed by serious complications and a gloomy outcome. Removal of blood by continuous drainage seems to make sense but, of course, a coagulated intraventricular haematoma cannot be evacuated by drainage. In a case of an intracerebral and intraventricular haemorrhage we installed a drainage through bilateral frontal burr-holes. During the next 2 days a few 100 ml blood-stained CSF escaped, but the intraventricular clot remained almost the same size. Sedimented and clotted blood was not removed. Intraventricular haematomas are dissolved only by fibrinolysis which should start a few days after the bleed. On theoretical grounds continuous CSF drainage should diminish fibrinolytic activity which is necessary to dissolve clots. Whether continuous drainage is capable of preventing an aneurysm from rebleeding by reducing fibrinolytic activity has not yet been proved. According to our experience, although continuous ventricular drainage may be of help in reducing intracranial pressure in obstructive hydrocephalus, it may also be hazardous.

8.5.5.1 Technical Note

J. Suzuki and A. Takaku, Sendai

Continuous ventricular drainage (CVD) has been accepted as a method for the relief of intracranial hypertension. However, this method is not always effective in cases with ventricular haemorrhage, because in such cases a drainage tube is apt to be occluded by clots.

We will describe our operative method of CVD in cases with ventricular haemorrhage (Figs. 1, 2). It seems to be important to perform the ventricular drainage bilaterally in all cases of ventricular haemorrhage, because one drainage tube is apt to be occluded by the clots. Two

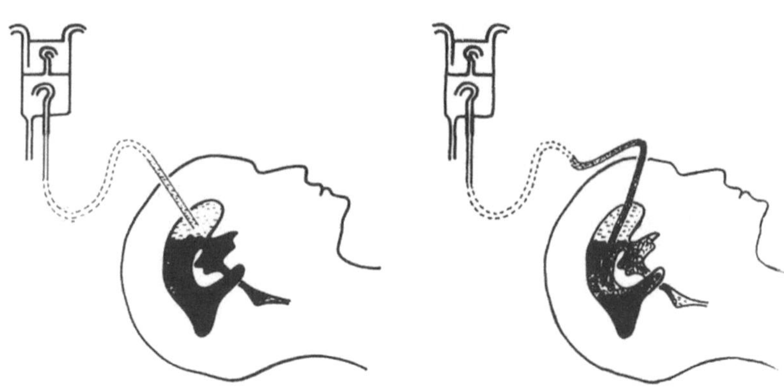

Fig. 1. Comparison of surgical procedures for ventricular haemorrhage. *Left,* the conventional method of continuous ventricular drainage; *Right,* our method of continuous ventricular drainage for ventricular haemorrhage

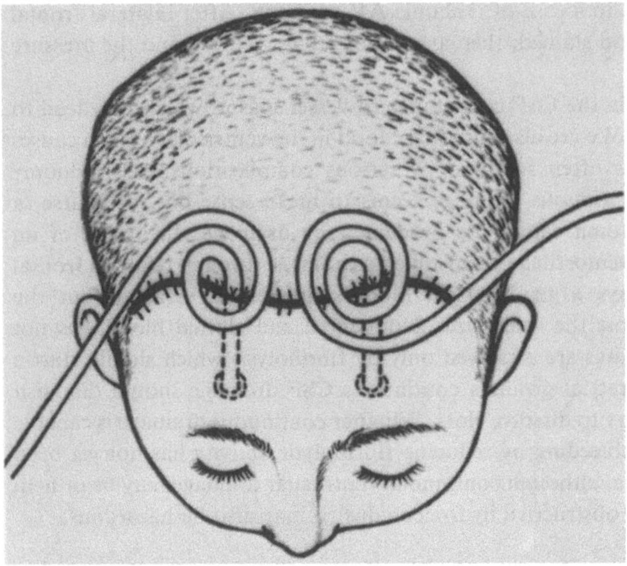

Fig. 2. Diagram of operative procedure for continuous ventricular drainage for ventricular haemorrhage

drainage tubes will be useful as an emergency measure in case one tube should become occluded by clots. A bilateral linear skin incision about 10 cm in length within the frontal hair line is performed. A flap of skin, muscle and periosteum is dissected in the direction of the orbital edges, and small burr-holes are then made bilaterally at the most anterior portion of the frontal bone. The drainage tubes should be inserted into the lateral ventricles from the frontal tip, as nearly parallel as possible to the body of the ventricles. By placing the tubing into the ventricles in such a direction we are able to aspirate a quantity of clots from the ventricles even as far back as the occipital horn. On the other hand, if the conventional direction of insertion is used from posterior point of frontal hair line, we will soon encounter the opposite ventricle wall and be unable to aspirate a sufficient quantity of clot. After the evacuation and frequent rinsing with saline solution, the tip of the drain must remain in the frontal horn in which the clots have disappeared completely. The drainage tube must then be fixed firmly to the scalp by several silk sutures, after which the drainage tube is connected to the drainage apparatus and allowed to drain at an appropriate pressure.

Discussion

To remove an adequate amount of ventricular haematoma, the cannula for aspiration of these haematoma must be inserted sufficiently deeply into the lateral ventricle. To achieve this we consider that the method described here is relatively easy to perform and can be used to aspirate haematoma from both lateral ventricles. However, in a few cases, the intraventricular clot is too hard to be aspirated. In such cases it is necessary that a small cortical incision is performed to the tip of the frontal horn and the haematoma is removed under direct vision.

Ventriculoperitoneal shunt should be promptly performed, if the intraventricular pressure is shown to be continuously high after the continuous ventricular drainage and the ventricular CSF has cleared and is no longer haemorrhagic. This method of continuous ventricular drainage will be useful not only in cases of primary ventricular haemorrhage, but also in secondary cases resulting from ruptured intracranial aneurysms and arteriovenous malformations.

8.5.6 Shunt Operations

J. Zierski, Giessen

In contrast to external ventricular drainage, which is occasionally employed in the acute phase in treating intracerebral haematoma with ventricular rupture, direct shunting during this stage has not been used and there is no rationale for doing it. The possible exceptions during the acute phase are the rare cases of isolated pontine and cerebellar haematomas which may produce obstruction of the fourth ventricle and aqueduct leading to acute hydrocephalus. It depends on the personal preference of the surgeon, whether to put an external drainage or a shunt and drain the ventricles before approaching the lesion directly. Taking into account the rarity of a correct pre-operative diagnosis of a pontine haematoma one may presume that there will be patients in whom a shunt was inserted as the only treatment of a pontine lesion suspected of being a tumour, but which was in fact a haematoma.

The other problem is the indication for shunting in patients who have survived their intracerebral haemorrhage and show some degree of ventricular enlargement. We do not have sufficient data to tell how many patients develop obstructive hydrocephalus after intracranial haemorrhage. Ventricular enlargement which progresses with the resorption or is found after evacuation of the haematoma should not be surprising in view of the loss of brain substance produced by the haemorrhage. The obstruction of the subarachnoid space with increased outflow resistance to CSF seems to occur in these patients much less frequently than in patients who have had a subarachnoid haemorrhage or a head injury. It has been shown that early ventricular enlargement after subarachnoid haemorrhage may subside spontaneously without requiring a shunt. Our shunting rate in the last 6 years for patients with subarachnoid haemorrhage from vascular malformations is around 1%, although in some centres the rate seems to be much higher. Of 135 patients with intracerebral haemorrhages of different aetiology, seven had external drainage at the acute stage but did not require conversion to shunt. In three patients a ventriculo-atrial shunt was employed between 1 and 3 months after the evacuation of a haematoma, because of hydrocephalus with increased intracranial pressure verified by ventricular pressure measurement.

One patient with clinical signs of classic "normal pressure hydrocephalus" verified by air and isotope study was a potential candidate for a shunt, but his family refused the operation.

Summary

Patients surviving spontaneous intracerebral haematoma caused by factors other then vascular malformations require a shunting procedure as an exceptional measure. The criteria for shunting should be considered very carefully and should include clinical evidence of secondary deterioration after recovery from the haemorrhage, detailed evaluation with computer tomography and an intracranial pressure study before the decision on placing a shunt is made.

9 Conclusions

9.1 Conservative and Surgical Management

F. John Gillingham, Edinburgh

In general it is remarkable how closely we are in agreement about what should be done. Patients with smaller haematomas who are alert, stable or improving, should be treated conservatively – probably with dexamethasone and other anti-oedema agents. The CT scan will almost certainly confirm that in these patients, the haematoma is small. Assuming that the cause of bleeding is not due to a structural lesion, we must then determine possible causes of bleeding with the broad screening of all possible factors, in particular, investigation of the dyscrasias and diagnosis of hypertension. This requires the help of a team, including haematologists and cardiovascular physicians.

Patients who have larger clots, but who are stable and with a reasonable level of consciousness should be investigated as soon as possible with CT scan and angiography and the clot evacuated. But when? I detect two schools of thought – those who favour operating on or about the 3rd day when most patients will have either improved to some extent or deteriorated hopelessly, and those who favour operating as soon as possible. Operation should be definitive and removal of clot fairly complete. Of course, those with blood dyscrasias or on anticoagulant therapy have to be properly protected to the point of normal coagulation before operation is carried out. So when do we evacuate spontaneous intracerebral haematomas? The CT scan and the operating microscope may have changed things, thus encouraging earlier intervention, but therefore a new evaluation is required to help us make this decision.

The results of evacuation of the clot in normotensive patients are certainly better than in hypertensive patients, and the risk of recurrent haemorrhage after operation is greater in hypertensive patients. However, a medical team must control vascular hypertension carefully and continuously and when this is carried out it may further improve the results of operation in these groups.

Patients with haematomas of the basal ganglia do better in the long run than in the short, and they should be treated surgically with patient optimism and good rehabilitation, waiting for the best results many months later. Patients with massive or bilateral haematomas and those deteriorating into deep coma with large clots should be left alone. The overall cost to the patients themselves, their relatives and to Health Services is too great. Cerebellar haematomas always need early operations unless they are small (2 cm in diameter or less). Open transcortical operations on thalamic haematomas are contra-indicated because of high morbidity, but stereotactic aspiration may help, particularly after a few days when the haematoma has become more fluid. The trans-Sylvian technique described by Suzuki may well offer the possibility of decreased morbidity and improved results.

Patients over 60 years of age have to be considered carefully before operation is performed and by an interview with their relatives, their physiological age has to be estimated in the light of their physical and intellectual performance before the ictus. In addition one has to consider the severity of the haemorrhage and its site, and the association with hypertension and other diseases such as diabetes mellitus. If they are young for their age, normotensive and in a reasonably high grade (of consciousness and neurological deficit), operation is then worthwhile. The aim of surgery is not only to save life, but rather to save its quality.

The possibility of trauma as a factor in all "spontaneous" intracerebral haematomas has to be thought of and a clear history always obtained. The CT scan helps greatly because it shows the size, shape and site of the clot. If it lies closely adjacent to the lesser wing of the sphenoid and in the temporal polar area, or inferior part of the frontal lobe, then it may well be traumatic in origin.

Further help in deciding what to do and when to do it may come from advances in cerebral blood flow studies, circulation times, and the newer Positron Emission Scanner which one hopes will show the functional activity and potential of the brain surrounding the clot. Above all, there is little doubt that we need to establish cooperative studies with larger series and to do this, we have to establish some system of grading of conscious level and neurological deficit. A few have already been put forward – two from our Japanese colleagues and one of my own. With respect to grading of consciousness, it is important to record evidence of primary or secondary midbrain involvement as shown by early or late signs of decerebrate rigidity which of course may arise from primary haematomas adjacent to the midbrain or from secondary displacement from a more distant clot. The lesions in the second group of patients may be reversible if handled early and effectively.

9.2 Prospects

The Editors

Introduction

The present workshop provided a review of the attitudes toward the problem of spontaneous intracerebral bleeding caused by conditions other than demonstrable vascular malformations. The subject has been extensively studied and analysed in detail from the anatomical, clinical and pathological viewpoint and it seemed there was little further one could add to the enormous amount of work already done. The existing knowledge was impressively reviewed here by Zülch and Jellinger in their opening contributions.

On the other hand the therapeutic attitude still undergoes changes and, although as Gillingham mentioned, "a remarkable degree of agreement has been achieved", there are different opinions concerning such important points as indications for operative treatment, timing and the comparison between surgical and conservative management.

Such differences in the approach to treatment and in the evaluation of results have their obvious causes:

The first is the paucity of stroke centres, in which both medical and surgical care are available and where patients with stroke can be admitted directly. Thus, the vast majority of neurosurgical units has no control over the system of referral so that effectively the decision upon conservative or operative treatment has already been made before the patient is seen by a neurologist or neurosurgeon. The neurosurgical centres, therefore, are dealing with a selected group of patients and have no possibility of comparing the results of surgical and conservative treatment. The same is true in the opposite direction.

The second is the lack of a uniform grading system, which would permit reasonable comparison of the effects of treatment in different units.

The third is the lack of a uniform and exhaustive anatomical classification of intracerebral haemorrhages in patients surviving the bleeding.

A coordinated effort to overcome these difficulties in the form of a cooperative study was suggested during the workshop by Gillingham and Pia. The need of it arises from the impact which the management of haemorrhages has received since the introduction of CT, a fact which was repeatedly stressed during the workshop. It is felt that now that the majority of larger neurological and neurosurgical centres have a CT at their disposal a *prospective* study is feasible.

The Aim of the Study

The aim is to evaluate the present state of management of ICH, to analyse the factors influencing the mortality and morbidity under standardized uniform aspects and to provide enough statistical data to permit unbiased conclusions with the best possible significance as to the mode of management.

In contrast to any existing surveys on cerebral stroke the present study will concentrate only on spontaneous cerebral haemorrhage, its management and follow-up. A comprehensive epidemiological survey is outside the scope of this project, and a detailed pathological study does not seem to be necessary in view of the data already accumulated.

Participation

It is indispensable that only centres in which neurological and neurosurgical units are closely linked and collaborating and which have CT facilities should take part in the study.

Organization

A central unit will prepare the necessary protocols, decide upon admission to the study and evaluate the accumulated data. The evaluation will be controlled by

1) Principal Neurological Investigator;
2) Principal Neurosurgical Investigator.

Further medical staff will incorporate

1) Principal Neuroradiological Adviser;
2) Principal Medical Adviser;
3) Principal Epidemiological Adviser;
4) Principal Rehabilitation Adviser.

In each centre participating in the study a surgical and neurological investigator will be appointed and will be responsible for the collection of data. They will of course collaborate closely with the corresponding neuroradiologist and other medical staff in their own centre. The mode of management of patients and the choice of treatment will be left absolutely to the discretion of the physician/surgeon treating. Whether the patient fulfils the criteria of admission to the study will be decided by the principal investigators.

The following protocols will be used:

1) General clinical protocol;
2) Neurological protocol;
3) CT and neuroradiological protocol;

4) Treatment protocol (medical);
5) Treatment protocol (surgical);
6) Follow-up and rehabilitation protocol.

Remarks Concerning the Classification and Evaluation of the Results

The necessity for uniformity in grading and classification has clearly emerged from the workshop. The grading systems as presented by Gillingham, Frowein, Kanaya and Suzuki vary slightly, but have many features in common with the established grading systems already in use for cerebral vascular diseases such as those of Botterell, Hunt, VanderArk and Kahn. From the papers presented at the workshop it is apparent that the level of consciousness and responsiveness is the single most important factor in deciding the choice of treatment on the one hand and the further fate of the patient on the other. It seems therefore that the scoring system used in the Glasgow Coma Scale, which has already been tested and proved to be useful for comparison of patients with cerebral trauma may also be used in patients with spontaneous intracerebral haemorrhage. It is recommended that a five-grade system be used for the level of consciousness, neurological deficit and, with some modification, for the follow-up, as proposed by Gillingham during the workshop. For scoring purposes it would be extended by three-grade scale of decerebration (primary and secondary) and five-point scale of medical factors (hypertension, diabetes, coagulation disorders, vascular disorders, cardiac and renal disorders). The weight of the score in relation to the further progress of the patients will be tested in the study.

It is obvious that a detailed CT classification taking into account the data presented in the literature and at the workshop (New, Kazner, Kitamura) should be the basis upon which further evaluations will be made. The evaluation of CT data will include, apart from the anatomical points, changing phenomena such as accompanying oedema (Nagai), progress of absorption (Laun) and volume measurement (Matsukado).

Duration of Study

The workshop showed that the number of patients with spontaneous ICH due to other conditions than vascular malformations treated surgically varies from centre to centre and even in large centres does not exceed 100 – 200 patients treated over a span of 10 – 20 years. The number of such patients treated conservatively in non-surgical centres is much higher.

Depending on the number of centres participating in the study it will be aimed to take in 1000 – 1500 patients within the period of 2 years. The follow-up period should be at least 3 years and, if the study is successful, a 5-year evaluation can take place.

Final Remarks

The editors of the proceedings of the workshop felt obliged to present this project to adhere to the direct conclusions achieved at the meeting in Bad Nauheim. They have chosen this perhaps unusual form of announcing the study in the hope of appealing to a much larger number of neurosurgeons and neurologists than the participants in the workshop and readers of specialized journals. Their comments on the feasibility of the study and participation will be welcomed.

We have little to add to the statement by Gillingham expressed in Bad Nauheim:

"If we spend resources on the irretrievable by determined intervention, then help may have to be withheld from the retrievable, those who could make much of it. If, therefore, we can define with reasonable clarity the groups of patients in which we can achieve a good quality of life by immediate or delayed operation or other treatment, then we shall have made a significant contribution."

Comments, inquiries and declarations to participate in the study should be sent to:

Cooperative Study on Spontaneous ICH
c/o Department of Neurosurgery
University of Giessen
Klinikstr. 29
6300 Giessen
Federal Republic of Germany

10 References

Abrams IF, Yessayan L, Shillito J, Barlow CF (1971) Spontaneous intracerebral haemorrhage in patients suspected of multiple sclerosis. J Neurol Neurosurg Psychiatry 34:157 – 162

Adams RD, van der Eecken HM (1953) Vascular diseases of the brain. Ann Rev Med 4:213 – 249

Agnoli AL, Cristante L, Busse O, Feistner H (1979) Brain herniation by cranial tomography: clinical, radiological correlations. VIII. Congress of the European Society of Neuroradiology, Strasbourg, 7. – 8. Sept. 1979

Amano S (1977) Vascular changes in the brain of spontaneously hypertensive rats: Hyaline and fibrinoid degeneration. J Pathol 121:119 – 128

Ambrose J (1973) Computerized transverse axial scanning (tomography): Part 2. Clinical application. Br J Radiol 46:1023 – 1047

Ameli NO (1957) Delayed post-traumatic haemorrhage of the brain. Acta Med Iran 1:267 – 291

Ameli NO (1968) Brain angiomata and intracerebral haematoma. Prog Brain Res 30:427 – 431

Anders HE, Eicke WJ (1941) Die Gehirngefäße beim Hochdruck. Arch Psychiatr Nervenkr 112:1 – 44

The Annual of Pathological Autopsy Cases in Japan, The Japanese Pathological Society, 1970 – 1975

Arana-Iniguez R, Wilson E, Basfarrica E, Medici M (1976) Cerebral hematomas. Surg Neurol 6:45 – 52

Aring CD, Merrit H (1935) Differential diagnosis between cerebral haemorrhage and cerebral thrombosis. Arch Intern Med 56:438 – 456

Armstrong MC, Warner ED, Connor WE (1970) Regression of coronary atheromatosis in rhesus monkeys. Circ Res 27:59 – 67

Arseni C, Oprescu I (1959) Cerebellar hematomas. J Neurosurg 16:503 – 507

Arseni C, Stancin M (1973) Primary haematomas of the brain stem. Acta Neurochir (Wien) 28:323 – 330

Arseni C, Ionescu S, Maretsis M, Ghitescu M (1967) Primary intraparenchymatous hematomas. J Neurosurg 27:207 – 215

Arseni C, Constantinescu A, Cioloca C (1971) Tumori cerebrale cu debut ictal. Neurol Psihiatr Neurochir 26: 16:193 – 199

Arsenjo A, Fierro J (1958) Surgical treatment of medical cerebral hemorrhages. Zentralbl Neurochir 18:234 – 238

Astrup J, Symon L, Branston NM, Lassen NA (1977) Cortical evoked potential and extracellular K^+ and H^+ at critical levels of brain ischemia. Stroke 8:51 – 57

Auer LM (1978) The pathogenesis of hypertensive encephalopathy. Acta Neurochir [Suppl] 27

Austrarheiv K (1956) Delayed traumatic intracerebral haemorrhage: report of one case with necropsy. Acta Pathol Microbiol Scand 38:177 – 185

Backlund EO (1978) Controlled sub-total evacuation of intracerebral hematomas by stereotactic technique. Surg Neurol 9:99 – 101

Bailey P (1904) Traumatic apoplexy. Med Rec 66:528 – 529

Baker HL, Campbell JK, Houser DW, Reese DF, Sheedy PF, Holman CB (1974) Computer assisted tomography of the head – An early evaluation. Mayo Clin Proc 49:17 – 27

Baratham G, Dennyson WG (1972) Delayed traumatic intracerebral haemorrhage. J Neurol Neurosurg Psychiatry 35:698 – 706

Barnes BD, Winestock DP (1977) Dynamic radionuclide scanning in the diagnosis of thrombosis of the superior sagittal sinus. Neurology (Minneap) 27:656 – 661

Becker DH, Silverberg GD (1978) Successful evacuation of an acute pontine hematoma. Surg Neurol 4:263 – 265

Becks J, Marguth F (1974) Zur Diagnose und operativen Therapie der intrazerebralen Massenblutung. MMW 116:717 – 722

Bender MB (1960) Resolution of subdural haematoma. Trans Am Neurol Assoc 85:192 – 194

Beneš V, Koukolik F, Obrovska D (1972) Two types of spontaneous intracerebral hemorrhage due to hypertension. J Neurosurg 37:509 – 513

Bergman PS (1950) Hemangioma of the pons. J Mt Sinai Hosp NY 17:119–131
Bergström M, Ericson K, Levander B, Svendsen P, Larsson S (1977) Variation with time of the attenuation values of intracranial hematomas. J Comp Assoc Tomogr 1:57–63
Bethke CC (1797) Über Schlagflüsse und Lähmungen oder Geschichte der Apoplexie, Paraplegie und Hemiplegie. Fleischer, Leipzig
Betz E, Schlote W (1977) Development and regression of experimental local carotid atheromatosis in rabbits. In: Zülch KJ, Kaufmann W, Hossmann K-A, Hossmann V (eds) Brain and heart infarct. Springer, Berlin Heidelberg New York
Binet EF, Loken MK (1970) Scintiangiography of cerebral arteriovenous malformations and aneuryms. AJR 109:707–713
Blackwood W (1963) The central nervous system in hypertensive vascular disease. In: Greenfield's neuropathology. William & Wilkins, Baltimore, pp 120–127
Böhne C (1931) Über die Bedeutung der Hirnerweichung in der Pathogenese der kompakten apoplektischen Hirnblutung. Z Gesamte Neurol Psychiatr 137:610–620
Bollinger O (1891) Über traumatische Spätapoplexie; ein Beitrag zur Lehre von der Hirnerschütterung. Int Beitr z Wiss Med 2:457–470
Botterell EH (1958) On brain injury. Presidential Address. Canadian Neurological Society, Toronto
Boysen G (1973) Cerebral hemodynamics in carotid surgery. Acta Neurol Scand [Suppl 52] 49:43–46
Branston NM, Symon L, Crockard HA, Pasztor E (1974) Relationship between the cortical evoked potential, blood flow and local cortical flow following acute middle cerebral artery occlusion in the baboon. Exp Neurol 45:195–208
Brennan RW, Bergland RM (1977) Acute cerebellar hemorrhage: Analysis of clinical findings and outcome in 12 cases. Neurology (Minneap) 27:527–532
Brewer DB, Fawcett FJ, Horsfield GI (1968) A necropsy series of non-traumatic cerebral hemorrhages and softenings, with particular reference to heart weight. J Pathol Bacteriol 96:311–320
Brihaye J, Frowein RA, Lindgren S, Loew F, Stroobandt G (1978) Report on the meeting of the W.F.N.S. Neuro-Traumatology Committee. Acta Neurochir (Wien) 40:181–186
Browder J (1942) Intracerebral hemorrhage of traumatic origin, its surgical treatment. NY State J Med 42:2230–2235
Brown FD, Mullan S, Duda EE (1978) Delayed traumatic intracerebral hematomas: report of three cases. J Neurosurg 48:1019–1022
Brown-Séquard CE (1861) Diagnosis of haemorrhage in the cerebellum. Lancet II:391
Brunner HR, Laragh JH, Baer L, Newton MA, Goodwin FT, Krakoff LR, Bard RH, Bühler FR (1972) Essential hypertension: renin and aldosterone, heart attack and stroke. N Engl J Med 286:441–449
Budzilovich GN (1976) On pathogenesis of primary lesions in blunt head trauma with special reference to the brain stem injuries. In: McLaurin RL (ed) Head injuries. Grune & Stratton, New York, pp 39–43
Buonanno FS, Moody DM, Ball MR, Laster DW (1978) Computed cranial tomographic findings in cerebral sinovenous occlusion. J Comp Assoc Tomogr 2:281–290
Burger PC, Vogel FS (1977) Hemorrhagic white matter infarction in three critically ill patients. Hum Pathol 8:121–132
Butler AB, Partain RA, Netsky MG (1972) Primary intraventricular hemorrhage. Neurology (Minneap) 22: 675–687
Butzer JF, Cancilla PA, Cornell SH (1976) Computerized axial tomography of intracerebral hematoma. Arch Neurol 33:206–214
Cervos-Navarro J, Iglesias Rozas J (1976) Untersuchungen der Hirnarteriolen bei normalen und hypertensiven Menschen. Sympos. Neuropath. Praha June 8–10, 1976
Charcot JM, Bouchard C (1868) Nouvelles recherches sur la pathogénie de l'hémorrhagie cérébrale. Arch Physiol (Paris) 1:110–127, 643–675, 725–734
Chodkiewicz JP, Vedrenne C, Radondo A (1973) Brain stem lesions following head injury. Gkc Med Int. Congr Ser 299:69
Cole FM, Yates PO (1967a) Pseudo-aneurysms in relationship to massive cerebral haemorrhage. J Neurol Neurosurg Psychiatry 30:61–66
Cole FM, Yates PO (1967b) Intracerebral microaneurysms and small cerebrovascular lesions. Brain 90:759–767
Cole FM, Yates PO (1967c) The occurrence and significance of intracerebral micro-aneurysms. J Pathol Bacteriol 93:393–411
Collomb H, Dumas M, Girard PL, Lemercier G, Tap D (1973) Hémorrhagies primitives du tronc cérébral. Rev Neurol (Paris) 129:185–210
Courville CB (1950) Pathology of the central nervous system, 3rd ed. Mountain View

Courville S, Blomquist O (1940) Traumatic intracerebral hemorrhage with particular reference to its pathogenesis and its relation to delayed traumatic apoplexy. Arch Surg 41:1 – 28
Courville CB, Friedman AP (1942) Hemorrhage into the lateral basal ganglia region. Bull Los Angeles Neurol Soc 7:137 – 149
Craig WM, Adson AW (1936) Spontaneous intracerebral hemorrhage. Etiology and surgical treatment, with a report of nine cases. Arch Neurol Psychiatry 35:701 – 716
Crompton MR (1971) Brainstem lesions due to closed head injury. Lancet I:669 – 673
Cruveilhier J (1829) Apoplexie. Dictionnaire de médecine et de chirurgie pratiques, tome III. Paris, Gabon, Méquignon-Marvis, Baillière, pp 201 – 297
Cuatico W, Adib S, Gaston P (1965) Spontaneous intracerebral hematomas. A surgical appraisal. J Neurosurg 22:569 – 575
Cushing H (1903) The blood-pressure reaction of acute cerebral compression, illustrated by cases of intracranial hemorrhage. Am J Med Sci 125:1017 – 1044
Dandy W (1959) The brain. In: Lewis D (ed) Practice of surgery, vol 12. Hagerstown, Prior, p 613
David M, Hecaen H (1945) Nouvelle contribution à l'étude clinique et thérapeutique des hématomes intracérébraux spontanés. Presse Med 27:371 – 372
Davidoff LM (1958) Intracerebral hemorrhage associated with hypertension and arteriosclerosis. J Neurosurg 15:322 – 328
Dejong RN (1942) Delayed traumatic intracerebral haemorrhage. Arch Neurol Psychiatry 48:257 – 266
De Vet AC (1965) Middle fossa traumatic intra- and extracerebral lesions, their treatment and prognosis. In: Proceedings of the Third International Congress of Neurological Surgery. pp 236 – 241
Dietrich H-J (1967) Mikroangiome als Ursache sogenannter "spontaner" intracerebraler Blutungen. Med Dissertation, University of Würzburg
Dietz R, Schömig A, Haebara H, Mann JF, Rascher W, Lüth JB, Grünherz N, Gross F (1978) Studies on the pathogenesis of spontaneous hypertension of rats. Circ Res [Suppl I] 43:98 – 106
Dinsdale HB (1964) Spontaneous hemorrhage in the posterior fossa. Arch Neurol 10:200 – 217
Doe FD, Shuangshoti S, Netsky MG (1972) Cryptic angioma of the choroid plexus. Neurology (Minneap) 22:1232 – 1239
Dolinskas CA, Bilaniuk LT, Zimmerman RA, Kuhl DE (1977a) Computed tomography of intracerebral hematomas. I. Transmission CT observations on hematoma resolution. AJR 129:681 – 688
Dolinskas CA, Bilaniuk, LT, Zimmerman RA, Kuhl DE, Alavi A (1977b) Computed tomography of intracerebral hematomas. II. Radionuclide and transmission CT studies of the perihematoma region. Am J Roentgenol 129:689 – 692
Donaghy RMP, Numoto M, Wallman LJ (1965) Reduction of post-traumatic neurological residual on the day of injury. In: Proceedings of the Third International Congress of Neurological Surgery. pp 174 – 180 (Amsterdam)
Doughty RG (1938) Post-traumatic delayed intracerebral hemorrhage. South Med J 31:254 – 256
Dublin AB, French BN, Rennick JM (1977) Computed tomography in the trauma. Radiology 122:365 – 369
Duffner PK, Klein DM, Cohen ME (1978) Calcification in brainstem gliomas. Neurology (Minneap) 28:832 – 834
Durand-Fardel M (1854) Traité clinique et pratique des maladies des vieillards. Paris
Eicke WJ (1952) Gehirngefäßveränderungen bei Hypertonie. Atti del Primo Congr. Internat. di Istopat. del Sistema Nervoso, Rome
Ellis AG (1909) The pathogenesis of spontaneous cerebral hemorrhage. Proc Pathol Soc Philad 12:197
Endo H, Larsen B, Lassen NA (1977) Regional cerebral blood flow alteration remote from the site of intracranial tumors. J Neurosurg 46:271 – 282
Eppinger H (1888) Die miliaren Hirnarterienaneurysmen (Charcot-Bouchard). Virchows Arch [Pathol Anat] 111:405
Epstein AW (1951) Primary massive pontine hemorrhage. J Neuropathol Exp Neurol 10:426 – 438
Evans JP, Scheinker IM (1946) Histological studies of the brain following head trauma, II Post traumatic petechial and massive intracerebral hemorrhage. J Neurosurg 3:101 – 113
Fahr T (1937) Apoplexie und Erweichung. Vergleichende statistische Untersuchungen. Zentralbl Allg Pathol 66:84 – 93
Fang HGH, Foly JM (1954) Hypertensive hemorrhages of the pons and cerebellum. Arch Neurol Psychiatry 72:638
Fasano AV, Broggi G (1956) Aspect clinique et chirurgical de l'hémorrhagie cérébrale (à propos de 9 cas, d'hématomes intracérébraux spontanés), Neurochirurgie 2:357 – 386

Fazio C, Sacco G, Bugiani O (1973) The thalamic hemorrhage. Eur Neurol 9:30 – 43

Fieschi C, Agnoli A, Battistini (1968) Derangements of regional cerebral blood flow and of its regulatory mechanisms in acute cerebrovascular lesions. Neurology (Minneap) 18:1166 – 1179

Fisher CM (1969) The arterial lesions underlying lacunes. Acta Neuropathol (Berl) 12:1 – 15

Fisher GM (1971) Pathological observations in hypertensive cerebral hemorrhage. J Neuropathol Exp Neurol 30:536 – 550

Fisher CM (1972) Cerebral miliary aneurysms in hypertension. Am J Pathol 66:313 – 330

Fisher CM, Adams RD (1951) Observations on brain embolism with special reference to the mechanism of hemorrhagic infarction. J Neuropathol Exp Neurol 10:92 – 93

Fisher CM, Picard EH, Polak A, Dalal P, Ojemann RG (1965) Acute hypertensive cerebellar hemorrhage: Diagnosis and surgical treatment. J Nerv Ment Dis 140:38 – 57

Freeman RE, Onofrio BM, Okazaki H, Dinapoli RP (1973) Spontaneous intracerebellar hemorrhage: Diagnosis and surgical treatment. Neurology (Minneap) 23:84 – 90

French BN, Dublin AB (1977) The value of computerized tomography in the management of 1000 consecutive head injuries. Surg Neurol 7:171 – 183

Freytag E (1968) Fatal hypertensive intracerebral haematomas: a survey of the pathological anatomy of 393 cases. J Neurol Neurosurg Psychiatry 31:616 – 620

Friedman AP, Nielsen JM (1941) Cerebellar hemorrhage. Bull Los Angeles Neurol Soc 6:135

Frowein RA, Steinmann HW, auf der Haar K, Terhaag D, Karimi-Nejad A (1978) Limits to classification and prognosis of severe head injury. Adv Neurosurg 5:16 – 26

Gänshirt H, Wolfram A, Haak G (1979) Die sogenannten spontanen intrazerebralen Hämatome. Nervenarzt 50:411 – 414

Galbraith S, Smith J (1976) Acute traumatic haematoma with skull fractures. Lancet I:501 – 503

Garraway M (1976) The size of the problem of stroke in Scotland. In: Gillingham FT, Mawdsley C, Williams AE (eds) Stroke. Churchill Livingstone, Edinburgh London New York, pp 72 – 82

Globus JH, Epstein JA, Green MA, Marics M (1949) Focal cerebral hemorrhage experimentally induced. J Neuropathol Exp Neurol 8:113 – 116

Globus JH, Epstein JA (1953) Massive cerebral hemorrhage: Spontaneous and experimentally induced. J Neuropathol Exp Neurol 12:107 – 131

Gögler E (1968) Chirurgie und Verkehrsmedizin. Klinik, Mechanik und Biomechanik des Unfalls. In: Wagner K, Wagner H-J (eds) Handbuch der Verkehrsmedizin. Springer, Berlin Heidelberg New York

Goldberg JD, Kurland LT (1962) Mortality in 33 countries from diseases of the nervous system. World Neurol 3:444 – 465

Goodman SJ, Hayes M (1974) Values of cerebral isotope flow studies in timing of surgery for ruptured aneurysm when there is vasospasm and neurologic deficit. J Nucl Med 15:1113 – 1116

Goutelle A, Lapras C, Trillet M (1969) Les hématomes intracérébraux. Revelateurs d'une tumeur cérébrale. Neurochirurgia (Stuttg) 12:218 – 227

Gowers WR (1892) Handbuch der Nervenkrankheiten. Cohen, Bonn

Gowers WR (1893) Diseases of the nervous system. Philadelphia

Gros C, Giraud G, Lafon H (1948) Hématome spontané de la calotte protuberantielle opéré et guéri. Presse Med 73:890

Grote E, Walther C, Wenker H (1969) Protrahierte Hirnmassenblutung bei hyperfibrinolytischer Hypofibrinogenämie. Nervenarzt 40:285 – 389

Grote E, Geletneky CL, Rompel K, Zorbas K, Meyer E, Prill A, Heene D (1970) Atypische intracerebrale Massenblutung. Dtsch Z Nervenheilkd 197:66 – 76

Grote E, Geletneky CL, Rompel K, Zorbas K, Meyer E, Prill A, Heene D (1971) Some unusual forms of intracerebral haematoma. In: Pia HW, Grote E, Mundinger F, Gleave JRW (eds) Modern aspects of neurosurgery. Excerpta Medica, Amsterdam, pp 264 – 267

Grotts BF (1950) Spontaneous hemorrhage from a haemangioma of the pons. J Pediatr 37:98 – 101

Grumme T, Lanksch W, Wende S (1976) Diagnosis of spontaneous intracerebral hemorrhage by computerized tomography. In: Lanksch W, Kazner E (eds) Cranial computerized tomography. Springer, Berlin Heidelberg New York, pp 284 – 290

Gudmundson G, Hallgrímsson J, Jónasson TA, Bjarnason O (1972) Hereditary cerebral haemorrhage with amyloidosis. Brain 95:387 – 404

Guillaume J, Joinville R (1945) Les hématomes spontanés intracérébraux. Presse Med 45:606 – 607

Guillaume J, Mazars G, Roge R, Pansini A (1957) Les accidents circulatoires du cerveau. Traitement chirurgical de l'hémorrhagie et de l'ischémie. Presses Universitaires de France, Paris

Gurdjian ES, Thomas LM (1965) Organization of services for the treatment of acute head injury in community and industrial practice. In: Proceedings of the Third International Congress of Neurological Surgery. pp 20–26 (Amsterdam)
Haebara H, Dietz R, Mann JFE, Lüth JB (1977) Gefäßveränderungen beim genetischen Hochdruck der Ratte. Verh Dtsch Ges Kreislaufforsch 43:15–19
Hamel E, Karimi-Nejad A (1978) Traumatic intracerebral haematomas. Adv Neurosurg 5:56–61
Hazama F, Amano S, Ozaki T (1978a) Pathological changes of cerebral vessel endothelial walls in spontaneously hypertensive rats. With special reference to the role of these cells in the development of hypertensive cerebrovascular lesions. Adv Neurol 20:359–369
Hazama F, Amano S, Haebara H, Yamori Y, Okamoto Y (1978b) Pathology and pathogenesis of cerebrovascular lesions in spontaneously hypertensive rats. In: Cervos-Navarro J (ed) The cerebral vessel wall. Raven, New York
Heiss W-D, Hayakawa T, Waltz AG (1976) Pattern of changes of blood flow and relationship to infarction in experimental cerebral ischemia. Stroke 7:454–459
Hemmer R (1965) The time factor in extradural haematoma. In: Proceedings of the Third International Congress of Neurological Surgery. pp 288–290 (Amsterdam)
Hier DB, Davis KR, Richardson EP Jr, Mohr JP (1977) Hypertensive putaminal hemorrhage. Ann Neurol 1:152–159
Hillbom E, Anttinent EE (1957) On the apopletic conditions occurring as delayed symptoms after brain injuries. Acta Psychiatr. Neurol Scand 52:103–116
Hiller F (1936) Die Zirkulationsstörungen des Gehirns und Rückenmarks. In: Bunke O, Foerster O: Handbuch Neurologie Vol. 11/3, Springer, Berlin, pp 178–465
Hirayama A, Kowada M, Fukasawa H (1974) Cerebrovascular Moya-moya disease. A case report and review of 12 autopsy cases in Japan. Brain Nerve (Tokyo) 26:1215–1225
Hollin SA, Decker RE, Gross SW (1977) Spontaneous cerebellar hematomas. Mt Sinai J Med (NY) 41:396–406
Hossmann K-A (1977) Total ischemia of the brain. In: Zülch KJ, Kaufmann W, Hossmann K-A, Hossmann V (eds) Brain and heart infarct. Springer, Berlin Heidelberg New York, pp 107–122
Hossmann V (1977) Coagulation disturbances in cerebrovascular disorders. In: Zülch KJ, Kaufmann W, Hossmann K-A, Hossmann V (eds) Brain and heart infarct. Springer, Berlin Heidelberg New York, pp 81–90
Housepian EM, Pool JL (1958) A systematic analysis of intracranial aneurysms from the autopsy file of the Presbyterian Hospital 1914–1956. J Neuropathol Exp Neurol 17:409–423
Huckman MS, Weinberg PK, Kim KS, Davis DO (1970) Angiographic and clinico-pathologic correlations in basal ganglionic hemorrhage. Radiology 95:79–92
Huhn A (1965) Die Thrombosen der intrakraniellen Venen und Sinus. Schattauer, Stuttgart
Huhn A (1972) Die Klinik der venösen Abflußstörungen des Gehirns. In: Gänshirt H (ed) Der Hirnkreislauf. Thieme, Stuttgart
Huk W, Schiefer W (1976) Computerized tomography (Siretom) of acute cerebrovascular events. In: Lanksch W, Kazner E (eds) Cranial computerized tomography. Springer, Berlin Heidelberg New York, pp 264–272
Humphreys RF (1975) Cerebral hemorrhage following heart surgery. J Neurosurg 43:671–675
Humphreys RP (1978) Computerized tomographic definition of mesencephalic hematoma with evacuation through pedunculotomy. J Neurosurg 49:749–752
Hunt WE, Hess RM (1968) Surgical risk as related to time of intervention in the repair of intracranial aneurysms. J Neurosurg 28:14–20
Hurtig HI, Reivich M (1977) Clinical aspects of cerebrovascular disease. In: Goldensohn ES, Appel SA (eds) Scientific approaches to clinical neurology. Lea & Febiger, Philadelphia, pp 292–295
Hyland HH, Levy D (1954) Spontaneous cerebellar hemorrhage. Can Med Assoc J 71:315–323
Ingvar DH (1976) Functional landscapes of the dominant hemisphere. Brain Res 107:181–197
Isherwood I, Occleshaw JV (1976) Stroke Proceeding of the 9th Pfizer International Symposium. Churchill Livingstone, Edinburgh London New York, pp 214–229
Istrati C (1975) Hematomul intracerebral primar. Master's Thesis, University of Bucureşti
Ito Z, Yamaguchi K, Matsuoka S, Sakurai Y, Kutsuzawa T (1973) Hypertensive intracerebellar hemorrhage with extravasation of contrast material. Report of a case (in Japanese). Brain Nerve 25:1727–1731
Jaffe ME, McHenry LC, Goldberg HI (1970) Regional cerebral blood flow measurement with small probes. II. Neurology (Minneap) 20:225–237
Jamieson KG, Yelland JDN (1972) Traumatic intracerebral haematoma. Report of 63 surgically treated cases. J Neurosurg 37:528–532

Janny P, Montrieul B, Tournilhac M, Chabannes J, Jourde J (1966) Les hématomes intra-cérébraux rompus dans le ventricule. Neurochirurgie 12:459 – 472

Janny P, Colnet G, Poppi M (1976) Intracranial pressure in the course of intracerebral hematomas in patients suffering from arterial hypertension. J Neurol Sci 20:224 – 225

Janny P, Colnet G, Georget A-M, Chazal J (1978) Intracranial pressure with intracerebral haemorrhages. Surg Neurol 10:371 – 375

Jellinger K (1971) Pathologie zentralnervöser Störungen bei internen Erkrankungen. Wien Z Nervenheilkd 29:1 – 37

Jellinger K (1972) Zur Ätiologie und Pathogenese der spontanen intrazerebralen Blutung. Therapiewoche 22:1440 – 1448

Jellinger K (1975) The morphology of centrally located angiomas. In: Pia HW, Gleave JRW, Grote E, Zierski J (eds) Cerebral angiomas. Springer, Berlin Heidelberg New York, pp 9 – 17

Jellinger K (1977a) Pathology of intracerebral hemorrhage. Zentralbl Neurochir 38:29 – 42

Jellinger K (1977b) Morphologie und Genese traumatischer Hirn- und Rückenmarksschäden. Aktuel Neurol 4:1 – 21

Jellinger K (1977c) Cerebrovascular amyloidosis with cerebral hemorrhage. J Neurol 214:195 – 206

Jellinger K (1979) Intracranial aneurysms: Pathology and aetiology. In: Pia HW (ed) Intracranial aneurysms. Springer, Berlin Heidelberg New York, pp 5 – 19

Jennett WB (1975) Epilepsy after non-missile head injuries. Year Book Medical Publishers, Chicago

Jochheim KA, Merkel K, Pampus I, Schüle K, Schüle-Hein K, Weck-Arnold S (1977) Einrichtungen der medizinischen Rehabilitation. Kohlhammer, Stuttgart Berlin Köln Mainz

Johansson S, Melin HS (1960) Spontaneous cerebral hemorrhage and encephalomalacia. Acta Psychiatr Scand 35:457 – 479

Kamisasa A, Hiratsuka H, Inaba Y (1972) Aneurysm arising from the abnormal vascular network at the base of the brain – case report and etiological study. Brain Nerve (Tokyo) 24:463 – 468

Kanaya H, Handa H (1974) The surgical treatment of hypertensive intracerebral hemorrhage on the cooperative study in Japan. Thirty-nineth Annual Meeting of the Japan Neurosurgical Society

Kanaya H, Yukawa H, Itoh Z, Kagawa M, Kanno T, Kuwabara T, Mizukami M (1978) A neurological grading for patients with hypertensive intracerebral hemorrhage and a classification for hematoma location on computed tomography. In: Proceeding of the 7th Conference of Surgical Treatment of Stroke. pp 265 – 270

Kane WC, Aronon SM (1969) Cerebrovascular disease in an autopsy population. Arch Neurol 20: 514 – 526

Kaneko M, Koba T, Yokoyama T (1977) Early surgical treatment for hypertensive intracerebral hemorrhage. J Neurosurg 46:579 – 583

Katzman R, Clasen R, Klatzo I, Meyer JS, Pappius HM, Waltz AG (1977) Brain edema in stroke. Stroke 8:509

Kawada M, Ito Z, Matsuoka S, Yamaguchi K (1971) Primary pontine haemorrhage revealed by pneumoencephalo-roulette tomography, and a report on surgically treated cases. Acta Neurochir (Wien) 25:269 – 276

Kawakami H, Kutsuzawa T, Uemura K, Sakurai Y, Nakamura T (1974) Regional cerebral blood flow in patients with hypertensive intracerebral hemorrhage. Stroke 5:207 – 213

Kazner E, Kubicki S, Kunze S, Schiefer W, Wende S (1969) Die Bedeutung der klinischen Zusatzuntersuchungen für die Differentialdiagnose zerebrale Massenblutung Hirninfarkt. Fortsch Neurol Psychiatr 37:511 – 520

Kazner E, Lanksch W, Steinhoff H, Wilske J (1975) Die axiale Computer-Tomographie des Gehirnschädels – Anwendungsmöglichkeiten und klinische Ergebnisse. Fortschr Neurol Psychiatr 43: 487 – 574

Kazner E, Klein W, Stochdorph O (1978) Möglichkeiten und Aussagewert der Computertomographie bei nicht tumorbedingten raumfordernden intrakraniellen Prozessen. Roentgenblätter 31:181 – 198

Kempe LG (1964) Surgical removal of an intramedullary haematoma simulating Wallenberg's syndrome. J Neurol Neurosurg Psychiatry 27:78 – 80

King AB, Chambers JW (1952) Delayed onset of symptoms due to extradural haematomas. Surgery 31:839 – 844

Kinkel WR, Jacobs L (1976) Computerized axial transverse tomography in cerebrovascular disease. Neurology (Minneap) 26:924 – 930

Klingler M (1966) Intrakranielle Blutungen bei Antikoagulantientherapie. Schweiz Arch Neurol Neurochir Psychiatr 98:20 – 25

Kodama N, Suzuki J (1974) Cerebrovascular Moya-moya disease. Third report – The study on the aging of the perforating branches and the possibility of a collateral pathway. Neurol Med Chir (Tokyo) 14:55–67
Kodama N, Suzuki J (1978) Moya-moya disease associated with aneurysm. J Neurosurg 48:565–569
Koos WT, Sunder-Plassman M, Salah S (1969) Successful removal of a large intrapontine haematoma. J Neurosurg 31:690–694
Kozniewska H, Wronski J, Zderkiewicz E (1965) Results of treatment in 226 cases of acute head injury. In: Proceedings of the Third International Congress of Neurological Surgery. p 247 (Amsterdam)
Krayenbühl HA (1975) The Moya-moya syndrome and the neurosurgeon. Surg Neurol 4:353–360
Krayenbühl H, Siegfried J (1964) Der neurochirurgische Beitrag zur Behandlung der intrazerebralen Blutung. Wien Klin Wochenschr 76:401–404
Krayenbühl H, Siebenmann R (1965) Small vascular malformations as a cause of primary intracerebral hemorrhage. J Neurosurg 22:7–20
Krayenbühl H, Yasargil MG (1972) Angiome and Aneurysmen. In: Gänshirt H (ed) Der Hirnkreislauf. Thieme, Stuttgart, pp 465–511
Kreindler A, Voiculescu V (1963) Hemoragia cerebralå. St. şi Cerc. de Neurol 1:15
Krenkel W (1970) Traumatische und nicht-traumatische Hirnblutungen. Langenbecks Arch Chir 327:949–954
Krücke W (1971) Pathologie der cerebralen Venen- und Sinusthrombosen. Radiologe 11:370–377
Kudo T (1967) A disease with abnormal intracranial vascular networks. Igakushoin, Tokyo, p 66
Kurtzke JF (1976a) The distribution of cerebrovascular disease. In: Gillingham FJ, Mawdsley C, Williams AE (eds) Stroke. Churchill Livingstone, Edinburgh London New York, p 5–20
Kurtzke JF (1976b) An introduction to the epidemiology of cerebrovascular disease. In: Scheinberg P (ed) Cerebrovascular disease. Raven, New York, pp 239–263
Laine E, Delandtsheer JM, Galibert P, Delandtsheer G (1956) Hématomes intracérébraux spontanés profonds en rapport avec des malformations angiomateuses. Neurochirurgie 2:340–355
Laine E, Lopez-Pinto C, Delandtsheer JM, Pruvot P et al. (1962) Considérations, étiologiques, anatomiques, électroencephalographiques, radiologiques et thérapeutiques tirées de l'étude d'une importante série d'hémorragies cérébrales operées. Neurochirurgie 8:208–215
Lampert H, Müller W (1926) Bei welchem Druck kommt es zu einer Ruptur der Gehirngefäße. Z Pathol 33:471–477
Landman S, Ross P (1974) Radionuclides in the diagnosis of arteriovenous malformations. J Nucl Med 15:953–958
Langerhans R (1903) Die traumatische Spätapoplexie. Hirschwald, Berlin
Langfitt, TW (1969) Increased intracranial pressure. Clin Neurosurg 16:436–471
Lanksch W, Grumme T, Kazner E (1978) Schädelhirnverletzungen im Computertomogramm. Springer, Berlin Heidelberg New York
Lassen NA, Ingvar DH (1963) Regional cerebral blood flow measurement in man. Arch Neurol 9:615–622
Lassen NA, Ingvar DH (1972) Radioisotopic assessment of regional cerebral blood flow. Prog Nucl Med 1:376–409
Laun A (1978) Traumatic aneurysms. Adv Neurosurg 5:124–129
Laurent JP, Molinari GF, Oakley JC (1976) Primate model of cerebral hematoma. J Neuropathol Exp Neurol 35:560–568
Lavin PJM, Bone I, Lamb JT, Swinburne LM (1978) Intracranial venous thrombosis in the first trimester of pregnancy. J Neurol Neurosurg Psychiatry 41:726–729
Lazorthes G (1956) L'hémorrhagie cérébrale vue par le neurochirurgien. Rapport présenté à la réunion de la Societé de Neuro-Chirurgie de Langue Française. Masson, Paris
Lazorthes G (1959) Surgery of cerebral haemorrhage. Report on the results of 52 surgically treated cases. J Neurosurg 16:355–364
Lee J, Berry CL (1978) Cerebral microaneurysm formation in the hypertensive rat. J Pathol 124:7–12
Lee MLK, Cheung EMT (1973) Moya-moya disease as a cause of subarachnoid haemorrhage in Chinese. Brain 96:623–628
Lhermitte J (1949) Les hémorragies de l'encéphale. In: Traité de medecine, tome XV. Masson, Paris, pp 743–760
Lindheimer JH, Barrows HS (1962) Recurrent pontine hemorrhage incidental to venous angioma of the pons. Bull Los Angeles Neurol Soc 27:128–133
Litner R (1965) Intracerebral haemorrhage of traumatic origin: a case report. Boston Med Q 12:13–19
Little RJ, Blomquist GA Jr, Ethier R (1977) Intraventricular hemorrhage in adults. Surg Neurol 8:143–149
Little RJ (1978) Cerebellar hemorrhage in adults. J Neurosurg 48:575–579

Luessenhop AJ, Shevlin WA, Ferrero AA, McCullough DC, Barone BM (1967) Surgical management of primary intracerebral hemorrhage. J Neurosurg 27:419–427
Luginbühl H (1966) Vascular disease in animals: comparative aspects of cerebrovascular anatomy and pathology in different species. In: Siekert RG, Whisnant JP (eds) Cerebral vascular diseases. Grune & Stratton, New York London, pp 3–27
Luyendijk W (1972) Intracerebral haematoma. In: Vinken FG, Bruyn GW (eds) Handbook of clinical neurology, vol 11. North Holland, Amsterdam, pp 660–719
Luyendijk W, Schoen JHR (1964) Intracerebral haematomas. A clinical study of 40 surgical cases. Psychiatr Neurol Neurochir 67:445–468
Lyager T (1955) Dødsarsager ved apoplexia cerebri. Nord Med 54:1315–1317
Mandybur TI, Bates SRD (1978) Fatal massive intracerebral hemorrhage complicating cerebral amyloid angiopathy. Arch Neurol 35:245–248
Mandybur TI (1977) Intracranial hemorrhage caused by metastatic tumors. Neurology (Minneap) 27:650–655
Margolis G, Odom GL, Woodhall B, Bloor BM (1951) The role of small angiomatous malformations in the production of intracerebral hematomas. J Neurosurg 8:564–575
Margolis G, Abraham J, Erbengl A, O'Loughlin J, MacCarty WC (1968) Pathogenesis of hypertensive intracranial hemorrhage: a hypothesis with supporting data. Prog Brain Res 30:453–462
Marin PH, Noterman L (1971) L'hematome bulbo protuberantiel opérable. Acta Neurol Belg 71:261–268
Marks JS (1960) Apoplectic death due to intracerebral hemorrhage. An anatomic study. Neurology (Minneap) 10:278–280
Mastaglia FL, Edis B, Kakulas BA (1969) Medullary haemorrhage. Report of two cases. J Neurol Neurosurg Psychiatry 32:221–225
Matsuoka S (1952) Histopathological studies on the blood vessels in apoplexia cerebri. Atti del primo congresso internazionale di istopatologia del sistema nervosos, vol III. Rom, pp 221–231
Mauersberger W (1976) Intracerebrale Massenblutung bei M. Nishimoto-Takeuchi-Kudo (Moyamoya-Krankheit). J Neurol 212:46–54
Mauersberger W, Fuchs EC, Ebhardt G (1977) Spontane intrazerebellare Hämatome im Kindesalter. Acta Neurochir (Wien) 36:255–264
McCormick WF, Rosenfield DB (1973) Massive brain hemorrhage: a review of 144 cases and an examination of their causes. Stroke 4:946–954
McDowell FH, Millikan CH (1978) Summary of 11th Princeton conference on cerebrovascular disease. Stroke 9:429
McKissock W, Richardson A, Walsh R (1960) Spontaneous cerebellar hemorrhage. A study of 34 consecutive cases treated surgically. Brain 83:1–9
McKissock W, Richardson A, Taylor J (1961) Primary intracerebral haemorrhage. A controlled trial of surgical and conservative treatments in 180 unselected cases. Lancet II:221–226
McLaurin RL, McBride BH (1956) Traumatic intracerebral haematoma, review of 16 surgically treated cases. Ann Surg 143:294–305
Meienberg O, Regli F, Wurster K (1972) Spontane Kleinhirnblutungen. Schweiz Med Wochenschr 102:166–171
Melicher LJ (1840) Die Apoplexia. Med. Dissertation, Universität Wien
Merino de Villasante J, Taveras JM (1976) Computerized tomography (CT) in acute head trauma. Am J Roentgenol 126:765–778
Meriwether RP, Barnett HG, Echols DH (1976) Moya-moya disease as a cause of subarachnoid hemorrhage in a negro patient. J Neurosurg 44:620–622
Messina AV, Chernik NL (1975) Computed tomography: the "resolving" intracerebral hemorrhage. Radiology 118:609–613
Meyer JS (1975) Medical and surgical treatment of cerebrovascular disease. In: Meyer JS (ed) Modern concepts of cerebrovascular disease. Spectrum, New York
Meynert T (1867) Der Bau der Großhirnrinde und seine örtlichen Verschiedenheiten, nebst einem pathologisch-anatomischen Corollarium. Vierteljahresschr Psychiatr 1:77–93
Michael JC (1932) Cerebellar apoplexy. Am J Med Sci 183:687
Miller JD, Adams H (1972) Physiopathology and management of increased intracranial pressure. In: Critchley M, O'Leary JL, Jennett B (eds) Scientific foundations of neurology. Heinemann, London, pp 308–326
Mitchell DE, Adams JH (1973) Primary focal impact damage to the brainstem in blunt head injuries. Does it exist? Lancet II:215–218
Mitsuno T (1971) Surgical mangement of apoplexy. The 18th General Assembly of the Japanese Medical Congress. Tokyo

Mitsuno T, Kanaya H, Shirakata S, Ohsawa K, Ishikawa Y (1966) Surgical treatment of hypertensive intracerebral hemorrhage. J Neurosurg 24:70 – 76

Molinari GF, Smith L, Goldstein MN, Satran R (1973) Pathogenesis of cerebral mycotic aneurysm. Neurology (Minneap) 23:325 – 332

Monakow C von (1905) Gehirnpathologie. In: Nothnagels Specielle Pathologie und Therapie, 1897, 2nd ed. Wien

Montgomery OOB, Muirhead EE (1954) A characterization of hyaline arteriolar sclerosis by histochemical procedures. Am J Pathol 30:521 – 531

Moossy J (1966) Cerebral infarcts and the lesions of intracranial and extracranial atherosclerosis. Arch Neurol 14:124 – 128

Moossy J (1971) Cerebral atherosclerosis: intracranial and extracranial lesions. In: Minckler J (ed) Pathology of the nervous system, vol II. McGraw Hill, New York, pp 1423 – 1432

Morawetz RB, Crowell RH, DeGirolami U, Marcoux FW, Jones TH, Halsey JH (1979) Regional cerebral blood flow thresholds during cerebral ischemia. Fed Proc 38:2493 – 2494

Morgagni JB (1960) The seats and causes of diseases investigated by anatomy. London, 1769. Reprint: Hafner, New York

Morin MA, Pitts FW (1970) Delayed apoplexy following head injury. J Neurosurg 33:542 – 547

Müke R, Heienbrock W, Kühne D (1978) Spontane intrazerebrale Hämatome. Neue Gesichtspunkte seit Einführung der Computertomographie. Zentralbl Neurochir 39:135 – 144

Müller H, Wiggli V (1977) Cerebral, cerebellar and pontine haemorrhages. In: du Boulay G, Moseley IF (eds) Computerized axial tomography in clinical practice. Springer, Berlin Heidelberg New York, p 249

Müller HR, Wüthrich R, Hünig R, Elke M, von Hochstetter A (1974) A graphical reporting system for computerized axial x-ray tomography (EMI scanning). Eur Neurol 11:197 – 207

Muirhead EE, Turner LB, Grollman A (1951) Hypertensive cardiovascular disease. Nature and pathogenesis of the arteriolar sclerosis included by bilateral nephrectomy as revealed by a study of its tinctorial characteristics. Arch Pathol 52:266 – 279

Murphy MG (1972) Successful evacuation of acute pontine hematoma. Case report. J Neurosurg 37:224 – 225

Mutlu N, Berry RG, Alpers BJ (1963) Massive cerebral hemorrhage, clinical and pathological correlations. Arch Neurol 8:644 – 661

Myers J, Scott M, Silverstein A (1961) Cystic hemangioblastoma of pons. J Neurosurg 18:694 – 697

Naffziger HC, Jones OW (1928) Late traumatic apoplexy; report of 3 cases with operative recovery. Calif West Med 29:361 – 364

Nag S, Robertson DM, Dinsdale HB (1977) Cerebral cortical changes in acute experimental hypertension. Lab Invest 36:150 – 161

Nakajima K, Ito Z, Hen R, Suzuki A, Fukasawa H (1977a) Clinicopathological study of pontile hemorrhage. I Clinical aspects (in Japanese). Brain Nerve 29:1047 – 1058

Nakajima K, Ito Z, Hen R, Suzuki A, Fukasawa H (1977b) Clinicopathological aspects of pontile hemorrhage. II Pathological aspects (in Japanese). Brain Nerve 29:1157 – 1165

Nayrac P, Laine E, Delandtsheer JM, Delandtsheer G (1953) Quelques remarques étiologiques à propos d'une série de vingt hématomes spontanés du cerveau ou du cervelet. Rev Neurol (Paris) 89:591

Nelson JS, Case MES, Gold J (1973) Extensive intracerebral hemorrhage during open heart surgery. Acta Neuropathol (Berl) 25:163 – 165

Neubürger K (1930a) Beiträge zur Histologie, Pathogenese und Einteilung der arteriosklerotischen Hirnerkrankung. Veroeff Kriegs- und Konstit Path 6

New PFJ, Aronow SPD (1976) Attenuation measurements of whole blood and blood fractions in computed tomography. Radiology 121:635 – 640

New PFJ, Scott WR, Schnur JA, Davis KR, Taveras JM (1974) Computerized axial tomography with the EMI scanner. Radiology 110:109 – 123

Nishimoto A, Takeuchi S (1968) Abnormal cerebrovascular network related to the internal carotid arteries. J Neurosurg 29:255 – 260

Noetzel H, Jerusalem F (1965) Die Hirnvenen- und Sinusthrombosen. Springer, Berlin Heidelberg New York

Nornes H, Hauge T (1972) Spontaneous intracerebellar hemorrhage. Acta Neurol Scand [Suppl] 48:253 – 255

Norris JW, Eisen AA, Branch CL (1969) Problems in cerebellar hemorrhage and infarction. Neurology (Minneap) 19:1043 – 1050

Nothnagel H (1879) Topische Diagnostik der Gehirnkrankheiten. Hirschwald, Berlin (1928)

Obrador S, Dierssen G, Odoriz BJ (1970) Surgical evacuation of a pontine-medullary haematoma. J Neurosurg 33:82–84

Odom GL, Bloor BM, Woodhall B (1952) Intracerebral hematomas. South Med J 45:936

Odom GL, Tindall GT, Dukes HT (1961) Cerebellar hematoma caused by angiomatous malformations. Report of four cases. J Neurosurg 18:777–782

Odom GL, Tindall GT, Cupp HB Jr, Woodhall B (1966) Neurosurgical approach to intracerebral hemorrhage. Res Publ Assoc Nerv Ment Dis 41:145–168

Ojemann RG, Mohr JP (1975) Hypertensive brain hemorrhage. CNS 21:220–244

Ojemann RG, New PFJ (1963) Spontaneous resolution of an intraventricular hematoma. J Neurosurg 20:899–902

Okamoto K, Yamori Y, Nagaoka A (1974) Establishment of the stroke-prone spontaneously hypertensive rat (SHR).Circ Res [Suppl I] 34/35:143–153

Olesen J (1971) Contralateral focal increase of cerebral blood flow in man during arm work. Brain 94:635–646

Ooneda G (1970) Pathology of cerebral hemorrhage (in Japanese). Trans Soc Pathol Jpn 59:27–56

Ooneda G, Yoshida Y, Suzuki K, Sekiguchi T (1973) Morphogenesis of plasmatic arterionecrosis as the cause of hypertensive intracerebral hemorrhage. Virchows Arch [Pathol Anat] 361:31–38

Ooneda G, Yoshida Y, Suzuki K, Shinkai H (1976) Plasmatic arterionecrosis and its thrombotic occlusion. Thrombos Res [Suppl II] 8:357–364

Opitz E, Schneider M (1950) Über die Sauerstoffversorgung des Gehirns und den Mechanismus von Mangelwirkungen. Ergeb Physiol 46:126–260

Ott KH, Kase CS, Ojemann RG, Mohr JP (1974) Cerebellar hemorrhage: Diagnosis and treatment: A review of 56 cases. Arch Neurol 31:160–167

Overgaard J (1978) Chroma-memo-flow technique for rapid sequential analysis of regional cerebral blood flow (rCBF) responses. Can J Neurol Sci 5:1–7

Pabelick W-H (1967) Die Veränderungen der Hirnarterien bei den Massenblutungen im Striatum. Klinische und pathologisch-anatomische Untersuchungen an 70 Fällen. Med Dissertation, Universität Köln

Padt JP, de Reuck J, van der Eecken H (1973) Intracerebral hemorrhage as initial symptom of a brain tumor. Acta Neurol Belg 73:241–251

Pagni CA, Bernasconi V, Bollati A, de Santis S (1969) Risultati del trattamento chirurgico di 71 casi di emorragia cerebrale. Minerva Neurochir 13:47–52

Paillas J (1968) Traitement chirurgical de l'hémorrhagic cérébrale. Evol Med 12:469–480

Paillas JE, Alliez B (1973) Surgical treatment of spontaneous intracerebral hemorrhage. Immediate and long-term results in 250 cases. J Neurosurg 39:145–151

Paillas JE, Bonnal J, Vigouroux R, Gastaut Y (1952) Les hématomes intracérébraux spontanés. Marseille Med 89:323–330

Paillas JE, Lesbros A, Bonnal J, Lavielle J, Jaffre M (1963) Syndrome alterné par hématome de la protuberance. Rev Otoneuroophtalmol 35:100–101

Papo I, Pasquini U, Salvolini U (1976) Subependymal brain stem hematomas: A report of two cases. Neuroradiology 11:279–282

Parkinson D, Chochinov H (1960) Subdural haematomas – some observations on their post-operative course. J Neurosurg 17:901–904

Parkinson D, Hunt B, Shields C (1971) Double lucid interval in patients with extradural haematoma of the posterior fossa. J Neurosurg 34:534–536

Paulson OB (1971) Cerebral apoplexy (stroke). Pathogenesis, pathophysiology and therapy as illustrated by regional blood flow measurements in the brain. Stroke 2:327–360

Paxton R, Ambrose J (1974) The EMI scanner. A brief review of the first 650 patients. Br J Radiol 47:530–565

Penfield W (1933) The operative treatment of spontaneous intracranial haemorrhage. Can Med Assoc J 28:369–372

Perret G, Nishioka H (1966) Cerebral angiography. J Neurosurg 25:98–114, 467–490

Pestalozzi R (1849) Über Aneurysmata spuria der kleinen Gehirnarterien und ihren Zusammenhang mit der Apoplexie. Med Dissertation, Universität Würzburg

Peters G (1969) Morphologie der traumatischen Veränderungen des Gehirns und seiner Häute. In: Kessel FK (ed) Neurotraumatologie, vol 1. Urban & Schwarzenberg, Berlin München Wien, pp 37–91

Petrovici I (1960) Hematomul cerebral intraparenchimatos spontan, Culegere de studii şi monografii de neurologie. Ed A Acad R.P.R., Bucureşti

Pia HW (1956) Die Einwirkungen der Hirndrucksteigerung auf den Hirnstamm, ihre Klinik und Behandlung. Munch Med Wochenschr 47:1609–1613

Pia HW (1959a) Ursachen und chirurgische Behandlung der nichttraumatischen Hirnblutungen. Ther Ggw 98:49 – 59
Pia HW (1959b) Diagnose und Behandlung der spontanen intracerebralen Massenblutungen. Acta Neurochir (Wien) 7:425 – 439
Pia HW (1961) Die neurochirurgische Behandlung der spontanen Hirnblutungen. Z Aerztl Fortbild (Jena) 50:329 – 337
Pia HW (1964) Die traumatischen Hirnblutungen des Kindesalters. Acta Neurochir (Wien) 11:583 – 600
Pia HW (1966) Diagnose und Therapie intraventriculärer Blutungen. In: Klinische Erfahrungen bei Hirnstammprozessen. Acta 25, Conventus Neuropsych. et EEG Hungarici, Budapest 1966
Pia HW (1968a) Diagnose und Therapie der Hirnblutungen im Kindesalter. Beitr Neurochir 15:245 – 251
Pia HW (1968b) Diagnose und Therapie der Hirnblutungen im Kindesalter. Tijdschr Geneesk 24: 765 – 770
Pia HW (1968c) The diagnosis and treatment of intraventricular haemorrhages. Prog Brain Res 30:463 – 470
Pia HW (1969) Vasculäre Mißbildungen und Erkrankungen der hinteren Schädelgrube und ihre Behandlung. HNO 17:165 – 171
Pia HW (1970) Therapie der Subarachnoidalblutungen. Dtsch Med Wochenschr 95:700 – 702
Pia HW (1972) The surgical treatment of intracerebral and intraventricular haematomas. Acta Neurochir (Wien) 27:149 – 164
Pia HW (1972) The surgical treatment of intracerebral hematomas. In: Fusek J, Kunc Z (eds) Present limits of neurosurgery. Avicenum, Prague, pp 323 – 328
Pia HW (1975) The acute treatment of cerebral arteriovenous angiomas associated with hematomas. In: Pia HW, Gleave JRW, Grote E, Ziersky J (eds) Cerebral angiomas – Advances in diagnosis and therapy. Springer, Berlin Heidelberg New York, pp 155 – 177
Pia HW (1979) Die operative Behandlung der spontanen intrazerebralen Blutungen. Neurol Psychiatr 5:356 – 364
Pia HW (1977) Operative treatment of spontaneous intracerebral haemorrhages. Proc 10th Conf Pol Soc Neurosurg, Gdánsk, pp 267 – 283
Pia HW, Müller W (1953) Klinik und Ätiologie der Massenblutungen in Hypophysenadenomen. Dtsch Z Nervenheilkd 170:326 – 336
Pick L (1910) Über die sogenannten miliären Aneurysmen der Hirngefäße. Berl Klin Wochenschr 47:325 – 329
Pilcher C (1941) Subcortical hematoma. Surgical treatment with report of eight cases. Arch Neurol Psychiatry 46:416 – 430
Pineda A (1977) Computed tomography in intracerebral haemorrhage. Surg Neurol 8:55
Pitner SE, Mance CJ (1973) An evaluation of stroke intensive care: Results in a municipal hospital. Stroke 4:737 – 741
Pouyanne H, Got M, Julien G, Riemens V, Paoli M (1967) Deux cas d'hématomes infraprotubérantiels opérés. Étude critique. Neurochirurgie 13:738 – 742
Ramey IG, Coles AB, Gifford AJ, Hicks DJ, Jarcho LW, Keilhofer GT, Madden BW, Marshall AM, Martin N, Peabody SR, Regan P, Rothberg JS (1972) Guidelines for the nursing care of stroke patients. Stroke 3:633
Ransohoff J, Randt CT (1965) Profiles of fatal and non-fatal closed head injury. In: Proceedings of the Third International Congress of Neurological Surgery. pp 137 – 142 (Amsterdam)
Ransohoff J, Derby B, Kircheff I (1970) Spontaneous intracerebral haemorrhage. Clin Neurosurg 18:247 – 266
Rapoport SI (1976) Opening of the blood-brain barrier by acute hypertension. Exp Neurol 52:467 – 479
Reisner H (1954) Die Klinik und Therapie der cerebralen Gefäßerkrankungen des höheren Lebensalters. Wien Z Nervenheilkd 9:92 – 108
Reisner H (1972) Differentialdiagnose Hirninfarkt – Hirnblutung. Verh Dtsch Ges Inn Med 78:461 – 466
Reisner H (1975) Die zerebrale Blutung. Kassenarzt 8:1087 – 1096
Reisner T, Dal-Bianco P (to be published) Computed tomography in intracerebral haemorrhage. Cerebral vascular disease. 9th International Conference Salzburg 1978. Excerpta Medica, Amsterdam
Reisner H, Felger GP, Scherzer E (1961) Das weitere Schicksal von 1000 zerebralen Insulten. Wien Klin Wochenschr 73:397 – 402
Rey-Bellet J (1960) Cerebellar hemorrhage: A clinicopathologic study. Neurology (Minneap) 10:217 – 222
Reynolds AF Jr (1978) Aphasia and left thalamic hemorrhage. J Neurosurg 48:570 – 574
Richardson AE (1969) Surgical therapy of spontaneous intracerebral haemorrhage. Progress Neurol Surg 3:397 – 418

Richardson AE (1972) Spontaneous cerebellar hemorrhage. In: Vinken PJ, Bruyn GW (eds) Handbook of clinical neurology, vol 12. North Holland, Amsterdam, pp 54–67
Richardson AE (1976) Spontaneous intracerebral and cerebellar haemorrhage. In: Ross Russell RZ (ed) Cerebral arterial disease. Churchill Livingstone, Edinburgh London New York, pp 210–230
Riishede J (1967) Cerebral apoplexy: statistical and diagnostic considerations. Can Med Assoc J 97:151–160
Robertson WF (1900) A text-book of pathology in relation to mental diseases. Clay, Edinburgh
Robson GS, Anderson RM (1973) Central nervous system lesions in childhood leukaemia. Med J Aust 23:1134–1137
Rockett JF, Moinnuddin MA (1976) Dynamic cerebral imaging. Clin Nucl Med 1:166–177
Rokitanski C (1844) Handbuch der pathologischen Anatomie. Bd II. Braunmüller & Seidel, Wien
Roland PE, Larsen B (1976) Focal increase of cerebral blood flow during stereognostic testing in man. Arch Neurol (Wien) 33:551–558
Rosenberg GA, Kaufman DM (1976) Cerebellar hemorrhage: Reliability of clinical evaluation. Stroke 7:332–336
Rosenblath L (1918) Über die Entstehung der Hirnblutung bei dem Schlaganfall. Dtsch Z Nervenheilkd 61:10–143
Rosenblum WI (1977) Miliary aneurysms and "fibrinoid" degeneration of cerebral blood vessels. Hum Pathol 8:133–139
Rosenthal LA (1971) Intravenous and intracarotid radionuclide cerebral angiography. Semin Nucl Med 1:70–84
Rothemund E, Frische M (1973) Klinisch-pathologische Studie zur Entstehung der intracerebralen Gefäßhyalinose bei Hypertonie. Arch Psychiatr Nervenkr 217:195–206
Rouchoux JA (1814) Recherches sur l'apoplexie, 1st ed. Béchet, Paris
Rouchoux JA (1842) Du ramollissement de cerveau et de sa curabilité. Gaz Med 10:376
Russell DS (1954) The pathology of spontaneous intracranial haemorrhage. Proc R Soc Med 47:689–704
Russell RW (1963) Observations on intracerebral aneurysms. Brain 86:425–441
Russo RH, Dicks RE (1977) Arteriovenous malformations of the brain stem in childhood. Surg Neurol 8:167–170
Sahs AL (1975) Medical management of vascular diseases. In: Tower DB (ed) The nervous system, vol 2. Raven, New York, pp 167–172
Sanders E (1881) A study of primary, immediate or direct hemorrhage into the ventricles of the brain. Ann J Med Sci 82:85–128
Sano K (1965) Survey of the organization of services for the treatment of acute head injury in Japan. In: Proceedings of the Third International Congress of Neurological Surgery. pp 39–46 (Amsterdam)
Sano K, Yoshioka M, Masuzawa H (1964) Spontaneous intracerebellar hemorrhage. Clin Neurol (Tokyo) 4:511–512
Santos-Buch CA, Goodhue WW, Ewald BH (1976) Concurrence of iris aneurysms and cerebral hemorrhage in hypertensive rabbits. Arch Neurol 33:96–103
Schaafsma S (1968) On the differential diagnosis between cerebral hemorrhage and infarction. J Neurol Sci 7:83–95
Schiefer W (1972a) Symptomatologie und Klinik der infratentoriellen Blutungen. In: Gänshirt H (ed) Der Hirnkreislauf. Thieme, Stuttgart
Schiefer W (1972b) Klinik der intrazerebralen Massenblutungen und spontanen Haematome. In: Gänshirt H (ed) Der Hirnkreislauf. Thieme, Stuttgart, pp 680–714
Scholz W, Nieto D (1938) Studien zur Pathologie der Hirngefäße. I. Fibrose und Hyalinose. Z Neurol 162:675–693
Schuier FJ, Vise WM, Hossmann K-A, Zülch KJ (1978) Cerebral microembolization. II. Morphological studies. Arch Neurol 35:264–270
Schwartz P (1972) Apoplectic lesions of the brain in adults. In: Vinken JP, Bruyn GW (eds) Handbook of clinical neurology, vol 11. North Holland, Amsterdam, pp 578–659
Scott BB, Seeger JF, Schneider RC (1973) Successful evacuation of a pontine hematoma secondary to rupture of a pathologically diagnosed "cryptic" vascular malformation: Case report. J Neurosurg 39:104–108
Scott M (1975) Spontaneous intracerebral hematoma caused by cerebral neoplasms. Report of eight verified cases. J Neurosurg 42:338–342
Scott WR, New PFJ, Davis KR, Schnur JA (1974) Computerized axial tomography of intracerebral and intraventricular hemorrhage. Radiology 112:73–80
Scoville WB, Poppen JL (1949) Intrapeduncular hemorrhage of the brain. Arch Neurol Psychiatry 61:688–694

Seeler RA, Imana RB (1973) Intracranial hemorrhage in patients with hemophilia. J Neurosurg 39:181 – 185
Severingshaus JW (ed) (1975) Coupling mechanisms, flow to function and metabolism in brain, a general discussion. In: Ingvar DH, Lassen NA (eds) Alfred Benzon Symposium VIII, Brain York. Munksgaard, Copenhagen, pp 503 – 517
Shinkai H, Yoshida Y, Ooneda G (1976) An electron microscopic study of plasmatic arterionecrosis in the human cerebral arteries. Virchows Arch [Pathol Anat] 369:181 – 190
Silverstein A (1972) Primary pontine hemorrhage. In: Vinken PJ, Bruyn GW (eds): Handbook of clinical neurology, vol 12. North Holland, Amsterdam, p 37
Skinhøj E (1965) Bilateral depression of CBF in unilateral cerebral diseases. Acta Neurol Scand [Suppl] 14:161 – 163
Skinhøj E, Strandgaard S (1973) Pathogenesis of hypertensive encephalopathy. Lancet I:461 – 462
Slater R, Reichvich M, Goldberg H, Banka R, Greenberg J (1977) Diaschisis with cerebral infarction. Stroke 8:684 – 691
Smith KR Jr, Bardenheider JA (1968) Aneurysm of the pericallosal artery caused by closed cranial trauma. Case report. J Neurosurg 29:551 – 554
Sostre S (1976) Vein of Galen malformation. Clin Nucl Med 1:211 – 212
Spatz H (1939) Pathologische Anatomie der Kreislaufstörungen des Gehirns. Z Gesamte Neurol Psychiatr 167:301 – 357
Sreerama K (1973) Neurosurgical complication of anticoagulant therapy. Can Med Assoc J 108:305 – 307
Staemmler M (1958) Kreislaufstörungen und Gefäßerkrankungen des Zentralnervensystems. In: Kaufmann's Lehrbuch der speziellen pathologischen Anatomie, vol III/1. De Gruyter, Berlin
Stebbens WE (1972) Pathology of the cerebral blood vessels. Mosby, St. Louis
Stein MA, Winter J (1974) Delayed appearance of anterior cerebral arteries on isotopic cerebral flow study: A sign of bleeding anterior communicating artery aneurysm. J Nucl Med 15:1217 – 1219
Steiner L, Bergvall U, Zwetnow N (1975) Quantitative estimation of intracerebral and intraventricular hematoma by computer tomography. Acta Radiol [Suppl] (Stockh) 346:143 – 154
Stender A (1958) Die chirurgische Behandlung der spontanen intracerebralen Haematome. Zentralbl Neurochir 18:243 – 253
Stender A, Schulze A (1965) The surgical treatment of space-occupying contusions and intracerebral haematoma after blunt cerebral trauma. In: Proceedings of the Third International Congress of Neurological Surgery. pp 231 – 235 (Amsterdam)
Steudel WI, Schneider E, Becker H (1980) Management and prognosis of intraventricular haemorrhage. Adv Neurosurg 7
Stochdorph O, Meessen H (1957) Die arteriosklerotische und die hypertonische Hirnerkrankung. In: Handbuch der speziellen pathologischen Anatomie und Histologie, vol XIII, IB. Springer, Berlin Göttingen Heidelberg, pp 1465 – 1510
Sundt TM Jr, Waltz AG (1971) Cerebral ischemia and reactive hyperemia: Studies of cortical blood flow and microcirculation before, during and after temporary occlusion of middle cerebral artery of squirrel monkeys. Circ Res 28:426 – 433
Sussmann BJ, Barber JB, Goald H (1974) Experimental intracerebral hematoma. Reduction of oxygen tension in brain and cerebrospinal fluid. J Neurosurg 41:177 – 186
Suzuki J, Kodama N (1971) Cerebrovascular "Moya-moya" disease. Second report: Collateral routes to forebrain via ethmoid sinus and superior nasal meatus. Angiology 22:223 – 236
Suzuki K, Ooneda G (1972) Cerebral arterial lesions in experimental hypertensive rats. Exp Mol Pathol 16:341 – 352
Suzuki J, Sato T (1972) The new transinsular approach to the hypertensive intracerebral hematoma. Jpn J Surg 2:47 – 52
Suzuki J, Sato T (1976) Surgery for the hypertensive intracerebral hematoma – Trans-Sylvian approach. Neurol Med Chir (Tokyo) 16:115 – 119
Suzuki J, Takaku A (1969) Cerebrovascular "Moya-moya" disease; a disease showing abnormal net-like vessels in base of brain. Arch Neurol 20:288 – 299
Swank RL, Bartsch W (1971) Influence of aggregated blood cells on cerebrovascular disease. In: Zülch KJ (ed) Cerebral circulation and stroke. Springer, Berlin Heidelberg New York, pp 164 – 174
Symon L (1978) Disordered cerebro-vascular physiology in aneurysmal subarachnoid haemorrhage. Acta Neurochir 41:1 – 3, 7 – 22
Symon L, Pasztor E, Branston NM (1974) The distribution and density of reduced cerebral blood flow following acute middle cerebral artery occlusion: An experimental study by the technique of hydrogen clearance in baboons. Stroke 5:355 – 364
Symonds CP (1940) Delayed traumatic intracerebral haemorrhage. Br Med J I:1048 – 1051

Tandon PN, Kristensen K (1965) Clinical pathological observations on brain stem dysfunction in craniocerebral injuries. In: Proceedings of the Third International Congress of Neurological Surgery (Amsterdam) pp 126 – 129

Tedeschi G, Bernini FP, Cerillo A (1975) Indication for surgical treatment of intracerebral hemorrhage. J Neurosurg 43:590 – 595

Teilmann K (1953) Hemangiomas of the pons. Arch Neurol 69:208 – 223

Tenuto RA, Cruz OR (1958) Hematoma intraprotuberantial. Arq Neuropsiquiatr 16:201 – 204

Terao H, Hori T, Matsutani M, Okeda R (1979) Detection of cryptic vascular malformations by computerized tomography. Report of two cases. J Neurosurg 51:546 – 551

Toole JF, Truscott BL, Anderson WW, Aronson PR, Blaisdell RW, Dustan HP, Dyken ML, Folex AR, Halsey JH, Langfitt TW, Lowrence MS, Mullan JF (1973) Medical and surgical management of stroke. Stroke 4:273

Torack RM (1975) Congophilic angiopathy complicated by surgery and massive hemorrhage. Am J Pathol 81:349 – 366

Tovi D (1972) Studies on fibrinolysis in the central nervous system with special reference to intracranial haemorrhages and to the effect of antifibrinolytic drugs. Med Dissertations No 8, Umea University

Tyson JW, Witherspoon LR, Wilkison RH, Goodrich JK (1974) Accuracy of radionuclide cerebral angiograms in the detection of cerebral arteriovenous malformations. J Nucl Med 15:953 – 958

Ule G, Kolkmann FW (1972) Pathologische Anatomie. In: Gänshirt H (ed) Der Hirnkreislauf. Thieme, Stuttgart, pp 47 – 190

Van der Ark GD, Kahn EA (1968) Spontaneous intracerebral hematoma. J Neurosurg 28:252 – 256

Vedrenne C, Chodkiewicz JP (1975) Les lésions du tronc cérébral chez les traumatisés crâniens (étude anatomique). IIIe Symposium international de posturographie. Paris 23. – 26. septembre 1975 (1 – 8)

Verjaal A (1958) Het spontane intracerebrale haematoom. Ned Tijdschr Geneeskd 102:1935 – 1936

Virchow R (1856) Phlogose und Thrombose im Gefäßsystem. Thrombose und Embolie. In: Gesammelte Abhandlungen zur wissenschaftlichen Medizin. Meidinger, Frankfurt, pp 219 – 380

Voris HC (1945) Factors influencing mortality in head injury. Radiology 44:166 – 170

Vuia O, Alexianu M, Gabor S (1970) Hypoplasia and obstruction of the circle of Willis in a case of atypical cerebral hemorrhage and its relationship to Nishimoto's disease. Neurology (Minneap) 20:361 – 367

Vital Statistics, 1951 – 1976, Division of Health and Welfare. Statistics, Welfare Minister Secretariat, Japan

Walker AE (1957) Prognosis in post-traumatic epilepsy. A 10 year follow-up on craniocerebral injuries in world war II. JAMA 164:1636 – 1641

Walker AE, Black P (1960) The heroic treatment of acute head injuries; a critical analysis of the results. Am Surg 26:184 – 188

Walshe T, Hier D, Davis K (1977) The diagnosis of hypertensive intracerebral haemorrhage: the contribution of computed tomography. Comput Tomogr 1:63

Walter W, Schütte W (1965) Zur Klinik und Pathogenese des spontanen intrazerebralen Hämatoms. Dtsch Z Nervenheilkd 187:660 – 679

Watanabe R (1963) Clinicopathological study of primary massive pontine hemorrhage. Clin Neurol 3:94 – 112

Weber J (1963) Das intrazerebrale Hämatom. Schweiz Arch Neurol Neurochir Psychiatr 91:510 – 551

Weigel K, Ostertag CB, Mundinger F (1978) CT follow-up control of traumatic intracerebral hemorrhage. Adv Neurosurg 5:62

Wepfer JT (1658) Observationes anatomicae ex cadaveribus eorum, quos sustulit apoplexia, cum exerzitatione de ejus loco affecto. Suter, Schaffhusii

Westphal K, Bär R (1926) Über die Entstehung des Schlaganfalles: I. Pathologisch-anatomische Untersuchungen zur Frage der Entstehung des Schlaganfalles. Dtsch Arch Klin Med 151:1 – 30

The White House Conference on Handicapped Individuals (1978) Summary final report. Department of Health, Education, and Welfare Office for Handicapped Individuals, Washington, D.C. 20201

Wiedersberg H (1970) Die zentralen Todesursachen bei der essentiellen Hypertension. Dtsch Med Wochenschr 95:1271 – 1274

Wilson JL, Moseley IF (1977) A diagnostic approach to cerebellar lesions. In: Du Boulay GH, Moseley IF (eds) Computerized axial tomography in clinical practice. Springer, Berlin Heidelberg New York, pp 123 – 131

Wissler RW (1977) Coronary atherosclerosis and ischemic heart disease. In: Zülch KJ, Kaufmann W, Hossman K-A, Hossmann V (eds) Brain and heart infarct. Springer, Berlin Heidelberg New York, pp 206 – 223

Wissler RW, Vesselinovitch D (1975) Regression of atherosclerosis in experimental animals and man. Verh Dtsch Ges Inn Med 81:857 – 865
World Health Organisation Disability Prevention and Rehabilitation Programme (1976)
World Health Statistics Annual (1970, 1971)
Wüllenweber R, zum Winkel K, Grumme T, Lange S, Meese W (1976) Differentialdiagnose des Schlaganfalles im Computer-Tomogramm. Neurochirurgia 19:1 – 9
Wylie CM (1972) Epidemiology of stroke. In: Handbook of clinical neurology, vol 11. North Holland, Amsterdam, pp 183 – 207
Yamori J, Horie R, Handa L, Sato M, Fukase M (1976) Pathogenetic similarity of strokes in stroke-prone spontaneously hypertensive rats and humans. Stroke 7:46 – 53
Yates PO (1976) Vascular disease of the central nervous system. In: Blackwood W, Corsellis JAN (eds) Greenfield's neuropathology, 3rd ed. Arnold, London, pp 86 – 147
Yoshida S, Sasaki M, Oka H, Gotoh O, Yamada R, Sano K (1978) Acute hypertensive cerebellar hemorrhage with signs of lower brain stem compression. Surg Neurol 10:79 – 83
Zenker FAZ (1872) Über die Pathogenese der spontanen Hirnhämorrhagien. Verh Naturforsch Ges
Zimmerman HM (1949) Cerebral apoplexy: mechanism and differential diagnosis. NY State J Med 49:2153 – 2157
Zimmermann RD, Leeds NE, Naidich TP (1977) Ring blush associated with intracerebral hematoma. Radiology 122:707 – 711
Zülch KJ (1961a) Die Pathogenese von Massenblutung und Erweichung unter besonderer Berücksichtigung klinischer Gesichtspunkte. Acta Neurochir (Wien) [Suppl VII] 51 – 117
Zülch KJ (1961b) Zur Operation der intracerebralen Massenblutungen. Zentralbl Chir 86:350 – 395
Zülch KJ (1963) Zur Pathogenese des cerebrovaskulären Insultes. Internist (Berlin) 4:64 – 70
Zülch KJ (1966) Über die Möglichkeiten chirurgischer Therapie bei Erkrankungen der Hirngefäße. Krüger-Gedenk-Symposion, Bad Ischl
Zülch KJ (1968) Neuropathology of intracranial hemorrhage. Progr Brain Res 30:151 – 165
Zülch KJ (1971a) Pathological aspects of cerebral accidents in arterial hypertension. Acta Neurol Belg 71:196 – 220
Zülch KJ (1971b) Hemorrhage, thrombosis, embolism. In: Minckler J (ed) Pathology of the nervous system, vol 2. McGraw-Hill, New York, pp 1499 – 1536
Zülch KJ (1972) Does a neurology department need its own intensive care unit? Z Neurol 201:1 – 5
Zülch KJ (1977a) Clinical ischemia: In: Brain and heart infarct. Zülch KJ, Kaufmann W, Hossmann KA, Hossmann V (eds) Brain Infarcts. Springer, Berlin Heidelberg New York, pp 288 – 296
Zülch KJ (1977b) Transient ischemic attacks (TIA). In: III. Symp. Internacional de EEG, Practica sobre Accidentes Vasculares Transitorios (TAIT) y Epilepsias Tardias Vasculares (ETV), Valencia, pp 177 – 189
Zülch KJ, Gehlen W (1971) Die Intensiv-Überwachungs- und Behandlungsstation der neurologischen Klinik. Fortschr Med 89:1247 – 1251
Zülch KJ, Gessaga E (1972) Infarcts in the carotid system. Vasc Surg 6:114 – 119
Zülch KJ, Tzonos T (1964) Transsudationsphänomene an den tiefen Hirnvenen nach Blockade von Arteriolen oder Kapillaren der Rinde durch Mikroembolien. Naturwissenschaften 51:539 – 540
Zülch KJ, Tzonos T (1965) Transudation phenomena in the deep veins after blockage of arterioles and capillaries by micro-emboli. Bibl Anat 7:279 – 284
Zülch KJ, Einsiedel-Lechtape H, Hartmann W (1973) Der Mediahauptstamm-Verschluß. Klinisch-angiographische Korrelation. In: Fisiopatologia clinica e terapia del circolo. Atti delle gionate mediche Triestine. Tipografia Gaetano Coana, Trieste, pp 117 – 124
Zülch KJ, Pakula H, Schuier F (1976) Distant perivenous demyelination after microembolization of the brain. Neuropathol Appl Neurobiol 2:163
Zülch KJ, Hossmann KA, Rackl A, Pawlik G (1978) Multimethodological study of cerebral ischemic lesions with particular reference to regional EEG Fourier analysis. In: XX. Alpines EEG-meeting, Courchevel

11 Subject Index

Aetiology 13 ff
–, cerebellar haematoma 154
–, in India 100 ff
–, Japanese diet 99
–, primary and secondary factors 69 ff
–, supratentorial haematomas 131 ff
Alcohol 60, 65, 73
Aneurysms
–, aneurysma spuria 5
–, micro 21
–, miliary 3, 5
–, mycotic 23
–, pseudo- 14, 22
–, saccular 23
Angiography
–, diagnosis of ICH 171 ff
–, differential diagnosis of ICH 165 ff
– and CT-scan 171
– and infarct 173
–, micro- 85
Angioma, 23
–, cryptic, arteriovenosum 44
–, –, venosum (hamartoma) 41
–, intraventricular 145
–, malformations 22
–, micro- 41 ff, 43, 47
Anticoagulants, circulating 33
–, ICH and 40
Apoplexy, capillary 2
–, delayed traumatic (Spätapoplexie) 71, 74
–, striatum 133
Arterial disease, amyloidosis 52
–, arteriosclerosis 4, 52
–, atherosclerosis 4
–, hyalinosis 4

Bleeding disorders (dyscrasias) 31 ff
–, acquired 32
–, circulating anticoagulants 33
–, coagulation factors 31
–, consumption coagulopathy 32
Bleeding, diffuse intravascular coagulation 32
–, inherited 31
–, partial thromboplastin time 33
–, plasma prothrombin time 34
–, prothrombin complex 32
–, – time 33
Brain abscess 129 ff
Burr-hole evacuation 379 ff

Cerebral blood flow (CBF) 107 ff
– – –, cortical flow 115
– – –, haemodynamic investigations 37, 107
– – –, pathological flow pattern 114
– – –, regional flow 115
Clinical course 233
–, deterioration 236
–, initial spontaneous course 234
–, prognostic elements 237 ff
–, pseudotumoural course 235
Clotting disorders 35 ff
– –, coagulation factors 31, 32
– –, consumption coagulopathy 32
– –, diffuse intravascular coagulation 32
– –, haemophilia 37
– –, hyperfibrinolysis, generalized 37, 38, 39
– –, indications and prognosis 308, 309
– –, thrombocytopaenia 37
Computerized tomography (CT scan) 178 ff
– –, absorption coefficient 191
– –, attenuation of blood 178, 180
– –, basal ganglia haemorrhage, classification 336
Computerized tomography, brain stem hge., diagnosis 196 ff
– –, diagnosis, automatic and quantitative 190 ff, 202
– –, differential diagnosis 185
– –, haemoglobin level in blood 195
– –, indications 188
– –, intraventricular haemorrhage 195
– –, occlusion of cisterns 198
– –, perifocal low density 194
– –, putaminal haemorrhage, size 341 ff
– –, region of interest (ROI) 191
– –, thalamic haemorrhage, classification 336
Craniotomy 374 ff

Diet, japanese (in relation to hypertensive H) 99
Differentiation, arteriosclerotic H 168
–, brain stem haemorrhage 162
–, brain tumours 167
–, CT-scan 185
–, microangiomas 166
Duret haemorrhage 156

Epidemiology 91 ff
–, annual mortality rates 13
–, mortality in Germany 91
–, – in India 100 ff
–, – in Japan 96 ff
–, WHO-figures 1, 91, 103 ff
Epsilon aminocaproic acid (EACA) 38

Familial incidence 50 ff
Follow-up 216 ff

Goldblatt model 4
Grading and timing, operative treatment 264ff
– –, basal ganglia hge 268ff
– –, putaminal hge 274ff

Haematoma, aetiology 153
–, brain stem (pontine) 156ff, 160ff
–, cerebellar 152ff, 154ff
–, –, occurence 152
–, –, or haemorrhage 30
–, primary 161
–, –, intraparenchymatous 307
–, unknow aetiology 82ff
Haemorrhage, aetiology 14ff
–, alcohol in 60, 65, 73
–, atypical spontaneous 24
–, basal ganglia, prognosis 334ff
–, brain stem 196ff, 198, 357, 366, 368
–, cerebellar 348ff, 356, 358, 361, 365
–, childhood 48
–, familial incidence 50
–, – & haematoma 30
–, intraventricular 326ff, 330ff
–, microangioma 141
–, mortality rates (annual) 13
–, natural hiostory 13
–, pathogenesis 17, 30
–, putaminal 133
–, spontaneous 294ff
–, spreading 294ff
–, supratentorial 131ff
–, thalamic 133
–, tissue reaction 14
–, traumatic 22, 58ff, 77
–, – (minor) 58ff, 61
–, unknown aetiology 87
–, vascular malformations 77
Hamartoma, cryptic arteriovenous 41
–, venous 41
Hemisphere lobe ICH, prognosis 322ff
Hyalinosis 4, 20
Hypertension, and Japanese 99
–, renal 86
–, spontaneous, in rats 86

Indications 283ff
Intracranial pressure 116ff
Intracranial pressure, autoregulation (response) 116
– –, Monro-Kellie doctrine 116
– –, spatial compensation 116
Intraventricular haemorrhage,
– –, complete tamponade 142
– –, due to angioma 144
– –, in CT scan 195ff
– –, partial haematocephalus 142
– –, – tamponade 142
– –, rôle of plexus 142
– –, total haematocephalus 141
– –, ventricular haematocephalus in Moya-Moya disease 145ff

Kügelblutung (Hiller) 4

Leukaemia (myeloid) 48

Malformations, microangiomas 41
–, vascular 22
Microangiomas, angiographic differentiation 166
–, histopathological evaluation 254
Microcirculation disturbances 10
Moya-Moya disease 145ff

Natural history 13, 216ff

Operative treatment, results 247ff, 251ff, 260, 262, 262, 289, 294, 310
– –, in basal ganglia ICH 270ff
– –, contraindications 281ff, 294ff
– –, in hypertensive haemorrhage 257ff

Partial thromboplastin time (PTT) 33
Pathogenesis 17
Pathology 13ff
Perivascular bleeding 125
Phenprocoumon (Marcumar) 40
Plasma prothrombin time (Quick) 33
Prognosis, basal ganglia ICH 334
–, & CT-scan 331
–, clinical course and prognostic factors 223
–, haematocephalus totalis 330
–, – partialis 330
–, haemorrhage intraventricularis 330
–, hemisphere lobe hge 322ff
–, hydrocephalus 238
–, intraventricular haemorrhage 326
–, late 240ff
–, putaminal ICH 344ff
–, secondary extension of haematoma 238
–, site of haematoma 237
–, thalamus ICH 334
–, volume of haematoma 238
Putaminal ICH, operative technique 383
–, prognosis 341
–, trans-Sylvian approach 345ff

Quick test 33

Rehabilitation 228, 231ff
Renin-angiotensin system 87
Reptilase-thrombin coagulation time 34

Sinus, dural thrombosis 56
Spätapoplexie 71, 74
Streptokinase 37
Stroke 1ff
–, capillary apoplexy 2
–, cause and pathogenesis 1
–, immediate care 223
–, in hypertensive rats 86ff

Thalamic ICH, operative technique 283
– –, prognosis 334ff
Tissue reaction 14
– –, histological changes 123
– –, perivascular bleeding 122, 124

Tissue reaction, status spongiosus 122, 124, 126
– –, surrounding ICH in experimental hge 121 ff
Trans-Sylvian approach 384
Trauma 58, 71, 76
–, alcohol & 60, 65, 73
–, birth 63
–, head injury 76 ff
–, latency 67, 77
–, minor 58, 61
–, Spätapoplexie 71
Traumatic Haemorrhage; indications 317 ff
– –, CT scan 202 ff
– –, prognosis 319 ff
– –, results and location 310 ff, 314, 319
Treatment; conservative 223 ff, 225 ff
–, immediate care 223
Tumours; angiographic differentiation 167, 173
Tumours, intracranial 26, 136 chemotherapy in 26
–, –, haemorrhage in 26
Vascular disease 61
–, malformations 22 ff, 136
Ventricular drainage, continuous 386
–, –, bilateral 387
Ventricular shunt operations 389

WHO figures 1

MIX
Papier aus verantwortungsvollen Quellen
Paper from responsible sources
FSC® C105338

If you have any concerns about our products,
you can contact us on
ProductSafety@springernature.com

In case Publisher is established outside the EU,
the EU authorized representative is:
Springer Nature Customer Service Center GmbH
Europaplatz 3, 69115 Heidelberg, Germany

Printed by Libri Plureos GmbH
in Hamburg, Germany